Clinical Methods
in
Paediatrics
Physical Examination of Children

Clinical Methods in Paediatrics

Physical Examination of Children

Volume 2 (Part B)

ML Kulkarni

MD FIAP FAMS FIMSA FCPCC (LON) FRCPCH (UK)
MNAS (NY) PhD (Gen)
Professor and Head
Department of Paediatrics
JJM Medical College, Davangere
Karnataka

JAYPEE BROTHERS
MEDICAL PUBLISHERS (P) LTD.
New Delhi

Published by

Jitendar P Vij
Jaypee Brothers Medical Publishers (P) Ltd

Corporate Office
4838/24 Ansari Road, Daryaganj, **New Delhi** - 110002, India, +91-11-43574357

Registered Office
B-3 EMCA House, 23/23B Ansari Road, Daryaganj, **New Delhi** 110 002, India
Phones: +91-11-23272143, +91-11-23272703, +91-11-23282021,
+91-11-23245672, Rel: +91-11-32558559 Fax: +91-11-23276490, +91-11-23245683
e-mail: jaypee@jaypeebrothers.com, Visit our website: www.jaypeebrothers.com

Branches

- 2/B, Akruti Society, Jodhpur Gam Road Satellite **Ahmedabad** 380 015
  Phones: +91-79-26926233,   Rel: +91-79-32988717
  Fax: +91-79-26927094   e-mail: ahmedabad@jaypeebrothers.com

- 202 Batavia Chambers, 8 Kumara Krupa Road, Kumara Park East
  Bengaluru 560 001   Phones: +91-80-22285971, +91-80-22382956,
  +91-80-22372664,   Rel: +91-80-32714073
  Fax: +91-80-22281761   e-mail: bangalore@jaypeebrothers.com

- 282 IIIrd Floor, Khaleel Shirazi Estate, Fountain Plaza, Pantheon Road
  Chennai 600 008   Phones: +91-44-28193265, +91-44-28194897,
  Rel: +91-44-32972089 Fax: +91-44-28193231   e-mail: chennai@jaypeebrothers.com

- 4-2-1067/1-3, 1st Floor, Balaji Building, Ramkote Cross Road
  Hyderabad 500 095   Phones: +91-40-66610020,
  +91-40-24758498,   Rel:+91-40-32940929
  Fax:+91-40-24758499,   e-mail: hyderabad@jaypeebrothers.com

- No. 41/3098, B & B1, Kuruvi Building, St. Vincent Road
  Kochi 682 018, Kerala   Phones: +91-484-4036109, +91-484-2395739,
  +91-484-2395740   e-mail: kochi@jaypeebrothers.com

- 1-A Indian Mirror Street, Wellington Square
  Kolkata 700 013   Phones: +91-33-22651926, +91-33-22276404,
  +91-33-22276415,   Rel: +91-33-32901926
  Fax: +91-33-22656075,   e-mail: kolkata@jaypeebrothers.com

- Lekhraj Market III, B-2, Sector-4, Faizabad Road, Indira Nagar
  Lucknow 226 016   Phones: +91-522-3040553, +91-522-3040554
  e-mail: lucknow@jaypeebrothers.com

- 106 Amit Industrial Estate, 61 Dr SS Rao Road, Near MGM Hospital, Parel
  Mumbai 400012   Phones: +91-22-24124863, +91-22-24104532,
  Rel: +91-22-32926896 Fax: +91-22-24160828,
  e-mail: mumbai@jaypeebrothers.com

- "KAMALPUSHPA" 38, Reshimbag, Opp. Mohota Science College, Umred Road
  Nagpur 440 009 (MS)   Phone: Rel: +91-712-3245220,
  Fax: +91-712-2704275   e-mail: nagpur@jaypeebrothers.com

USA Office
- 1745, Pheasant Run Drive, Maryland Heights (Missouri), MO 63043, USA
  Ph: 001-636-6279734   e-mail: jaypee@jaypeebrothers.com,anjulav@jaypeebrothers.com

Clinical Methods in Paediatrics (Vol 2-Part B)

© 2005, ML Kulkarni

This book has been published in good faith that the material provided by author/contributors is original. Every effort is made to ensure accuracy of material, but the publisher, printer and author will not be held responsible for any inadvertent error(s). In case of any dispute, all legal matters are to be settled under Delhi jurisdiction only.

First Edition: **2005**
Reprint 2008

ISBN 81-8061-285-6

Typeset at   JPBMP typesetting unit
Printed at   Replika Press Pvt. Ltd. Kundli.

This book is dedicated
to the memory of my beloved father
Late Shri Laxmanrao Bhimrao Kulkarni
(5-12-1918 to 01-12-1999)
a dedicated, disciplined school teacher,
who practiced Gandhian Principles
throughout his life

PREFACE

The examination of children poses a special challenge, which should be tailored to their developmental achievements, situational adjustments and to their temperament. The most powerful tool for pediatric examination remains the **powerful observational skill** that has **breadth, depth, insight, intellect** and above all **gentleness.** There is no shortcut for development of this skill. It requires continued committed efforts in examining a large number of children all through one's professional career.

Several excellent works are available pertaining to different aspects of pediatric examination. I have scanned several such works and gratefully acknowledge them.

The Volume 2 of the *Clinical Methods in Paediatrics*, deals with examination of children. The volume is divided into eight sections with many chapters in each. The sections are:

1. Basics of Paediatric Examination.
2. Head to Foot Examination
3. Systemic Examination
4. General Scheme of Examination
5. Examination in Special Situations
6. Paediatric Records and Appendices
7. Neonatology
8. Author's Tips

This book should serve as a guide for clinical examination but the **"real books"** from where the clinical skills should be developed, include **"children both healthy and sick".**

ML Kulkarni

ACKNOWLEDGEMENTS

The author sincerely wishes to acknowledge the constant source of inspiration he has received from vast number of his students with whom he has intellectually interacted in the process of teaching and learning for the past two and a half decades. Many of my residents have actively participated in bringing out this book. I would like to place on record the help I have received from Dr Nilesh Lokeshwar, Dr Mohan GL, Dr Mradul Singhal, Dr Kiran Kumar BV, Dr Aninda Saha, Dr Anuradha Naik, Dr Aji Verghese, Dr Somendarnath Roy, Dr Rajan, Dr Shashidhar, Dr Tushar Jain and Dr Ramesh Dasari.

Several excellent works have been scanned for bibliographic purpose, which I gratefully acknowledge.

I think, it is befitting to appreciate my father, a dedicated and disciplined school teacher from whom I have inherited and imbibed few of his qualities and my mother, whose love and affection, has always encouraged in my endeavours.

The author acknowledges sincere contributions from Shri Manjunath P Gundal and Brothers, M/s Gundal Computers, Davangere in their meticulous computerized paging of this book.

The author specially acknowledges the help of Shri Jitendar P Vij, Chairman and Managing Director of Jaypee Brothers Medical Publishers Pvt. Ltd., New Delhi and their team in bringing out this book.

I specially appreciate my wife Dr(Mrs) Bhagyawati Kulkarni MD DMRD(Radiologist), my daughter Dr Preethi and my son Akhil for their patience and understanding without which publishing this book would have not possible.

Special Acknowledgement

The author would especially like to thank *Dr Bathini Srinivasulu* for the editorial assistance rendered to him.

ACKNOWLEDGEMENTS

CONTENTS

Section 1

Basics of Pediatric Examination

Section 2

Head to Foot Examination

Section 3

Systemic Examination

Section 4

General Scheme of Examination

Section 5

Examination in Special Situations

Section 6

Pediatric Records and Appendices

Section 7

Neonatology

Section 8

Author's Tips

SECTION 3

Systemic Examination

CHAPTER

24 Examination of the Abdomen

Anatomy

The abdominal cavity contains several of the body's vital organs (Figs 24.1A and B). The peritoneum, a serous membrane, lines the cavity and forms a protective cover for many of the abdominal structures. Double folds of the peritoneum around the stomach constitute the greater and lesser omentum. The mesentery, a fan shaped fold of the peritoneum, covers most of the small intestines and anchors it to the posterior abdominal wall.

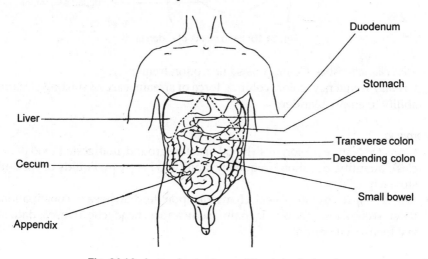

Fig. 24.1A: Anatomic structures of the abdominal cavity

Review of Related History (Present Problem)

Abdominal Pain

- *Onset and duration:* When it began; sudden or gradual; persistent, recurrent, intermittent.
- *Character:* Dull, sharp, burning, gnawing, stabbing, cramping, aching, colicky.
- *Location:* At onset, change in location over time, radiating to another area, superficial or deep.
- *Associated symptoms:* Vomiting, diarrhoea, constipation, passage of flatus, belching, jaundice, change in abdominal girth.
- *Relationship to:* Menstrual cycle, abnormal menses, urination, defecation, inspiration, change in body position, food or stress, time of day, trauma.

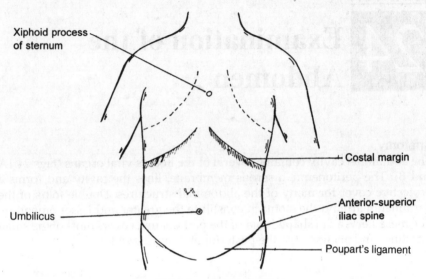

Fig. 24.1b: Land marks of abdomen

- *Stool characteristics:* Color, consistency, odor, frequency.
- Urinary frequency, color, volume, force of stream, ease of starting stream, ability to empty bladder.

Vomiting
- *Character:* Nature (Color, fresh blood or coffee ground, undigested food particles), quantity, duration, frequency, ability to keep any liquids or food in stomach.
- *Relationship to:* Previous meal, change in appetite, diarrhoea or constipation, fever, weight loss, abdominal pain, medications, headache, nausea, date of last menstrual period.

Diarrhea
- *Character:* Watery, copious, explosive; color, presence of blood, mucus, undigested food, oil, or fat; odor; number of times per day, duration; change in pattern.
- *Associated symptoms:* Chills, fever, thirst, weight loss, abdominal pain or cramping, fecal incontinence.
- *Relationship to:* Timing and nature of food intake, stress.
- *Medications:* Prescription or nonprescription; laxatives or stool softeners; antidiarrheals.

Constipation
- *Character:* Presence of bright blood, black or tarry appearance of stool; diarrhea alternating with constipation; accompanied by abdominal pain or discomfort.

- *Pattern:* Last bowel movement, pain with passage of stool, change in pattern or size of stool.
- *Diet:* Recent change in diet, inclusion of high-fibre foods.
- *Medications:* Prescription or nonprescription; laxatives, stool softeners, diuretics; iron.

Fecal Incontinence

- *Character:* Stool characteristics, timing in relation to meals, number of episodes per day; occurring with or without warning sensation.
- *Associated with:* Use of laxatives, presence of underlying disease (inflammatory bowel disease, diverticulitis, colitis, proctitis).
- *Relationship to:* Fluid and dietary intake, immobilization.
- *Medications:* Prescription or nonprescription; laxatives, stool softeners, iron, diuretics acetaminophen.
- *Jaundice:*
  - onset and duration
  - color of stools or urine
  - associated with abdominal pain, chills, fever
  - exposure to hepatitis.

Dysuria

- *Character:* Location (suprapubic, at end of urethra), pain or burning, frequency or volume changes.
- *Exposure to:* Tuberculosis, fungal or viral infection, parasitic infection, bacterial infection.
- Increased frequency of sexual intercourse.

Urinary Frequency

- Change in usual pattern and/or volume
- Associated with dysuria or other urinary characteristics: urgency, hematuria, incontinence, nocturia.
- Change in urinary stream; dribbling.
- Medications: Prescription or nonpresription; diuretics

Urinary incontinence

- *Character:* Amount and frequency, constant or intermittent, dribbling versus frank incontinence.
- Associated with dysuria or other urinary characteristics: Urgency, hematuria, incontinence, nocturia.
- Change in urinary stream; dribbling
- Medications: Prescription or nonprescription; diruetics

Hematuria.

- *Character:* Color (bright red, rusty brown, cola-colored); present at beginning, end, or throughout voiding.

- *Associated symptoms:* Flank or costovertebral pain, passage of worm like clots, pain on voiding.
- *Alternate possibilities:* Ingestion of foods containing red vegetable dyes (may cause red urinary pigment); ingestion of laxatives containing phenolpthalein.
- Medication: Prescription or nonprescription; aspirin.

Chyluria (Milky Urine)
- Exposure to parasitic infection through travel.
- Exposure to tuberculosis.
- Medications: Prescription or nonprescription.

Past Medical History
- *Gastrointestinal disorder:* Peptic ulcer, polyps, inflammatory bowel disease, intestinal obstruction, pancreatitis.
- Hepatitis or cirrhosis of the liver.
- Abdominal or urinary tract surgery or injury.
- Urinary tract infection: Number, treatment.
- *Major illness:* Arthritis (Steroids or aspirin use), kidney disease, cardiac disease.
- Blood transfusion.
- Hepatitis vaccine.

Family History
- Worm Infestations, amebiasis.
- Hereditary disease: Renal stones, polycystic kidney, renal tubular acidosis, renal or bladder carcinoma.
- Malabsorption syndrome: Cystic fibrosis, celiac disease.
- Hirschprung's disease, aganglionic megacolon.
- Polyposis—Peutz-Jeghers syndrome, familial multiple polyposis coli.
- Liver disorders—Wilson's disease, Alpha-1 antitrypsin deficiency, Indian childhood cirrhosis.
- Gallstones, galactosemia, spherocytosis.
- Birth weight (less than 1500 gm at higher risk for necrotizing enterocolitis).
- Passage of first meconium stool within 24 hours, meconium ileus in newborns may be the first manifestation of cystic fibrosis.
- Jaundice in newborn period, exchange transfusions, phototherapy, breast-fed infants, appearing later in first month of life.
- Vomiting: Increasing in amount or frequency, forceful or projectile, failure to gain weight, insatiable appetite, blood in vomitus.
- Bilious vomiting in newborns often suggests intestinal obstruction.
- Diarrhoea, colic, failure to gain weight, weight loss, steatorrhea (malabsorption syndrome).
- Apparent enlargement of abdomen (with or without pain) constipation, or diarrhoea.

Children
- Constipation: Toilet training methods; diet; soiling; diarrhoea; abdominal distention; pica, size, shape, consistency, and odor of last stool; rectal bleeding; painful passage of stool.
- Abdominal pain: Splinting of abdominal movement, resists movement, keeps knees flexed.

Examination and Findings: Equipments
- Stethoscope
- Centimeter ruler and nonstretchable measuring tape
- Marking pen
- Torch (Light source).

Preparation
To perform the abdominal examination satisfactorily, you will need a good source of light, full exposure of the abdomen, warm hands with short fingernails, and a comfortable, relaxed patient. Have the patient empty his or her bladder before the examination begins. A full bladder interferes with accurate examination of organs and makes the examination uncomfortable for the patient. Place the patient in a supine position with arms at sides. The patient's abdominal musculature should be as relaxed as possible to allow access to the underlying structures. It may be helpful to place a small pillow under the patients head and another small pillow under the slightly flexed knees. Drape a towel over the patients chest for warmth and privacy. Ask the patient to breathe slowly through the mouth. Make your approach slowly and gently, avoiding sudden movements. Ask the patient to point to any tender areas, and examine those last.

Landmarks
For the purpose of examination, the abdomen can be divided into either four quadrants or nine regions. To divide the abdomen into quadrants, draw an imaginary line from the sternum to the pubis, through the umbilicus. Draw a second imaginary line perpendicular to the first, horizontally across the abdomen through the umbilicus (Fig. 24.2). The nine regions are created by two imaginary horizontal lines, one across the lowest edge of the costal margin and the other across the edge of the iliac crest, and by two vertical lines bilaterally from the midclavicular line to the middle of the Poupart ligament, approximating the lateral borders of the rectus abdominis muscles (Fig. 24.3). Choose one of these mapping methods and use it consistently. Quadrants are the more common of the two methods. The box below lists the contents of the abdomen in each of the quadrants and regions. Become accustomed to mentally visualizing the underlying organs and structures in each of the zones as you proceed with the examination.

Certain other anatomic landmarks are useful in describing the location of pain, tenderness, and other findings. These landmarks are illustrated in Figure 24.1B.

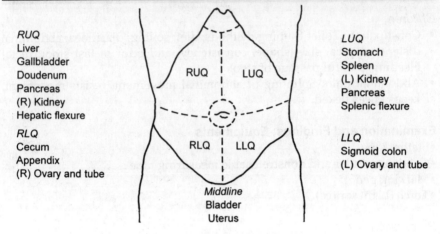

RUQ
Liver
Gallbladder
Doudenum
Pancreas
(R) Kidney
Hepatic flexure

RLQ
Cecum
Appendix
(R) Ovary and tube

LUQ
Stomach
Spleen
(L) Kidney
Pancreas
Splenic flexure

LLQ
Sigmoid colon
(L) Ovary and tube

Middline
Bladder
Uterus

Fig. 24.2: Superficial topography of the abdomen. Four quadrant system

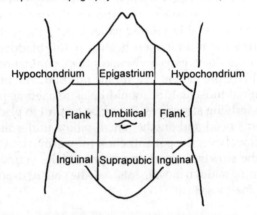

Fig. 24.3: Nine region system

Landmarks for abdominal examination (Tables 24.1 and 24.2)

Table 24.1: Anatomic correlates of the four quadrants of the abdomen

Right upper quadrant	Left upper quadrant
Liver and gallbladder	Left lobe of liver
Pylorus	Spleen
Duodenum	Stomach
Held of pancreas	Body of pancreas
Right adrenal gland	Left adrenal gland
Portion of right kidney	Portion of left kidney
Hepatic flexure of colon	Splenic flexure of colon
Portions of ascending and transverse colon	Portions of transvers and descending colon
Right lower quadrant	*Left lower quadrant*
Lower pole of right kidney	Lower pole of left kidney
Cecum and appendix	Sigmoid colon
Portion of ascending colon	Portion of descending colon

Contd...

Contd...

Right lower quadrant	Left lower quadrant
Bladder (if distended)	Bladder(if distended)
Ovary and salpinx	Ovary and salpinx
Uterus (if enlarged)	Uterus (if enlarged)
Right spermatic cord	Left spermatic cord
Right ureter	Left ureter

Table 24.2: Anatomic correlates of the nine regions of the abdomen

Right hypochondriac	*Epigastric*	*Left hypochondriac*
Right lobe of liver	Pyloric end of stomach	Stomach
Gallbladder	Duodenum	Spleen
Portion of duodenum	Pancreas	Tail of pancreas
Hepatic flexure of colon	Portion of liver	Splenic flexure of colon
Portion of right kidney		Upper pole of left kidney
Suprarenal gland		Suprarenal gland
Right lumber	*Umbilical*	*Left lumbar*
Ascending colon	Omentum	Descending colon
Lower half of right kidney	Mesentery	Lower half of left kidney
Portion of duodenum and jejunum	Lower part of duodenum Jejunum and ileum	Portions of jejunum and ileum
Right inguinal	*Hypogastric (Pubic)*	*Left inguinal*
Cecum	Ileum	Sigmoid colon
Appendix	Bladder	Left ureter
Lower end of ileum	Uterus (in pregnancy)	Left spermatic cord
Right ureter		Left ovary
Right spermatic cord		
Right ovary		

Inspection

Surface characteristics: Begin by inspecting the abdomen from a seated position at the right side of the patient. This position allows a tangential view that enhances shadows and contour.

Observe the skin color and surface characteristics.

Note the veins in standing position (Fig. 24.4). In infants with good subcutaneous tissue, veins are rarely visible. Visible but not distended veins are usually seen until puberty in healthy children and are especially noticeable in malnourished children. Distended veins are seen with heart failure, peritonitis and venous obstruction. Above the umbilicus, venous return should be towards the head; below the umbilicus it should be towards the feet (Figs 24.5A). To determine the direction of venous return, use the following procedure (Figs 24.6A to D). Place the index finger of each hand, side by side over a vein. Press laterally, separating the fingers and milking empty a section of the vein. Release one finger and time the refill. Release the other finger and time the refill. The flow of venous blood is in the direction of the faster filling. Flow patterns are altered in some disease states (Figs 24.5B and C). In portal hypertension, there are periumbilical engorged veins (caput mediusae) with flow of blood away from the umbilicus. In inferior vena cava obstruction, the direction of blood flow is from below upwards and in superior vena caval obstruction, it is from above downward. Bidirectional blood flow is seen in long-standing dilated veins (incompetence of venous valves) and in case of congenital absence of valves in the veins. In normal individuals, venous flow is away from umbilicus.

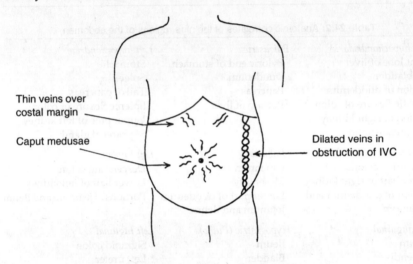

Thin veins over costal margin

Caput medusae

Dilated veins in obstruction of IVC

Fig. 24.4: Veins of abdominal wall

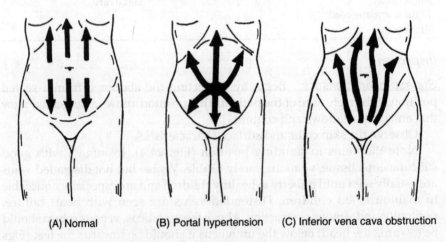

(A) Normal   (B) Portal hypertension   (C) Inferior vena cava obstruction

Figs 24.5A to C: Abdominal venous patterns

Unexpected findings include generalized color changes such as jaundice or cyanosis. A glittering appearance suggests ascites. Inspect for bruises and localized discoloration. Areas of redness may indicate inflammation. A bluish periumbilical discoloration (Cullen sign) suggests intra-abdominal bleeding.

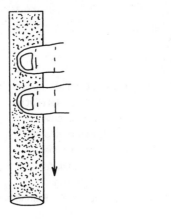

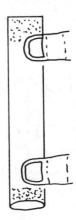

(A) Place two fingers side by side

(B) Move the lower finger away thus emptying part of the vein

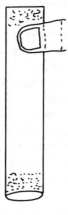

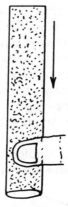

(C) Remove the lower finger and see whether vein remains empty or fills quickly. Here vein remains empty

(D) Replace the finger and remove the upper finger, blood will run down from above

Figs 24.6A to D: Detecting the direction of blood flow in a vein

Striae often result from weight gain or pregnancy. Striae of recent origin are blue in color but turn silvery white overtime. Abodminal tumor or ascites that stretches the skin also produces striae. The striae of Cushing's disease remain purplish.

Inspect for any lesions, particularly nodules. Lesions are of particular impor-tance since gastrointestinal disease often produces secondary skin changes. A pearl like enlarged umbilical node may signal intra-abdominal lymphoma.

Note any scars (Fig. 24.7) and draw their location, configuration. If the cause of a scar was not explained during the history, now is a good time to pursue that information. The presence of scarring should alert you to the possibility of internal adhesions.

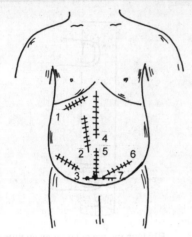

Fig. 24.7: Common abdominal incisions
1. Rt. subcostal (Kocher's)
2. Rt. paramedian
3. Appendicectomy
4. Upper midline
5. Lower midline
6. Left inguinal
7. Suprapubic (Pfannensteil)

Contour

Inspect the abdomen for contour, symmetry, and surface motion, using tangential lighting to illuminate contour and visible peristalsis. Contour is the abdominal profile from the rib margin to the pubis, viewed on the horizontal plane. The expected contours can be described as flat, rounded, or scaphoid (Figs 24.8A and B). The abdomen of the young child protrudes slightly, giving a potbellied appearance when the child is standing, sitting, and supine (Fig. 24.9). In the newborn, depressed or scaphoid abdomen may suggest a large diaphragmatic hernia with most of the abdominal contents in the chest. In older children, scaphoid abdomen occurs with marasmus, marked dehydration or high intestinal obstruction. In newborns, the abdomen is normally prominent, in toddler it is protruberant while in adolescents it is flat. Thin individuals have scaphoid abdomen while obese persons have prominent belly.

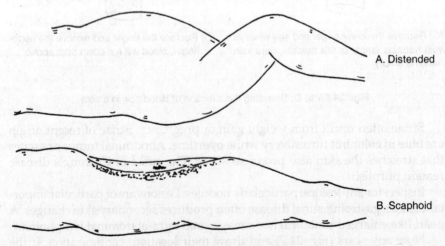

A. Distended

B. Scaphoid

Figs 24.8A and B: Contour of abdomen

Note the location and contour of the umbilicus. Normally it is closed and puckered, but hernia may be present as observed by protrusion of some abdominal contents. Umbilical remains are common in infants upto the age of two. Hernias are specially common in peritonitis, rickets, cirrhosis, mucopolysaccharidosis, hypotonic condition, children with hypothyroidism, Down syndrome, the chondrodystrophies; or large chronically distended abdomen. Granulomas, ulcers and drainage of the umbilicus can occur in the newborn.

Look for any distension or bulges. Real distention of the abdomen is usually caused by air (due to malabsorption, lactose intolerance, anticholinergic drugs, etc.) or fluid in the bowel or peritoneal cavity, but it may also be caused by atonic abdominal muscultaure, paralysis of the abdominal musculature, faces in the bowel, abnormal enlargement of organs, intestinal duplication, or tumors. Distention is frequently noted in children with pancreatic fibrosis, rickets, hypothyroidism, bowel obstruction, constipation, ileus, (following septicemia, drug intake, uremia, etc.), ascites or protein energy malnutrition. Localised bulge is seen in phantom hernia as seen in acute polio.

Ask the patient to take a deep breath and hold it. The contour should remain smooth and symmetric. This maneuver lowers the diaphragm and compresses the organ so that the abdominal cavity, which may cause previously

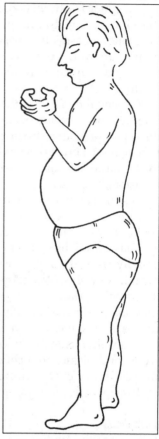

Fig. 24.9: Pot bellied stance in a toddler

unseen bulges or masses to appear. Next ask the patient to raise his or her head from the table. This contracts the rectus abdominis muscles, which produces muscle prominent in thin or athletic adults. Superficial abdominal wall masses may become visible. If a hernia is present, the increased abdominal pressure may cause it to protrude.

Observe Specifically for Hernia
An umbilical hernia protrudes through the umbilical ring. In the newborn a congenital umbilical hernia may result from improper closure of the abdominal wall; a hernia of the umbilical cord, also termed an omphalocele, is produced. In this, peritoneal sac is not covered by the skin of the abdominal wall.

True umbilical hernias are common during the first year of life. The maximum size is generally reached by 1 month of age, and the hernia will generally close spontaneously by 1 to 2 years of age. In this type the peritoneal sac is covered by skin. Increased intra-abdominal pressure due to trauma, cough, or constipation may contribute to their formation.

An epigastric hernia occurs through a weakness in the linea alba between the xiphoid and the umbilicus, usually due to a developmental defect. Pregnancy, obesity, trauma, or constipation may be contributing factors. These hernias are most common in young adult males. The hernial sac is usually small and may contain omentum but rarely intestine. Strangulation rarely occurs.

Incisional hernias, as the name indicates, occur through surgical incision. Infection, poor wound healing, faulty wound closure, postoperative vomiting, ileus, partial wound disruption, and obesity may be contributing factors. This type of hernia often reaches large size, and the intestines are usually adherent to the underside of the peritoneum. Strangulation is uncommon but may occasionally occur.

A spigelian hernia occurs at some point in the semilunar line at the lateral margin of the rectus muscle, usually in the lower abdomen at the linea semicircularis where the posterior rectus sheath is absent.

Diastasis of the rectus muscle may be noted as a protrusion in the midline, usually from the xiphoid to the umbilicus but occasionally down to the symphysis pubis. Ordinarly the protrusion is 1/2 to 2 inches size; it is usually a normal variant but may be caused by a congenital weakness of the musculature in a chronically distended abdomen. Diastasis of rectus abdominis ordinarily resolves by 6 years of age.

Transilluminate the abdomen with a strong light beam to differentiate cystic from solid masses in a child with an enlarged abodmen. Transillumination helps detect cystic tumors, bladder distention, and multicystic or hydronephrotic kidneys, as well as ascites.

Umbilicus
It lies opposite 4th lumbar ventra and aorta bifurcates below it.
1. Umbilical hernia is common in infants with rickets, Down syndrome, cretins and mucopolysaccaroidosis.
2. Look for omphalocele and gastrochisis.
3. Granuloma: Fleshy red granulation tissue at the base of umbilicus. In newborn it is due to infection or due to practice of putting talcum powder in umbilicus.
4. Polyp: Cherry red mass due to persistence of omphalomesenteric duct and patent urachus.
5. Discharge from umbilicus: Omphalitis, patent urachus (urinary discharge) patent vittelointestinal duct (fecal discharge).
6. Signs of omphalitis: Discharge, redness and erythema around umbilicus.
7. Transversly stretched umbilicus is seen in ascitis.

Movement of Abdominal Wall
1. Normally in inspiration abdomen moves upwards and during expiration inwards.
2. In diaphragmatic paralysis abdomen moves upwards in expiration and inwards in respiration (paradoxical respiration). This often occurs in

diaphragmatic paralysis due to phenic nerve injury in newborn and due to polio and Guillain-Barre syndrome in older children.

3. Bulging of abdominal wall during crying (phantom hernia) is seen in abdominal wall muscle paralysis in acute poliomyelitis.
4. Abdominal wall movements are severly restricted in peritonitis, tetanus and in strychnine poisoning.

With the patients head again resting on the table, inspect the abdomen for movement. Smooth, even movement should occur with respiration. Males exhibit primarily abdominal movement with respiration, whereas females show mostly costal movement. Respiration is largely abdominal in children upto 6 to 7 years of age, and even after this age the abdominal wall usually moves with respiration in children lying supine and in pregnant adolescents. Peritonitis, appendicitis, other acute surgical emergencies of the abdomen, paralytic ileus, diaphragmatic paralysis, a large amount of ascitic fluid, or a large amount of abdominal air may be present if the abdominal wall fails to move with respiration. If respiration is entirely abdominal in the young child or largely abdominal in the order child, suspect emphysema, pneumonia, or other pulmonary disorders.

Next look for *peristalsis* or *gastric waves*. Peristalsis is most easily seen if your eye is about at the level of the abdomen and a light is directed across the abdomen. Visible peristalsis is always a sign of obstruction until ruled otherwise. In infants upto 2 months of age, gastric visible peristalsis may indicate pyloric stenosis or pylorospasm. In older children, intestinal type (stepladder) of peristalsis may denote obstructions (due to round worm, volvulus, intussuception etc). It may be seen normally in thin, small infants, especially premature ones.

1. In the preterm babies, thin newborns, infants and children peristaltic waves may be normally seen.
2. There are 3 types of pathological peristaltic waves seen.
    a. Gastric visible peristalsis these waves travel from left hypochondrium to right hypochondrium and disappears under the right costal margin. These movements become prominent after a feed.

       The commonest cause in infants less than 6 months of age is congenital hypertrophic pyloric steonsis. Rarely duodenal bands, annular pancreas and other obstruction at pyloric region produce visible gastric peristalisis.
    b. Step ladder type (small intestinal type)

       Here the bowel loops are seen in the central portion of the abdomen and are one above the other like step ladder.

       The common causes in children include, round worm obstruction, congenital bands in general, whereas intususception, obstructed hernia are the causes in children below 2 years.
    c. Large bowel type-coils of intestine, are seen at the periphery of the abdomen, e.g. Hirschprung's disease, habitual constipation.

       Pulsations in the upper midline is often invisible in the adults. Marked visible pulsation over the epigastrium may be found in right ventricular hypertrophy, aneurysm of the abdominal aorta or due to the pulsatile liver of tricuspid incompetence.

Ausculation

Once inspection is completed, the next step is auscultation. Unlike the usual sequence, auscultation of the abdomen always precedes percussion and palpation because these may alter the frequency and intensity of bowel sounds. Moreover, the stethoscope itself may be used, concurrent with careful auscultation as the first instrument of light palpation. This technique is used to assess bowel sounds and to discover vascular sounds.

Bowel Sounds

Place the stethoscope firmly over the abdomen and listen carefully for bowel sounds. Note their frequency and character. They are usually heard as clicks and gurgles that occur irregularly and range from 5 to 35 per minute. bowel sounds should be present within 1 to 2 hours after birth. Sound can be increased in frequency and intensity simply by stroking the abdomen with a fingernail. Loud prolonged gurgles called borborygmi (stomach growling) are sometimes heard. High pitched and frequent bowel sounds may occur with early peritonitis, diarrhea from any cause, early intestinal obstruction, gastroenteritis, or hunger. Decreased bowel sounds occur with peritonitis and paralytic ileus. The absence of bowel sounds is established only after 5 minutes of careful listening. Auscultate all four quadrants to make sure that no sounds are missed and to localize specific sounds.

With outlet obstruction of the stomach, a succussion splash is at times detectable because of the presence of fluid and gas in the distended organ. This is easily appreciated by placing the stethoscope diaphragm over the epigastium and shaking the patient vigourously from side to side (Fig. 24.10). A characteristic splashing and gurgling sound is readily identified. It is important to determine the interval since the previous meal, as it is possible to elicit this sign in a normal person immediately after ingestion of a large quantity of fluid.

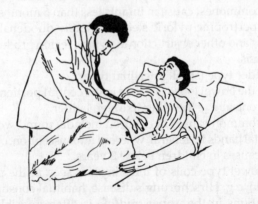

Fig. 24.10: Eliciting succussion splash

Auscultation may be employed for roughly gauging the size of the stomach or for detecting gastric dilatation. The chestpiece of the stethoscope being placed over the entire of the stomach, the skin of the abdomen is scratched with a fingernail along various lines radiating from the centre. A sudden change in intensity or character of the scratching sound is noted along each line. By joining three various points, the outline of the stomach can be roughly delineated. A tuning fork may be substituted for direct percussion with the finger.

Vascular Sounds

Listen with the bell of the stethoscope in the epigastric region and each of the four quadrants for bruits in the aortic, renal, iliac and femoral arteries. A murmur may be heard over the aorta in children with aortic aneurysm, aortitis or coarctation of aorta. Auscultate the area over the kidneys posteriorly with the bell to the stethoscope in children with hypertension. A murmur in this area may suggest renal artery stenosis, renal arteriovenous fistulae or vena caval thrombosis.

Friction Rubs

Listen with the diaphragm for friction rubs over the liver and spleen. Friction rubs are high pitched and are heard in association with respiration. Rubs may be heard over the liver in patients with hepatic tumor or infection and over the spleen in splenic infarction (chronic myeloid luekaemia, infectious mononucleosis, malaria, sickle cell anemia, subacute bacterial endocarditis), neoplasia and infection. Bruits heard over liver may suggest malignancy (e.g. as in hemangioma, vascular tumor, lymphosarcoma, hepatoma) or cirrhosis.

Auscultate with the bell of the stethoscope in the epigastric region and around the umbilicus for a venous hum, which is soft, low pitched and continous. A venous hum occurs with increased collateral circulation between portal and systemic venous systems. A bruit over umbilicus is heard in Cruvelier Bumgarten syndrome.(persistent patent umbilical artery)

Percussion

Percussion (generally indirect) is used to assess the size and density of the organs in the abdomen and to detect the presence of fluid (as with ascites), air (as with gastric distention), and fluid filled or solid masses.

First percuss all quadrants or regions of the abdomen for a sense of overall tympany and dullness (Table 24.3). Tympany is the predominant sound because air is present in the stomach and instestines. Dullness is heard over organs and solid masses (Figure 24.11 shows areas of dullness on abdominal percussion). A distended bladder produces dullness in the suprapubic area. Develop a systematic route for percussion, as shown in Figure 24.12.

Next percuss individually the liver, spleen, stomach and urinary bladder.

Liver Span

Begin liver percussion at the right midclavicular line over an area of tympany (always begin with an area of tympany and proceed to an area of dullness,

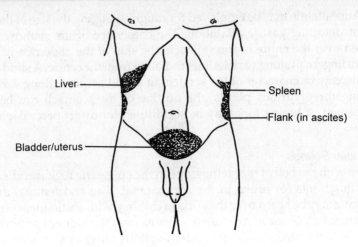

Fig. 24.11: Areas of dullness on abdominal percussion

Liver

Spleen

Flank (in ascites)

Bladder/uterus

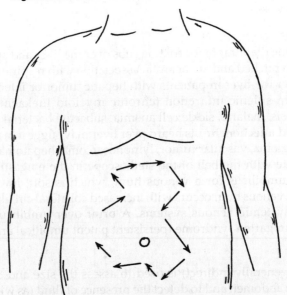

Fig. 24.12: Systematic route of abdominal percussion

Table 24.3: Percussion notes of the abdomen

Note	Location
Tympany	Over air filled viscera.
Hyperresonance	Base of left lung.
Resonance	Over lung tissue and sometimes over the abdomen.
Dullness	Over solid organs adjacent to air-filled structures.

because that sound change is easier to detect than the change from dullness to tympany) Percuss upward along the midclavicular line, as shown in Figure 24.13 to determine the lower border of the liver. The area of liver dullness is usually heard at the costal margin or slightly below it. Mark the border with a marking pen. A lower liver border that is more than 2 to 3 cm (¾ to 1 in) below the costal margin indicates organ enlargement or downward displacement of the diaphragm because of emphysema or other pulmonary disease.

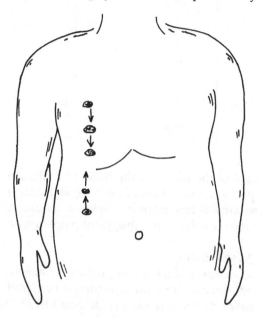

Fig. 24.13: Percussion of liver

To determine the upper border of the liver, begin percussion on the right midclavicular line at an area of lung resonance. Continue downwards until the percussion tone changes to one of dullness, which marks the upper border of the liver. Mark the location with the pen. The upper border usually begins at the fifth to seventh intercostal space. An upper border below this may indicate downward displacement or liver atrophy. Dullness extending above the fifth intercostal space suggests upward displacement from abdominal fluid or masses. the upper edge, in the liver should be detected within 1 cm of the fifth intercostal space at the right midclavicular line. It is normally placed in the seventh intercostal space along the right midaxillary line and at the ninth intercostal space along the right posterior axillary line.

Measure the distance between the marks to estimate the vertical span of the liver. the usual span is approximately 6 to 12 cm. A span greater than this may indicate liver enlargement, whereas a lesser span suggests atrophy, age and sex influence liver size. Obviously, the liver will be larger in adults than in children. Liver span is usually greater in males and tall individuals than in females and short people. Until 2 years of age females have a slightly larger liver span than males. The mean range of liver spans in infants and children is as follows (Table 24.4):

Table 24.4: Liver span in normal children (Mean ± SEM in cm)

Age	Boys		Girls	
	Liver span	SEM	Liver span	SEM
0.5	2.4	2.3	2.8	2.6
1	2.8	2.0	3.1	2.1
2	3.5	1.6	3.6	1.7
3	4.0	1.6	4.0	1.7
4	4.4	1.6	4.3	1.6
5	4.8	1.5	4.5	1.6
6	5.1	1.5	4.8	1.6
8	5.6	1.5	5.1	1.6
10	6.1	1.6	5.4	1.7
12	6.5	1.8	5.6	1.8
14	6.8	2.0	5.8	2.1

Liver Descent

To assess the descent of the liver, ask the patient to take a deep breath and hold it while you percuss upward again from the abdomen at the right mid-clavicular line. The area of lower border dullness should move downward 2 to 3 cm. This maneuver will guide subsequent palpation of the organ.

Additional Liver Assessment

If liver enlargement is suspected, additional percussion maneuvers can provide further information. Percuss upward and then downward over the right midaxillary line. Liver dullness is usually detected in the fifth to seventh intercostal space. Dullness beyond those limits suggests a problem. One can also percuss along the midsternal line to estimate the midsternal liver span. Percuss upward from the abdomen and downward from the lungs, marking the upper and lower borders of dullness. the usual span at the midsternal line is 4 to 8 cm (1½ to 3 in). Spans exceeding 8 cm suggest liver enlargement.

It is best to report the size of the liver in two ways by liver span as determined from percussing the uppper and lower borders and by the extent of liver projection below the costal margin.

Spleen

The spleen is behind the 9th, 10th and 11th ribs, with its long axis along the level of the 10th rib. Anteriorly, it extends to the midaxillary line, while posteriorly its superior angle is one and half inches lateral to the 10th thoracic spine.

The spleen is percussed just posterior to the midaxillary line on the left side. Percuss in several direction, beginning at areas of lung resonance.

A small area of splenic dullness may be heard from the sixth to the tenth rib. A large area of dullness suggests spleen enlargement; however, a full stomach or feces filled intestine may mimic the dullness of splenic enlargement. Remember that it is not possible to distinguish between the dullness of the posterior flank and that of the spleen. In addition, the dullness of a healthy spleen is often obscured by the tympany of colonic air.

Gastric Bubble

Percuss for the gastric air bubble in the area of the left lower anterior rib cage and left epigastric region. The tympany produced by the gastric bubble is lower in pitch than the tympany of the instestine.

Urinary Bladder

Move to the suprapubic area and outline the upper border of the urinary blader if possible. Watch carefully for evidence of tenderness while percussing. Percussable enlargement of the urinary bladder may or may not be of pathological signicance, depending on other factors.

Ascites Assessment

Ascites may be suspected in patients who have protuberant abdomen or who have flanks that bulge in the supine position. Percuss for areas of dullness and resonance with the patient supine. Since ascites fluid settles with gravity, expect to hear dullness in the dependent parts of the abdomen and tympany in the upper parts where the relatively lighter bowel has risen. Mark the borders between tympany and dullness.

Shifting Dullness

Then test for shifting dullness to help ascertain the presence of fluid. Make the patient lie on one side and again percuss for tympany and dullness and mark the borders. In the patient without ascites, the borders will remain relatively constant. In ascites, the border of dullness shifts to the dependent side (approaches the midline) as the fluid resettles with gravity (Fig. 24.14). The distribution of ascitic dullness is horseshoe shaped (Fig. 24.15).

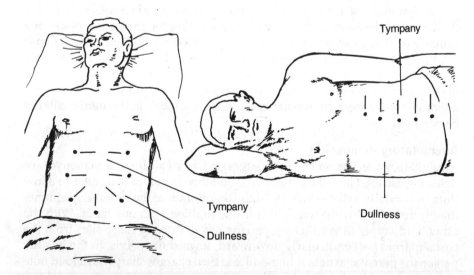

Fig. 24.14: Testing for shifting dullness. Dullness shifting to the dependent side

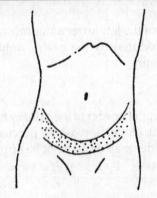

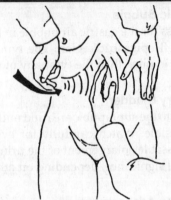

Fig. 24.15: Distribution of ascitic fluid (Horseshoe shaped)

Fig. 24.16: Demonstration of the fluid wave

Fluid Wave (Fluid Thrill)

Another maneuver is to test for a fluid wave. This procedure requires three hands, so you will need assistance from the patient or another examiner (Fig. 24.16). With the patient supine, ask him or her or another person to press the edge of the hand and forearm firmly along the vertical midline of the abdomen. This positioning helps to stop the transmission of a wave through adipose tissue. Place your hands on each side of the abdomen and strike one side sharply with your fingertips. Feel for the impulse of a fluid wave with the fingertips of your other hand. An easily detected fluid wave suggests ascites, but be cautioned that the findings of this maneuver are not conclusive. A fluid wave can sometiems be felt in people without ascites and, conversely, may not occur in people with early ascites.

A fluid wave may not be obtained if the volume of ascites is only moderate and abdominal distention is slight. In such a case it may be possible to elicit a fluid wave if the examination is performed during the expiratory phase of a cough or during a Valsalva maneuver. This produces contraction of the abdominal muscles, reduces the volume of the abdominal cavity, and temporarily puts the ascites under enough tension to elicit a wave. This sign may be obtained in the presence of intra-abdominal cysts or fluid filled intestines, although under these circumstances 'shifting dullness' in the flanks will not be obtained.

Auscultatory Percussion

Auscultatory percussion has been suggested as an additional maneuver for detecting ascites. Have the patient void and then stand for 3 minutes to allow fluid to gravitate to the pelvis. Hold the diaphragm of the stethoscope immediately above the symphysis pubis in the midline with one hand. With the other hard, apply finger flicking percussions to three or more sites from the costal margin perpendicularly downward, toward the pelvis. In the healthy person the percussion note is first dull and then charges sharply to a loud note at the pelvic border. In patients with ascites, the percussion note changes above the pelvic border at the fluid level.

Puddle Sign

Another maneuver allows you to test for fluid pooling (puddle sign). Ask the patient to assume the knee chest position and maintain that position for several minutes to allow any fluid to pool by gravity. Percuss the umbilical area for dullness to determine the presence of fluid (Fig. 24.17). The area will remain tympanic if no fluid is present.

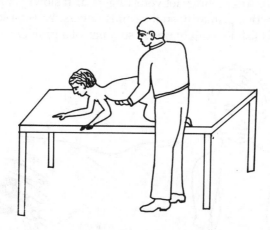

Fig. 24.17: Puddle sign

Fluid in the abdomen (ascites) is found in children with chronic liver disease (for example, cirrhosis), chronic kidney disease (for example, Nephrosis), tuberculous peritonitis, and rarely, heart failure, rupture or leak of the abdominal lymphatics (chylous ascites).

"Hydatid thrill" should be looked for whenever there is gross isolated hepatomegaly. In case of suspected hydatic cyst of the liver, when the middle finger of the left hand is placed over the lump and percussed, a peculiar quivering vibration of the finger is experienced. The displaced scolices and hydatid 'sand' touch the pleximeter finger soon after the tap.

Palpation

Palpation is used to assess the organs of the abdominal cavity and to detect muscle spasm, masses, fluid and areas of tenderness. The abdominal organs are evaluated for size, shape, mobility, consistency and tension. Stand at the patient's right side with the patient in the supine position. Make certain that the patient is comfortable and that the abdomen is as relaxed as possible; bending the patients knees may help relax the muscles. You can also ask the patient to breath with his mouth open. Your hands should be warm to avoid producing muscle contraction.

The ticklishness of a patient can sometimes make if difficult for you to palpate the abodmen satisfactorily. Here are some ways to overcome this problem.

- Distract the child with a toy, or question the child about a favourite activity as you begin palpating.
- Palpate the abdomen of a child who is ticklish with a firm rather than a feathery touch.
- If that is unsuccessful, ask the child to perform self palpation, and place your hands over the childs fingers, not quite touching the abdomen itself (Fig. 24.18A). After a time, let your fingers drift slowly onto the abdomen while still resting primarily on the childs fingers. You can still learn a good deal, and ticklishness might not be so much of a problem.

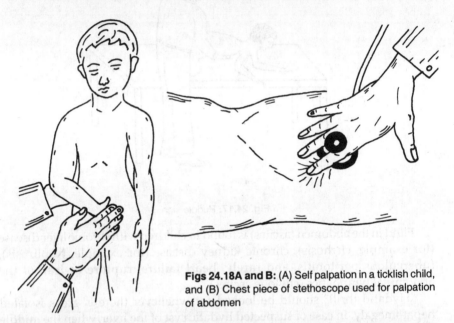

Figs 24.18A and B: (A) Self palpation in a ticklish child, and (B) Chest piece of stethoscope used for palpation of abdomen

- You might also use the diaphragm of the stethoscope (making sure it is warm enough) as a palpating instrument. This serves as a starting point, and again your fingers can drift over the edge of the diaphragm and palpate without eliciting an excessively ticklish response.
- Applying a stimulus to another, less sensitive part of the body with your nonpalpating hand can also divert a ticklish repsonse.
- Piecemeal examination or examination under mild sedation can also be resorted to, if the situation warrants. Sedation can also be resorted to, if the situation warrants. Sedation is sometimes essential in the detailed evaluation of abdominal mass, Trichlofos syrup is the best sedative. The so called nipple to knee exposure advocated in the examination of adults may be frightening to children and may be unwarranted.

Doll to baby: Apprehension in toddlers can be reduced by palpating and ascultating over a doll and then over the patient.

The abdomen of an infant can seem very silly in relation to the size of your hand. One technique for palpating a very small abdomen is as follows:

Place your right hand gently on the abodmen with the thumb at the right upper quadrant and the middle finger at the left upper quadrant. Press very gently at first, only gradually increasing pressure as you palpate the entire abdomen. The thumb feels for liver and the middle finger the spleen both at the same time, then bring the hand downwards to palpate other parts of abdomen (Fig. 24.19).

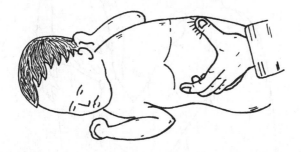

Fig. 24.19: Palpation of liver and spleen simultaneously unimanual method

Infants are generally apprehensive and often cry and strain thus tensing the abdomen. It is best to examine an infant in the mothers lap. Breastfeeding is the best soother to elicit cooperation (Fig. 24.20).

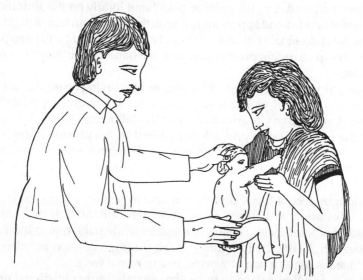

Fig. 24.20: Palpation of child's abdomen while he is breastfeeding

Toddlers often will allow you to palpate their abdomen while standing, but object voiceferously once you lie them down (Fig. 24.21).

Light Palpation

Palpate gently and superficially, using the upper hand for most of the palpatory sensation. Begin in the left lower quadrant and then proceed to the left upper,

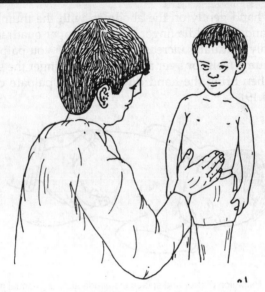

Fig. 24.21: Palpating the abdomen of the toddler standing on a couch

right upper, right lower quadrants and middle. If a localized site of pain or tenderness is found. Palpate this area after the other parts of the abdomen have been palpated. Lay the palm of your hand lightly on the abdomen with the fingers extended and approximated with the palmar surface of your fingers, depress the abdominal wall no more than 1 cm, using a light and even pressing motion. When changing position, remove the hand rather than drag it across the surface.

Light palpation is particularly useful in identifying muscular resistance, warmth and areas of tenderness. If resistance is present, try to determine whether it is voluntary or involuntary in the followings way: place a pillow under the patients knees and ask the patient to breath slowly through the mouth as you feel for relaxation of the rectus abdominis muscles on expiration. If the tenseness remains, it is probably an involuntary response to localized or generalized rigidity.

A doughy feel of the abdomen is found in protein energy malnutrition, worm infestation and tuberculous abdomen. Indentation on pressure is suggestive of fecal mass. Feeling of crepitus while palpation is indicative of trichobezoar. A sensation of gurgle is felt during palpation of colon, round worm mass is felt as a bag of worms (bag of worm feel).

Edema of abdominal wall can be demonstrated either by digital pressure, which leads to the phenomenon of pitting or by picking up a fold of skin and subcutaneous tissues in which case the thickening of tissues through edema becomes obvious (Fig. 24.22A) Edema of the abdominal wall may be associated with generalised edema or anasarca, as in cases of nephritis or cardiac failure, or with massive ascites.

Skin turgor is elicited by pinching a fold of skin with underlying subcutaneous tissue in lower abdomen. Normally the fold of skin goes back slowly and in severe dehydration very slowly.

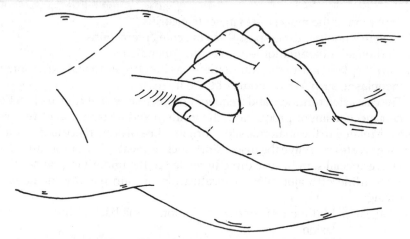

Fig. 24.22A: Skin pinch for loss of turgor in dehydration. This test can also be used for noting abdominal wall edema

Hyperesthesia should be tested for routinely. Specific zones for peritoneal irritation may be identified through cutaneous hypersensitivity (Fig. 1.22b). To evaluate hypersensitivity, gently lift a fold of skin away from the underlying muscle or stimulate the skin with a pen or other object and have the patient describe the local sensation. In the event of hypersensitivity, the patient will perceive pain or an exaggerated sensation in response to this manuever.

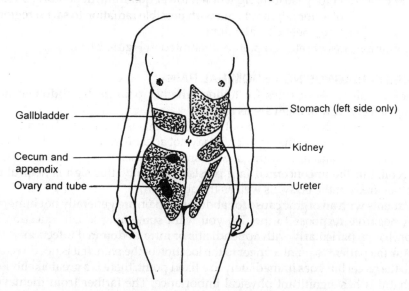

Fig. 24.22b: Areas of cutaneous hypersensitivity

Pain Assessment

Pain of gastrointestinal origin varies greatly depending on its underlying cause. The major pain mechanism include:
1. Capsular stretching-as in liver congestion due to heart failure.

2. Irritation of the mucosa—as in acute gastritis.
3. Severe smooth muscle spasm—as in acute enterocolitis
4. Peritoneal inflammation—as in acute appendicitis.
5. Direct splanchnic nerve stimulation—as in retroperitoneal extension of a neoplasm, such as carcinoma of the pancreas.

The character, duration, and frequency of gastrointestinal pain are functions of their mechansim of production; the location and distribution of refrerred pain are related to the anatomic site of origin. Time of occurrence and elements that aggravate and relive the discomfort, such as meals, defecation, and sleep, also have special significance directly related to the underlying cause.

An outline of major sites of localization of pain usually includes the following:

Esophageal : Midline retrosternal; radiation to the back at the level of the lesion.

Gastric : Epigastric, radiation occasionally to back, paricularly left subscapular.

Duodenal : Epigastric; radiation to back, particularly right subscapular.

Gallblader : Right upper quadrant or epigastric; radiation to right subscapular or midback.

Pancreatic : Epigastric; radiation to midback or left lumbar area. Small Intestinal Periumbilical.

Appendiceal : Periumbilical, migrating later to right lower quadrant.

Colonic : Hypogastrium, right or left lower quadrant, depending on site of lesion; sigmoid pain with possible radiation to sacral region.

Rectal : Deep pelvic localization.

Common sites of referred pain is illustrated in Figure 24.23.

CLUES IN DIAGNOSING ABDOMINAL PAIN

There are all types of rules for telling whether pain in the abdomen has significance. A few of them are as follow:

- Patients may give a touch me not warning—that is, not to touch in a particular area; however, these patients may not actually have pain if their faces seem relaxed and unconcerned, even smiling. When you touch they might recoil, but the unconcerned face persists (Actually, this sign is helpful in other areas of the body, as well as the abdomen).
- Patients with an orgnic cause for abdominal pain are generally not hungry. A negative response to the 'Do you want something to eat' question is probable, paricularly with appendicitis or intra-abdominal infection.
- Ask the patient to point a finger to the location of the pain. If it is not directed to the navel but goes immediately to a fixed point, there is a great likelihood that this has significant physical importance. The farther from the navel the pain, the more likely it will be organic in origin (Apley's rule). If the finger goes to the navel and the patient seems otherwise well to you, you should include psychogenic causes in the list of differential diagnosis.
- Patients with nonspecific abdominal pain may keep their eyes closed during abdominal palpation, whereas patients with organic disease usually keep their eyes open.

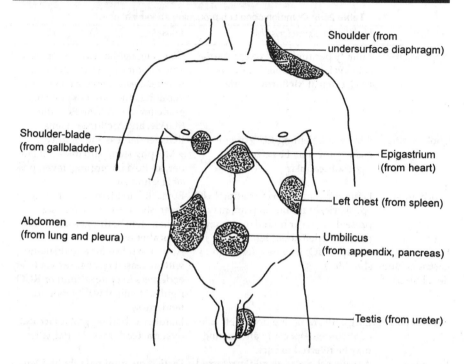

Fig. 24.23: Common sites of referred pain

- Pain that is severe enough to make the patient unwilling to move, accompanied by nausea and vomiting, and marked by areas of localized tenderness generally has an underlying physical cause.
- You can determine the site of tenderness by watching the patient's face, noting whining, cry, and change of pitch of cry as the really tender area is touched. Note the pupils when palpating when a truly tender area is touched, the pupils will dilate.
- When child is continuously crying because of apprehension, to determine the tenderness over abdomen, try pressing over thigh and then over abdomen and see the difference in the intensity of cry.
- If a child is kicking his/her legs, then possibly an abdominal surgical condition can be ruled out.
- If a child has significant watery diarrhea, it almost rules out an acute surgical abdomen.
- In a crying child, distinguish between a soft and hard abdomen by feeling immediately on inspiration when the child may relax for a moment. If the child is tense and does not relax even during inspiration, peritoneal irritation should be suspected.
- Intra-abdominal tenderness can be distinguished from muscle tenderness by asking the child to raise the head and then palpate. Intra-abdominal tenderness is lessened, whereas superficial tenderness is increased by this maneuver.

Table 24.5: Common condition producing abdominal pain

Conditions	Usual pain characteristics	Possible associated findings
Appendicitis	Initially periumbilical or epigastric; colicky; later becomes localized to RLQ, often at McBurney point	Guarding tenderness; + iliopsoas and + obturator signs, RIQ skin hyperesthesia; anorexia, nausea or vomiting after onset of pain; low-grade fever; + Aaron, Rovsing, Markle, and McBurney signs
Cholecystitis	Severe, unrelenting RUQ or epi-gastic pain; may be referred to right subscapular	RUQ tenderness and rigidity, + Murphy sign, palpable gallblad-der, anorexia, vomiting, fever, pos-sible jaundice
Pancreatitis	Dramatic, sudden excruciating LUQ, epigastric, or umbilical pain; may be present in one or both flanks; may be referred to left shoulder	Epigastric tenderness, vomiting, fever, shock;+ Grey Tuner sign; + Cullen sign: both signs occur 2-3 days after onset
Perforated gastric or duo-denal ulcer	Abrupt RUQ; may be referred to shoulders	Abdominal free air and distention with increased resonance over liver; enderness in epitgastrium or RUQ; rigid abdominal wall, rebound tenderness
Diverticulitis	Epigastric, radiating down left side of abdomen especially after eating; may be referred to back	Flatulence, borborygmi, diarrhea, dysuria, tenderness on palpation
Intestinal obstruction	Abrupt, severe, spasmodic; referred to epigastrium, umbilicus	Distention, minimal rebound ten-derness, vomiting, localized tender-ness, visible peristalsis; bowel sounds absent (with peristaltic obstruction)
Volvulus	Referred to hypogastrium and umbilicus	Distention, nausea, vomiting, guarding; sigmoid loop volvulus may be palpable
Leaking abdo-minal aneu-rysm	Steady throbbing midline over aneu-rysm; may radiate to back, flank	Nausea, vomiting, abdominal mass, bruit
Biliary stones colic	Episodic, severe, RUQ, or epigas-trium lasting 15 min to several hours; may be referred to subscapular area, especially right	RUQ tenderness, soft abdominal wall, anorexia, vomiting, jaundice, subnormal temperature
Salpingitis	Lower quadrant, worse on left	Nausea, vomiting, fever, suprapubic tenderness, rigid abdomen, pain on pelvic examination
Ecotpic pregnancy	Lower quadrant; referred to shoulder; with rupture is agonizing	Hypogastric tenderness, symptoms of pregnancy, spotting, irregular menses, soft abdominal wall, mass on bimanual pelvic exam. Ruptured: shock, rigid abdominal wall, distention; + Kehr, Cullen signs
Pelvic inflam-matory disease	Lower quadrant, increases with activity	Tender adnexa and cervix, cervical discharge, dyspareunia
Ruptured ovarian cyst	Lower quadrant steady, increases with cough or motion	Vomiting, low-grade fever, anorexia, tenderness, on pelvic examination

Contd...

Contd...

Conditions	Usual pain characteristics	Possible associated findings
Renal calculi	Intense; flank, extending to groin and genitals, may be episodic	Fever, hematuria + kehr sign
Splenic rupture	Intense, LUQ, radiating to be the shoulder, may worsen with foot of bed elevated	Shock, pallor, lowered temperature
Peritonitis	Onset sudden or gradual; pain generalized or localised, dull or severe and unrelenting; guarding; pain on deep inspiration.	Shallow respiration; + Blumberg, Markle, Ballance signs; reduced bowel sounds, nausea and vomiting + obturator and Iliopsoas Tests.

Table 24.6: Quality and onset of abdominal pain

Characteristic	Possible-related condition
Burning	Peptic ulcer
Cramping	Biliary colic, gastroenteritis
Colic	Appendicitis with impacted feces; renal stone
Aching	Appendiceal irritation
Knifelike	Pancreatitis
Gradual onset	Infection
Sudden onset	Duodenal ulcer, acute pancreatitis, obstruction, perforation.

Table 24.7: Causes of acute abdominal pain perceived in anatomical regions

a. **Right upper quadrant**
   Acute cholecystitis
   Duodenal ulcer
   Hepatitis
   Congestive hepatomegaly
   Pyelonephritis
   (R) Pneumonia

b. **Left upper quadrant**
   Ruptured spleen
   Gastric ulcer
   Pyelonephritis
   (L) Pneumonia

c. **Right lower quadrant**
   Appendicitis
   Salpingitis
   Tubo-ovarian abscess
   Ruptured ectopic pregnancy
   Renal/ureteral stone
   Incarcerated hernia
   Mesenteric adenitis
   Meckel's diverticulitis
   Regional ileitis
   Perforated cecum
   Psoas abscess

d. **Left lower quadrant**
   Sigmoid diverticulitis
   Salpingitis
   Tubo-ovarian abscess
   Ruptured ectopic pregnancy
   Incarcerated hernia
   Perforated colon
   Regional ileitis
   Ulcerative colitis
   Renal/ureteral stone

e. **Periumbilical region**
   Intestinal obstruction
   Acute pancreatitis
   Early appendicitis
   Mesenteric thrombosis
   Diverticulitis

Table 24.8: Findings in peritoneal irritation

- Involuntary rigidity of abdominal muscles
- Tenderness and guarding
- Absent bowel sounds
- Positive obturator test
- Positive iliopsoas test
- Rebound tenderness (Blumberg sign)
- Abdominal pain on walking
- Positive heel jar test (Markle sign)
- Positive rousing sign.

  Mnemonics: Features of peritonitis: 'PERITONITIS'

  P   Pain: front, back sides, shoulders
  E   Electrolytes fall, shock ensues
  R   Rigidity or rebound tenderness of anterior abdominal wall
  I   Immobile abdomen and patient
  T   Tenderness (rebound)
  O   Obstruction
  N   Nausea and vomiting
  I   Increasing pulse, decreasing blood pressure
  T   Temperature falls and then rises
  I   Increasing girth of abdomen
  S   Silent abdomen (no bowel sounds)

- It is sometimes difficult to differentiate an acute upper abdominal process from intrathoracic disease. In this situation, deep pressure on the opposite side of the abdomen directed towards the affected side will produce pain if the basic process is intra-abdominal; however, it will not elicit pain if the disease is intrathoracic.
- In gastroenteritis, vomiting is followed by pain abdomen. The reverse is true in acute appendicitis.

Common causes of abdominal pain are described in Table 24.5. Careful assessment of the quality (Table 24.6) and location of pain (Table 24.7) can usually narrow the possible causes, allowing you to select an additional diagnostic studies with greater efficiency. Findings associated with peritoneal irritation are summarized in Table 24.8. Some of the tests mentioned in Table 24.8 are now being elaborated.

Rebound Tenderness

The following maneuver is considered crude and unnecessary by many examiners, since light percussion produces a mild localized response in the presence of peritoneal inflammation. If the patient is experiencing abdominal pain, this maneuver can be used to determine peritoneal irritation. Place the patient in the supine position. Hold your hand at a 90 degrees angle to the abdomen with the fingers extended, then press gently and deeply into a region remote from the area of discomfort. Rapidly withdraw your hand and fingers (Fig. 24.24). The return to position (rebound) of the structures that were compressed by your fingers causes a sharp stabbing pain at the site of peritoneal inflammation (positive Blumberg sign). Rebound tenderness over the McBurney point in the lower right quadrant suggests appendicitis (positive McBurney sign). The maneuver for rebound tenderness should be performed at the end of the examination, because a positive response produces pain and muscle spasm that can interfere with any subsequent examination.

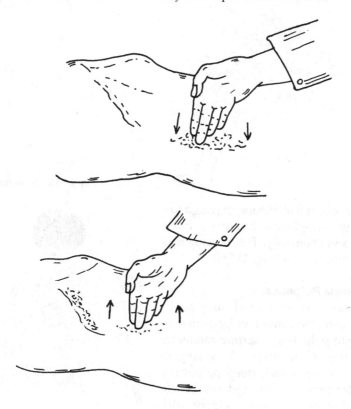

Fig. 24.24: Rebound tenderness

Iliopsoas Test

A patient with a positive iliopsoas sign will experience lower quadrant pain. Perform this test when you suspect appendicitis. An inflamed appendix may cause irritation of the lateral ileopsoas muscle. Ask the patient to lie supine and then place your hand over the lower thigh. Ask the patient to raise the leg, flexing at the hip, while you push downward against the leg (Fig. 24.25).

An alternate technique is to position the patient on the left side and ask that the right leg be raised from the hip while you press downwards against it.

A third technique is to hyperextend the leg by drawing it backward while the patient is lying on the right side.

Obturator Test

If the inflammatory process is adjacent to the obturator internus muscle, as in the presence of pelvic abscess or a ruptured appendix, lower abdominal pain

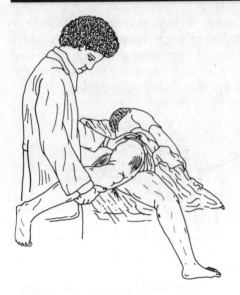

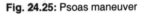

Fig. 24.25: Psoas maneuver

may be elicited by flexing the thigh to a 90 degree angle and rotating it internally and externally. This is known as the obturator test (Fig. 24.26).

Moderate Palpation

Continue palpation of all four quadrants with the same hand position as for light palpation, exerting moderate pressure as an intermediate step to gradually approach deep palpation. Tenderness not elicited on gentle palpation may become evident with deeper pressure. An additional maneuver of moderate palpation is performed with the side of your hand. This

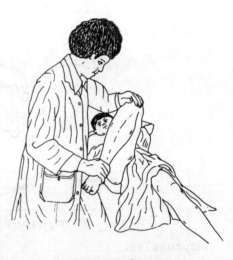

Fig. 24.26: Obturator test

maneuver is useful in assessing organs that move with respiration, specifically the liver and spleen. Palpate during the entire respiratory cycle; as the patient inspires, the organ is displaced downward, and you may be able to feel it as it bumps gently against your hand (Fig. 24.27).

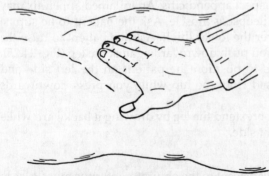

Fig. 24.27: Moderate palpation using side of hand

Deep Palpation

Deep palpation is necessary to thoroughly delineate abdominal organs and to detect less obvious masses. Use the palmar surface of your extended figners pressing deeply and evenly into the abdominal wall (Fig. 24.28). Palpate all four quadrants, moving the fingers back and forth over the abdominal contents (The abdominal wall may also

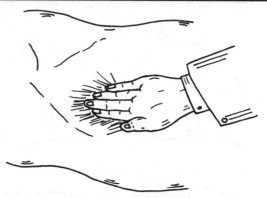

Fig. 24.28: Deep palpation. Press deep with palmal surface of extended fingers

slide back and forth as you do this). Often you are able to feel the borders of the rectus abdominis muscles, the aorta, and portions of the colon. Tenderness not elicited with light or moderate palpation may become evident. Deep pressure may also evoke tenderness in the healthy person over the cecum, sigmoid colon, aorta, and in the midline near the xiphoid process.

Bimanual Palpation

If deep palpation is difficult because of obesity and muscular resistance, you can use bimanual technique with one hand atop the other as shown in Figure 24.29. Exert pressure with the top hand while concentrating on sensation with the other hand.

Palpation by Ballotment

In children with ascites, it may be difficult to feel any masses directly. Under these circumstances, it is sometimes possible to detect such a mass by ballotment. To perform abdominal ballotment with one hand, place your extended figners, hand, and forearm at a 90 degree angle to the abodmen. Push in forward the mass with the finger tips (Fig. 24.30A). If the mass is freely movable, a rebound sensation will be felt in the flickeing hand, as if a ball has been thrown forward and has came back (Dipping method).

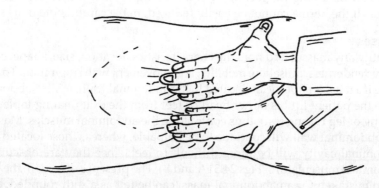

Fig. 24.29: Bimanual palpation

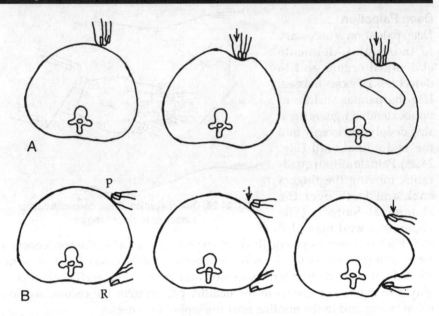

Figs 24.30A and B: Ballottement technique. (A) Single-handed ballotterment. Push inward at a 90° angle. If the object is freely movable, it will float upward to touch the finger tips, (B) Bimanual ballottement: P, pushing hand; R, receiving hand

To perform *Bimanual ballotment*, place one hand on the anterior abdominal wall and one hand against the flank. Push inward on the abdominal wall while palpating with the hand at the flank to determine the presence and size of the mass (Fig. 24.30B).

Umbilical Ring

Palpate the umbilical ring and around the umbilicus. The area should be free of bulges, nodules, and granulation. The umbilical ring should be round and free of irregularites. Note whether it is incomplete or soft in the center, which suggests the potential of herniation. Palpate the umbilical hernia, if noted previously. Note the presence of bowel in the hernia by palpating a gas filled loop and obtaining the feeling of silk rubbing against silk on replacing the viscus. If the hernia cannot be easily reduced, make careful note of its size.

Masses

Identify any masses and note the characteristics: location, size, shape, consistency, tenderness, pulsation, mobility, and movement with respiration. To determine if a mass is superficial (located in the abdominal wall) or intra-abdominal, have the patient lift his or her head or feet from the examinating table (head raising or leg raising test), thus contracting the abdominal muscles. Masses in the abdominal wall will continue to be palpable, whereas those located in the abdominal cavity will be more difficult to feel, since they are obscured by abdominal musculature (Figs 24.31A and B). The presence of feces in the colon, often mistaken for an abdominal mass, can be felt as a soft, rounded, boggy mass in the cecum and in the ascending, descending, or sigmoid colon. Fecal mass indents on pressure. Other structures that are sometimes mistaken for masses are the lateral borders of the rectus abdominis muscles, the uterus, aorta, sacral promontory, and common iliac artery (Fig. 24.32). If you can mentally visualize the placement of the abdominal structures it will be easier to distinguish between what you know ought to be there and an unexpected finding. For example, a midline suprapubic mass suggests Hirschsprung's disease, in which feces fill the rectosigmoid colon. A sausage-shaped mass in the left or right upper quadrant may indicate intussusception.

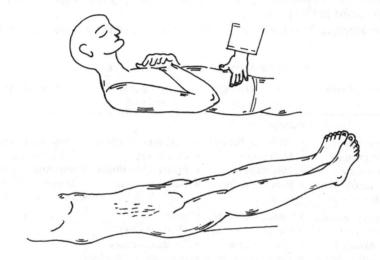

Figs 24.31A and B: (A) Neck rising test, and (B) leg rising test

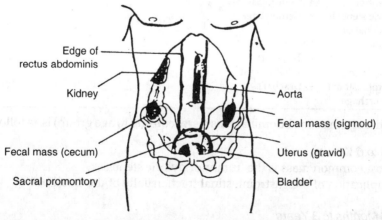

Fig. 24.32: Some normal abdominal "masses"

Abdominal masses can also have pulsation. Pseudopancreatic cyst, for example, may give rise to transmitted pulsation. Liver, on the other hand, can have expansile pulsation secondary to tricuspid regurgitation or hemangioma.

The "head raising test" is used to differentiate between an upper intra-abdominal mass from an intra-abdominal one whereas the "leg raising test" is used to determine whether a lower abdominal mass is intra-abdominal or extra-abdominal.

Intra-abdominal masses tend to move freely with respiration. Liver, spleen and stomach have good movement with respiration, kidney, however, moves less with respiration. In a crying child, an extra-abdominal lump will become more prominent compared to an intra-abdominal lump.

To know whether a mass is intraperitoneal or retroperitoneal, put the patient in a knee chest position and palpate for the lump. An intraperitoneal lump falls forward in this position.

Common abdominal masses (region wise) have been delineated in Table 24.9.

Table 24.9: Abdominal mass: a physical examination

Upper abdomen	Mid-abdomen and flanks	Lower abdomen and pelvis	Variable location
Liver	*Kidneys*	*Uterus*	
• Hepatomegaly	• Hydronephrosis	• Hydrometrocolpos	• Mesenteric cyst
• Subcapsular-hematoma	• Multicystic	• Ovarian cyst	• Omental cyst
• Ruptured spleen	• Polycystic	• Presacral teratoma	• Intestinal duplication
• Hemangioma	• Renal vein thrombosis	• Neuroblastoma	• Meconium ileus
			• Abscess
• Hepatoblastoma	• Congenital meso-blastic nephroma	*Bladder*	
• Neuroblastoma (metastatic)	• Wilms' tumor	• Urethral valves	
• Choledocal cyst	• Horseshoe kidney	• Urethral stenosis	
		• Neurogenic bladder	
		• Ectopic kidney	
Gastric	*Adrenal glands*		
• Distention	• Neuroblastoma		
• Pyloric stenosis	• Hemorrhage		
• Duodenal obs-truction			
	Retroperitoneal		
	• Teratoma		
Adrenal glands	• Vitelline cyst		
• Neuroblastoma	• Urachal cyst		
• Hemorrhage			

A list of common abdominal masses (according to age group) is as follows:

Age 3 to 6 Weeks
1. Most common mass is the 'tumor' of pyloric stenosis.
2. Duplication of the gastrointestinal tract, usually of the small bowel.

Age 6 Months to 3 Years
1. Intussuccseption is the most common mass.
2. Mesenteric cyst.
3. Appendiceal abscess.
4. Abscesses and fistulas secondary to granulomatous colitis.

5. Most common tumors are Wilms' tumor (about 60 percent occur before the age of 5 years) and neuroblastoma (about 50 percent occur within the first 2 years of life).

Older Infant and Child
 a. Renal malformations.
 b. Hydronephrosis.
 c. Left lower quadrant
      Bladder distention
      Pregnancy in adolescent
      Ovarian cyst
      Urachal cyst
      Hydrometrocolpos.
 d. All four quadrants
      Hydronephrosis
      Multicystic dysplastic kidney
      Polycystic kidney disease
      Intestinal duplication
      Teratoma
      Abscess
      Anterior meningocele
      Mesenteric cyst
      Omental cyst
      Retroperitoneal lymphangioma
      Hard masses of the abdomen are the following
      Neuroblastoma
      Nephroblastoma
      Hepatoma
      Nodular masses of the abdomen consist of
      Mesenteric lymph nodes (tuberculosis, lymphoma, leukemia)
      Tabes mesenterica.
      Adominal masses with extreme mobility side to side include
      Mesenteric cyst
      Duplication of intestine
      Roundworm mass
      Fecolith
      Ovarian cyst with peduncle
      Rarely, hydatid cyst with peduncle.

Palpation of Specific Structures

Liver

Place your left hand under the patient at the eleventh and twelfth ribs, pressing upward to elevate the liver toward the abdominal wall. Place your right hand on the abdomen, fingers pointing towards the head and extended so the tips rest on the right midclavicular line below the level of liver dullness, as shown

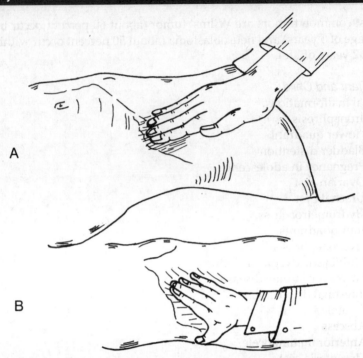

Figs 24.33A and B: (A) Palpation of liver, and (B) alternative method of palpation of liver

in Figure 24.33A. As an alternative, you can place your right hand parallel to the right costal margin, as shown in Figure 24.33B. In either case, press your right hand gently but deeply in and up. Have the patient breathe regularly a few times and then take a deep breath. Try to feel the liver edge as the diaphragm pushes it down to meet your fingertips. Ordinarily, the liver is not palpable, although it may be felt in some thin persons even when no pathologic condition exists. If the liver edge is felt, it should be firm, smooth, even, and nontender. Feel for nodules, tenderness, and irregularity. If the liver is palpable, repeat the maneuver medially and laterally to the costal margin to assess the contour and surface of the liver.

Alternate techniques An alternate technique is to hook your fingers over the right costal margin below the border of liver dullnes, as shown in Figure 24.34. Stand on the patient's right side facing his or her feet. Press in and up towards the costal margin with your fingers and ask the patient to take a deep breath. Try to feel the liver edge as it descends to meet your fingers.

If the abdomen is distended or the abdominal muscles tense, the usual techniques for determining the lower liver border may be unproductive. At such a point, the scratch test may be useful (Fig. 24.35). This technique uses auscultation to detect the differences in sound transmission over solid and hollow organs. Place the stethoscope over the liver and with the finger of your other hand scratch the abdominal surface lightly, moving toward the liver border. When you encounter the liver, the sound you hear in the stethoscope will be intensified.

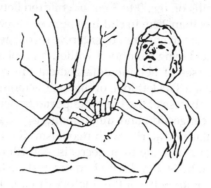

Fig. 24.34: Palpation of the liver (see text) hooking

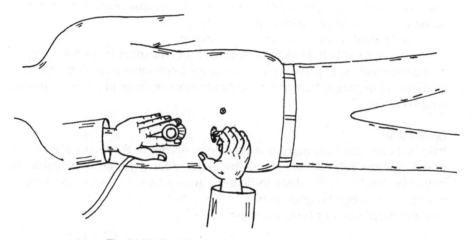

Fig. 24.35: Scratch technique for auscoltating the liver

To check for liver tenderness when the liver is not palpable, use indirect fist percussion. Place the palmar surface of one hand over the lower right rib cage, and then strike your hand with the ulnar surface of the fist of your other hand as shown in Figure 24.36. The healthy liver is not tender to percussion.

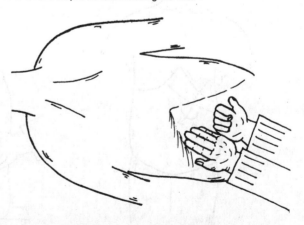

Fig. 24.36: Fist percussion of the liver

If the liver edge is palpated, measure the size below the costal margin at the midclavicular line using a ruler or tape measure. Normal values are: 2 to 3 cm below the costal margin up to 9 months of age: 0 to 3 cm in children between six month and four years of age: less than 2 cm in children between four years and ten years of age and less than 1cm in children over ten years of age. However, the liver may remain palpable during childhood without pathologic significance.

The principal causes of hepatic enlargement are congestion, cirrhosis, hepatitis and neoplasm. The left lobe of the liver is more prominent than the right lobe in amebic abscess of the liver and portal hypertension. Tenderness is more likely with congestion and inflammations, a hard consistency with cirrhosis and irregular nodularity with neoplasm. Rapidly decreasing liver size may be diagnostic of acute liver necrosis. A thrill felt over an enlarged liver or a gurgling sound is found with hydatid cysts in the liver. Friction rub over the liver occurs with pelvic inflammatory disease. Pulsation of the liver best felt by bimanual palpation, usually results from transmission of the impulse from the aorta, but quite rarely it may be because of tricupsid regurgitation or stenosis or constrictive pericarditis.

Bimanual palpation of liver for liver pulsations.

With one hand behind right lumbar area and the other in the Right hypochondrium feel the expansile pulsation of the liver. Liver pulsations are seen in tricupsid regurgitation and vascular tumors of liver like hemangioma, lymphangioma.

Gallbladder

Palpate below the liver margin at the lateral border of the rectus abdominis muscle for the gallbladder. A healthy gallbladder will not be palpable. A palpable, tender gallbladder indicates cholecystitis, whereas non tender enlargement suggests common bile duct obstruction.

Position of gallbladder is shown in figure 24.37A.

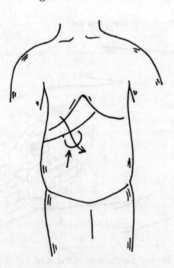
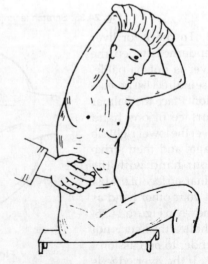

Fig. 24.37A: Position of gallbladder (small arrow)

Fig. 24.37B: Eliciting Murphy's sign. In Moynihan's method the patient lies down

If you suspect cholecystitis, have the patient take a deep breath during deep palpation. As the inflamed gallbladder comes in contact with the palpating fingers, the patient will experience pain and abruptly halt respiration-Murphy sign (Fig. 24.37B).

Spleen
The spleen, though not physiologically part of the gastrointestinal system is, because of its location in the abdomen, examined here. The patient is supine, arms at side, and knees flexed slightly. Outline the area of splenic dullness as a first step. This should be done not so much to delineate the splenic size but rather to loosen the abdomen. Percussion may outline a greatly enlarged spleen, directing initial palpation to the left lower portion of the abdomen. Figure 24.38A shows the position of the examiners hand. Note that pressure is light. Press the tips of the index and middle figners of the right hand to a point just beneath the costal margin, then ask the patient to turn his head to the side away from you and take a long, deep breath through his mouth. Do not move the hand as the patient inhales. The edge of an enlarged spleen will then brush against the fingers, lifting them slightly upward. As the patient exhales, probe the left upper quadrant more deeply, moving the fignertips in a slightly rotary motion. If nothing is felt, drop the hand about 1cm and repeat. Do not dig. This will cause spasm of the muscles, making palpation difficult. Furthermore, slight splenic enlargement can be missed because the fingertips may be below the splenic edge, which will glide over the backs of the fingers.

Two special maneuvers may be helpful. First, have the patient slip his left forearm under the small of his back (Fig. 24.38B); this position will tend to thrust the spleen upward. Second, roll the patient on his right side with the right leg straight and the left knee flexed (Fig. 24.38C). The tips of the palpating figners should be placed 1 or 2 cm below the costal margin with this maneuver.

To detect minor degrees of splenic enlargement, hooking method may be used, standing on the left side of the patient, similar to liver palpation. Do not forget to percuss the spleen, as, for palpation, the spleen has to enlarge 2 to 3 times. The tip of the normal spleen is purcussed at mid axillary line in the 10th left intercostal space. Any dullness beyond mid axillary line indicates enlargement (Table 24.10).

Summary of liver examination
1. Size below right costal margin in midclavicular line and midline.
2. Edge of liver (Conventional method, dipping method in presence of ascites).
3. Surface.
4. Consistency.
5. Tenderness.
6. Pulsations.
7. Fist percussion for tenderness.
8. Intercostal pressure for tenderness.
9. Auscultation for bruit, rub.
10. Liver span (by percussion).
11. Ascultopercussion for size.

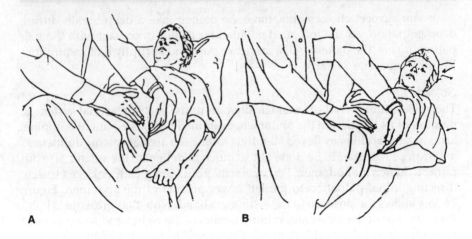

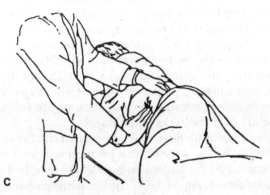

Figs 24.38A to C: Palpation of the spleen (A) positioning of examiner's hands, (B) patient's hand under his back, and (C) patient rolled to right side

Table 24.10: Differentiating an enlarged spleen from an enlarged left kidney

Spleen	Kidney
1. A characteristic notch	• No notch
2. Angular poles	• Rounded poles
3. Superficial	• Deep
4. Fingers cannot be pushed between spleen and costal margin	• Possible to push fingers between kidney and costal margin
5. Dull on percussion	• Vertical band of colonic resonance in front
6. Bimanually not palpable	• Bimanually palpable
7. Moves freely with response	• Movement with response not so marked
8. Moves early on inspiration	• Moves late on inspiration
9. Direction of movement on respiration downward and to the right	• Moves directly downward on respiration
10. Tendency to bulge forward	• Tendency to bulge into the loin and inward
11. The loin (posteriorly) is resonant on percussion	• No area of resonance between the mass and the spine, the whole loin being dull
12. Cannot be pushed back into the loin	• Can be pushed backward into the loin
13. Fingers can be dipped into space between lump and erotor spinae muscles posteriorly.	• No space between lump and erector spinae muscles posteriorly.

Normally the spleen is not palpable in the adult. It must be two or three times the normal size before it becomes palpable. however, it may be palpable 1 to 2 cm below the left costal margin in newborns (because of extramedullary hematopoiesis) and in normal infants and young children. The direction of splenic enlargement is usually vetically downwards in infancy unlike in adults.

Splenomegaly is common to many different and unrelated types of disease. It may be due to hyperplasia, congestion, or infiltrative replacement of the splenic pulp by neoplasm, meyloid elements, lipid, or amyloid. An unusually large spleen may be bimanually palpable and this should not be confused with kidney.

A classification of splenomegaly ascending to the degree of enlargement is listed in Table 24.11 and illustrated in Figure 24.39.

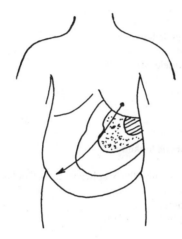

Fig. 24.39: Direction of enlargement of spleen

Kidneys

To assess each kidney for tenderness, ask the patient to assume a sitting position. Place the palm of your hand over the right costovertebral angle and strike your hand with the ulnar surface of the fist of your other hand (Fig. 24.40). Repeat the maneuver over the left costovertebral angle. Direct percussion with the fist over each costovertebral angle may also be used. The patient should perceive the blow as a thud, but it should not cause tenderness or pain. For efficiency of time and motion, assessment for kidney tenderness is usually performed while examining the back rather than the abdomen.

Left kidney Ask the patient to lie supine. Standing on the patient's right side, reach across with your left hand as you do in spleen palpation and place it over the left flank. Place your right hand at the patient's left costal margin. Have the patient take a deep breath and then elevate the left flank with your left hand and palpate deeply because of the retroperitoneal position of the kidney with your right hand. Try to feel the lower pole of the kidney with your fignertips as the patient inhales. The left kidney is ordinarily not palpable.

Table 24.11: Some causes of splenomegaly

Slight enlargement (1-2 cm)
  Typhoid
  Subacute bacterial endocarditis
  Miliary tuberculosis
  Septicemia
  Rheumatoid arthritis
  Syphilis, rickets, iron deficiency and megaloblastic anemia in infants
  Brucellosis
  Congestive heart failure
  Acute hepatitis
  Acute malaria
  Pernicious anemia
  Acute viral infection in infants
Moderate enlargement (3-7 cm)
  Cirrhosis of the liver
  Acute leukemia
  Chronic lymphocytic leukemia
  Lymphoblastoma
  Infectious mononucleosis
  Polycythemia vera
  Hemolytic anemia
  Sarcoidosis
  Rickets
Great enlargement (7+ cm):
  Chronic granulocytic leukemia
  Chronic malaria
  Hemolytic anemia (Hereditary spherocytosis, Thalassemia)
  Portal hypertension
  T-cell acute leukemia
  Congenital syphilis in the infant
  Amyloidosis
  Rare causes include
  Gaucher's disease, Niemann-Pick disease, kala azar,
  trophical splenomegaly, splenic cysts (congenital and hydatid).

Another approach is to 'caputre' the kidney. Move to the patients left side and position your hands as before, with the left hand over the patients left flank and the right had at the left costal margin. Ask the patient to take a deep breath. At the height of inspiration, press the fingers of your two hands together to caputre the kidney between the fingers. Ask the patients to breathe out and hold the exhalation while you slowly release your fingers. If you have captured the kidney you may feel it slip beneath your fingers as it moves back into place. Although the patient may feel the capture and release, the maneuver should not be painful. Again, a left kidney is seldom palpable.

Right kidney Stand on the patients right side, placing your left hand under the patients right flank and your right hand at the right costal margin. Perform the same maneuvers as you did for the left kidney (Fig. 24.41). Because of the anatomic position of the right kidney, it is more frequently palpable than the left kidney. If it is palpable, it should be smooth, firm, and nontender. It may

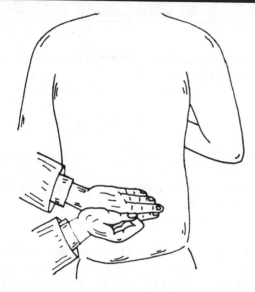

Fig. 24.40: First percussion for renal angle tenderness

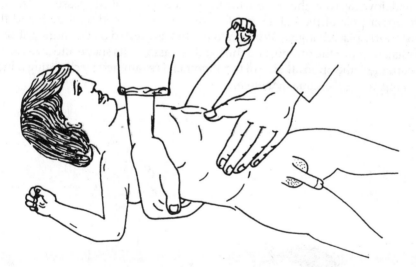

Fig. 24.41: Palpating for right kidney

be difficult to distinguish the kidney from the liver edge. The liver edge tends to be sharp, whereas the kidney is more rounded. The liver also extends more medially and laterally and cannot be captured.

In the newborn, the unimanual technique is preferred (Fig. 24.42), and will permit the examiner to ascertain, in addition to the presence of masses, the presence of kidneys and their size. It is most reliably performed in the first three days of life, when the abdominal muscles are still hypotonic and the abdominal cavity is easily palpated. The abdomen is relaxed by flexing the legs of the prone infant while lifting the buttocks off the bed. The fingers of the opposite hand support the matching loin posteriorly while the thumb

Table 24.12: Common causes of renal rulargement

Unilateral kidney mass
1. Tumor
   a. Renal: Wilms' tumor, renal cell carcinoma, congenital mesoblastic nephroma.
   b. Non-renal: Neuroblastoma, adrenal cell carcinoma.
2. Hydronephrosis
3. Hypertrophied solitary kidney.
4. Renal cyst
5. Renal vein thrombosis.

Bilateral kidney masses
1. Polycystic kidney disease (infantile-autosomal recessive; adult type-autosomal dominant)
2. Hydronephrosis: Posterior urethral valves, vesico-urethral reflux, neurogenic bladder.
3. Tumour-Wilms', leukemia, lymphoma, tuberous sclerosis.
4. Metabolic: Glycogen storage disease type 1(A and B).

searches at the side of the abdomen systematically, first superficially and then deeply. Deep palpation is performed by applying a gentle, steadily increasing pressure subcostally in a superior and cephalad direction. The thumb is then slid downward without reducing the posteriorly applied pressure. Usually, the upper pole of the kidney is felt between the descending thumb and the posteriorly placed fingers. While mild traction is exerted on the kidney, it slips cephalad under the thumb, and during this passage, its shape and size can be ascertained. the opposite side of the abdomen is examined by changing hands and repeating the same maneuver.

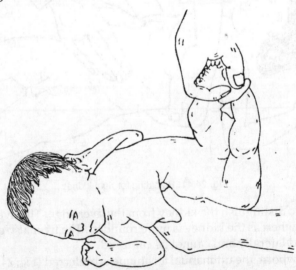

Fig. 24.42: Unimanual technique of abdominal palpation in the newborn. The legs of the prone infant are fiexed while the buttocks are lifted off the bed to relax the abdomen

While palpating the kidney, minimal palpation is recommended for suspected malignant mass.

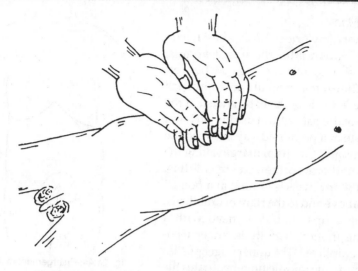

Fig. 24.43: Palpation of abdominal aorta and para-aortic nodes

The common cause of renal enlargement are listed in Table 24.12.

Aorta

With the patient in the supine position, palpate deeply, slightly to the left of the midline and feel for the aortic pulsation. If the pulsation is prominent, try to determine the direction of pulsation. A prominent lateral pulsation suggests an aortic aneurysm. Although the aortic pulse may be felt, particularly in thin adults, the pulse should be in an anterior direction. Aortic aneurysm is rare in children. Palpation for aortic pulsation is important in non-specific aortitis or Takayashu's disease.

If you are unable to feel the pulse on deep palpation, an alternate technique may help (Fig. 24.43). Place the palmar surface of your hands with fingers extended on the midline. Press the fingers deeply inward on each side of the aorta and feel for the pulsation. In thin individuals, you can use one hand, placing the thumb on one side of the aorta and the fingers on the other side. Feel for the para-aortic glands after you have palpated the aorta, by the same technique.

Urinary Bladder

The urinary bladder is not palpable in a healthy adult patient unless the bladder is distended with urine, when the bladder is distended, you can feel it as a smooth, round, tense mass (Fig. 24.44). You can determine the bladder outline with percussion; a distended bladder will elicit a lower percussion not than the surrounding air filled intestines. Bladder enlargement may be attributable to anatomic urinary tract obstruction, voluntary control, embarrassment of the patient, or low spinal cord lesions. pressure produces desire to micturate while palpating a distended bladder. In infants and young children a normal bladder is palpable.

Pyloric Mass

The tumor of pyloric stenosis is best felt on deep palpation after the infant vomits, mother should put the baby at her left breast. The examiner should now approach from the left side of the baby and sit at the left side of the patient and use his left hand to palpate at a point midway between the umbilicus and the costal margin along the right lateral border of the rectus muscle (Fig. 24.45). Pyloric mass is located at a point 2 to 3 cm above and to the right of umbilicus. The finger tips should be used with a kneading motion. The three finger technique is employed. The upper finger pushes the liver up, the middle finger palpates the

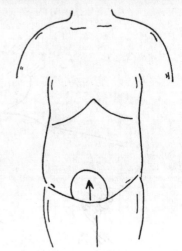

Fig. 24.44: Enlargement of bladder

mass while the lower finger pushes the coils of intestine downwards. The mass has firm cord like feel.

Abdominal Reflexes

With the patient supine, stroke each quadrant of the abdomen with the end of a reflex hammer or tongue blade edge. The upper abdominal reflexes are elicited by stroking upwards and away from the umbilicus, and lower

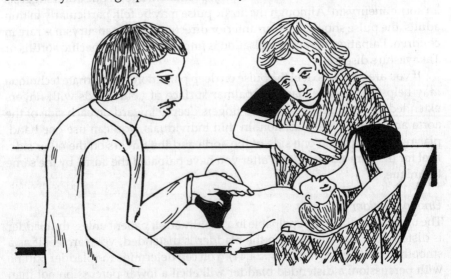

Fig. 24.45: Palpation for pyloric mass

1. Doctor in left side of patient
2. Baby feeding on left breast
3. Doctor's left hand for palpation
4. Doctor, mother and baby all relaxed !
5. Doctor's index finger of left hand lifts liver
6. Doctor's ring finger of left hand pushes intestines down
7. Doctor's middle finger of left hand kept on lateral side of rectus feels the firm card like pyloric mass with kneeding movement

abdominal reflexes are elicited by stroking downwards and away from the umbilicus.

With each stroke, expect to see the contraction of the rectus abdominis muscles and pulling of the umbilicus towards the stroked side. This skin reflex is absent in normal children under one year of age and in children with early poliomyelitis, multiple sclerosis, or other central or pyramidal disorders.

Palpation of Femoral Area

It is important to examine the sites of possible external herniation as a routine measure. Particular attention should be paid to the femoral canal to rule out the presence of a small hernia or Richter's hernia. Incarcerated or strangulated hernias are so often the cause of or associated with intra-abdominal processs, that this observation should be performed without fail in all cases. the femoral artery should be palpated during this part of the examination, since absence of its pulsations or inequality between the two sides may suggest embolic disease or the presence of a ruptured or dissecting aneurysm or coarctation of the aorta (Fig. 24.46).

Table 24.13 enlists unexpected abdominal findings associated with common abnormalities.

Table 24.14 delineates symptoms found in other body system that help direct the abdominal examination.

Acute Abdomen

Acute abdomen is an abdominal condition of sudden onset requring immediate attention. Acute pain is an important manfestation in many disorders (Table 24.15).

Apley's Rule

"Farther the pain from the umbilicus, more likely to have an organic cause."

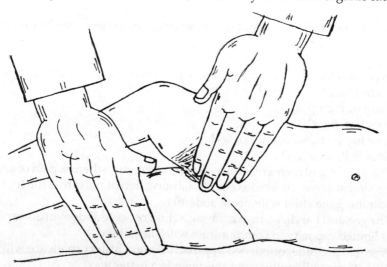

Fig. 24.46: Palpation of femoral area for femoral pulse

Table 24.13: Unexpected abdominal findings associated with common abnormalities

Signs	Descriptions	Asscoiated conditions
Cullen	Ecchymosis around umbilicus	Hemoperitoneum; pancreatitis; ectopic pregnancy
Grey turner	Ecchymosis of flanks	Hemoperitoneum, pancreatitis
Kehr	Abdominal pain radiating to left shoulder	Spleen rupture; renal calculi; ectopic pregnancy
Murphy	Abrupt cessation of inspiration on palpation of gallbladder.	Cholecystitis
Dance	Absence of bowel sounds in right lower quadrant	Intussusception
Romberg-Howship	Pain down the medial aspect of the thigh to the knees	Strangulated obturator hernia
Blumberg	Rebound tenderless	Peritoneal irritation; appendicits
Markle (heel jar)	Patient stands with straightened knees, then raises up on toes, relaxes, and allows heels to hit floor, thus jarring body. Action will cause abdominal pain if positive.	Peritoneal irritation; appendicitis
Rovsing	Right lower quadrant pain intensified by left lower quadrant abdominal pressure	Peritoneal irritation; appendicititis.
Ballance	Fixed dullness to percussion in left flank, and dullness in right flank that disappears on change of position	Peritoneal irritation
Aoron	Pain or distress occurs in the area of the patients heart on palpation of McBurney point	Appendicitis
McBurney	Rebound tenderness and sharp pain when McBurney point is palpated	Appendicitis

Significant diarrhoea, as defined by large volume rather than by frequency, rarely points to a surgical lesion.

The history of the pediatric patient with acute abdominal distress should focus on the character of the pain and associated symptoms. Is pain constant or intermittent?

- Sharp or crampy?
- Does it radiate?
- How has it changed since onset?
- What is its location?

The pain of gastroenteritis follows onset of emesis, whereas pain of appendicitis almost always precedes emesis. Observation of posture is the first step in examining the child with acute abdomen.

The greatest handicap in examining a child of acute abdomen is the physicians limited capacity to communicate with the patient.

A seat at bed side, unhurried approach, careful history, patience will help in evaluating a child with acute abdomen in a better way.

Table 24.14: Symptoms or signs elicited in other systems that may relate to the abdominal examination

Symptom or sign	Possible pathologic condition
Shock	Acute pancreatitis, ruptured tubal pregnancy obstruction
Mental status deficit	Hemorrhage-duodenal ulcer
	Aortic dissection
Hypertension	Abdominal aortic aneurysm
	Renal infarction
	Glomerulonephritis
	Vasculitis, acute intermittent porphyria
Orthostatic hypotension	Hypovolemia—blood loss, fluid loss
Pulse deficit	Aortic dissection
	Aortic aneurysm or thrombosis
Bruits	Aortic dissection
	Aoric aneurysm, dissection or aneurysm of arteries—splenic, renal, or iliac artery stenosis
Atrial fibrillation	Ischemia of the mesentery
Valvular disease, congestive heart failure	Embolus
Pleural effusion	Esophageal rupture
	Pancreatitis
	Ovarian tumor
Flank tenderness	Renal inflammation, pyelonephritis
	Renal stone
	Renal infarct
	Renal vein thrombosis
Leg edema	Iliac vein obstruction, pelvic mass
	Renal disease
	Renal vein thrombosis
Lymphadenopathy	Hepatitis
	Lymphoma
	Infectious mononucleosis
Jaundice	Hepatobiliary disease
	Excessive hemolysis
Dark yellow to brown urine	Hepatobiliary disease
	Blood as a result of kidney stone, infarct, glomerulonephritis, or pyelonephritis
Fever (103°F) and chills	Peritonitis
	Pelvic infection
	Cholangitis
	Pyelonephritis
White blood cell count >10000/mm³ or shift to left, > 20000/mm³	Appendicitis
	Acute cholecystitis
	Localized peritonitis
	Bowel strangulation
	Bowel infarction
Clues in history and general examination (symptom/sign)	
Toxaemia	Appendicular abscess,
	Perinephric abscess,

Contd...

Contd...

Symptom or sign	Possible pathologic condition
	Pelvic abscess, pyonephrosis,
	Hepatic abscess (amebic, non-specific), pyometrocolpos.
Jaundice	Choledochal cyst, hepatitis
	Cirrhosis, cholecystitis
	Late stage of hepatoma
Tuberculous allergy (Phlycten, erythema nodosum)	Tabes mesenterica, Tuberculosis of liver
Lymph nodes	Lymphoma, tuberculosis, leukaemia
Alopecia	Trichobezoar
Hemangioma	Hemangioma of liver
Aniridia, hemihypertrophy	Wilms' tumor
Proptosis	Neuroblastoma
Hypertension	Hydronephrosis, renal vein thrombosis, nephroblastoma, pheochromocytoma, neuroblastoma, acute intermittent porphyria (AIP)
Severe anaemia	Leukemia, nephroblastoma, malignancy
Down syndrome	Leukemia
Contact with dogs	Hydatid cyst
Hematuria	Wilms' tumor, renal vein thrombosis, hydronephrosis
Florid herpes labialis/zoster	Hydronephrosis Immunodeficiency, in leukaemia/lymphoma
Hypoglycemia	Glycogen storage disease
Petechiae	Leukemia (ALL, CML), hypersplenism
Adenoma sebaceum, Shagreen patch, hypopigmented patch renal cysts	Tuberous sclerosis.
Chloroma eye, skull, pelvic bones	Neuroblastoma
Liver mass	Glycogen storage disease-I
Prune belly syndrome	Renal mass (hydroneprhosis) bladder mass.

Total examination of the child is the cornerstone in arriving at proper diagnosis.

Warm hand, urine examination, rectal examination and a willingness to reconsider the doubtful cases are of a paramount importance.

Severe abdominal pain without any abdominal signs should suggest the possibility of acute intermittent porphyria, diabetic ketoacidosis, abdominal epilepsy and psychogenic pain.

Severe abdominal pain without any abdominal findings, associated with disorientation with similar history in the past and family history of epilepsy may be suggestive of abdominal epilepsy.

Repeated examinations are important.

When to suspect surgical condition in children.

Surgical evaluation is mandatory in the following conditions:

1. Presence of free abdominal air.
2. Rebound tenderness
3. Bowel obstruction

Table 24.15: Causes of acute abdomen in children

Condition	Newborn	Infant	Older child
Intestinal	– Infantile colic – Gastroenteritis – Constipation – Primary peritonitis – Necrotising enterocolitis	– Infantile colic – Gastroenteritis – Constipation – Primary peritonitis – Hemolytic uremic syndrome	– Gastroenteritis – Constipation – Parasitic infection – Mesentetric adenitis – TB – Intramural hematoma
Genitourinary	Urinary infection	Urinary infection	Urinary infection Ovarian and uterine pathology
Hepatobiliary	Biliary atresia	—	– Infectious hepatitis stones
Pancreatic systemic	Birth trauma Ileus	— Ileus Henochs purpura	– Pancreatitis – Rheumatic fever – Diabetes – Porphyria – Abdominal epilepsy, – Herpes – Henoch's purpura – Psychogenic

4. Enteric bleeding with acute abdomen.
5. Surgeon should be kept informed about any child's admission who is admitted for undiagnosed acute abdominal pain.

Atypical and complicated cases to be referred to the centre with more experienced pediatric and surgical personnel (Table 24.16).

Table 24.16: Outline of physical findings that have gastrointestinal significance

Signs	Diseases
Skin	
1. Color (Pigmentation)	Adrenogenital syndrome Addison's disease Neurofibromatosis Wilson's disease Hartnup disease
2. Pallor	Gastrointestinal bleeding from oesophagus to anus Gastrointestinal allergy
3. Jaundice	Hepatobiliary diseases, pancreatic diseases, tumors; genetic, metabolic and endocrinal entities
4. Carotenemia	Anorexia nervosa, hypervitaminosis A, hypothyroidism, diabetes mellitus, nephrosis
5. Periorbital edema	Wilson-Lahey syndrome, protein losing enteropathies
6. Perioral rash	Acrodermatitis enteropathica, malabsorption states, syphilis
7. Rose spots	Typhoid fever
8. Diaper dermatitis	Deprivation syndrome, dysgammaglobulinemia, disaccharidase deficiencies
9. Spider angioma	Cirrhosis

Contd...

Contd...

	Signs	Diseases
10.	Petechiae	Portal hypertension, Henoch-Schonlein purpura, hemolytic-uraemic syndrome
11.	Ecchymosis	Portal hypertension, Henoch-Schonlein purpura, malabsorption syndromes
12.	Cafe-au-lait spots	Neurofibromatosis
13.	Urticaria	Lymphomas, mastocytosis
14.	Erythema nodosum	Chronic ulcerative colitis, regional enteritis
15.	Telangiectasia	Rendu-Osler-Weber disease, ataxia-telangiectasia
16.	Hemangiomas	Rendu-Osler-Weber diseases, hamartomas (capillary type) of liver
17.	Lipomas	Gardner's syndrome
18.	Vesicles	Reye's syndrome
19.	Bullae	Dermatitis herpetiformis, epidermolysis bullosa
20.	Tanning of the dorsum of hands	Hartnup disease
21.	Tanning of the anterior tibial skin	Wilson's disease
22.	Scratch marks	Hepatobiliary disease (intrahepatic or extrahepatic)
23.	Xanthoma	Biliary obstruction (intrahepatic or extrahepatic)
24.	Webbing of neck	Turner's syndrome

Nails

1.	Clubbing	Regional enteritis, liver disease, celiac disease, cystic fibrosis
2.	Pitting, spooning	Anemia

Hair

1.	Color change	Protein calorie malnutrition, marasmus, protein-losing enteropathies
2.	Texture	Hypothyroidism, malasoroption states, protein-losing enteropathies, Menke's kinky hair syndrome
3.	Sparseness	Protein-calorie malnutrition, trichotillomania, acrodermatitis enteropathica

Lymph nodes

1.	Adenopathy	Infectious mononucleosis, typhoid fever
2.	Lymphoid hypoplasia	Dysgammaglobulinemia, intestinal lymphangiectasia

Head

1.	Microcephaly	Failure to thrive, congenital disease, rubella, toxoplasmosis, cytomegalic inclusion (Neonatal hepatitis), inborn errors of metabolism.
2.	Hydrocephalus	Failure to thrive, diencephalic syndrome, syphilis
3.	Craniotabes	Malabsorption syndromes, hypervitaminosis A.
4.	Bruits	Rendu-Osler-Weber syndrome, chronic liver disease
5.	Bulging fontanel (Pseudotumour cerebri)	Hypervitaminosis A, Rapid protein renutrition

Eyes

1.	Corneal ulcer	Familial dysantonomia (Riley-Days syndrome)
2.	Telangiectasia	Atania-telangiectasia
3.	Iritis	Crohn's disease, chronic ulcerative colitis
4.	Uveitis	Crohn's disease, chronic ulcerative colitis

Contd...

Contd...

Signs	Diseases
5. Xerophthalmia	Malabsorption syndromes
6. Kayser-Fleischer rings	Wilson's disease
7. Cataracts	Bassen-Kornzweiz syndrome, Wilson's disease, galactosemia
8. Papilledema	Hypervitaminosis A, cystic fibrosis
9. Defects in field of vision	Diencephalic tumors

Nose and Sinuses

1. Polyps	Cystic fibrosis
2. Sinusitis	Hypogammaglobulinemia

Mouth

1. Pigmentation of the lips	Peutz-Jeghers syndrome
2. Pigmentation of the gums	Adrenogenital syndrome, plumbism, adrenal insufficiency
3. Cheilosis	Malabsorption syndrome
4. Rhagades	Syphilis
5. Moniliasis(thrush)	Immunity defects
6. Hemangioma	Rendu-Osler-Weber disease
7. Stomatits	Regional enteritis
8. Gingival inflammation	Wilson's disease, regional enteritis
9. Absence of taste buds	Dysautonomia
10. Fetor	Hepatic coma
11. Glossitis	Vitamin B_{12} deficiency, regional enteritis

Chest

1. Increased anteroposterior	Cystic fibrosis, immunity defects
2. Increased respiratory rate	Ascites, tracheoesophageal fistula, anaemia, chronic liver disease
3. Gynecomastia	Cirrhosis
4. Costal rosary	Malabsorption syndromes, Deprivation syndromes
5. Asymmetrical expansion	Diaphragmatic hernia, Cystic fibrosis, pleural fluid
6. Abnormal breath sounds (rales, rhonchi, wheezes, with or without diminished transmission of sound)	Cystic fibrosis, pancreatitis pleural effusion, chylothorax, protein-losing enteropathy, immunity defects
7. Bowel sounds	Diaphragmatic hernia
8. Bruits	Rendo-Osler-Weber disease, cirrhosis
9. Murmurs	Liver disease, anaemia
10. Kussmaul's respiration	Reye's syndrome, diabetic ketoacidosis

Heart

1. Shift of mediastinum	Diaprhagmatic hernia
2. Signs of pericardial effusion	Lymphangiectasia, protein-losing enteropathy
3. High output murmurs	Cirrhosis, anaemia
4. Cardiomegaly	Protein-losing enteropathy, anaemia

Abdomen

1. Scaphoid abdomen (Newborn)	Diaphragmatic hernia
2. Distention (after 5 yr of age)	Malabsorption syndromes, masses, aerophagy, constipation

Contd...

Contd...

Signs	Diseases
3. Visible peristalsis	Pyloric stenosis, antral ulcers, Hirschsprung's disease, partial obstructions
4. Venous pattern	Portal hypertension
5. Differential percussion note	Celiac disease, cystic fibrosis
6. Bruits (Cruveilhier Baumgarten murmur)	Portal hypertension
7. Cullen's sign	Pancreatitis
8. Turner's sign	Pancreatitis
9. Hepatomegaly	Hepatic tumors, hepatobiliary disease, tumors, cysts, storage disease, abscesses
10. Splenomegaly	Portal hypertension, infectious mononucleosis, cysts, hepatitis, storage diseases
11. Mass	Duplications, liver abscess cysts
12. Ascites	Cirrhosis, lymphangiectasia protein-losing enteropathy, pancreatitis
13. Peritoneal signs	Peritonitis, polyserositis, pneumonia
14. Abnormal bowel sounds	Peritonitis, obstruction, gastroenteritis

Inguinal Regions and Genitilia

Signs	Diseases
1. Clitoral enlargement	Adrenogenital syndrome
2. Scrotal edema	Chylous ascites, protein-losing enteropathy
3. Testicular mass	Cystic fibrosis
4. Rectovaginal fistula	Imperforate anus

Limbs and Joints

Signs	Diseases
1. Asymmetry	Lymphangiectasia
2. Lymphedema	Lymphangiectasia
3. Pitting edema	Protein-losing enteropathy
4. Thrombophlebitis	Chronic ulcerative colitis
5. Arthritis	Regional enteritis, chronic ulcerative colitis, chronic active hepatitis, hepatitis virus B disease
6. Widened epiphyses	Malabsorption syndrome
7. Pigmentation (hands, anterior tibial skin)	Hartnup disease Wilson's disease
8. Clubbing of nails	Regional enteritis, celiac disease, cirrhosis, cystic fibrosis

Nervous System

Signs	Diseases
1. Sucking and swallowing disorders	Brainstem tumors
2. Ataxia	Malabsorption syndromes, Hartnup disease, abetalipoproteinaemia (Bassen-Kornzweig syndrome)
3. Tremors	Wilson's disease
4. Dystonia	Wilson's disease
5. Dysarthria	Wilson's disease, ataxia-telangiectasia
6. Confusion	Reye's sydrome, hepatic coma
7. Posturing (decerebrate, decorticate)	Reye's syndrome
8. Papilledema	Cystic fibrosis, anaemia, hypervitaminosis A
9. Hyperreflexia	Hepatic coma, Reye's syndrome
10. Babinski's reflex	Reye's syndrome, hepatic coma
11. Asterixis	Hepatic coma.

CHRONIC DIARRHEA COMMONLY ENCOUNTERED IN PEDIATRIC PRACTICE

Chronic Diarrhea (Table 24.17)

Definition

Includes 3 important aspects:
1. Watery or bloody diarrhea
2. Lasting more then 14 days
3. Associated with weight loss.

Chronic Diarrhea: Synonyms
1. Protracted diarrhea
2. Persistent diarrhea.

Chronic Diarrhea: Etiology
I. **Persistent intestinal infection**
   — *E. coli*
   — *Salmonella*
   — *Shigella*
   — Superinfection
   — Contamination of upper gastrointesntinal tract
   — Rotavirus
II. **Parasitic infection**
   — Amebiasis
   — Giardiasis
III. **Bad treatment of acute diarrhea**
   — Antidiarrheals
   — Antibiotics
   — Starvation
IV. **Sugar intolerance**
   — Lactose
   — Sucrose/isomaltose
   — Glucose
V. **Dietary protein intolerance**
   — Cow's milk allergy
   — Soya milk allergy.
VI. **Extraintestinal infection**
   — Urinary tract infection
   — Pneumonia
   — Tuberculosis (?)
VII. **Mucosal damage**
   — PEM
VIII. **Bile acid malabsorption.**

Chronic Diarrhea: Pathophysiology
— Maldigestion (pancreatic, bile acid deficiency)
— Selective diasaccharidase deficiency.

Table 24.17: Two categories of chronic diarrhea

Osmotic	Secretory
1. Stop after starvation	1. Does not stop
2. Often stops at night	2. Day and night
3. Low sodium in stool (<50 mEq/l)	3. High sodium (90 mEq/l)
4. Increased osmotic gap (>160 mosm/l)	4. Decreased osmotic gap (< 20 mosm/l)

— Defect in enterocytic absorption (Acrodermatitis enteropathica (ADE), Wolman's disease)
— Excessive sorbitol ingestion.
— Enteric infection
— Noninfectious small bowel mucosal inflammation (Henoch purpura, systemic lupus erythematosus).
— Noninfection colonic mucosal inflammation (Inflammatory bowel disease)
— Obstruction of intestinal lymphatics.

Chronic Diarrhea (Causes) (Table 24.18)
— Disorders of intestinal motility (Irritable bowel syndrome).
— Drugs
— Endocrine causes (hyperthyroidism)
— Multiple causes.

Table 24.18: Chronic diarrhea: etiology—age related

Infancy	After infancy	Any age
– Milk protein intolerance	– Lactose deficiency	– Enteric infection
– Parenteral infection	– IBD	– PEM
– Cholestasis	– IBS	– Bacterial overgrowth
– Congenital lactose	– HSP	– Celiac disease
deficiency	– Lymphoma	– Eosinophilic gastroenteritis
– Other sugar intolerance	– Tropical sprue	– Lymphocytic disease colitis
– Galactosemia	– Coll vascular	– Drugs
– Acrodermatitis entero-		– Primary immune deficiency
pathica		– Hyperthyroidism
– Lymphangiectasia		– GVH reaction
– AB lipoproteinemia		
Wolman's diseases		
Menke's syndrome		
CAH		
– Enterokinase deficiency		

Osmotic Diarrhea: Presentation
1. After acute enteric infection.
2. Diet and dirrhea (milk, wheat canesugar, sorbitol).
3. Risk factors (Malnutrition, immunodeficiency, drugs).
4. Symptoms of malabsorption.
5. Symptoms of IBD.
6. Symptoms of functional diarrhea.

Secretory Diarrhea: Congenital Transport Defects
— Congenital chloride diarrhea.
— Congenital sodium diarrhea.
— Primary bile acid malabosrption.

Intestinal Obstruction
— Hirschsprung's disease
— Partial small bowel obstruction.
  Neural crest tumor
  Enteric infection (bacterial overgrowth *E. coli*)
  Idiopathic villous atrophy (AIDS, congenital immunodeficiency).

Chrjonic Diarrhea: Work-up
1. Weight, birthweight, progress of weight.
2. Feeding   — Milk (dilution, amount, bottle)
           — Solids
           — Cows milk (milk allergy)
           — Cereals (celiac disease)
           — Fruits (sucrose/isomaltase deficiency)
           — Appetite
           — Feeding behavior.
3. Stool macro — Bulky foul, fatty stools in steatorrhea
           — Clay colored stools in cholestasis
           — Blood and mucus in amebiasis, *Shigella* infecttion and IBD
           — Green, watery in giardiasis
           — Watery explosive with flatus in sugar intolerance.
4. Nutritional deficiency
           — Pallor (Anemia)
           — Night blindness (Vit A)
           — Ataxia (Vit E)
           — Bruise (Vit K)
           — Rash (Zinc, Vit B)
           — Pigmentation (Folate).

Chronic Diarrhea: Work-up Specific Clues
1. Chest infection   — Cystic fibrosis
2. Infections   — HIV, congenital immunodeficiency, Schwachman's
3. Arthralgia   — Crohn's disease
4. Erythema nodosum, multiforme — Crohn's disease
5. Perineal tag, abscess   — Regional ilitis
6. Family history   — Cystic fibrosis, celiac, Crohn's lactose intolerance
7. Past history   — Surgery, necrotising enterocolitis.

Investigations: Others
1. Sweat test: Cystic fibrosis
2. Small bowel biopsy: Inflammatory bowel disease, oeliac disease, lymphangiactasia.
3. Radiology: contrast (IBD, obststruction) bone age (Schwachman's).
4. Breath test: Lactose intolerance.
5. Pancreatic function test.
6. Serum carotene and 1 hr xylose test.

Investigation: Blood
1. CBC, PS, ESR
2. HbF (Shwachman's)
3. Pancreatic isoamylase (Shwachman's)
4. Anti gliadin antibodies (Coeliac)
5. Anti endomysial antibodies (Coeliac)
6. LFT (Chronic liver disease, IBD)
7. Ig (Immuno deficiency, SCS and others)
8. HIV

Investigations: Stool
1. Macro
   Blood and mucus: Amebiasis, *Shigella*, IBD.
   Watery, profuse, flatus: Osmotic diarrhea.
   Green, watery, frothy: Giardiasis,
   Clay colored: cholestatic,
   Large, pale and foul: Steatorrhea.
2. Micro
   Pus cells-Infection, IBD.
   Eosinophils-Cow's milk allergy
   Cyst/Tropozoite-Giardia, amoebiasis
   Fat globules: Cystic fibrosis, Schwachman's disease
   Fatty acid crystals, Cystic fibrosis
3. Reducing substances: Lactose intolerance
4. Alpha-1-antitrypsin: Protein loosing enteropathy
6. Culture: Infection
7. Three day fecal fat: Steatorrhea, cystic fibrosis.

General Therapy
1. Diet
2. Fluid therapy
3. Special diet
4. Antibiotics
5. Bowel cocktail (oral gentamicin, metronidazole and cholestyramine)
6. Loperamide
7. Aspirin.

Chronic Diarrhea: Management (Table 24.19)

Table 24.19: Diet management

Diet A	Diet B	Diet C
— Low milk diet — Cereal + milk (or curd) — Cereal + legume + oil	— Animal milk free diet — Low starch diet — Cereal + legume + oil	— Starch and disaccharide free diet. — Glucose + oil + protein — Eggs (puree, chicken)

Outline of Abdominal Examination

Inspection
1. Contour
2. Veins
3. Skin
4. Scars
5. Umbilicus
6. Peristaltic waves
7. Localised distention
8. Swellings
9. Diastasis of recti
10. Pulsations
11. Movement with respiration
12. Hernial sites

Palpation
1. Light palpation for:
   a. Guarding and rigidity
   b. Doughy feel
   c. Edema of abdominal wall
   d. Crepitus
   e. Gurgle
   f. Skin turgor
   g. Hyperesthesia
   h. Reboud tenderness
2. Deep palpation
   a. Palpation of liver
   b. Palpation of spleen
   c. Gall bladder
   d. Other abdominal masses
3. Palpation of kidneys
   a. Bimanual palpation
   b. Unimanual palpation
   c. Ballotments
4. Palpation of aorta
5. Palpation of bladder
6. Palpation of para aortic lymphnodes

7. Palpation of pyloric mass
8. Palpation of femoral area
9. Abdominal reflexes
10. Iliopsoas test
11. Obturator test
12. Palpation of umbilical ring.

Percussion
1. Overall percussion
2. Liverspan for liver descent
3. Percussion for spleen
4. Percussion of the gastric bubble
5. Percussion of the urinary bladder
6. Ascitis
   a. Shifting dullness
   b. Fluid thrill
   c. Auscultatory percussion
   d. Puddle sign
7. Fist percussion for liver tenderness and renal angle tenderness

Auscultations
1. Bowel sounds
2. Vascular sounds
3. Friction rubs.

25 Examination of the Respiratory System

Anatomy

Knowledge of the underlying anatomy of the lungs is essential to a properly conducted examination.

The chest or thorax is a cage of bone, cartilage and muscle capable of movement, as the lungs expand. It consists anteriorly of, the sternum, manubrium, xiphoid process and costal cartilages; laterally of 12 pairs of ribs; and posteriorly of, the 12 thoracic vertebrae. All the ribs are connected to the thoracic vertebrae, the upper 7 are attached anteriorly to the sternum by the costal cartilage (Figs 25.1A to E).

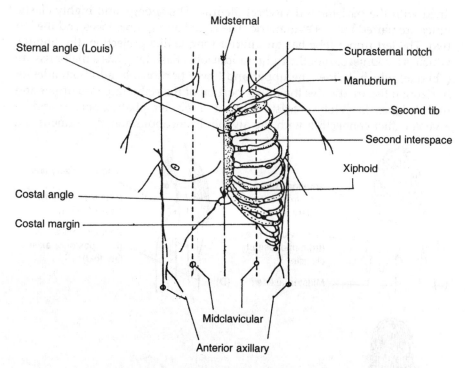

Fig. 25.1A: Landmarks on the chest wall (anterior)

The interior of the chest is divided into 3 major spaces; right and left pleural cavities and mediastinum. The mediastinum, situated between the lungs, contains all of the thoracic viscera except the lungs. The pleural cavities are

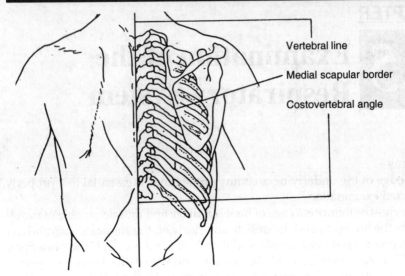

Fig. 25.1B: Landmarks on the chest wall (posterior)

lined with the parietal and visceral pleurae. The spongy and highly elastic lungs are paired but not symmetric. The right having three lobes and the left two. The left upper lobe has an inferior tongue like projection, the lingula, which is a counterpart of the right middle lobe. Each lung has a major fissure (oblique) which divides the upper and lower portions. In addition, a lesser horizontal fissure divides the upper portion of the right lung into upper and middle lobes. Each lobe consists of blood vesels, lymphatics, nerves, and an alveolar duct connecting with the alveoli. Bronchopulmonary segment is a

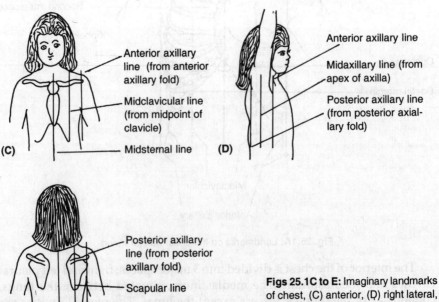

Figs 25.1C to E: Imaginary landmarks of chest, (C) anterior, (D) right lateral, and (E) posterior

Table 25.1: Division of broncho pulmonary segments

	Right Lung	Left Lung
Upper		Upper
	Apical	Apical
	Posterior	Posterior
	Anterior	Anterior
Middle		Superior lingual
	Lateral	Inferior lingual
	Medial	Lower
Lower		Apical
	Apical	Anterior basal
	Anterior basal	Posterior basal
	Posterior basal	Lateral basal
	Lateral basal	
	Medial basal	

wedge of lung tissue supplied by a single bronchus and corresponding pulmonary artery and vein.

Right lung and left lung are divided into 10 and 9 bronchopulmonary segments each (Fig. 25.2), respectively (Table 25.1).

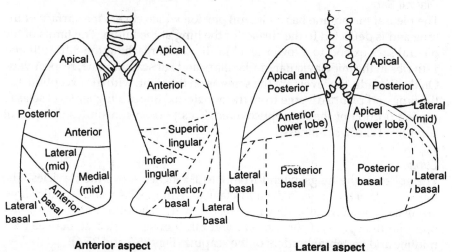

Anterior aspect   **Lateral aspect**

Fig. 25.2: The respiratory segments supplied by the segmental bronchi

Anatomic Landmarks

1. The nipples.
2. *Angle of Louis* It is a transverse bony ridge at the junction of body of the sternum and manubrium sterni. It corresponds to (a) bifurcation of trachea, (b) 2nd costal cartilage, (c) Arch of aorta, (d) left atrium.
3. *Suprasternal notch* A depression at the base of the ventral aspect of the neck just superior to the manubristernal junction.
4. *Costal angle* Formed by the blending together of the costal margins at the sternum. Usually not more than 90°, with the ribs inserted at approximately 45°

5. *Vertebrae*   Better seen and felt with the patients head bent forward. Two prominences are felt, the upper is that at the spinous process of C7 and the lower is that of T1. It is difficult to count the ribs posteriorly because the spinous process from T4 down project obliquely, thus overlying the ribs below the number of it's vertebra.

Imaginary landmarks of chest are illustrated in Figs 25.1C to E).

Surface Marking

Lung Fissures

The main fissure on each side is indicated by drawing a line from the spine of the second dorsal vertebra, downward and outward along the fifth rib as it leaves the vertebral column, to the 6th costochondral junction in front. When the scapula is tilted, by putting the hand on the head, the vertebral border lies along the line of fissure. The extratransverse fissure on the right side is indicated by drawing a horizontal line from the sternum, at the level of the fourth costal cartilage, to meet the line of main fissure laterally, in the mid axillary line, at the level of fifth rib or interpace.

Pleural Sac

The pleural membrane has a visceral portion which covers the surface of the lung and is deflected to the surface of the lung at the hilum. The limits of the pleural sacs extend to a lower level in the chest, reaching the 8th, 10th and 12th ribs in the midclavicular, midaxillary and subscapular line, respectively. On the left side, the levels are the same as on the right, with the exception that the lung and pleura diverge from the midsternal line at a higher level so as to leave a portion of the heart uncovered. This portion constitutes the area of superficial cardiac dullness.

Lungs

The apices of the lungs extend from 1 to 1½ inches above the clavicles. The lower levels of the lungs in the mid-clavicular, midaxillary and scapular lines are usually the 6th, 8th, 10th ribs, respectively. The hilum of the lung lies opposite the spines of the 4th, 5th and 6th thoracic vertebrae between the midline and vertebral borders of the scapula (Figs 25.3 and 25.4)

Chemical and Neurologic Control of Respiration

The purpose of respiration is to keep the body adequately supplied with oxygen and protect from excess accumulation of carbon dioxide. It involves the movement of air back and forth from the deepest reach of the alveoli to the outside (ventilation), gas exchange across the alveolar-pulmonary capillary membranes (diffusion and perfusion), and circulatory system transport of oxygen to, and carbon dioxide from the peripheral tissues. Control of this complex process is not yet fully understood.

Chemoreceptors in the medulla oblongata are exquisitely sensitive and respond quickly to changes in hydrogen ion concentration in the blood and spinal fluid. Peripherally, the chemoreceptors of the carotid body at the

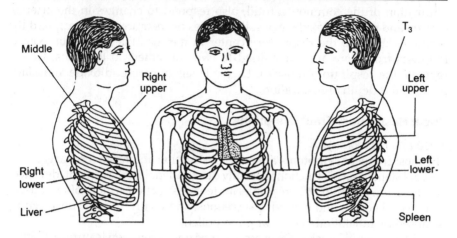

Fig. 25.3: Surface markings of the lungs and underlying viscera
(A) Right lateral, (B) Anterio-position, and (C) Left lateral

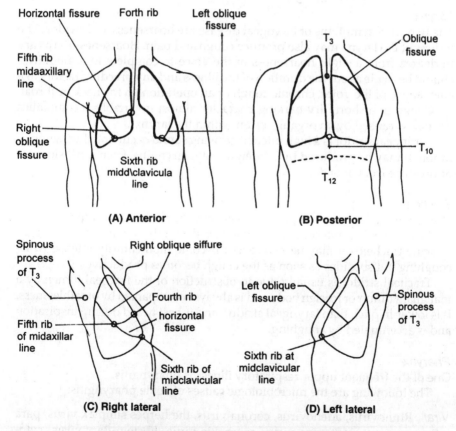

Fig. 25.4: Surface markings of the lungs (A) anterior,
(B) posterior, (C) right lateral, and (D) left lateral

bifurcation of the common carotid, also respond to changes in the arterial oxygen and carbon dioxide levels. Both types of chemoreceptors respond by sending signals to the respiratory center in the medulla oblongata. Nerve impulses from here are transmitted to two subcenters in the pons, which regulate the respiratory muscles. Excess levels of carbon dioxide stimulate the rate and depth of respiration.

Upper Respiratory Tract Symptoms

Nose and Nasopharynx

The most frequent symptoms are nasal obstruction and nasal discharge.

Persistent nasal obstruction is usually due to adenoid enlargement, deviated nasal septum or polyp. Whereas intermittent obstruction is more often caused by mucosal edema and excessive secretions, and recurrent nasal obstruction is caused by inhalation of dust or grain pollen.

History should be asked for excessive sneezing, a common feature of allergic rhinitis and headache which may accompany acute infection of the nasal sinuses.

Larynx

The two chief symptoms of laryngeal disease are hoarseness and stridor. The lesions of the larynx may also produce cough and pain. Hoarseness may vary in degree from a slight hoarseness of the voice to complete loss. Enquiries should be made about the duration of the illness and any precding factors like cold, abuse of the voice, chronic cough or an operation on the neck or throat.

Cough of a short, dry barking character almost invariably accompanies hoarsness caused by an organic lesion within the larynx.

Laryngeal stridor is a high pitched crowing sound occurring during inspiration. It may be produced by a foreign body, laryngitis, from intrinsic mass or pressure from outside.

Trachea

Disease of the trachea may produce pain, cough, stridor and dyspnea.

Tracheal pain is referred behind the sternal manubrium. In the early stages of acute tracheitis it may be severe and become momentarily intense while coughing but subsides as soon as the cough becomes productive.

Tracheal stridor is usually due to obstruction of the tracheal lumen by a malignant tumor or foreign body and is always accompanied by breathlessness. It is lower in pitch than laryngeal stridor, and is best heard during inspiration and is accentuated by coughing.

Pharynx

One of the frequent upper respiratory illness is pharyngitis.

The following are the microbiologic causes of acute pharyngitis:

Viral Rhinovirus, adenovirus, corona virus, the herpes simplex virus, para influenza virus, influenza virus, coxsackie virus, Ebstein-Barr virus, cytomegalovirus, respiratory syncytial virus.

Bacterial *Streptococcus pyogens*, groups C and G betahemolytic Streptococcus, *H. influenza*, *Morarcella catarrhalis*, *Acenobacter haemolyticum*, anarobes, *Corynebacterium diphtheriae*, *Corynebacterium ulcerans*, *Neisseria gonorrhoea*, *Staphylococcus aureus*.

Fungus *Candida albicans* The following are the non infectious causes of pharyngitis: Foreign body, allergy, gastroesophageal reflux trauma, chemical burns, thermal injury, toxins.

Dysphagia

A normal respiratory tract is necessary for normal deglutition and protection of the lung, in addition to the cough reflex and laryngeal closure mechanism to prevent aspiration during the swallowing process (Table 25.2).

A child with dysfunction of the swallowing mechanism presents a complex and often challenging problem. In some instances the dysphagia is temporary and is due to either immaturity or a temporary central nervous system aberration that spontaneously subsides. A search for the cause is necessary in all cases.

Etiological classification of dysphagia

- Prematurity
- Congenital defect of the upper airway
- Acquired anatomic defects
- Inflammatory conditions and manifestation of systemic diseases
- Neoplastic conditions
- CNS diseases
- Neuromuscular disease
- Gastrointestinal disease.

History of Previous Illness

When the present illness appears to involve the respiratory system, information of considerable value in diagnosis, prognosis and treatment may be obtained from the past medical history (Table 25.3).

Family History

Eliciting the history of certain diseases in the family is mandatory in evaluating the respiratory system disorders.

History regarding tuberculosis, bronchial asthma, atopic dermatitis, cystic fibrosis should be elicited in detail.

Other hereditary diseases of the lungs are listed in Table 25.4.

Occupational History

Not important in the pediatric history taking.

Both past and present occupation are important in assessing the lung disease.

Numerous chemicals, moulds, organic dust and animal proteins can cause asthma and allergic alveolitis.

Table 25.2: Differential diagnosis of dysphagia in children

Prematurity/Developmental Delays	Acquired Anatomic Defects Trauma	Central Nervous System Conditions
Birth weight < 1500gm or < 32 weeks gestation	External	Head trauma
Oral aversion/poor conditioning	Internal (Intubation injury)	Hypoxia and anoxia
Hypoxia and anoxia	Iatrogenic (surgical injury to mucosa or nerves)	Cortical atrophy, hypoplasia, agenesis
Associated "intensive care unit factors"	**Foreign body**	Arnold-Chiari malformation
Congenital Defects of Upper Airway Nasal and Nasopharyngeal	Hypopharynx and oral cavity	Infection (Meningitis, brain abscess)
Choanal atresia or stenosis (CHARGE) association	Esophagus	**Neuromuscular Diseases**
Septal deformity	Airway	Amyotonia (Duchenne muscular dystrophy)
NOWCA	**Chemical Ingestion**	Cerebral palsy
Piriform aperture defect	Acids, alkalies, catalysts	Guillain-Barre syndrome
Anotia	Medication-induced	Poliomyelitis (Bulbar paralysis)
Anosmia	**Postsurgical Effects**	Botulinum toxin
Oropharynx and Oral Cavity	Tracheostomy	Riley-Day syndrome
Defects of lips and alveolar processes	Laryngotracheal reconstruction	**Behavioral/Psychological Factors**
Defects of palate(cleft and submucous cleft)	Stricture	Globus
Craniofacial defects (e.g., Treacher Collins, Goldenhar)	Colonic or jejunal interposition	Food Vsnonfood dysphagia
Defects of tongue or floor of mouth (e.g., Beckwith, Wiedemann, congenital ranula)	**Inflammatory Conditions and Manifestations of Systemic Disease Infection**	Anorexia
	Streptococcal and nonstreptococcal pharyngitis	Bulimia
	Fungal (esophagitis)	Munchausen by proxy
	Protozoal (Chaga's disease)	**Primary Gastrointestinal Disease Upper Esophagus**

Contd ...

Contd....

Prematurity/Developmental Delays	*Acquired Anatomic Defects Trauma*	*Central Nervous System Conditions*
Hypopharynx and Supraglottic Larynx	Viral (AIDS)	Cricopharyngeal dysfunction
Craniofacial defects (Pierre Robin sequence)	**Connective Tissue Disorders**	Nonsphincteric esophageal spasm
Laryngomalacia	Scleroderma	Achalasia
Congenital cysts	Lupus	Zenker diverticulum
Congenital Defects of Larynx, Trachea, and Esophagus Larynx	Rheumatoid arthritis	**Lower esophagus**
Vocal cord paralysis	Sjogren syndrome	Gastroesophageal reflux (chalasia)
Glottic and subglottic stenosis	**Manifestations of systemic diseases**	Barrett esophagus
Laryngeal cleft	Diabetes	Esophagial varices
Tracheoesophageal fistula (H-type) with associated atresia Esophageal anomalies, atresia, and strictures Vascular anomalies causing compression ("Vascularring")	Thyroid disorders	**Stomach**
	Neoplastic Conditions	Peptic ulcer
	Benign (e.g., cystic hygroma, hemangioma, papilloma)	Gastritis
	Malignant (e.g., adenocarcinoma, lymphoma)	**Small and Large Intestine**
Aberrant right subclavian artery	Double aortic arch	Crohn disease
		Ulcerative colitis
Right aortic arch with left ligamentum		

* NOWCA : Nasal obstruction without choanal atresia.

Note: Details of cough, dyspnea, wheeze, stridor etc are discussed in vol-I of this book.

Table 25.3: Consequences of past medical history

History	Consequneces
Tuberculosis	May have relapsed, caused bronchiectasis or aspergilloma may have formed in an old TB lung cavity.
Pneumonia,	May have caused bronchiectasis.
pleurisy	Recurrent pneumonia and pleurisy may be caused by bronchiectasis, bronchial tumors, aspiration of esophageal contents.
Measles, whooping cough	Can be complicated by pneumonia, and later bronchiectasis
Wheezy bronchitis/recurrent bronchitis	Recurrence of asthma in adults who have a history of childhood asthma is common
Chest injuries	Traumatic hemothorax can give rise to gross pleural thickening which splints the lung.
Recent general anesthetic or loss of consciousness	Aspiration of oropharyngeal secretions or foreign body can give rise to aspiration pneumonia or lung abscess.
Chest X-ray	Comparison of a recent chest X-ray with one taken in the past.

Nonorganic particles like silica, coal dust and asbestos are important cause of pneumoconioses and malignant diseases in adults.

Social History

Enquire about pets (animals and birds) and cigarette smoking by parents, sometimes in adventurous adolescents.

PHYSICAL EXAMINATION

External Features of Respiratory Disease

Initial Impression

A number of features may have become evident during the course of history taking and should immediately cause the observer to suspect respiratory disease. These are cough, wheeze, stridor and labored breathing. Attention should be paid to any abnormality of the voice, sounds produced by children (wheeze, stridor, croup, hoarseness, aphonia, type of cough, type of cry, etc), and fetor of the breath. The state of nutrition should be roughly assessed, any suggestion of anemia or polycythemia should be noted. Note signs of respiratory distress, tachypnea, chest indrawing, suprasternal recession, use of accessory muscles of respiration and flaring of alae nasi. Note also rate and type of respiration.

Cyanosis

Cyanosis is the bluish or violet discoloration of the skin or mucous membrane due to an excessive amount of deoxygenated hemoglobin (> 5 gm/dl) in the peripheral blood vessels associated with inadequate oxygenation of systemic tissues.

Table 25.4: Hereditary diseases of the lungs

Mendelian diseases and modes of inheritance

Agammaglobulinemia (Bruton's disease)	Sex-linked recessive/Autosomal recessive
Ataxia-telangiectasia syndrome	Autosomal recessive
Chronic granulomatous disease	Sex-linked recessive
Cystic fibrosis	Autosomal recessive
Familial dysautonomia	Autosomal recessive
Familial emphysema (homozygous deficiency of alpha-1-antitrypsin)	Autosomal recessive
Familial interstitial fibrosis	Autosomal dominant
Familial pulmonary alveolar microlithiasis	Autosomal recessive
Familial spontaneous pneumothorax	Autosomal dominant
Hunter syndrome	Sex-linked recessive
Hurler's syndrome	Autosomal recessive
Kartagener's syndrome	Autosomal recessive
Lung in Marfan syndrome	Autosomal dominant
Primary pulmonary hypertension	Autosomal recessive
Pulmonary arteriovenous fistulas	Autosomal dominant
Tuberous sclerosis	Autosomal dominant

Intermediate diseases (Familial aggregation with genetic contribution to etiology)

Chronic bronchitis and bronchiectasis	Susceptibility to repeated infection and to action of irritants
Familial emphysema	Heterozygous alpha-1-antitrypsin deficiency and possibly other producing "susceptibility of lung to action of an irritant"

Miscellaneous rare diseases

Obesity-hypoventilation syndrome	**Data on inheritance meager**
Potter's syndrome	some may be simple Mendelian disorders
Pulmonary cystic lymphangiectasis	
Scimitar syndrome	
Tracheobronchomegaly	
Wolman's disease	
Williams-Campbell syndrome (bronchial cartilage deficiency)	
Letterer-Siwe disease	

Polygenic Diseases (with mixed genetic and environmental factors

Allergic respiratory disease diathesis (asthma, rhinitis)	Inherited allergic
Sarcoidosis	Unknown, but familial aggregation reported
Tuberculosis	Increased susceptibility to bacterial invasion
Other communicable diseases	Increased susceptiblity or genetically determined "low resistance"

Pathophysiology of Cyanosis in Pulmonary Diseases

Upper airway obstruction results in cyanosis by alveolar hypoventilation due to reduced pulmonary ventilation. Obstruction may occur from the nares to carina. Intrapulmonary disease such as hyaline membrane disease, atelectasis and pneumonitis cause inflammation, collapse and fluid accumulation in alveoli, which result in completely deoxygenated blood in the systemic circulation.

Causes of (respiratory) cyanosis.

- *Acute hypoxia*
  Foreign body
  Respiratory distress syndrome
  Tension pneumothorax
  Acute severe asthma
  Pulmonary embolism
- *Chronic hypoxia*
  Interstitial pneumonia
  Chronic obstructive airway disease
  Types of cyanosis
- *Peripheral*
- *Central*

Peripheral cyanosis—is due to excessive extraction of oxygen from the blood, when the circulation is impaired from vasoconstriction, low cardiac output or stasis. It is visible only in the skin. It occurs in healthy people, when the extremities are cold and warmth abolish it. Clubbing at the fingers and polycythemia do not occur.

Central cyanosis—is due to oxygen undersaturation of the arterial blood from poor gaseous exchange in the lungs resulting from respiratory failure or pulmonary edema or when there is a right to left shunt as in congenital heart disease.

Differences between central and peripheral cyanosis are discussed in Table 25.5.

Vasomotor instability and peripheral circulatory sluggishness are revealed by deep redness or purple lividity in a crying infant whose color may darken promptly with closure of the glottis. Preceding a vigorous cry and by harmless cyanosis (acrocyanosis) of the hands and feet.

Clubbing

Clubbing is bulbous enlargement of soft parts of the terminal phalanges with both transverse and longitudinal curving of the nails but less obviously affect the toes. It is due to interstitial edema and dilatation of the arterioles and capillaries.

Clubbing in children is one of the important clinical signs indicating chronic pulmonary insufficiency. The manifestation of clubbing denotes the underlying chronic anoxemia due to primary respiratory or cardiac problems.

Pathophysiology

- Clubbing occurs due to interstitial edema and dilatation of the arterioles and capillaries

Table 25.5: Difference between central and peripheral cyanosis
on the basis of characteristics

Characteristics*	Central*	Peripheral*
1. Visible in	• Warm areas and skin.	Skin
2. Cause—	• Venous admixture-and defective ventilation, perfusion/diffusion	Vasoconstriction low cardiac output.
3. Pathophysiology	• Decreased arterial O_2 saturation	• Increased arteriovenous oxygen difference
4. Deoxygenated Hb	• > 5 gm/dl	• Normal
5. Clubbing	• Present	• Absent
6. Relief	• O_2 useful in cyanosis of pulmonary origin.	• Warming and cardiovascular support.

*Factors that determine the degree of cyanosis—
1. The amount of reduced hemoglobin in the arterial blood.
2. The degree of utilization of capillary oxygen by the tissues.
3. The total hemoglobin concentration.

- Swelling of the subcutaneous tissues over the base of the nail, causes the overlying skin to become tense, shiny and red with obliteration of skin creases
- Later on the swelling involves the curvature of the nail especially in its long axis
- Finally, swelling of the pulp of the finger occurs in all dimensions
- In a few cases, there may also be hypertrophic pulmonary osteoarthropathy causing pain and swelling of the hands, wrist, knees, feet and ankles.

Mechanism

Although mechanism of clubbing is not clear, it is believed that the stimulus of clubbing is hypoxia. Hypoxia leads to opening up of deep arteriovenous fistula which increases the blood supply of the fingers and toes causing it to undergo hypertrophy.

Another hypothesis is that when reduced ferritin in venous blood escapes oxidation in the lungs and enters systemic circulation, it causes dilatation of arteriovenous anastamosis and hypertrophy of terminal phalanges resulting in clubbing.

Grading

Grade I : Softening of nailbed.
Grade II : Obliteration of the angle of the nailbed.
Grade III : Swelling of subcutaneous tissue over the base of nail, resulting in parrot beak or drumstick appearance.
Grade IV : Swelling of fingers in all dimensions with hypertrophic pulmonary osteoarthropathy.

Respiratory Causes of Clubbing

- Bronchiectasis
- Lung abscess
- Empyema

- Intrathoracic tuberculosis (cavitatory)
- AV fistula.

Special Forms of Clubbing

— Unilateral clubbing—aneurysmal dilatation of aorta and its branches, bronchial arteriovenous fistula, pancoast tumor, erythromelalgia and lymphangitis.
— Unidigital—may be hereditary, if bilateral and involving the thumbs. Other causes are median nerve injury, local trauma, tophaceous gout, sarcoidosis.
— Differential clubbing—only in upper limbs-Heroin addicts, due to chronic obstructive phlebitis.
— Only in lower limbs—patent ductus arteriosus with reversal of blood flow.

Pseudoclubbing

In hyperparathyroidism excessive bone resorption may result in disappearence of terminal phalanges with telescoping of soft tissues and drumstic appearence of the fingers resembling clubbing. However, the curvature of the nail is not present.

Edema

The presence of peripheral edema in patients with chronic obstructive airway disease suggests right ventricular failure or may simply be due to associated malnutrition. Edema of a different distribution is seen in obstruction of the superior vena cava. This is most commonly a complication of mediastinal masses like lymph nodes as in lymphomas, leukemias or due to tumors like neuroblastoma, teratoma, etc.

Jugular Veins

These may be overfilled in superior mediastinal obstruction. Filling of the jugular veins during expiration and emptying during inspiration may result from raised intrathoracic pressure in patients with expiratory airway obstruction (e.g. asthma).

Accessory Respiratory Movements

Inspiratory contraction of the sternomastoid muscle may occur with respiratory distress of any kind, but is particularly associated with overinflation of the lungs due to chronic airway obstruction.

Head-bobbing

In synchrony with each inspiration, the head is noted to bob forward owing to neck flexion. This phenomenon is probably explained by contraction of scalene and sternocledomastoid muscle, which are accessory muscles of inspiration.

This is a sign of dyspnea, best observed in an exhausted or sleeping infant lying in its mother's arm. The head must be unsupported except for the suboccipital area.

Pulsus Paradoxus

When the systolic pressure falls more than 10 mmHg during inspiration, the pulse is referred to as pulsus paradoxus.

In normal individuals the systolic BP drops by 2-4 mmHg during inspiration, it is increased in heart failure, cardiac tamponade, bronchiolitis, asthma and cystic fibrosis.

The phenomenon has been explained physiologically as the result of lowering intrathoracic pressure. Which increases the systemic venous return to the right heart, increases the force required of the left ventricle to maintain the previous arterial pressure.

Flapping Tremors

Seen in respiratory failure.

Flaring of the Alae Nasi

Flaring of the alae nasi exists when an enlargement of both nares occurs during inspiration. It is due to contraction of the anterior and posterior dialators nares muscle. The appearance of flaring indicates that accessory muscles are being required for inspiration. It is an excellent sign of dyspnea.

Unilateral flaring is a sign of facial paralysis on the opposite side.

Eyes

It is important to examine the eyes in patients suspected of having respiratory disease (Table 25.6).

Table 25.6: Examples of eye conditions in respiratory disorders

Condition	Disease
Horner's syndrome	Carcinoma of the bronchus
Phlyctenular keratoconjunctivitis	Primary tuberculosis
Iridocyclitis	Tuberculosis
	Sarcoidosis
Choroidal tubercles	Miliary tuberculosis
Chemosis, conjunctival and retinal vein dilatation	Hypercapnia, superior vena caval obstruction.

Neck

In patients with possible respiratory disease the scalene lymph nodes require careful examination. These are involved when lymphoma, sarcoidosis or tuberculosis are present.

Skin

Examination of the skin may yield information of considerable value in the diagnosis of the respiratory disease.

Skin lesions which may yield information of diagnostic importance are discussed in Table 25.7.

Table 25.7: Skin lesions and their corresponding condition

Disease	Condition
Erythema nodosum	May be initial clinical manifestations of tuberculosis and sarcoidosis.
Cutaneous sarcoidosis and lupus pernio	May occur in association with intrathoracic sarcoidosis.
Rash of lupus erythematosus	May accompany pulmonary or pleural manifestation of this connective tissue disorder.
Herpetic vesicles	May identify the case of unilateral chest pain
BCG scar	Immunization status

Examine upper respiratory tract—ear, nose, throat and para nasal sinuses

Inspection of Chest

Cardinal Points for Inspection
1. Shape of the chest
2. Tracheal position
3. Apical position
4. Respiratory movements

Additional Points for Inspection
1. Spine
2. Shape and contour of chestwall
3. Pulsations over chest wall.
4. Veins
5. Respiratory sounds like type of cough, wheeze, stridor, whoop, grunt, croup, etc.

Cardinal Points

Shape of the Chest
In infancy and early childhood, the cross-section of the chest is almost circular, the anteroposterior and lateral diameters being about equal. The general shape of the thorax tends to be cylindrical. The shape of the chest in childhood may be greatly modified by hypertrophied adenoids or rickets.

The shape of the chest changes as the age advances (Fig. 25.5).

Abnormal chest Any abnoramality of contour, size or shape of the chest must be noted carefully, as it may explain the nature of present or past diseases.

An abnormal chest may be either symmetrically or asymmetrically abnormal.
   a. **Normal contour** (Fig. 25.6A)
   b. **Barrel shaped chest** The anteroposterior diameter is increased relative to lateral diameter. The normal ratio is 5:7. This is seen in emphysema (Fig. 25.6B).
   c. **Pectus excavatum** (Funnel shaped chest) There is a depression in the lower part of the sternum or less commonly depression of the whole length of the body of sternum. Which may be congenital, following rickets in

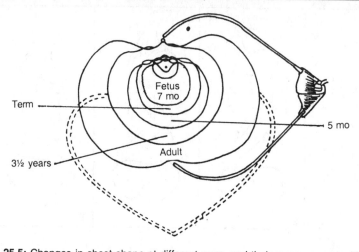

Fig. 25.5: Changes in chest shape at different ages, and their measurement with obstetrical calipers. The relatively round chest of the fetus and term infant gradually flattens dorsoventrally with age. Measurements should be made in either the recumbent (infants) of standing (chindren) position, never in the sitting position. Maximum dimensions are measured in both cases without regard to the level or phase of respiration, but care must be taken to place the calipers in a .... plane. The distance between the caliper .... then measured with a steel centimeter rule

childhood or an occupational deformity (in cobblers). Usually asymptomatic, but when there is a very marked degree of depression, the heart may be displaced to the left and the ventilatory capacity of the lungs restricted (Fig. 25.6C).

d. **Pectus carinatum** This is a common sequale to chronic respiratory disease in childhood. It consist of a localised prominence of the sternum and adjacent costal cartilages, often accompanied by indrawing of the ribs to form symmetrical horizontal grooves (Horrison's sulci) above the costal margin, which are themselves usually everted. These deformities are thought to result from lung hyperinflation with repeated strong contractions of the diaphragm while the bony thorax is still in a pliable state. This deformity may also be caused by rickets (Fig. 25.6D).

e. **Thoracic kyphoscoliosis** This ranges in degree from the minor changes in spinal curvature to grossly disfiguring and disabling deformities. Severe kyphoscoliosis may have profound effect on pulmonary functions, as the chest deformity reduces the ventilatory capacity of the lungs and increases the work of breathing. Many such patients develop hypoxemia, hypercapnea and heart failure at an early stage (Figs 25.6E to G).

Tracheal Position
By noting the position of trachea, the shift of the mediastinum can be detected. Always comment about position of trachea after both inspection and palpation.
Normally the trachea may be slightly shifted to right or central.

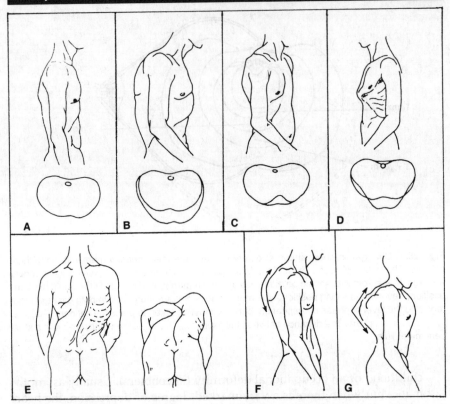

Figs 25.6A to G: Chest wall contours (A) Normal contour, (B) Barrel shaped chest (emphysema), (C) Pectus excavatum (funnel shaped chest), (D) Pectus carinatum (pigeon breast), (E) Scoliosis, (F) Kyphose, and (G) Gibbus kyphoscoliosis

Trail sign Undue prominence of the clavicular head of the sternomastoid muscle on one side, is usually indicative of tracheal displacement to that side.

Mechanism The pretracheal fascia encloses the sternomastoid muscle and is in close contact with the tendon of the muscle. Tracheal displacement is reflected therefore in an increased tension of the sternomastoid muscle on the same side as that to which the mediastinum is pulled or pushed.

Apical Position
It is important to locate the exact position of the cardiac apex in all cases of respiratory disease, as it may be displaced to one or other side by disease of lung or pleura. Like commenting on tracheal position always combine inspectory and palpatory finding while localizing the apex.

Position of the mediastinum in respiratory diseases is given in Table 25.8.

Respiratory Movement
- Respiratory rate
- Rhythm

Table 25.8: Position of mediastinum in respiratory diseases

Central	Shifted to same side (pull)	Shifted to opposite side (push)
Bronchitis	Collapse Consolidation	Pleural effusion empyema
Bronchial asthma	Fibrosis	Pneumothorax
Bronchiectasis	Pleural Thickening	Hydropneumothorax
Emphysema	Long-standing	Diaphragmatic hernia
Pneumonia	Bronchiectasis	Huge thoracic mass
Lung abscess	lung abscess and empyema, due to	
Insterstitiae fibrosis	associated collapse and fibrosis.	

- Character
- Equality
- Accessory muscles of respiration
- Intercostal retractions

Respiratory rate The physician should reach a conclusion as to whether the respiratory rate for this patient is normal or abnormal.

Respiratory rate varies with the age (Table 25.9).

Table 25.9: Respiratory rate corresponding to increasing age (rate per minute)

Age	Sleeping		Awake	
	Mean	Range	Mean	Range
6-12 months	27	22-31	64	58-75
1-2 years	19	17-23	35	30-40
2-4 years	19	16-25	31	23-42
4-6 years	18	14-23	26	19-36
6-8 years	17	13-23	23	15-30
8-10 years	18	14-23	21	15-31
10-12 years	16	13-19	21	15-28
12-14 years	16	15-18	22	18-26

The rate increases in a variety of physiological and pathological conditions.

Physiological
- Excessive crying
- Exertion
- Excitement

Pathological
- Fever
- Anemia
- Acidosis
- Poisoning

The rate decreases in the following conditions.
- Narcotic poisoning
- Brain tumor
- Increased Intracranial pressure.

Respiratory rhythm Normal respiration has regular rhythm with inspiration longer than expiration. Abnormal/irregular respiratory rhythm is due to pathological conditions (Fig. 25.7) .

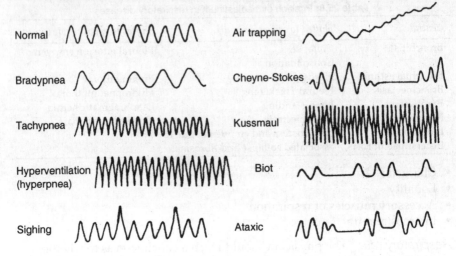

Fig. 25.7: Patterns of respiration. The horizontal axis indicates the relative rates of these patterns. The vertical swings of the lines indicate the relative depth of respiration

- *Cheyne-Stoke respiration* It consists of rhythmic alteration of apnea and hyperpnea due to anoxemia seen in left ventricular failure, increased intracranial pressure with damage to both cerebral hemisphere, diencephalon, poisoning, uremia.
- *Kussmaul's respiration* It is characterised by deep and rapid respiration (air hunger), and is seen in diabetic ketoacidosis and in uremia.
- *Biot's respiration* Irregularly irregular respiration seen in meningits.

Additional points for inspection
1. **Spine** Spinal deformities due to any cause may lead to asymmetry and may decrease the size of thoracic cage and restrict lung movementis.
   a. *Scoliosis* Is an abnormal lateral curvature of the spine. Causes are as follows:
      - Congenital
      - Positional—carrying heavy weight on one side.
      - Compensatory—reduced length of arm or one lower limb.
      - Reflex—to relieve pain as in sciatica or renal colic.
      - Neurological—poliomyelitis, syringomyelia, muscular dystrophy, hereditary ataxia.
      - Rickets
      - Functional.
   b. *Kyphosis* Is an abnormal anteroposterior curvature of the spine with foward concavity and dorsal prominence. Causes are as follows:
      - Congenital—wedge shaped vertebra.
      - Postural—carrying weights on the back
      - Diseases of bones and joints—tuberculosis, rheumatoid arthritis, rickets, osteoarthritis, osteitis deformans, fracture of the vertebral body, new growth of spine, mucopolysaccharoidosis and other skeletal dysplasias.

- Neurological—muscular dystrohy, hereditary spastic paraplegia, Friedreich's ataxia, syringomyelia, poliomyelitis, cerebral palsy, neurofibromatosis.
  c. *Lordosis* Is an abnormal anteroposterior curvature of the spine with forward convexity. Causes are the following:
  — secondary to hip disease and congenital dislocation of the hip.
  — muscular dystrophy.
  — large abdominal tumors.
2. **Chest wall** Normally the chest wall is bilaterally symmetrical, with smooth contours and slight recession below the clavicles.
   - Bulging—one side or a part of it may bulge in pleural effusion, pneumothorax, tumors, aneurysm, empyema necessitans, cardiomegaly, pericardial effusion or scoliosis.
   - Depression—one side of the chest or a part of it may be depressed or flattened in fibrosis, collapse or pleural adhesion.
3. **Pulsations** Visible and pulsating subcutaneous vessels along the interspaces and over the back are characteristic of the anastomotic circulation of coarctation of the aorta.

   Pulsating swelling anywhere over the chestwall (especially anteriorly) may be caused by an aortic aneurysm, vascular new growth or empyema necessitans.
4. **Distended chest veins** Prominent or engorged veins over the front of the chest are suggestive of superior vena caval obstruction, they furnish an early and important sign of mediastinal new growth, enlarged mediastinal lymph nodes or aortic aneurysm. Small venules along the costal margin (emphysematous girdle), although regarded once as indicative of emphysema, are of no clinical importance.

Palpation
Cardinal points:
1. Tracheal position
2. Position of apex
3. Vocal fremitus
4. Movements of chest wall.

Additional points:
- Intercostal tenderness
- Pulsations
- Spine
- Palpable rhonchi, rub, crepitations
- Subcutaneous emphysema (crepitus).

Cardinal Points
Position of trachea and apex gives valuable and reliable information about position of the mediastinum. Careful evaluation of these two should be carried out.

Position of Trachea

In normal subjects the upper 4-5 cm of the trachea can be felt in the neck between the cricoid cartilage and the suprasternal notch.

Methods of palpation of trachea   With a little experience in tracheal palpation it is possible to detect relatively small degrees of mediastinal shift.

Patient is made to sit or stand with head in midline and neck is slightly extended. Left hand of the examiner is used to fix the head in the mid line. The tip of right index finger is placed in the suprasternal notch and gently slide in the midline which normally encounters trachea. In case of tracheal shift finger consistently slides off to the side of shift (Fig. 25.8A).

An alternative method of detecting tracheal deviation is to measure the space between the sternomastoid and trachea (Tracheosternomastoid space) by introducing index finger. This space is decreased to the side of tracheal deviation. This method is more suitable in children (Fig. 25.8B).

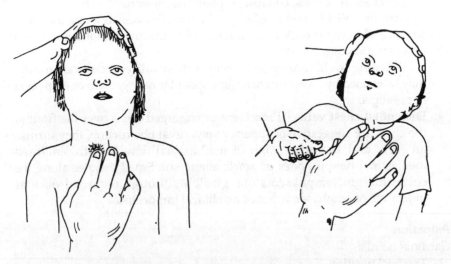

Figs 25.8A and B: Techniques of determining tracheal position in—(A) an older child. Inspection of the suprasternal area may show asymmetry of the fossae bounded laterally by the sternoclei-domastoid muscles and medially by the trachea. In this case the fossa on the right is larger than that on the left as indicated by its larger shadow. It is concluded that the trachea has been shifted to the left, (B) technique of determining tracheal position in an infant. The index-finger of the pulpating band is placed in the suprasternal notch and gently .... in the midsagittal plane. It is essential that the head be fixed in a neutral position and the neck be slightly extended. If the finger consistently slides off one side of the trachea. It can be concluded that the trachea is deviated in the opposite direction. In the illustration, the trachea is shifted to the left. This method can also be applied in older children

Apex

In all the cases of respiratory disorders it is important to locate the position of apical impulse. Value of apical impulse in respiratory system examination is, it gives us the information about position of mediastinum.

Apical impulse after inspection should be located accurately by palpation. Palm of the hand is used initially to feel the apex. The localisation should be done with single digit. Relation of this to midclavicular line should be noted. Normally apex beat is in the 5th intercostal space, just inside the midclavicular line (Fig. 25.9).

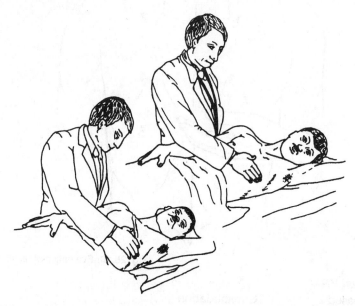

Fig. 25.9: Palpation of the precordium. The morphology of the apical impulse can often be appreciated best in the left decubitus position. The impulse may be amplified in placing a tongue blade over the impulse

In pathology involving upper lobes only, tracheal position will be altered, whereas apical impulse may remain in normal position, in lower lobe pathology only apical position may be altered with trachea remaining in its normal position.

Tactile Vocal Fremitus

Vocal fremitus (VF) is palpation of vibration of chest wall produced by asking the patient to say one-one-one and in small children this can be done during crying. The medial side of the hand is used to palpate VF symmetrically on either side (Fig. 25.10).

Proceed symmetrically downwards from apices to the bases.

Mechanism of TVF: TVF occurs when sounds vibrations from larynx pass down the bronchi and cause the lungs and the chest wall to vibrate. Intensity of fremitus tends to parallel the breath sound intensity.

Variation of TVF   Normal Even in normal healthy subjects marked variation of VF are common. Degree of fremitus depends upon age, sex, thickness of chest wall, volume and pitch of voice. Normally fremitus is less marked in children than adults.

The intensity of tactile fremitus varies considerably from front (strong) to back and from apex (stronger) to lung base in normal persons. Thus, the key comparison is between symmetric points.

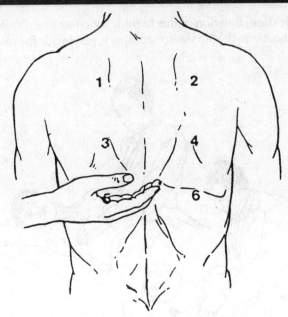

Fig. 25.10: Evaluation of tactile fremitus

Abnormal VF

Increased   — Consolidation

Decreased   — Pneumothorax, pleural effusion

Collapse

Fibrosis

Bronchial obstruction.

Movements of Chest Wall

Comparative palpation of the two sides of chest in an orderly manner from above downward is the best important method for evaluation of the degree and symmetry of expansion with respiration.

Method Apical area To test the movements of apical area patient is made to sit on a stool with head bent forward. Examiner's two hands are placed over the apical regions from behind. The degree of up and down movements are noted as the patient breaths (Fig. 25.11).

Infraclavicular area Patient is made to sit. Place both palms over the chest each on either side of

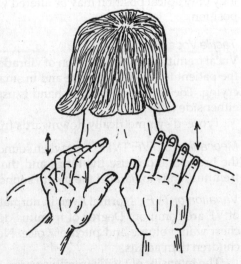

Fig. 25.11: Palpation for up and down movement of apices of lung (supraclavicular area) from back

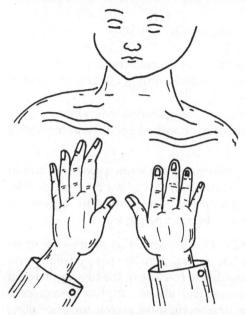

Fig. 25.12: Palpation for to and fro movement of chest in infraclavicular area

chest in the infraclavicular area. The degree of to and fro movements are noted as patient takes breath (Fig. 25.12).

Mammary and inframammary areas Patient is made to sit. The examiner faces the patient and with both hands encircle the chest while thumbs are actively stretched in order to just meet in the midline. As the patient breaths, side to side movements are noted by amount of thumb separation.

Scapular and infrascapular movements are checked by standing behind the patient. Two hands are placed symmetrically on either side of patient's chest, so as to grip the two sides with the palms, whilst the thumbs are actively stretched in order to just meet in the midline. The movement of thumbs from the midline during deep inspiration are noted (Fig. 25.13).

Additional points

Tenderness over the chest Intercostal tenderness should be elicited by slight pressure with finger in the inter costal spaces and over the ribs. Tenderness can also be elicited by gentle percussion with the ulnar side of a fist.

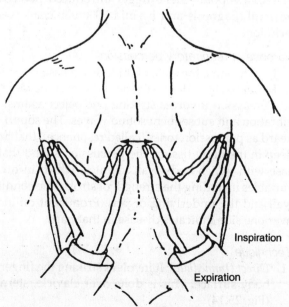

Inspiration

Expiration

Fig. 25.13: Palpation for scapular and infrascapular movements

Causes
— Diseases of skin and subcutaneous tissues like-cellulitis.
— Muscular affection-myositis
— Affection of nerves—herpes zoster neuritis neurofibromatosis.
— Diseases of bones and joints costochondral arthritis (Tietz's syndrome), fracture of rib.
— Pulmonary causes Pleurisy, pneumonia, lung abscess, empyema.
— Tender hepatomegaly as in viral hepatitis, amoebic hepatitis and congestive cardiac failure.

Palpable rhonchi, rub, crepitations   Rhonchi are dry sounds produced within the chest due to bronchospasm. When sufficiently loud, these may be palpable.
Rub—when pleural surfaces are roughened by inflammation, it gives rise to friction sounds which sometimes may become palpable.

Subcutaneous emphysema (crepitus)   This is a sensation of presence of air in the subcutaneous tissues which has a characteristic spongy feeling and usually results from injury to the lung due to fracture of the ribs, drainage of a pneumothorax or in bronchopneumonia with alveolar rupture as in cases of postmeasles bronchopneumonia. The air from ruptured alveoli, traverses along perilymphatic space to mediastinum and then to subcutaneous space of neck and chest.

Spine   (Kyphosis and Scoliosis). The spine should be palpated for any abnormality.

Percussion
In 1761 Leopold Auenbrugger introduced percussion as a corner stone of physical diagnosis and by mid 1800 clinicians were using it as a bed side technique.

Purpose of respiratory percussion
• To determine the state of underlying tissues.
• To delineate or define the boundaries or border of the lung.
    Percussion involves striking one object against another, thus producing vibration and subsequent sound waves. The sound waves thus produced are heard as percussion tones (called resonance), that arise from vibration 4-6 cm deep in the body tissue. The percussion sound that is produced reflects the ease with which body wall vibrates, which in turn is influenced by many variables including the strength of stroke, the condition and state of the body wall and the underlying organs. Prominent dullness or unusual resonance over one side indicates disease in that part.

Technique
1. *Direct (Immediate):* It involves striking the finger or hand directly over the body surface. This is done over clavicle, sternum and in infant's chest (Fig. 25.14).

2. *Indirect (Mediate):* The finger of one hand acts as hammer (plexor) and a finger of the other hand acts as the striking surface (pleximeter). The distal phalynx of the middle finger should be placed firmly on the body surface with the other fingers slightly elevated off the surface. Snap the wrist of your other hand downwards and with the tip of the middle finger, sharply tap the interphalyngeal joint of the finger that is on the body surface (Figs 25.15A and B).

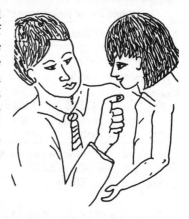

Fig. 25.14: Direct percussion over clavicle

The degree of percussion note is classified in Table 25.10.

Precautions

1. The downward snap of the striking finger should originate from the wrist and not from the forearm or shoulder.
2. The tap should be sharp and rapid.
3. Once the finger strikes, lift the finger to prevent dampening of the sound.
4. The tip and not the pad of plexor finger is used, hence trim the nails !.
5. Do not percuss one location several times.
6. Practice is important for the skill of percussion. Percuss your own body parts! percuss objects in your room !! or you can even percuss your friend's head !!!.
7. Fist percussion is used in eliciting tenderness over liver, gallbladder or kidneys.

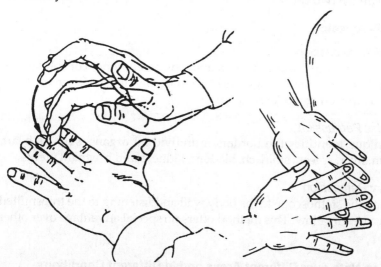

Figs 25.15A and B: (A) Direct percussion of the chest, and (B) indirect percussion

Table 25.10: Resonance of sound waves with respect to percussion notes

Tone	Intensity	Pitch	Duration	Quality	Example
Tympanic	Loud	High	Moderate	Drum like	Gastric bubble
Hyperresonant	Veryloud	Low	Long	Boom like	Emphysematous lung
Resonant	Loud	Low	Long	Hollow	Healthy lung tissue
Dull*	Soft to moderate	Moderate high	Moderate	Thudlike	Over liver
Flat**	Soft	High	Short	Very dull	Over muscle

*Impaired — Bronchopneumonia
Woodydull — Consolidation
**Stony dull — Effusion

Peculiarities of pediatric percussion
- Percussion should be done at the end of examination as it might frighten the children
- The stroke of percussion should vary depending on the thickness of the chest wall and the age of the child. It is learned by practice
- The best position for percussion is when the child is on mothers shoulder
- In infant direct percussion can be done over the chest
- Percuss on either side starting from supposed to be normal side. Quickly interpret
- Slap percussion with four fingers may be used in young children.

Rules of Percussion
1. Always percuss from the resonant area to the expected dull area.
2. Keep the plexor parallel to the expected dull area.
3. Compare the two sides.

Types of Percussion

Comparative Percussion
Detects most large pleural effusions and few pneumonic consolidations. Shifting dullness is a reliable and fairly accurate sign for detection of ascites and pleural effusion of moderate quantity.

Topographic Percussion
This technique identifies the borders in individual organs, such as heart, diaphragm, liver, spleen, stomach, bladder, kidneys and pregnant uterus.

Ascultatory Percussion
By applying the stethoscope to the body wall and listening to the transmitted note from a nearby blow. This method offers no special advantage over other methods.

Percussion Note over Different Areas and in Different Conditions
1. Percuss upper border of dullness and mark 'S shape curve of Ellis' which will be noted in pleural effusion. Here, the level of dullness is higher in

axilla as compared to front and back of chest. This is due to capillary action where in, fluid rises in the axillary area. In case of hydro pneumothorax the upper band of dullness is horizontal.

2. Percuss shifting dullness, which is present in moderate effusions and is absent in massive or encysted effusions. To do this make the patient sit up, percuss both anteriorly and posteriorly from above downward and mark the upper level of dullness. Then ask the patient to bend forward and percuss the back. If shifting dullness is present, the dull area becomes resonant as the pleural fluid moves forward. The otherway to elicit this sign is to ask the patient lie down supine after noting dullness at upper border of fluid in sitting position, when the dull area become resonant due to movement of fluid backward.

3. Traube's area becomes dull in left sided pleural effusion.

   Traube's area is a triangular space bound medially by left lobe of liver, above by left lung and below by costal margin and is normally occupied by fundus of stomach and hence the percussion note is tympanic.

4. Skodiac note (subtympanic note) over pleural effusion is due to relaxed lung above the fluid. It is a kind of hyperresonant note.

5. Grocco's triangle—Is a right angle triangle of dullness over the posterior part of the chest opposite a pleural effusion.

6. Garland's triangle—Is a small area of relative resonance on the side with pleural effusion, near the top of the effusion and next to spine.

7. About 500 ml fluid is required for eliciting dullness in pleural effusion.

Special Techniques
Besides the customary or classical method of percussion, the following are the special techniques for percussion.

Flicking Percussion
This is a special form of light percussion, the surface to be percussed being flicked with the finger and thumb. It is useful for percussion of the abdomen, topographical percussion of cardiac borders and for eliciting metallic resonance in case of pneumothorax, while normally a flick on one side of the chest is heard as a dull sound on the opposite side; in the case of pneumothorax the sound heard has metallic, ringing or chimming quality.

Threshold Percussion
This is sometimes useful when the degree of resonance over the chest is in doubt. The area of suspected impairment is percussed progressively more lightly until a note is no longer obtained. The corresponding area over the opposite lung is then percussed with equal intensity. If a note is then obtained, it affords additional evidence of impairment on the side originally suspected.

Direct or Indirect Palpatory Percussion
It is done with a view of determining the sense of resistance to percussion, may be used to advantage for detecting the presence of fluid or consolidation within the chest. For this purpose direct percussion with the pads of the three middle

fingers of the right hand usually prove most effective, particularly when employed over the back of the chest.

Limitations of Percussion

1. It is not possible to percuss deeper than 5 cm. Hence, it is not possible to detect a lung lesion covered by a layer of air more than 5 cm thick or fluid 1cm thick.
2. A lesion less than 2 cm in diameter does not cause any change in the percussion note.
3. Free fluid less than 200 ml in the pleural cavity may not be detected on percussion.

Types of Percussion Notes

1. Normal percussion notes
2. Abnormal percussion notes

Normal Percussion Notes

The normal percussion note of the chest is due to the underlying lung tissue, containing a normal amount of air in the air vesicles, air sacs and air passages. The percussion note over the healthy lung tissue has a distinctive and clear character with a low pitch.

As a rule, the front wall of the chest yields more resonant note than the back, because of the lesser bulk of musculature is in front than at the back.

Abnormal Percussion Notes

Abnormal types of percussion notes may be either—

1. Quantitatively different from normal lung resonance as in case of tympany, subtympany, hyperresonance, impairment of note, dullness and stony dullness.
2. Qualitatively different as cracked pot resonance, amphoric resonance and bell tympany.

Abnormal Types of Percussion Notes (Table 25.11)

1. *Tympany* A drum-like note, elicited normally over the stomach, intestine, larynx or trachea, is referred to as tympanic note. When such a note is heard over a region of the chest wall it indicates.
   a. Pneumothorax
   b. Subcutaneous emphysema
   c. Superficial cavity.
2. *Subtympany (Skodiac)* A hyperresonant note, with a boxy quality, usually heard just above the level of pleural effusion or pneumonic consolidation.
3. *Hyperresonant* A note intermediate in pitch between normal lung resonance and tympany can be elicited, over normal lung tissue, by keeping the chest in full inspiration during percussion.
   Pathologically:
   • Bilaterally in case of emphysema
   • Unilaterally in case of pneumothorax, lung cyst, large bullae, diaphragmatic hernia, compensatory emphysema, obstructive emphysema.

4. *Impaired note* When a part of a lung becomes comparatively airless, it fails to vibrate sufficiently to the percussion stroke and gives rise to an impairment of note or slight loss of resonance and found in:
   a. Consolidation
   b. Collapse
   c. Fibrosis

5. *Dull note* An impairment of note, of greater degree than the impaired note, is referred to as dullness and is found in:
   a. Consolidation
   b. Collapse
   c. Thickened pleura
   d. Extensive tuberculous infiltration of lung.
   Basal dullness as a consequence of diaphragm elevation can be confused with pleural fluid, but the diaphragmatic dullness will move downwards on deep inspiration (unless muscle is paralysed).

6. *Stony dullness or Flatness* A percussion note completely devoid of resonance or displaying absolute dullness is referred to as flat or stony dull note, can be elicited normally percussing on the thigh of the patient. Found in:
   a. Pleural effusion (Volume > 200 ml)
   b. Empyema: In these conditions, the fluid dampens the vibration of both chest wall and underying retracted tissue. A feeling of resistance to the percussion blow within the finger used for stroking is, also present in
   c. Solid intrathoracic tumour
   d. Fibrosis with pleural thickening.

7. *Cracked pot resonance* This is special variety of tympanic resonance, which can be elicited normally over the chest of an infant or child during the act of crying.
   Pathologically, cavity communicating with a bronchus.

8. *Amphoric resonance* A low pitched and hollow note, can be artifically reproduced by percussing the normal trachea or cheeck (moderately distended with air). May be found in pneumothorax, and in large cavity.

9. *Bell tympany* High pitched note with a tympanic or metallic sound over the chest in case of massive pneumothorax. When a silver coin is placed flat on the affected side and percussed with a second coin, the stethoscope applied directly over the opposite side of the chest detects a clear bell like sound (Hammer on an anvil or chiming of a church bell). This is also known as "coin test".

Table 25.11: Characteristic features of percussion

Type of tone	Intensity	Pitch	Duration	Quality
Resonant	Loud	Low	Long	Hollow
Hyperresonant	Very loud	Very low	Longer	Booming
Dull	Medium	Medium high	Medium	Thud like
Tympanic	Loud	High	Medium	Drum like
Flat	Soft	High	Short	Extremely dull

Percussion

Percussion

Cardinal points

1. Lung fields percussion
2. Shifting dullness
3. S-shaped curve of Ellis
4. Liver dullness

Additional

- Skodiac dullness
- Traube's area
- Cardiac dullness
- Splenic dullness
- Tidal percussion
- Coin test
- Grocco's triangle
- Garland's triangle
- Percussion Myokymia

Cardinal Points (Some details)

Topographic Percussion of the Lungs

Percussion of the chest to determine the boundaries of lungs. This is of parti-cualr value in determining the upper or apical border of the lungs (apical percussion), lower border (basal percussion), and anterior border of the left lung (Fig. 25.16).

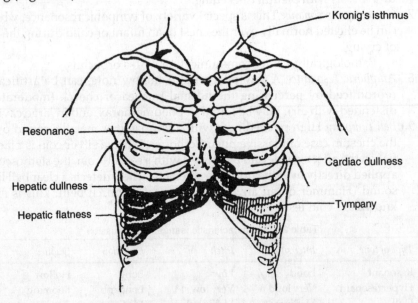

Kronig's isthmus

Resonance

Cardiac dullness

Hepatic dullness

Tympany

Hepatic flatness

Fig. 25.16: Percussion notes over the normal chest

Apical percussion This can be carried out in the supraclavicular fossa anteriorly, by determining the upper borders of the lung resonance on the two sides.

Normally, the upper border is from 3 to 5 cm above the clavicle, on either side, being at times somewhat higher on the right side.

Diminition or absence of the supraclavicular zone of resonance is good evidence of pulmonary tuberculosis. On the other hand an increased extent of resonance bilatreally, suggests emphysema.

An alternative method of percussion of the apical regions is percussion over the Kronig's isthmus on either side. It is a band of resonance, which corresponds roughly to the apex of the lung, is usually 5-7 cm in width and is bounded medially by a dull zone corresponding to the structures of the neck and laterally by the dullness of the shoulder region.

Basal percussion Normally, during quiet breathing, the lower border of the lung resonance corresponds to the fifth rib in midclavicular line, eighth rib in the midaxillary line and 10th rib in the scapular line.

Percussion of the lower border of the lung necessiates light percussion anteriorly and heavy percussion at the back (because of the thicker musculature).

The lower border of the lung resonance tends to be depressed in case of emphysema or pneumothorax, and raised in case of lung fibrosis, collapsed lung, consolidations, ascites, massive abdominal tumor or pleural effusion.

Shifting Dullness

In case of hydropneumothorax, in sitting position there is hyperresonant note above followed by dullness below. On changing the posture to supine, this area of dullness of the field changes.

This shifting dullness always signifies presence of both air and fluid. Also found in moderate size pleural effusion but never with interlobar or loculated effusion.

S-shaped Curve of Ellis

In moderate sized effusion within the pleurla sac, the upper border of the dullness or flatness, which is highest in the axilla and lowest at the spine; tends to assume the shape of the letter "S". This is due to capillary action where in the fluid rises to a higher level in the axillary area as compared to front and back.

Liver Dullness

Over the lower part of the right side of the chest, anteriorly and laterally one can map out an extensive area of dullness, corresponding to the position of the underlying liver. Normally liver dullness lies at the 5th space in midclavicular line, 7th space in anterior axillary line and 9th space in scapular line.

Liver dullness is present in 4th space in the following conditions; amebic or pyogenic abscess of the liver, diaphragmatic paralysis, collapse of the lower lobe of the lung.

Liver dullness is pushed to 6th space in emphysema, right sided pneumothorax, air in the peritoneal cavity.

Additional points

1. *Skodiac dullness* A hyperresonant note with a boxy quality which occurs due to the relaxed lung just above the level of pleural effusion.
2. *Traubes area* At the lower border of the left lung anteriorly, pulmonary resonance is replaced by a drum like tympanic note over a semilunar area (Traubes area) due to the presence of fundus of stomach.

   This area is bounded above by pulmonary resonance, on the right by liver dullness, on the left by spleenic dullness, below by left costal margin.

   Obliteration of Traube's area Traube's semilunar area of tympany may be partially obliterated in case of a large left sided pleural effusion.
3. *Cardiac dullness* Cardiac dullness extends in triangular fashion from the sternum (on the right) to the junction of the midclavicular line with the 5th left intercostal space.
4. *Splenic dullness* A smaller area of dullness or diminished resonance, in the eight interspace in the midaxillary line, is similarly attributed to the presence of spleen on that side.
5. *Tidal percussion* Percussion of the upper border of the liver dullness on the right side anteriorly, at the height of deep inspiration and expiration. Serves to determine the extent of diaphragmatic movement. Is restricted in pulmonary fibrosis, empyema, subdiaphramatic abscess.
6. *Coin test* At the junction of fluid and air, the metallic quality of the coin, sounded on one side of the chest can be appreciated at the diametrically opposite side of the chest wall.
7. *Grocco's triangle* An area of relative dullness roughly triangular in shape, can sometiems be mapped out by percussion in cases of large or medium sized pleural effusion on the opposite side.

   The triangular area is bounded medially by mid-spinal line from above the level at effusion to the level of the tenth dorsal vertebra, below by a horizontal line extending outward from the 10th dorsal vertebrae along the lower limit of lung resonacne for a distance of about 3-7 cm, and laterally by a somewhat curved line connecting these two lines.
8. *Garland's triangle* It is an inconstant sign of little or no value.

   In the case of a moderate sized or large pleural effusion the lung on the side of the effusion floats upward and backward, its lower part being released. The roughly triangular area, with a sligthly tympanic note or skodiac resonance that may be elicited in such a case by percussion over the released area at lung, is referred to as Garland's triangle.
9. *Percussion myokymia* In a chronically wasted individual as in pulmonary tuberculosis, a percussion stroke over mid front of the chest, close to the sternum, may cause a transient twitching of the muscle which is more marked on the side of the pulmonary affection. This is called percussion myokymia.

Auscultation

Auscultation with a stethoscope provides important clues to the condition of the lungs and pleura. Following points should be kept in mind before and while auscultating the chest.

1. The patient and examiner must be mentally and physically relaxed and comfortably placed at the examination.
2. For auscultation of the lungs the ideal posture for the patient is upright, either sitting or standing (Fig. 25.17). In younger children auscultation, should be carried out with child on mothers shoulder (Fig. 25.18).

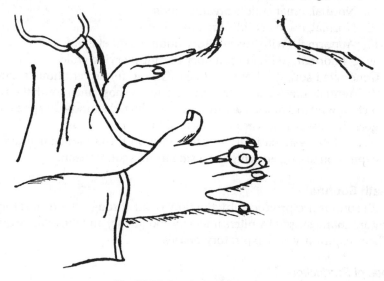

Fig. 25.17: Ascultation of chest

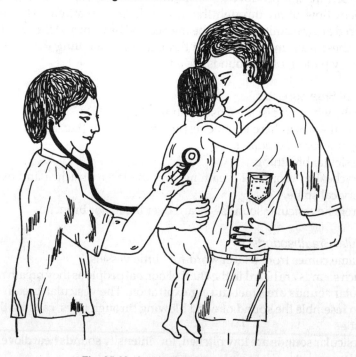

Fig. 25.18: Ascultation of chest in infant

3. In an uncooperative or crying children auscultation should be carried out while sleeping.
4. Practice pediatric auscultation in one of the following situations to appreciate adventitious sounds when children are crying. This practice has to be done throughout life.
    i. Normal, quiet child's breathsounds.
    ii. Normal, crying child's breathsounds.
    iii. Abnormal, (with auscultatory findings) quiet child.
    iv. Abnormal, (with auscultatory findings) crying child.
5. Conducted sounds should not be mistaken for adventitious sounds. To differentiate one from another auscultate overnose and mouth then slowly inch downward at the base of lung. Conducted sounds disappear as one goes downwards towards the base of the lungs.
6. Auscultate systematically at each position throughout inspiration and expiration taking advantge of a side to side comparison.

Breath Sounds

Breath sounds are produced by the flow of air through the respiratory tree. They are characterised by pitch, intensity and quality and the relative duration of their inspiratory and expiratory phases.

Mode of Production

Breath soudns are produced by vibration of the vocal cords caused by the turbulent flow of air through the larynx during breathing. The sounds so produced are transmitted along the trachea and bronchi and through the lungs to the chest wall. In their passage through a normal lung the intensity and frequency pattern of the sounds are altered.

Types of Breathsounds

Normal—when no disease exists in lungs (Fig. 25.19).
Abnormal—when there is some respiratory problem (Fig. 25.19).

Types of normal breathsounds
1. Vesicular breathing
2. Tracheal or bronchial breathing over the larynx trachea and over lower cervical spine.
3. Bronchovesicular sounds—heard over the major bronchus.

Vesicular Breathsounds

The name comes from a latin word for "little vessels."

Such sounds are heard in the chest of normal people as they breath normally. Vesicular sounds are quiet during expiration. The vesicular breath sound is said to resemble the sound of wind blowing through trees, causing the leaves to rustle.

Vesicular sounds are low pitched, low intensity sounds heard over healthy lung tissue.

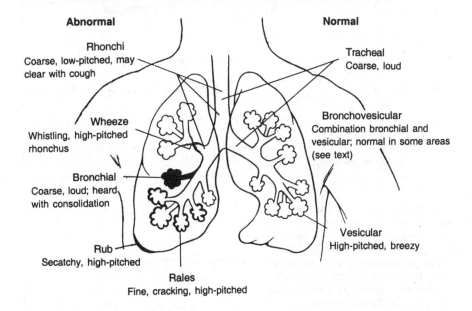

Fig. 25.19: Representation of normal breath sounds and abnormal sounds in the chest

This is characterised by active inspiration due to inflow of air into bronchi and alveoli, followed by shorter expiration due to elastic recoil of the alveoli without a pause between inspiration and expiration (Figs 25.20A and B).

Distribution Typical of normal aerated lung parenchyma, is heard all over the chest in heatlh except.

1. Over larynx, trachea, lower cervical vertebrae.
2. Over and around the upper part of the sternum and third and fourth dorsal vertibrae.

Bronchial Breath Sounds

Can be heard in normal subjects in certain area but they are considered abnormal when they are heard over the peripheral lung tissue (Table 25.12).

Table 25.12: Charactersitic features of vesicular and bronchial breathing

Vesicular breathing	*Bronchial breathing*
• Normal breath sounds	Can be normal or abnormal
• Heard all over the chest in health except over larynx trachea, lower cervical vertebra	Normally heard over larynx, trachea lower cervical vertebrae
	Anormal when heard over peripheral lung tissue
• Rustling or breezy quality	Blowing quality
• Low pitched	High pitched
• Inspiration is longer being three to five times as the expiration	Expiratory phase is equal or longer than inspiration phase
• No pause between inspiration and expiration	Definitive pause between inspiration and expiration

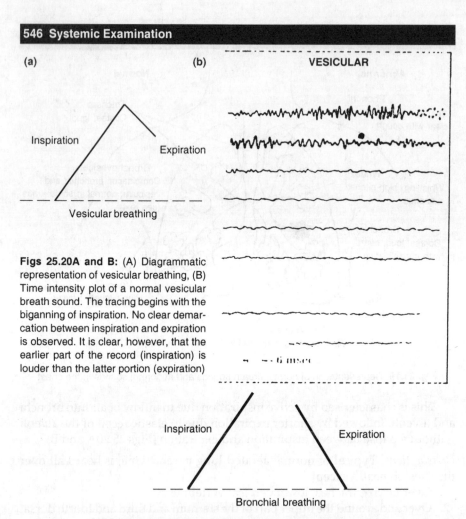

(a)

(b)

VESICULAR

Inspiration

Expiration

Vesicular breathing

Figs 25.20A and B: (A) Diagrammatic representation of vesicular breathing, (B) Time intensity plot of a normal vesicular breath sound. The tracing begins with the biganning of inspiration. No clear demarcation between inspiration and expiration is observed. It is clear, however, that the earlier part of the record (inspiration) is louder than the latter portion (expiration)

Inspiration

Expiration

Bronchial breathing

Fig. 25.21: Diagrammatic representation of bronchial breathing

This is characterised by active inspiration due to the passage of air in to the bronchi. The alveolar phase is absent. There is no rustling quality to the sound (Fig. 25.21).

Mode of Production of Bronchial Breathing

Normally the laryngotracheal sounds are modified by the air cells of normally functioning lung tissue into the characteristically rustling vesicular sound. When normally aerated lung is replaced by consolidation of lung the glotic sounds are conducted to the chest wall without modification through the solid lung tissue.

Bronchial Breath Sounds are Further Classified into Three Types

1. *Tubular* High pitched sound, therefore better heard with the diaphragm of stethoscope. They are heard over consolidated area, when the lung has become solid due to exudate in alveoli and the tracheal sounds are directly transmitted to chest wall without alteration.

2. *Cavernous* Low pitched bronchial sound. Therefore, better heard with the bell of the stethoscope. They are normally heard over the occipital area. Pathologically they are heard over the cavities in the lung and in early pneumonias and bronchopneumonias.
3. *Amphoric* High pitched and has a peculiar metallic quality. It resembles the sound produced by blowing through an empty bottle with a narrow neck. It is heard in hydropneumothorax, just above the fluid level. Also heard over the large pulmonary cavity with patent bronchus.

Adventitious Sounds

Adventitous sounds are the sounds which are unexpected in normal individuals. They are of 2 types.
1. *Continuous*: Sounds last for more than a small fraction of the respiratory cycle, e.g. rhonchi.
2. *Discontinuous*: Also called as intermittent, they occur in relatively brief bursts, similar to popping of bubbles or cracking sounds of a fire. They are called rales sometimes crepitations or crackles.

The adventitious sounds vary in their pitch, intensity, quality and site of production and is shown in Figures 25.22A and B.

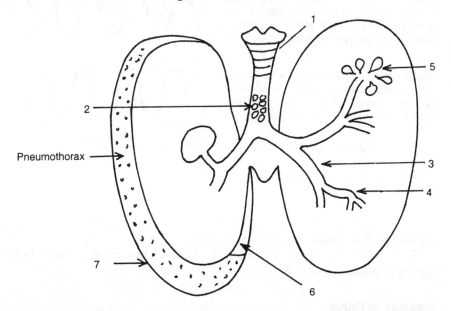

Fig. 25.22A: Adventitions sounds: site of origin–(1) stridor (laryngeal or tracheal), (2) death rattle (tracheal secretions), (3) coarse and leathery crepitations (bronchi), (4) rhonchi (bronchi and bronchioles), (5) fine crepitations (alveoli and bronchioles), (6) succusion splash (air and fluid in pleura), and (7) pleural rub

— Wheezes (Rhonchi) As mentioned earlier these are continuous, dry, musical sounds originating from the respiratory tract.
Mode of production They are produced by the passage of air through an airway obstructed by thick secretions, muscular spasm, newgrowth, or external pressure (Fig. 25.23).

Fine crackles: High-pitched, discrete, discontinuous crackling sounds heard during the end of inspiration; not cleared by a cough

Medium crackles: Lower, more moist sound heard during the midstage of inspiration; not cleared by a cough

Coarse crackles: Loud, bubbly noise heard during inspiration; not cleared by a cough

Rhonchi (sonorous wheeze): Loud, low, coarse sounds like a snore most often heard continuously during inspiration or expiration; coughing may clear sound (usually means mucus accumulation in trachea or large bronchi)

Wheeze (sibilant wheeze): Musical noise sounding like a squeak; most often heard continuously during inspiration or expiration; usually louder during expiration

Pleural friction rub: Dry, rubbing, or grating sound, usually caused by inflammation of pleural surfaces; heard during inspiration or expiration; loudest over lower lateral anterior surface

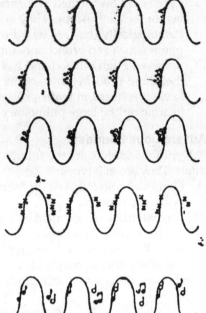
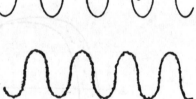

Fig. 25.22B: Charecterstic features of adventitious breath sounds

Two types of rhonchi are:
1. Sonorus rhonchus.
2. Sibilant rhonchus.

Sonorus rhonchus: They are deeper, more rumbling more pronounced during expiration. Resembles the sound of snoring.

Sibilant rhonchus They are continuous, high pitched musical sound, heard during inspiration and expiration.

Crackles or Rales

These are interupted, short, sharp, nonmusical sounds heard more often during inspiration.

They are caused by disruptive passage of air through the small airways in the respiratory tree (Fig. 25.24).

Crackles are classified into:
1. Fine
2. Medium
3. Coarse.

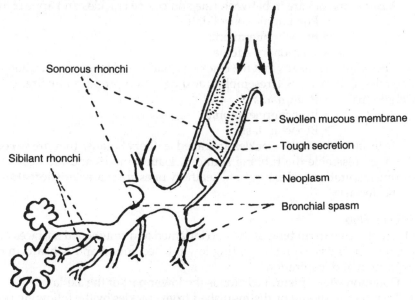

Fig. 25.23: Mode of productrion of rhonchi

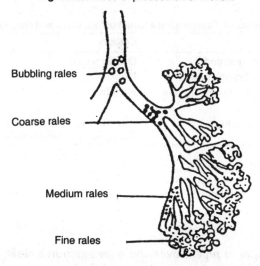

Fig. 25.24: Sites of production of rales

Fine crackles are short in duration and are less louder than coarse crackles, they resemble rubbing of hairs between fingers.

Conditions • Pneumonia
• Pulmonary edema
• Bronchiolitis
• Bronchitis
• Atlectasis
• Fibrosis.

Medium crackles are in between fine and coarse crackles and appear in:
- Pneumonic consolidation
- Bronchopneumonia
- Pulmonary edema.

Coarse crackles means that the crackle is louder and longer in duration than fine rales. Coarse crackle resemble crackling sound produced by fire.

Conditions
- Pneumonia ·
- Bronchopneumonia
- Bronchiectasis.

In bronchiectasis the crackles are called leathery because they are so coarse that they resemble the rubbing sound of leather pieces and are heard both during inspiration and expiration. Leathery rales are characteristic features of bronchiectasis.

Friction Rub

Originates due to rubbing of the two inflamed and roughened surfaces of the pleura. It is a dry. Crackly, grating low pitched sound and is heard in both expiration and inspiration.
- Common site of pleural friction is the lower part of the axilla
- Friction rub should be distinguished from crackles by the following points (Table 25.13).

Table 25.13: Comparative account of friction rub and crackles

Friction rub	Crackles
• Superficial, scratchy sound	Deeper sound
• Associated with pleuritic pain	No pain
• Intensify with pressing stethoscope over the chest	No effect
• Does not alter with cough	Alteration with cough is seen. They either disappear or intensify following coughing

Vocal Resonance

Auscultatory analog of tactile fremitus is vocal resonance. Vocal resonance means sounds heard with stethoscope over various parts of the chest during the act of phonation.

Technique

The patient is made to repeat over and over again in a slow, loud, uniform voice, some syllables like "one-one-one", while the examiner auscultates the chest over symmetric areas of the two sides of the chest.

Vocal resonance of normal intensity generally, conveys the impression of being produced just at the chest piece of the stethoscope. Various pulmonary pathologies alter the vocal resonance.

Increased VR When the vocal resonance is increased, it gives an impression that sound is nearer to the ear than at chest piece.
- VR is increased in
  1. Over areas of consolidation (Solidified lung is a good conductor of sound vibrations).
  2. Small superficial lung cavity.

- Decreased VR is seen in:
  - Pleural effusion
  - Pneumothorax
  - Thicked pleura
  - Emphysema.

Bronchophony

This is an increased vocal resonance, where in, spoken sounds appear loud and clear and close to the ear. However, the individual syllables remain indistinguishable.

Normally audible over the larynx and trachea. However, presence of bronchophony over the chest or lung parenchyma is always pathological.

Consolidation is the most common cause.

Whispering Pectoriloquy

If bronchophony is extreme even a whisper can be heard, clearly through stethoscope as if uttered directly into the examiner's ear and is called as whispering pectoriloquy. It, is heard in:

1. Consolidation.
2. Large cavity communicating with bronchus.

Egophony

When the intensity of spoken voice is increased and there is a nasal quality, the auditory quality is called egophony. It has the quality of sound produced by bleeting of a goat.

Heard above the level of pleural effusion and pneumothorax.

The site where the breath sounds are better perceived while auscultating yields valuable information as shown in Figure 25.25.

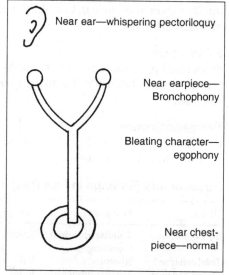

Fig. 25.25: Breath sounds: where better heard?

Post-tussive Crepitations

These crepitations are audible after making the patient cough, while they are not audible during normal respiration.

It signifies presence of cavity which is filled with thick material which gets dislodged during coughing allowing air to bubble through the remaining fluid producing the crepitation. In small children Crepitations that are not heard during quiet breathing may be heard after a bout of cry (post crying crepitations). They have the same significance as post-tussive crepitations.

Mediastinal Crunch (Hamman Sign)

It is found with mediastinal emphysema. There is great variety of noisy loud crackles and clicking and gurgling sounds. These are synchronous with the heart beat and not particularly so with respiration, but sounds can be more pronounced towards the end of expiration. They are easier to hear when the patient leans to the left or lies down on the left side.

Succussion Splash

Air and fluid in the pleural cavity simultaneously or in large cavities within the lungs are suspected if one listens over the possible involved area and gently shakes the patient from side to side. This can be achieved with patient sitting. First place a hand on the patients shoulder and then with your hand, move the patient from side to side, not brosquely but with a bit of vigor. The fluid will splash, and in the presence of air, a succussion splash will be heard.

Coin Test

It is a special test done in a case of hydropneumothorax. A silver coin is placed flat on the affected side and percussed with a second coin, the stethoscope is applied directly on the opposite side of the chest. A high pitched, tympanic or metallic sound is heard over the chest.

d'Espian's Sign

The presence of bronchial breathing and increased vocal resonance in the midline over the back below the level of 5th thoracic vertebra in cases of mediastinal mass.

Ewart's Sign

Bronchial breath sounds, heard over left lower interscapular area in a patient with pericardial effusion due to compression of left main bronchus leading to collapse.

Peristaltic Sounds

If peristaltic sounds are heard in left chest, they indicate diaphragmatic hernia, eventeration of diaphragm.

Auscultatory Findings in Few Respiratory Disorders

Disease	Breath sounds	Foreign findings	VR	Special sounds
Consolidation	Tubular bronchial breathing	Rales	Increased	WP +
Total collapse	Absent	Nil	Absent	—
Partial collapse	Tubular bronchial breathing	Rales Ronchi	Increased	WP +
Cavity	Cavernous breathing	Rales	Increased	WP +
Pleural effusion	Absent or decreased	Absent	decreased	
Pneumothorax	Absent or	Absent amphoric	Absent	

Contd...

Contd...

Disease	Breath sounds	Foreign findings	VR	Special sounds
Hydropneumo-thorax	Absent	—	Absent	Succusion splash, + coin test
Bronchial asthma	Vesicular with prolonged Expiration	Rhonchi	Normal	
Bronchiectasis	Vesicular	Coarse leathery Crepitations	Normal	
Lt. sided diaphra-gmatic hernia or eventeration.	Decreased	Nil	Decreased	Peristaltic sounds in left chest

WP = Whispering pectoriloquy

General Physical Examination Findings which can Aid to the Diagnosis of Disorders of Respiratory System

Signs	Diseases
	Head and Neck
1. Phlycten	Tuberculosis
2. Sinusitis	Suppurative lung disease, bronchial asthma, cystic fibrosis, Kartagener's syndrome
3. Potter facies	Pneumothorax
4. Allergic salute	Bronchial asthma
5. Caries	Suppurative lung disease
6. Swollen nasal mucosa	Allergic rhinitis
7. Retinal venous dilatation	Hypercarbia
8. Cleft palate	Aspiration pneumonia
9. Lymphadenopathy	Tuberculosis
10. Bulbar palsy	Aspiration pneumonia
11. Audible slap and palpable thud	Foreign body in trachea
12. Halitosis	Bronchiectasis and other supurative lung disease
13. Excessive oral secretions	Tracheoesophageal fistula
14. Allergic shrines	Allergic disorder
15. Drooling with hyperextended neck	Supralaryngeal obstruction
16. Hoarse voice, stridor	Laryngotracheobronchitis
17. Nasal polyp	Cystic fibrosis, allergy, bronchiectasis
18. Meningismus	Pneumococcal pneumonia
19. Herpes labialis	Pneumonia
20. Face-'Ex-premmie'	Bronchopulmonary dysplasia
21. Dysmorphic facies	Pierre Robin sequence
22. Ear discharge	Serous otitis media
23. *Chlamydia/Mycoplasma* conjuctitivitis	Interstitial pneumonia
	Chest
1. Harrison's sulcus	Chronic respiratory infection
2. Increased AP diameter of chest	Hyperinflation
3. Asymmetry of chest	Hypoplastic lung, congenital lobar emphysema
4. Paradoxical respiration	Pneumothorax
5. Pectus excavatum	Chronic adenoidal hypertrophys

Contd...

Contd...

Signs	Diseases
6. Pectus carinatum	Cystic fibrosis, chronic lung disease
7. Scar on chest	Previous pneumothorax, lobectomy, heart-lung transplant
8. Wheeze	Bronchial asthma
9. Use of accessory muscles, intercostal recession, tracheal tug	Respiratory failure
10. Tachypnea	Restrictive or parenchymal lung disease
11. Lymphocytic interstitial pneumonia	HIV infection
Upper Limbs	
1. Flapping tremor	Carbon dioxide retention
2. Pulsus paradoxus	Severe airway obstruction
3. Bounding pulses	Hypercarbia
4. Hypertrophic pulmonary osteoar-thropathy	Cystic fibrosis
5. Tachycardia	Hypoxia
6. Clubbing	Chronic suppurative lung diseases, cystic fibrosis, cavitating tuberculosis, AV fistula
7. Cyanosis	Hypoxia
Skin	
1. Erythema nodosum	Tuberculosis
2. Ecthyma gangrenosum	*Pseudomonas pneumoniae*
3. Urticaria	Bronchial asthma
4. Sarcoid nodules	Sarcoidosis
5. SLE rash	Pleural effusion
6. Scleroderma rash	Pleural effusion
7. Eczema	Allergic disorder
8. Measles rash	Interstitial pneumonia
9. Pityriasis simplex	Atopy
10. Cutaneous strawberry haemangiomata	Subglotic hemangioma
11. Hairy leukoplakia	HIV infection
12. Tuberous sclerosis	Pneumothorax
13. Skin lesions	Staphyloccal pneumonia
14. Face and neck edema	Superior vena caval obstruction
15. Peripheral edema	Cor pulmonale CCF

Outline of Clinical Examination of the Respiratory System in the Pediatric Age Group

• Clinical Regions	— Anterior
	— Lateral
	— Posterior
Anterior	— Supraclavicular
	— Infraclavicular
	— Mammary
	— Inframammary
Lateral	— Axillary
	— Infra-axillary
Posterior	— Suprascapular
	— Interscapular
	— Infrascapular

Contd...

Contd...

- Anatomical regions
  - — Rt. lung   Lt. Lung
  - — Upper lobe   Upper Lobe
  - — Middle lobe   Lower Lobe
  - — Lower lobe
- Radiological zones
  (Roentgenological)   — Zones
  Above 2nd anterior rib   — Rt. lung   Lt. Lung
  2nd-4th anterior rib   — Upper zone   Upper zone
  below the 4th anterior rib   — Middle zone   Middle zone
     — Lower zone   Lower zone
- Bronchopulomonary
  segments   — Rt. lung   Lt. lung
     Upper   — Superior (Apical)   Superior
     — Anterior   Anterior
     — Posterior   Posterior
     Middle   — Lateral   Superior lingular
     — Medial   Inferior lingular
     Lower   — Superior   Superior
     — Anterior   Anterior
     — Posterior   Posterior
     — Lateral   Lateral
     — Medial
- General physical examination
- Opening statement   — Consisting of the following points
  - Sex of the child
  - Age of the child
  - Build and nourishment
  - General impression   — Sickness
     — Decubitus
     — Dehydration
     — Respiratory distress
- Vital signs   — Temperature
     — Respiratory rate and rhythm
     — Blood pressure
     — Pulse
- Respiratory rate and type   — Indicating respiratory distress
  Any noise e.g: — Grunt, stridor, cough, wheeze
     Decubitus   — Note the position of the child
     Cyanosis   — Peripheral
     — Central
- Upper Respiratory Tract
  Examination   — Ears, nose, paranasal sinuses, throat
  Lymph node examination   — Detailed description
  Clubbing
     Grade I   — Softening of the nailbed and obliteration of the angle
  b/w the nail base and adjacent skin of the finger
     Grade II   — Drumstick appearance
     Grade III   — Parrot beak apppearance
     Grade IV   — Hypertrophic pulmonary osteoathropathy
  Evidence of TB   — Glands
     — Absence of BCG scar
     — Phlycten
     — Erythema nodosum
     — Gibbus

Contd...

Contd...

Anthropometry	— Hepatomegaly — Splenomegaly — Head circumference — Chest circumference — Mid-arm circumferance — Height for age — Weight for age	
• Nutritional status	— IAP classification — Wellcome classification — Aggarwal's charts — Plotting on NCHS charts.	

• Head to foot examination
  systemic examination — "The rule of 4" i.e., 4 cardinal and 4 additional points to be taken into consideration while examining the patient

• Inspection: Cardinal — Shape of the chest
  — Movement of the chest
  — Tracheal position (Trail sign)
  — Apical position

  Additional — Spine
  — Pulsations over the chest
  — Veins
  — Signs of distress (Movement of alae nasi, tachypnea, suprasternal indrawing, intercostal indrawing, use of accessory muscles of respiration)

• Palpation: Cardinal — Tracheal position
  Apical position —Palmar palpation
  —Digital palpation
  — Movements —Infraclavicular (To and from)
  —Supraclavicular (Up and down)
  —Mammary (To and fro)
  —Interscapular (Side to side movements)
  —Infrascapular (Side to side movements)
  — Vocal fremitus —All areas

  Additional — Tenderness (intercostal)
  — Rubs
  — Rhonchi   } Palpable
  — Crepitations

Percussion: Cardinal — Lung field
  — Liver border
  — Heart border
  — Shifting dullness (mild to moderate pleural effusion and hydropneumothorax)

  Additional — Coin test
  — Level of dullness rising in Axilla (Ellis Curve) in pleural effusion, horizontal in hydopneumothorax)
  — Tidal Percussion
  — Traube's area (obliterated in Lt. Pl. Effusion).

Contd...

Contd...

Region to be percussed	:	Types of percussion notes
Posterior — Suprascapular		Imapired-Patchy consolidation
— Interscapular		Woody Note-Established consolidation
— Infrascapular		Stony Dullness-Presence of fluid
Anterior — Supracavicular		Hyperresonant-Emphysema
— Clavicular (direct		Tympanitic-Pneumothorax
percussion)		
— Infraclavicular		
— Mammary		
— Inframammary		
Lateral — Axillary		
— Infra-axillary		

Auscultation

Cardinal	—	Breath sounds
	—	Adventitious sounds
	—	Vocal resonance
	—	Succussion splash (hydropneumothorax)
Additional	—	Whispering pectoriloquy (consolidation)
	—	Bronchophony
	—	Aegophony (above pleural effusion)
	—	Post-tussive and postcrying crepitations
Breath sounds	—	Vesicular
	—	Broncho Vesicular
	—	Bronchial
Bronchial breath sounds	—	Hollow blowing character
	—	Expiratory phase harsh and prolonged, definite gap between inspiration and expiration

Types			Conditions
1. Tubular	—	High pitch (Better heard with diaphragm of stethoscope)	Consolidation
2. Cavernous	—	Low Pithc (better heard with bell of stethoscope)	Cavity and early consolidation
3. Amphoric	—	High Pitch with a metallic quality (Better heard with diaphragm of stethoscope)	Large cavity, hydropneumo-thorax

Adventitious sounds

Creptations (Crackles)	—	Fine	
	—	Medium	
	—	Coarse	
	—	Leathery	— (Bronchiectasis)
	—	Death Rattle	— (Tracheal secretions)
Rhonchi	—	Sonorous, sibilant	
Rub	—	Pleural	

26 Examination of Cardiovascular System

INTRODUCTION

This chapter discusses the methodical physical examination of a child with cardiac disease and certain particular points are emphasized in detail for better understanding. Before proceeding to cardiovascular examination a full general physical examination is mandatory. While examining children, the examiner should look for anticipated positive physical findings after evaluating history. Findings that may point to cardiac disease include abnormal vital signs, presence of cyanosis, anemia, edema, clubbing, dismorphic features, skin change, etc. To avoid missing positive physical findings it is better to examine the cardiovascular system in the following order.

Before discussing physical examination a review of history taking is given below.

SYMPTOMATOLOGY: EVALUATION OF CARDIOVASCULAR SYMPTOMS

Dyspnea

- Dyspnea is difficult breathing
- In cardiac disorders dyspnea is an important feature.

Evaluation of Dyspnea

- Note onset (abrupt, insidious), progression, duration, relation to activity and position
- Grade dyspnea according to NYHA grading
- Whether it is progressive
- Note if there is orthopnea
- Note if there is any PND
- Note associated features like cough, palpitation, chest pain, sweating, edema, etc.

Hemoptysis

Hemoptysis may be an important but a rare presentation of cardiac disorders. It may be seen in severe pulmonary hypertension, ususally in children with rheumatic mitral stenosis. The other causes of hemoptysis in mitral stenosis include pulmonary infarcts, intercurrent bronchitis. In acute left ventricular failure the patient may expectorate large, pink frothy sputum. In primary pulmonary hypertension and in cyanotic congenital heart diseases with severe pulmonary hypertension and collaterals, hemoptysis may occur. Occasionally hemoptysis may be seen in infective endocarditis.

But most cases of hemoptysis are due to respiratory illnesses like bronchiectasis, foreign body, pulmonary hemosiderosis, bronchial adenoma, sequestration of lung, Good Pasture's syndrome, etc.

Palpitation

Awareness of one's own heart beat is known as palpitation. It may be due to fast, slow or irregular heart beat.

Elicit the following details.
1. *Onset*   – Abrupt—SVT, extrasystoles and other arrhythmias.
                                – Insidious—anemia, CHD.
2. *Mode of termination* – Abrupt—SVT.
                                – Insidious—anemia, RHD, CHD.

With vagal maneuver (vomiting, Valsalva phenomenon, pressure over eyeballs, induction of vomiting, etc)—SVT.

With passage of large volume of urine—SVT (due to increased secretion of atrial natriureteric protein (ANP).

Rest

Drugs—(Beta-blockers, digoxin).

Precipitating Factors
- Exertion
- Drugs (stimulants, β-agonists, aminophylline)
- Excessive coffee.
- Emotions, etc.

Associated Features
- Sweating—angina, thyrotoxicosis, emotions.
- Chest pain—angina
- Neck choking—SVT
- Vomiting.

In small children excessive pulsation observed over chest are interpreted as palpitation by the mother. These are common in hyperdynamic circulation states like anaemia, PDA, etc.

Evaluation of Cyanosis

Onset

Cyanosis present at birth: Transposition of great arteries (TGA), pulmonary atresia, critical pulmonary stenosis, hypoplastic left heart syndrome (HLHS).
Cyanosis appearing in the first week: Tricuspid atresia, Ebstein's anomaly, pulmonary atresia, Total anamolous pulmonary venous circulation (TAPVC) (obstructive type), severe TOF.
Cyanosis appearing after 3 months: TOF, tricuspid atresia, pulmonary hypertension, AV malformation.
Later age: Eisenmenger syndrome.

Course

Cyanosis decreases for some weeks and reappears—Ebstein's anomaly.

Acyanotic heart showing cyanosis after few years—Eisenmenger syndrome.

Cyanosis—Increases with crying in cardiac cyanosis.

Decreases with crying in respiratory cyanosis

Cyanosis—Increasing during crying, feeding is seen in cyanotic CHD.

Cyanosis associated with cyanotic spells (bouts of excessive crying in infants, usually in the early hours of morning, precipitated by cold, intercurrent infection, associated with severe cyanosis, sometimes ending in fits and fainting). They indicate obstructive pulmonary CHD with decreased pulmonary circulation, e.g. TOF, TGA with pulmonary stenosis, etc.

Cyanotic spells are due to sudden obstruction of right ventricular outflow tract (RVOFT). Cyanosis associated with squatting indicates TOF. Squatting increases peripheral resistance by muscular compression over the arteries in the lower limbs and causing increase in peripheral resistance which decreases right to left shunt. At the same time squatting pools venous blood in the lower limbs and causes decreased right ventricular venous return thus causing decrease in right to left shunt. Both these mechanisms by decreasing right to left shunt relieves the patient of his symptoms.

Cyanosis appearing only in lower limbs in PDA indicates differential cyanosis which is due to reversal of shunt.

Importance of Age in Cardiac Disorders

Age

Age of presentation of cyanosis:
- First week: Ebstein's anomaly, obstructive TAPVC
- Birth to 1 month: TGA, pulmonary atresia, tricuspid atresia
- 3 to 6 months: TOF.

Age of presentation of CHD:
- At birth: TGA, HLHS, Aortic stenosis, tricuspid atresia, coarctation of aorta, VSD
- One week: VSD, PDA, common AV cannal
- 1 month: VSD, pulmonary stenosis
- 6 months to 1 year: TOF
- 4 to 5 years: ASD.

Age of presentation of rheumatic fever:
- 5 to 15 years.
- Earlier the age of onset, more likely that severely the heart is involved
- Mitral stenosis can occur in Indian setting as early as 6 years (Juvenile mitral stenosis).

H/o Suggestive of CCF
- Feeding difficulty
- Tachypnea
- Dyspnea   — (Pulmonary venous congestion)
- Wheeze
- Basal crepitation

- Hepatomegaly   — (Systemic venous congestion)
- Edema
- Tachycardia   — (Low cardiac output)
- Pallor, sweating, poor pulses, cold extremities
- Abnormal weight gain,   — (Fluid retension)
  decreased urine output.

Symptoms Associated with Cardiac Disease

Features Suggestive of Infective Endocarditis
1. Persistent fever
2. Progressive pallor
3. Stroke
4. Petechiae
5. Arthralgia
6. Clubbing
7. Sphinchter hemorrhages
8. Janeway nodules
9. Osler's nodules
10. Roth's spots in retina
11. Microscopic haematuria
12. Splenomegaly
13. Changing and/or musical murmurs.

Chest Pain in Cardiac Disorders
Cardiac origin of chest pain is rare in children. Among cardiac causes of chest pain in children.
  a. Most common: Pericarditis (viral, rheumatic and rheumatoid arthritis). Retrosternal pain, increases on deep breathing.
  b. Next common: A sort of dull, heavy sensation due to enlarged heart of any cause (RHD, cardiomyopathy and pericardial effusion).
  c. Anginal pain is rare in children—occasionally seen in Kawasaki disease (aneurysm of coronary artery). Severe AS, severe PS, anomalous origin of left coronary artery, rupture of sinus of Valsalva, familial hyper-cholesterolemia, premature aging syndromes like progeria, Werner's syndrome, etc.
  d. Suffocating sensation in neck and retrosternal area sometimes seen in SVT.
  e. Dysphagia misinterpreted as chest pain: cardiomegaly causing dysphagia includes large left atrium in MS of rheumatic etiology, abnormal vessels.

CHD Presenting with Collapse
- 0-2 days   — HLHS
- 7-10 days   — Coarctation of aorta, aortic stenosis and complex defects
- Any age   — Myocardial disease, arrhythmias.

CHD with Asymptomatic Murmurs
- 0-2 days   — AS, PS, TOF (mild)
- > 3 days   — VSD, PDA (small)

- > 3 months — ASD
- Any age — Innocent murmur, ASD.

Features of Left to Right Shunt
- Frequent chest infections
- Feeding problems
- Increase sweating
- Absence of cyanosis
- Precordial bulge
- Hyperkinetic precordium
- Flow murmur
- Pulmonary plethora on X-ray, e.g. ASD, VSD, PDA.

Features of Right to Left Shunt
- Cyanosis
- Clubbing
- Polycythemia.

Features Suggestive of RHD
1. Acute migratory polyarthritis in children between 5 and 15 years from lower socioeconomic background living in crowded places.
2. Repeated sore throat.
3. Previous h/o arthritis (which may be absent in 50% of cases)
4. Recurrent abdominal pain and epistaxis.
5. Rheumatic nodules around joint, along tendons.
6. Rheumatic chorea.
7. Penicillin prophylaxis.

Feature Suggestive of Carditis in Rheumatic Fever
1. Persistent tachycardia (sleeping pulse rate to be taken).
2. Muffled heart sound.
3. Gallop rhythm, arrhythmia, changing and muscial murmur or new murmurs.
4. Pericardial rub.
5. Features of CCF.
6. Presence of subcutaneous nodules indicates that in about 75 percent of cases there is an underlying carditis.
7. Persistent dry cough.
8. ECG changes, increased ESR, presence of CRP, vegetations and or pericardial effusion or echo.

Other Historical Details

Present History
Ask the following questions:
1. History of frequent lower respiratory tract infections, e.g. left to right shunts.
2. Symptoms of congestive cardiac failure such as excessive sweating, feeding problems, decreased urine output, frequent respiratory infections,

poor growth, failure to thrive and facial puffiness. Conditions to be suspected are VSD, PDA, coarctation of aorta, TAPVC.

3. History of bluish discoloration of skin and mucous membrane, e.g. cyanotic heart disease depending on age of presentation. Rt. to Lt. shunts,
   - Cyanosis and palpitation—Ebstein's anomaly.
   - Cyanotic spells associated with crying, feeding—TOF.
   - Differential cyanosis—Rt. to Lt. shunting across PDA with coarctation or interrupted aortic arch.

4. History of squatting episodes—TOF, tricuspid atresia.

5. History of syncope or faintness, e.g. aortic stenosis, pulmonary stenosis, primary pulmonary hypertension, coarctation of aorta, arrhythmias.

6. Symptoms of infective endocarditis (Fever, bleeding spots, hematuria, tender fingers, weakness of one side of body, prolonged treatment with high dose of penicillin).

7. History of chest pain, e.g. severe aortic stenosis, pulmonary stenosis, Kawasaki disease.
   Anomalous origin of (Lt.) coronary artery from the pulmonary artery.

8. In older child assess the degree of dyspnea. New York Heart Association has classified dyspnea into functional and therapeutic.

   Class I   : Patient is asymptomatic or symptoms occur on extraordinary exertion.

   Class II   : Symptoms occur on ordinary exertion.

   Class III : Symptoms occur on less than ordinary exertion.

   Class IV : Symptoms occur at rest or on slight exertion.

   Therapeutic Classification

   Class A : No restriction.

   Class B : Severe effort restricted.

   Class C : Ordinary effort moderately restricted.

   Class D : Ordinary effort markedly restricted.

   Class E : Confined to chair.

9. Leg fatigue, leg pain after exercise, claudication pain—coarctation of aorta. Competitive exercises may be dangerous in children with pulmonary hypertension, aortic stenosis, and in hypertrophic cardiomyopathies.

10. History of dysphagia—coarctation with the right subclavian artery passing behind the esophagus.

11. An observant mother may give history of infants heart beating against chest wall, or the vibration of a thrill, e.g. Conditions associated with overactive precordium.

12. Awareness of pulsation in the neck, e.g. coarctation, venous pulsations of giant a waves in primary pulmonary hypertension, severe pulmonary stenosis and congenital complete heart block.

13. History of weakness of one side of the body with dizziness, visual disturbances, headache, fever. Then consider the following conditions:

- Cerebral abscess due to cyanotic congenital heart disease with Rt. to Lt. shunt.
- Emboli from endocardial fibroelastosis.
- Emboli from idiopathic cardiomyopathy.

14. History of weakness and incoordination.
    Cardiomyopathy of Friedreich's ataxia or muscular dystrophy.
15. History of mental retardation.
    Down's syndrome—endocardial cushion defect.
    William's syndrome—supravalvular aortic stenosis.
16. History of hoarseness of voice, e.g. large PDA.
    Primary pulmonary hypertension.
17. History of swelling pain warmth and tenderness of lower extremities, e.g. hypertrophic osteoarthropathy suggests PDA with Eisenmenger's syndrome.
18. Recurrent bleeding from the nose, lips, or mouth, with hemoptysis or melena, multiple cerebral symptoms such as dizziness and visual disturbances, and a family history of epistaxis? (This complex of symptoms comprises hereditary hemorrhagic telangiectasis or Rendu-Osler-Weber disease, and suggests a pulmonary arteriovenous fistula, especially if the patient is cyanotic).
19. History of disease impact on child, e.g. growth development, schooling (academic performance, sports restrictions, school days lost, teachers attitude, peer attitude). In many congenital cyanotic heart diseases, there is a delay in attainment of puberty. The details about other issues like sexual performance, contraception and pregnancy should be asked in adolescent and young adults.
20. Previous history of medications, hospitalization, surgical procedures and catheterization, should be asked for.
21. Previous infections and immunisation: Gastroenteritis may cause dehydration and precipitate intracranial thrombosis in congenital cyanotic heart diseases. Further dehydration may be associated with hypokalemia which is dangerous in patients on digoxin and diuretics.

Viral and other respiratory infection and fever often cause cardiac decompensation by increasing the metabolic needs of the body and by causing hypoxic effect on the pulmonary vascular resistance.

Immunisation   There is no contraindication for immunisation except in associated immunodeficiency state like Asplenia, Digeorge syndrome, etc. Children with congenital heart disease should be immunised like any other child at appropriate age.

Family History
In family history questions should be asked regarding:
1. Diabetes mellitus in family members—TGA.
2. History of congenital heart disease in family—endocardial fibroelastosis.
3. Parental consanguinity-Autosomal recessive conditions with heart diseases, e.g. Friedreich's ataxia.

Antenatal History
1. History of maternal illness during pregnancy.
   - Rubella—PDA, Pulmonary artery branch stenosis.
   - Mumps—Endocardial fibroelastosis.
   - Diabetes—TGA
   - PKU—VSD, ASD, PDA, COA
   - SLE—Congenital heart block.
2. History of drug consumption during pregnancy:
   - Alcohol—TGA, VSD, PDA
   - Amphetamines—TGA, VSD, ASD, PDA
   - Phenytoin—PS, AS, COA, PDA
   - Lithium—Ebstein's anomaly
   - Sex hormone—TGA, TOF, VSD

Birth History
History of high birth weight-TGA.

GENERAL PHYSICAL EXAMINATION
1. Position of child: Decubitus.
2. Vital signs.

Pulse
Assessment of the arterial pulses is a vital part of cardiovascular examination. Ordinarily the radial artery is studied in detail, but other peripheral pulses also should be palpated. The location of peripheral arteries are given in Table 26.1.

Table 26.1: Locations of palpable pulses

Pulse	Location
Carotid	In the neck, just medial to and below angle of the jaw (do not palpate both sides simultaneously)
Brachial	Just medial to biceps tendon
Radial	Medial and ventral side of wrist (gentle pressure)
Femoral	Inferior and medial to inguinal ligament; if patient is obese, midway between anterior superior iliac spine and pubic tubercle (press harder here than in most areas)
Popliteal	Popliteal fossa (press firmly); the patient should be prone with the knee flexed
Dorsalis pedis	Medial side of dorsum of foot with foot slightly dorsiflexed (pulse may be hard to feel and may not be palpable in some well persons)
Posterior tibial	Behind and slightly inferior to medial malleolus of ankle (pulse may be hard to feel and may not be palpable in some healthy children)

The following observation should be made with regard to cardiac function. **Rate:** The pulse should be counted when child is resting and for one full minute, because of possible irregularities in rhythm. Normal pulse rate in various age groups are provided in Table 26.2.

Table 26.2: Pulse rate at rest

Age	Range	Average
Newborn	70-190/min	125/min
1-11 months	80-160/min	120/min
2 years	80-130/min	110/min
4 years	80-120/min	100/min
6 years	75-115/min	100/min
8 years	70-110/min	90/min
10 years	70-110/min	90/min

Tachycardia
- Resting pulse >160 in newborns
- Resting pulse >120 beats in children <2 years
- Resting pulse >100 beats in older children and adults.

Causes
Exercise, fever, thyrotoxicosis, infections, tachyarrhythmias.

Bradycardia
- Resting pulse <100 beats/min in newborn
- Resting pulse <80 beats/min in children <2 years
- Resting pulse <60 beats/min in older children.

Causes
- Athletes, familial or hereditary myxedema
- Following infections like pneumonia and influenza
- Jaundice, raised ICT
- Metabolic causes such as hypocalcemia, metabolic acidosis and hyperkalemia
- Cardiac causes such as heart block, corrected TGA
- Digitalis toxicity.

Rhythm
Decide rhythm is regular or irregular. If it is irregular, decide whether it is regularly irregular or irregularly irregular.

Causes of irregular rhythm Sinus arrhythmias is a physiologic variation in impulse discharges from within the sinus node related to respirations. It is characterised by increase in heart rate with inspiration and decrease with expiration due to vagal inhibition. Sinus arrhythmias are commonly seen in premature infants, especially bradycardia associated with periodic apnea. It is exaggerated during convalescence from febrile illness and drugs such as digitalis. It is usually abolished by exercise or by atropine.

Other causes include: Extrasystoles, atrial fibrillation, paroxysmal atrial tachycardia with block; Atrial flutter with varying block; partial heart block with irregularly dropped beats.

Causes of regularly irregular rhythms
- — Heart blocks.
- — Extrasystoles.

Causes of irregularly irregular rhythms
- — Atrial Fibrillation.

Pulse deficit In atrial fibrillation, the auscultated heart rate is faster than the palpated pulse rate. This is due to the poor contraction of ventricles, which is not strong enough to open the aortic valve or to transmit an arterial pressure wave through the peripheral artery. Pulse deficit is obtained by simultaneously counting heart rate and radial pulse rate.

Volume
This denotes the amplitude of movement of the vessel wall. It is estimated by the amount of lift produced by the arterial wall. Volume of pulse is a direct indicator of pulse pressure. Depending on pulse volume, there are two types of pulses:

a. **Hypokinetic Pulse (Weak Pulse)** This is due to reduced cardiac output and pulse pressure will be in narrow range (Fig. 26.1).

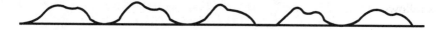

Fig. 26.1: Small, weak pulse

Causes Shock, CCF, Hypovolemia, Cardiac tamponade, Chronic constrictive pericarditis, myocarditis, cardiomyopathy, mitral stenosis, aortic outflow tract obstruction, co-arctation or aortic arch syndrome.

b. **Hyperkinetic Pulse (Bounding Pulse):** Due to increase cardiac output and decrease peripheral resistance (Fig. 26.2).

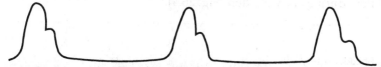

Fig. 26.2: Large, bounding pulse

Causes Anxiety, Exercise, Complete heart block, AR.

Fever, anemia, thyrotoxicosis, hyperkinetic heart syndrome, AV fistula, Beriberi, cirrhosis of liver, coarctation of aorta.

Equality of Pulses
A comparison of radial and femoral pulses should be done to detect presence of radio-femoral delay. If present, clinical diagnosis of coarctation of aorta should be considered.

Next compare both radial artery pulsation and look for weak or absent pulsation of one or both radial arteries. Cardiac conditions associated with this are:

— Anomalous or aberrant course of radial artery.
— Aneurysm of aorta.
— Dissecting aneurysm of the aorta.
— Coarctation of aorta.
— Supra valvular aortic stenosis.

Character A careful study of the character of the pulse is an important step in the physical diagnosis of cardiac disease. A normal contour of arterial pulse is illustrated in Figure 26.3.

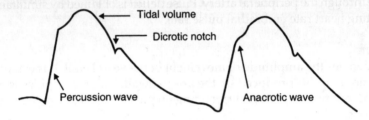

Fig. 26.3: Normal arterial pulse

The different characters of abnormal pulses and associated conditions are as follows.

Abnormal Pulse—Different Characters

Anacrotic Pulse
This is a slow rising pulse of smaller amplitude seen in conditions like aortic stenosis. The term anacrotic means an upbeating pulse and refers to the exaggerated anacrotic notch found in aortic stenosis. It is related to a jet effect produced by ejection across the abnormal valve or to decreased velocity of blood flow during early ejection (Fig. 26.4).

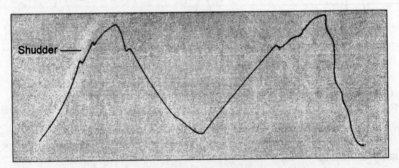

Fig. 26.4: Anacrotic pulse

Double Beating Pulses
A double beating or twice beating pulse occurs when there are two palpable arterial pulses per cardiac cycle. The different types of double beating pulses and associated cardiac conditions are given in Table 26.3.

Table 26.3: Types of double beating pulses and their related conditions

Type of pulse	Causes
Bisferiens pulse	Combined AR and AS, high output states
Bifid pulse (Spike and dome)	Hypertrophic cardiomyopathy
Dicrotic pulse	Cardiomyopathy or severe LV dysfunction
	Typhoid fever

Bisferiens Pulse

The pulse form shows two positive peaks during systole. This is felt best in carotid arteries. The following diagram shows contour of bisferiens pulse (Figs 26.5A to C).

Bifid Pulse

This type of pulse is commonly recorded than palpated. The initial spike is followed by a mid systolic pulse collapse and then by a late systolic impulse. It is illustrated in Figures 26.5A to C.

Dicrotic Pulse

In this waveform the second palpable component is a diastolic reflection wave. The detectable delay between two palpable peaks is much longer than in the bisiferens pulse.

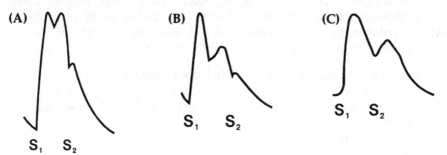

Figs 26.5A to C: Double beating pulses: (A) Bisferiens pulse, (B) Spike and dome arterial pulse, and (C) Dicrotic pulse

Pulsus Alternans

This is characterised by a strong and weak beat occuring alternatively. This phenomenon is related to a beat to beat alternation in developed LV pressure caused by changing ejection dynamics. This can be objectively confirmed by recording blood pressure. While recording the blood pressure, once systolic pressure is recorded and the mercury column is lowered, there is a abrupt doubling of Korotkoff's sound. The wave form is illustrated in Figure 26.6.

Pulsus alternans is an important sign of left ventricular dysfunction.

Pulsus Paradoxus

Pulsus paradoxus refers to a marked and exaggerated inspiratory fall in systolic blood pressure in which the palpable arterial pulse and audible Korotkoff

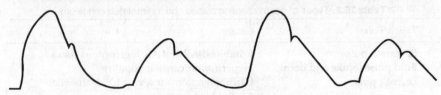

Fig. 26.6: Pulsus alternans

sounds disappear during inspiration. Normally, inspiration reduces systolic arterial pressure less than 6-8 mm Hg, if the inspiratory fall is more than 10 mm Hg, pulsus paradoxus is said to be present (Fig. 26.7).

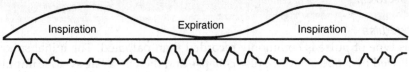

Fig. 26.7: Pulsus paradoxus

Mechanism of pulsus paradoxus Normally during inspiration, due to decrease in intrathoracic pressure, the lung capacity increases and pulmonary vascular bed expands. This reduces the amount of blood reaching the left heart and in turn reduces the systolic pressure by 6-8 mm Hg, which is considered as normal phenomenon. Whereas in cardiac tamponade, due to raised intrapericardial pressure, the left atrial and left ventricular pressure increases, which further reduces the amount of blood returning to left heart. Hence, reducing the blood pressure >10 mm Hg during inspiration.

Determination of a paradoxic pulse (sphygmomanometer)
— Ask the child to breathe as easily and comfortably as possible.
— Apply the sphygmomanometer and inflate it until no sounds are audible.
— Deflate the cuff gradually until sounds are audible only during expiration.
— Note the pressure.
— Deflate the cuff further until sounds are also audible during inspiration.
— Note the pressure.
— The difference in systolic pressure between expiration and inspiration is greater than 10 mm Hg, paradoxic pulse is present.

Causes of pulsus paradoxus
— Pericardial tamponade.
— Constrictive pericarditis.
— Emphysema.
— Asthma, severe congestive heart failure.

Collapsing Pulse (Water Hammer Pulse)
The term 'Water Hammer' refers to a popular victorian toy comprising of a glass vessel partially filled with water which produced a slapping impact on

being turned over. Thus, a collapsing pulse is characterised by a sudden thrust and receeding back sensation of the pulse wave. The abrupt upstroke is due to the greatly increased stroke volume. The collapsing character is caused by two factors: First, the diastolic run off into the left ventricle; and secondly, the rapid run off to the periphery because of a low systemic vascular resistance.

Method of palpating collapsing pulse   Palpate radial artery above wrist, through the muscles of forearm. Then lift arm above the level of childs head. If collapsing pulse is present, a sudden thrust and collapsing sensation is felt. The raising of arm above the level of heart brings in the factor of gravity, thus exaggerating the leak at aortic level as in AR (Fig. 26.8).

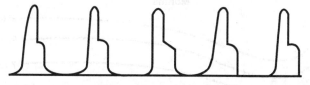

Fig. 26.8: Collapsing pulse

Causes
- Physiological-Exercise, heat.
- Hyperkinetic circulatory state-Beri-beri, hepatic disease, anemia.
- Leak in the arterial side of circulation AR, PDA, AV fistula, large VSD, MR, Truncus arteriosus, Blalock-Taussig Shunt, rupture of coronary sinuses.

Respiratory Rate
The normal respiratory rate is inversely related to age; it is rapid in neonates, then decreases in older infants and children. The normal respiratory rate according to age is described in Table 26.4.

Table 26.4: Respiratory rates in relation to age

Age	Respiratory rate
Newborn	40-60/min
Infants	Upto 30/min
1-4 years	24-26/min
4-8 years	20-22/min
> 8 Years	18-20/min

Type of Respiration
- Thoraco abdominal—Adult women
- Abdomino thoracic or diaphragmatic—Children and adult males.

Tachypnea
- Physiological—Excitement or exertion.
- Pathological—Fever, disease of lungs or heart.

Decreased RR
- Narcotic poisoning.
- Endocrine disease associated with hypometabolism.

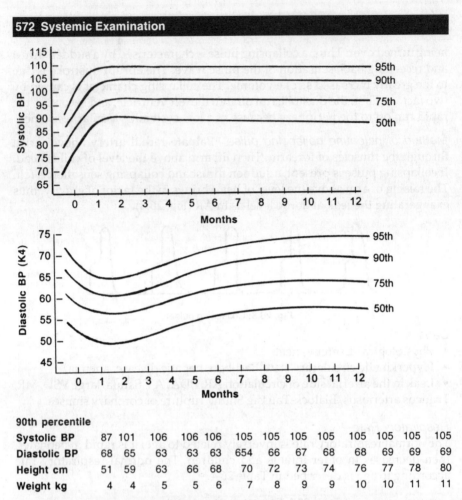

Figs 26.9A and B: Age specific percentile of BP measurements in boys—birth to 12 months of age

90th percentile

Systolic BP	87	101	106	106	106	105	105	105	105	105	105	105	105
Diastolic BP	68	65	63	63	63	654	66	67	68	68	69	69	69
Height cm	51	59	63	66	68	70	72	73	74	76	77	78	80
Weight kg	4	4	5	5	6	7	8	9	9	10	10	11	11

Uremia, Diabetic Coma.

Raised intracranial pressure.

Temperature

Blood Pressure Blood pressure is determined by cardiac output and systemic vascular resistance. Normal blood pressure varies with the age of the child and is closely related to height and weight. The median (50th percentile) systolic blood pressure for children older than 1 year may be approximated by the following formula (Figs 26.9A and B):

$$90 \text{ mm Hg} + (2 \times \text{Age in years})$$

The lower limit (5th percentile) of systolic blood pressure can be estimated by following formula:

$$70 \text{ mm Hg} + (2 \times \text{Age in years})$$

Normal values of blood pressure according to age is provided in Table 26.5.

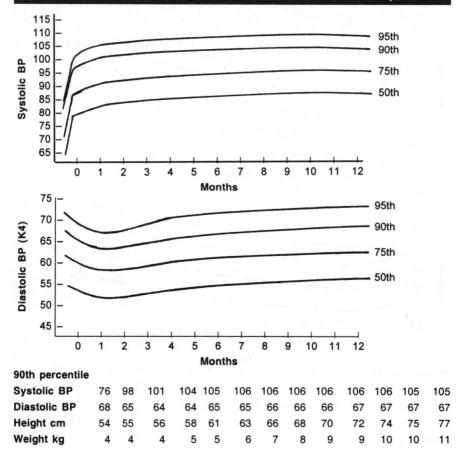

90th percentile

Systolic BP	76	98	101	104	105	106	106	106	106	106	106	105	105
Diastolic BP	68	65	64	64	65	65	66	66	66	67	67	67	67
Height cm	54	55	56	58	61	63	66	68	70	72	74	75	77
Weight kg	4	4	4	5	5	6	7	8	9	9	10	10	11

Figs 26.10A and B: Age specific percentile of BP measurements
in girls—birth to 12 months of age

Table 26.5: Normal values of blood pressure with respect to age

Age	Systolic pressure (mmHg)	Diastolic pressure (mmHg)
Birth (12 hr, <1000 g)	39-59	16-36
Birth (12 hr, 3 kg)	50-70	25-45
Neonate (96 hr)	60-90	20-60
Infant (6 months)	87-105	53-65
Toddler (2 years)	95-105	53-66
School Age (7 years)	97-112	57-71
Adolescent (15 Years)	112-128	66-80

Age specific percentile charts of BP measurements are given in the Figures 26.10 to 26.14.

Different methods of examining BP in children
1. Conventional sphygmomanometry
2. Doppler method

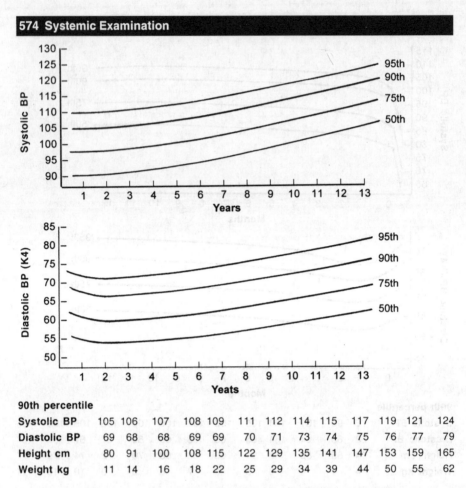

90th percentile													
Systolic BP	105	106	107	108	109	111	112	114	115	117	119	121	124
Diastolic BP	69	68	68	69	69	70	71	73	74	75	76	77	79
Height cm	80	91	100	108	115	122	129	135	141	147	153	159	165
Weight kg	11	14	16	18	22	25	29	34	39	44	50	55	62

Figs 26.11A and B: Age specific percentile of BP measurements in boys—1 to 13 years of age

3. Oscillometric method
4. Flush method used in infants.

Guidelines for Measuring BP

1. **Position of child**   Ideally patient should be sitting or lying at ease with limb to be recorded kept at level of heart.
2. **Using appropriate sized cuff**   The most important factor in accurately measuring blood pressure is by using appropriate sized cuff:
   — The cuff size refers to inner inflatable bladder and not the cloth covering.
   — The cuff should cover approximately 75 percent of upper arm between top of shoulder and olecranon.
   — Enough room at antecubital fossa to place bell of stethoscope and enough room at upper edge of cuff to prevent obstruction of axilla.

   The various recommended bladder dimensions for blood pressure cuffs according to age are given in Table 26.6.

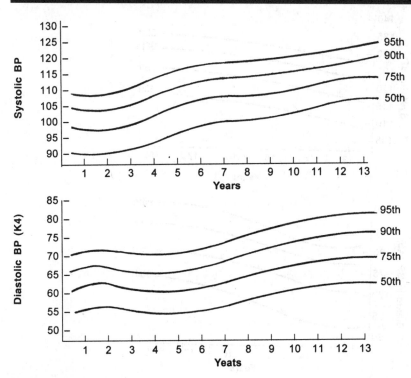

90th percentile													
Systolic BP	105	105	106	107	109	111	112	114	115	117	119	122	124
Diastolic BP	67	69	69	69	69	70	71	72	74	75	77	78	80
Height cm	77	89	98	107	115	122	129	135	142	148	154	160	165
Weight kg	11	13	15	18	22	25	30	35	40	45	51	58	63

Figs 26.12A and B: Age specific percentile of BP measurements in girls—1 to 13 years of age

Table 26.6: Bladder dimensions for blood pressure cuffs with respect to age

Arm circumference at midpoint (cm)	Cuff name	Bladder width (cm)	Bladder length (cm)
5—7.5	Newborn	3	5
7.5—13	Infant	5	8
13—20	Child	8	13
24—32	Adult	13	24
32—42	Large arm	17	34
42—50	Thigh	20	42

3. BP should be recorded in all four limbs. The different sites for measuring blood pressure is illustrated in Figures 26.15A to D.
4. Ordinarily, the BP recorded in the lower limbs with cuff technique is about 10 mm Hg higher than in the arms. This is due to the direct transmission

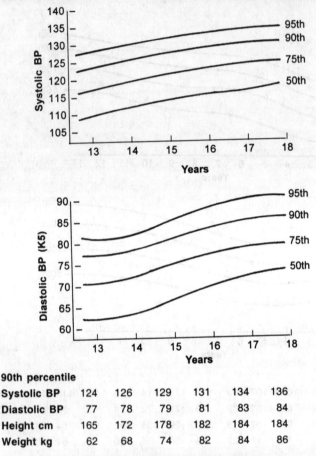

90th percentile						
Systolic BP	124	126	129	131	134	136
Diastolic BP	77	78	79	81	83	84
Height cm	165	172	178	182	184	184
Weight kg	62	68	74	82	84	86

Figs 26.13A and B: Age-specific percentile of BP measurements in boys—13 to 18 years of age

of pressure from the aorta to the larger descending aorta. The pressure is transmitted from aorta to the upper limb through comparatively narrow vessel. The other reason for high BP may be due to the use of same BP cuff for upper limb and lower limb.

5. Read mercury gravity manometer at eye level.
6. Record systolic value at onset of a clear tapping sound (First Korotkoff sound).
7. Record diastolic pressure at:
   — Fourth Korotkoff sound (Low pitched, Muffled sound) for children upto age 12 years.
   — Fifth Korotkoff sound (disappearance of all sound) for children 13 to 18 years.

Phase of Korotkoff sound is given in Table 26.7.

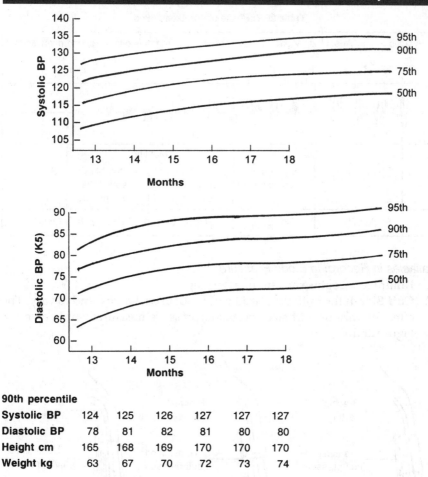

90th percentile						
Systolic BP	124	125	126	127	127	127
Diastolic BP	78	81	82	81	80	80
Height cm	165	168	169	170	170	170
Weight kg	63	67	70	72	73	74

Figs 26.14A and B: Age-specific percentile of BP measurements in girls—13 to 18 years of age

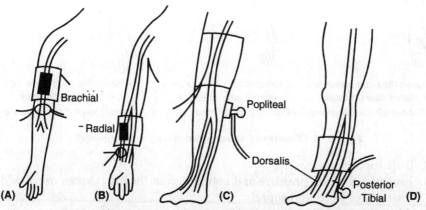

Figs 26.15A to D: Sites for measuring blood pressure: (A) Upper arm; (B) Lower arm or forearm; (C) Thigh; (D) Calf or ankle

Table 26.7: Phase of Korotkoff sound

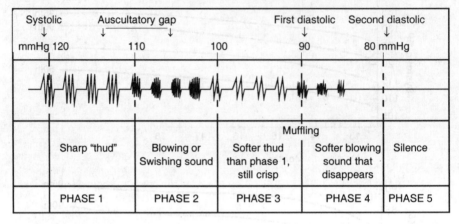

PHASE 1	PHASE 2	PHASE 3	PHASE 4	PHASE 5
Systolic ↓ mmHg 120	Auscultatory gap ↓ 110 ↓ 100		First diastolic ↓ 90	Second diastolic ↓ 80 mmHg
		Muffling		
Sharp "thud"	Blowing or Swishing sound	Softer thud than phase 1, still crisp	Softer blowing sound that disappears	Silence

Fallacies in Recording Blood Pressure

1. Failure to recognise an auscultatory gap.
2. **Cuff Size**-If the optimum sized cuff is not used, values tend to vary. The effect of various cuff sizes on blood pressure measurement is given in Figure 26.16.

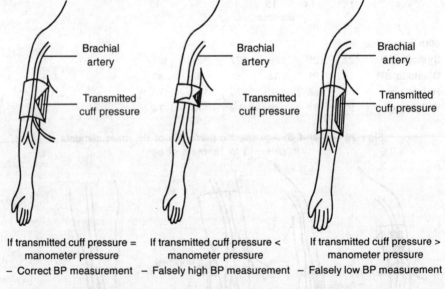

Fig. 26.16: Effect of cuff size on blood pressure measurement

3. Cuff applied too loosely.
4. Excessive venous pressure and congestion in the arm causes decreased intensity of Korotkoff sounds.
5. Arm above or below heart level.
6. Variable intensity of Korotkoff sounds during arrhythmias.

Abnormalities of Blood Pressure

Hypertension   Measured BP more than 95th centile for age and sex. It can be essential or due to secondary causes such as; vascular, kidney, endocrine, increased intracranial pressure, polycythemia vera.

Conditions associated with high BP in upper limbs
1. Non-specific aortitis.
2. Periarteritis nodosa.
3. SLE.
4. Peripheral artery disease.

Hypotension   A fall in blood pressure occurs in following conditions:
1. **Constitutional**-benign.
2. **Acute transitory:**
   • Vasovagal syndromes, orthostatic or postural.
   • Carotid sinus reflex.
   • Peripheral circulatory failure.
   • Acute myocardial failure, pericardial effusion.
   • Drugs-Nitrites.
3. **Chronic or persistant** Addison's disease, Simond's disease, chronic pulmonary TB, anaemia, myxedema, aortic regurgitation.

Pulse pressure   It is the difference between the systolic and diastolic pressures. The conditions associated with decreased and increased pulse pressures are given below:
a. **Increased pulse pressure**
   • Essential or other types of hypertension AR, PDA, AV fistula, complete heart block.
   • Fever, anemia, thyrotoxicosis, exercise, beri-beri.
b. **Narrow pulse pressure**
   • Shock, aortic stenosis.
   • Cardiac tamponade, constrictive pericarditis, severe paroxysmal tachycardia, tight MS with hypertension, CCF.

Capillary filling time   It is the time taken by the capillary bed to fill after it is occluded by pressure. To guage the capillary refill time, perform the following:
1. Blanch the nail bed with a sustained pressure of several seconds on a toe nail or finger nail.
2. Release the pressure.
3. Observe the time elapsed before the nail regains its full colour. If capillary system is intact, this should occur almost instantly i.e., within 3 seconds.

CYANOSIS

Cyanosis is a bluish colour of skin and mucous membrane due to presence of reduced hemoglobin in blood: Cyanosis is clinically apparent when approximately 5 g desaturated hemoglobin is present per deciliter of blood. Minimum cyanosis appear as a dusky hue when PO_2 is in between the range of 80-85, and it is easily visible when PO_2 is below 80 percent. Usually, cyanosis become more obvious during spells, cry, feeding and excitement.

There are two physiological type of cyanosis; central and peripheral cyanosis. The difference between the two are described in Table 26.8. Cardiac causes of cyanosis are described in Table 26.9.

Table 26.8: Characteristic difference between central and peripheral cyanosis

Characteristics	Central	Peripheral
1. Visible in	Warm areas (lips, tongue and conjunctivae and skin	Skin (nose, cheek and fingers)
2. Cause	Venous admixture and defective ventilation perfusion/	Vasoconstriction and low cardiac output diffusion
3. Pathophysiology	Diminished arterial O_2 saturation	Increased arteriovenous O_2
4. Deoxygenated hemoglobin	Increased	Normal
5. Clubbing of finger	Present	Absent
6. Relief	O_2 useful in cyanosis of pulmonary origin	Warmth and CVS support

Next step is to determine whether cyanosis is cardiac or pulmonary in origin. The difference between these two are given in Chapter 7 of this book.

Table 26.9: Cardiac causes of cyanosis

Age at presentation	Lesion
0-2 days	— Transposition of great arteries
	— Pulmonary atresia with/without VSD
	— Critical pulmonary stenosis
	— Tricuspid atresia with restricted blood flow
	— Hypoplastic left heart syndrome
3-28 days	— Complex mixing lesions
	— Ebstein's anomaly
	— Total anomalous pulmonary venous return
	— Severe TOF
28 days to 6 months	— TGA
	— Truncus arteriosus
	— TAPVC
	— Tricuspid atresia
	— Single ventricle
6 months to 1 year	— TOF, Truncus arteriosus
	— Pulmonary hypertension with reversal of shunt
	— AV malformation
Late onset	— Eisenmenger's syndrome

Differential Cyanosis

Is a clinical manifestation characterised by blue lower extremities and pink upper extremities. For demonstration of differential cyanosis, the patient is asked to sit and keep prewarmed hands on the dorsum of feet. Then a comparison of colour is made between the two. This clinical sign is typically seen with right to left shunting across a ductus arteriosus in the presence of a coarctation or interrupted aortic arch.

CLUBBING

Is thickening of tissues at base of the nail resulting in obliteration of angle between the nail base and adjacent skin of the finger. Cardiac conditions associated with clubbing include:

1. Congenital cyanotic heart disease.
2. Infective endocarditis.

Ordinarily, clubbing appears in cyanotic CHD, when child is one or two years old. But in severely cyanotic children, clubbing is seen as early as 2 to 3 weeks of age.

Clinical Grading of Clubbing

Grade
  I. Softening of nail bed.
 II. Obliteration of the angle of the nail bed.
III. Parrot beak or drum stick appearances.
IV. Hypertrophic pulmonary osteoarthropathy.

Signs of Clubbing

Fluctuation of nail bed and loss of angle between the nail and nail bed are the earliest signs of clubbing.

Shamroth Sign in Clubbing

Normally, a diamond shaped space is formed, when the two thumbs of the child are kept opposed on their dorsal aspect. But in clubbing this shape is oblitered. This is illustrated in Figure 26.17.

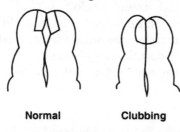

Normal   **Clubbing**

Fig. 26.17: Shamroth sign in clubbing

Next step is to look for extracardiac signs of CCF, infective endocarditis and cardiac lesions such as aortic regurgitation.

Congestive Cardiac Failure (Table 26.10)

Infants
— Tachypnoea (resting respiratory rate >50/min).
— Cool extremities, delayed capillary filling time, hepatomegaly.
— Poor weight gain.
— Excessive sweating of forehead.
— Periorbital edema.

Children
   Right heart failure.
   Left heart failure.

Table 26.10: Signs of congestive cardiac failure

Signs of systemic venous congestion	Signs of decreased myocardial function	Signs of pulmonary venous congestion
Hepatomegaly	— Diminished or widened arterial pulse pressure — Decreased capillary refill — Pulsus alternans — Peripheral cyanosis — Sweating	— Tachypnea basal — Basal rales — Central cyanosis

Physical Signs of Infective Endocarditis

Systemic Infection
Fever, pallor, weight loss, splenomegaly.

Intravascular Lesions
   a. *Petechiae*   They appear on plantar surface of toes, finger tips as well as conjuctival and buccal mucosa.
   b. *Splincter hemorrhages*   They are linear subungal hemorrhages, resembling tiny splincters of wood under the nail but not reaching the nail margin.
   c. *Roth's spots*   They are retinal hemorrhages with a white or yellow center surrounded by a bright red, irregular halo.
   d. *Osler's nodes*   They are painful tender, pea sized, bluish nodules on an erythematous base and appear in the pulp of fingers and toes due to small infective emboli, immune complex deposition.
   e. *Janeway lesions*   < 5 mm, non tender, pink macules with irregular out-line present over palms and soles and do not fade with blanching.
   f. New murmurs, changing murmurs.
   g. Signs of CCF.
   h. Meningeal signs, stroke, mycotic aneurysms.
   i. Infarction or ischemia of viscera or extremities.

Immunologic Features
— Arthritis
— Vascular phenomenon
— Finger clubbing

Peripheral Signs of Aortic Regurgitation
   1. Water hammer pulse—   Collapsing pulse.
   2. De Musset's sign   —   To and fro motion of the head synchronous with the cardiac cycle.

3.	Corrigan's sign	— Dancing carotids.
4.	Landolfi's sign	— Change in size of pupil synchronous with the cardiac cycle.
5.	Muller's sign	— Pulsations of the uvula.
6.	Quincke's sign	— Alternate paling and flushing of lightly compressed skin (nail bed, mucous membrane of mouth)
7.	Dancing brachials	— Visible pulsation over brachial artery.
8.	Rosenbach's sign	— Pulsations in the liver.
9.	Gerhardt's sign	— Pulsations in the enlarged spleen.
10.	Pistol shot femorals	— Booming sound synchronous with systole heard over the femoral arteries.
11.	Traube's sign	— Booming systolic and diastolic sounds over artery.
12.	Durozeizis sign	— Systolic and diastolic bruits heard if the femoral artery is lightly compressed with bell of the stethoscope
13.	Hill's signs	— Popliteal cuff BP exceeding brachial cuff BP by 20-100 mmHg

Peripheral Signs of Rheumatic fever such as subcutaneous nodules, erythema nodosum, chorea and signs suggestive of carditis should be looked for. (A detailed description about signs of Rheumatic fever is given in Chapter 14 of this book).

Signs suggestive of collagen vascular disease such as SLE, juvenile rheumatoid arthritis also should be looked for. Various dysmorphic syndromes associated with cardiac defects are shown in Table 26.11.

Table 26.11: Features of various syndromes associated with cardiac lesions

Syndromes	Features
1. 21 Trisomy (Down syndrome)	Endocardial cushion defect, VSD, TOF and PDA.
2. Fragile X syndrome	MVP, Aortic root dilatation
3. 18 Trisomy	VSD, ASD, PDA
4. 13 Trisomy	VSD, ASD, PDA
5. Noonan's syndrome	Pulmonary valve stenosis, obstructive cardiomyopathy
6. Turner's syndrome	Coarctation of the aorta, AS, VSD
7. Marfan's syndrome	MVP, MR, Aortic root dilatation, aortic dissection
8. Holt-Oram	ASD, VSD, First degree heart block
9. Rubinstein Taybi	PDA, VSD
10. William syndrome	Supravalvular aortic stenosis peripheral pulmonic stenosis
11. Congenital rubella	PDA, Peripheral pulmonary stenosis
12. Foetal hydantoin syndrome	Pulmonary and aortic stenosis Coarctation of aorta, PDA.
13. Fetal alcohol syndrome	ASD, VSD
14. Kawasaki disease	Coronary artery aneurysms, MR, arrhythmias, myocardial infarction

Contd...

Contd...

Syndromes	Features
15. VATER association	VSD, TOF, ASD, PDA
16. Leopard (Lenti ginosis)	Pulmonic stenosis, hyper-trophic cardiomyopathy, myxomas
17. Friedreich ataxia	Cardiomyopathy, dysarrhythmias

Note: An exhaustive list of syndromes associated with CHD is given in *Pediatric Cardiology* by Robert H Anderson, Vol 1, Page 42-59.

Presence of Scars of Previous Surgeries or Other Procedures should be Carefully Looked for

Scars

Medial sternotomy (all open heart corrections)

Lateral thoracotomy (e.g. coarctation repair, pulmonary artery banding, ligation of PDA or vascular ring, pulmonary artery reconstruction, shunts).

Groin (cardiac catheters).

Cardiovascular Examination

The heart should be examined in a systematic manner.

INSPECTION

Precordium

The anterior aspect of chest wall, which overlies the heart should be examined for **Precordial bulging**. This appears as lateral displacement and elevation of left nipple. If precordial bulging is present it indicates a long standing heart disease. Precordium should be viewed tangentially either from the foot end of bed or from side of the bed.

Conditions Associated with Precordial Bulging

1. Skeletal deformities—Scoliosis, Kyphoscoliosis, rickety deformity.
2. Diseases of CVS — Right ventricular hypertrophy, pericardial effusion
3. Disease of lungs — Pneumomediastinum.
   — Pleural effusion.
   — Mediastinal growth.

Conditions Associated with Flattened Precordium

1. Old pericarditis or adherent pericardium.
2. Fibrosis or collapse of lung.
3. Congenital deformity.

Pulsations

During inspection, apex beat should be localised and other precordial and extraprecordial pulsations should be looked for.

Apex Beat

Definition   Lower most, outer most, best felt, perpendicular thrust imparted to the chest wall by juxta-apical portion of the left ventricle.

Location   The position of apex beat varies according to the age of child and it is described in Table 26.12.

Table 26.12: Location of apex beat with respect to age of child

Age	Location
Birth to one year	Left 3rd intercostal space (ICS)
	Lateral to midclavicular line (MCL)
1 to 4 years	Left 3rd ICS in the MCL
4 to 8 years	Left 4th ICS in the MCL
8 to 12 years	Left 4th ICS medial to MCL
Puberty	Left 5th ICS medial to MCL

Conditions Associated with Displaced Apical Impulse
Cardiac Causes

Congenital	—	Dextrocardia
Acquired	—	Hypertension
		Aortic and mitral valve disease
LVH	—	Apex shifted downward and outward
RVH	—	Apex is usually shifted outward and is often diffuse.

Extracardiac Causes
1. *Extrathoracic*—scoliosis, funnel chest, straight back.
2. *Intrathoracic*—pleural effusion, pneumothorax, mediastinal tumors.
3. *Intra-abdominal*—ascites, abdominal tumor.

Conditions Associated with Invisible Apex Beat
   Anatomical—if apex beat is behind a rib or if chest wall is thick.
   Cardiac conditions—pericardial effusion, adherent pericardium.

Extent of Apex Beat
Depending on the extent of apex beat it is typed into diffuse and forcible apex beat.

Conditions Associated with Diffuse Apex Beat
— Thin chest wall.
— Hyperkinetic state.
— Severe valvular regurgitation.
— Left to Right shunt.
— Complete AV block.
— Hypertrophic cardiomyopathy.
— Retraction of the lung from fibrosis or collapse.

Conditions Associated with Forcible Apex Beat
— Thin chest wall.
— Retracted lung.
— Thyrotoxicosis, Fever or Exertion.
— LVH in diastolic overload as in MR, AR, PDA.

Precordial Pulsations

After localising apex beat; precordial pulsations should be looked in 2nd left ICS and 3rd left ICS. Various cardiac pulsations associated with precordial pulsations are given below.

Second Left ICS Pulsations
— Pulmonary hypertension due to dilated pulmonary artery.
— Enlarged left atrial appendages.
— PDA.

Third Left ICS Pulsations
— RVH
— VSD

Third and Fourth ICS Pulsations
— RVH, VSD

Extraprecordial Pulsations

In addition to the apex beat and precordial pulsations already described, pulsations may also be noted at the root of the neck, in the epigastrium and the right side of chest. The various cardiac conditions associated with these pulsation are:

Epigastric	Right ventricular hypertrophy. Aortic pulsations as in anxiety, thin abdomen, aneurysm of aorta, mass over aorta. Liver pulsations as in tricuspid regurgitation.
Suprasternal	Co-arctation of aorta. Aneurysm of aorta (AR). Hyperkinetic state.
Right side of the chest	Dextrocardia. Right atrial enlargement.
Back	Coarctation of aorta. Arteriovenous fistula.

Jugular Venous Pressure (JVP)

The JVP is studied on the level of pressure in the (Rt.) internal jugular vein, and this gives important information about right heart hemodynamics. The venous pulse has 3 positive waves 'a', 'c' and 'v' and two negative waves or descents 'x' and 'y'. A normal JVP tracing is given in Figures 26.18A and B.

The 'a' wave is due to atrial contraction. The 'c' wave is due to bulging of the A-V valve apparatus into the atrium during the onset of ventricular systole.

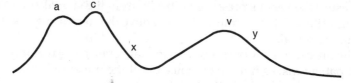

Fig. 26.18A: Jugular venous pulse waveform

The 'v' wave is due to venous inflow and rise in pressure in the atria during ventricular systole. The 'x' descent is due to atrial relaxation and also due to ventricular contraction pulling down the floor of atrium towards the ventricular aspect. The 'y' descent is due to rapid atrial emptying in the early part of ventricular diastole.

Examining Jugular Venous Pulse

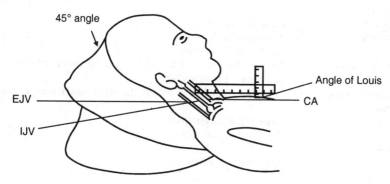

Fig. 26.18b: Measuring jugular venous pressure
EJV: External jugular vein; IJV: Internal jugular vein; CA: Carotid artery

1. Make sure light is good.
2. The patient should be lying at 45° to the horizontal.
3. Always look for the JVP on both sides of the neck as kinking of the jugular vein, pressure from the innominate artery or thrombosis may cause an erroneous conclusion that it is raised.
4. Distinguish the JVP from arterial pulsation. A detailed description is given in Table 26.13.

Table 26.13: A comparative account of JVP and carotid arterial pulsations with respect to different characteristics

	JVP	Carotid arterial pulsations
Position	More lateral	Medial
Visible or palpable	Better seen that felt	Better felt than seen.
Wave form	Multiple gentle pulse waves	Single brief pulsation.
Effect of respiration, posture and abdominal compression	Decreased with inspiration or sitting up and exaggerated with expiration, lying down or abdominal compression	Unaffected
Valsalva maneuver	Distention of neck vein increases	No effect

5. Measure the venous pressure vertically from the sternal angle (Junction of 2nd rib with the sternum); 4-5 cm above the sternal angle is the upper limit of normal.
6. If the pressure is low or if you wish to exaggerate the waveform, lowering the patient makes it more obvious; but if the pressure is high it may be necessary to make the patient sit up.
7. Press on the abdomen to elicit hepatojugular reflux, a sign of cardiac failure. This maneuver increases venous return which a failing heart unlike a normal heart, cannot eject. The result is a rise in JVP.

Abnormalities of Waves (Table 26.14)

Table 26.14: Abnormalities of different waves and the diseased conditions exhibited by them

Abnormalities of waves	Conditions
'a' Wave:	
Absent	— Atrial fibrillation.
Diminished	— Tachycardia.
	— Prolonged PR interval.
Giant 'a' waves	— Tricuspid stenosis, tricuspid atresia, pulmonary stenosis, pulmonary hypertension.
Cannon 'a' waves	— Complete heart block, ventricular tachycardia, ectopic beats.
'x' Wave:	
Absent	— Tricuspid regurgitation.
Large	— Constrictive pericarditis.
'v' Waves:	
Large	— Tricuspid regurgitation.
'y' Waves:	
Rapid 'y' descent	— Constrictive pericarditis. Severe heart failure. Tricuspid regurgitation.
Short 'y' descent	— Tricuspid stenosis.

Elevated JVP
— Right ventricular failure.
— Cardiac tamponade, tricuspid stenosis.
— Superior vena caval obstruction.
— Increased blood volume.
— Hyper kinetic circulatory state.
— Pulmonary causes-asthma, emphysema.

Kussmaul's Sign
Paradoxical increase in jugular venous pressure on inspiration in constrictive pericarditis.

PALPATION
After completing inspection, palpation is performed to confirm the location of apex beat, for palpable heart sounds, thrill and, for demonstrating parasternal heave.

Apex Beat

Once apex beat is localised, a combination of careful inspection and palpation will allow to distinguish different types of apex beat. By description there are 3 types of apex beat.

Technique of Palpating Apex Beat

For localising apex beat, the child is examined in supine position and then palmar palpation is done for approximate localisation of apex and digital palpation is done for precise location of apex beat. Then the character of apex beat is assessed by continuing palpation on left lateral position.

i. *Heaving (sustained)* Impulse resulting from systolic or pressure overload, e.g systemic hypertension, aortic stenosis.

ii. *Hyperdynamic (forceful)* Impulse due to diastolic or volume overload, e.g MR, AR, PDA, VSD.

iii. *Tapping apex* Mitral stenosis.

Heart Sounds

- Accentuated heart sounds and valve opening sounds.
- Mitral tap—palpable S_1 in mitral area; it is associated with mitral stenosis.
- Opening snap—just inside the apex.
- Diastolic shock—palpable P_2 in pulmonary area also with pulmonary hypertension.
- Ejection clicks—in pulmonary hypertension.
- Pericardial knock—constrictive pericarditis.
- Vibration produced by prosthetic valves.

Thrill

A palpable murmur is called a thrill and it transmits to the hand a sensation like the purring of a cat (Table 26.15).

Parasternal Heave

If parasternal heave is demonstrable, it indicates right ventricular hypertrophy or enlarged left atrium. A grading system is available for determining the severity of parasternal heave, accordingly there are 3 grades:

Grading

Grade I	:	Epigastric.
Grade II	:	Palpable lift.
Grade III	:	Visible lift.

PERCUSSION

Percussion of heart is now hardly carried out and adds little to the clinical assessment. But if it is performed, following 3 areas over precordium should be analysed.

Table 26.15: Systolic and diastolic thrills with respect to location and probable cause

Timing	Location	Probable cause
Systole	Suprasternal notch and/or second and third right intercostal spaces	• Aortic stenosis
	Suprasternal notch and/or second and third left intercostal spaces	• Pulmonic stenosis
	Fourth left intercostal space	• Ventricular septal defect
	Apex	• Mitral regurgitation
	Left lower sternal border	• Tricuspid regurgitation
		• Tetralogy of Fallot
	Left upper sternal border, often with extensive radiation	• Patent ductus arteriosus
Diastole	Right sternal border	• Aortic regurgitation
		• Aneurysm of ascending aorta
		• Apex
		• Mitral stenosis

Right Border of Heart

It normally correspond to the right sternal border. If dullness extends beyond right sternal border; it suggests.

• Right atrial enlargement.
• Pericardial effusion.
• Dextrocardia.

Left Border of Heart

It normally corresponds to the apex beat. If left border extends beyond apex beat, consider pericardial effusion.

II Left Intercostal Space

Percussion should be done in sitting position. If a dull note is elicited, consider the following conditions:

• Pulmonary hypertension.
• Left atrial enlargement.
• Pericardial effusion.
• PDA
• Pulmonary pathology.

Technique of Percussion

Percussion of heart is done in a systematic manner. Before percussing for borders of heart, the examiner should percuss for liver dullness. To locate liver dullness the examiner should start percussing from (Rt) infraclavicular region downwards till the liver dullness is reached. Liver dullness is defined first in order to make sure that the dullness produced over the right sternal region is not caused by enlarged liver and to confirm the location of liver.

Then the right border of the heart is defined by percussing from the right midclavicular line towards the sternum. For this the left middle finger (pleximeter finger) is placed parallel to the sternal edge on midclavicular line and then start percussing medially till the cardiac dullness is reached. Normally the right cardiac border coincides with the right sternal border. An enlarged right border of the heart may be due to right atrial enlargement or a generalised increase in the size of heart as in the case of cardiomyopathy or pericardial effusion.

After defining the right border of heart the examiner should percuss for the left border of heart. To obtain the left border of heart the examiner should start percussing from the left midaxillary line medially towards the left border of sternum. For this the pleximeter finger is kept vertically on the 3rd, 4th and 5th intercostal spaces and then start percussing medially till cardiac dullness is reached. Normally the left border of heart correspond to the apex beat. In pericardial effusion the left border of the heart is beyond the apex beat.

AUSCULTATION

Auscultation of heart often presents difficulties and often requires a great deal of practice and constant repetition. After inspection it is desirable to auscultate the heart in a sleeping infant before he is frightened or awakened by palpation and percussion. Apart from auscultating four classical areas, namely mitral area, tricuspid area, aortic area and pulmonary area; the stethoscope should be moved to four additional areas for auscultation, i.e. 2nd aortic area (left 3rd close to the sternum), axilla, back and neck.

Low and medium frequency sounds (e.g. S_3 and S_4, mid diastolic murmurs) are more easily heard with the bell applied lightly to the skin; the diaphragm is more appropriate for high frequency sounds (e.g. first and second heart sounds, opening snap, ejection and some regurgitant, murmurs and adventitious sounds).

Procedures for Auscultating the Heart

- Patient sitting up and leaning slightly forward and, preferably, in expiration, listen in all areas. This is the best position to hear relatively high-pitched murmurs with the stethoscope diaphragm.
- Patient supine: listen in all five areas.
- Patient left lateral recumbent, listen in all five areas. This is the best position to hear the low-pitched filling sounds in diastole with the stethoscope bell.
- Other positions depend on your findings. Patient right lateral recumbent: this is the best position for evaluating right rotated heart or dextrocardia. Listen in all five areas.
- Inch, don't jump, your way from area to area.

HEART SOUNDS

First Heart Sound (S_1)

S_1 marks the onset of systole and is produced mainly by mitral valve closure and to a lesser extent by tricuspid valve closure. It is best heard in the mitral area. The various factors affecting intensity of S_1 are described in Table 26.16.

Table 26.16: Factors affecting the intensity of S_1

LOUD S_1	Normally heard in children
	Sinus tachycardia
	Mitral and tricuspid stenosis
	Hyperdynamic state
	Short PR interval
	Left atrial myxoma
SOFT S_1	Long PR interval
	Pericardial effusion
	Emphysema
	Mitral stenosis with calcified valves
	Mitral and tricuspid regurgitation
	LBBB
	Myocarditis

Second Heart Sound (S_2)

Second heart sound is produced by closure of the aortic and pulmonary valves and it marks the end of systole and begining of diastole. S_2 is best assessed in the pulmonary area. A complete assessment of S_2 means, auscultating carefully for aortic and pulmonary components of second heart sound and appreciating splitting of second heart sound.

Normal Splitting of Second Heart Sound

A normal splitting of second heart sound means, wide splitting during inspiration and narrow split in expiration. It is illustrated in Figure 26.19A.

Pathophysiology

As described earlier, second heart sound is produced by the closure of aortic and pulmonary valves. In expiration the closure of both valves is almost synchronous thus producing a single sound. But in inspiration due to increased venous return and more right ventricular filling the pulmonary component is delayed, resulting in splitting of II heart sound.

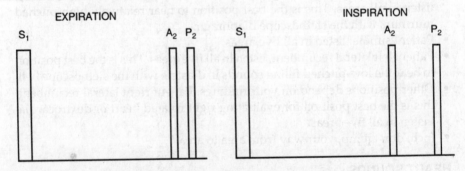

Fig. 26.19A: Normal splitting of second heart sound

Wide Inspiratory Splitting

Due to delay in P_2 (Fig. 26.19B).

Causes—pulmonic stenosis.

Pathophysiology

In pulmonary stenosis, the right ventricular blood is emptied slowly and thus further delaying the closure of pulmonary valve.

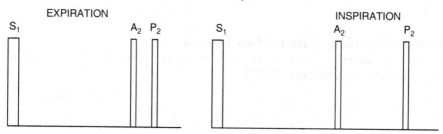

Fig. 26.19B: Wide inspiratory splitting

Due to early A_2
- Mitral regurgitation.
- Ventricular septal defect.

Pathophysiology

In VSD, the wide inspiratory split is due to the early closure of aortic valves as a result of rapid emptying of blood through the defect into the right ventricle and aorta. Whereas in mitral regurgitation, the blood is rapidly emptied into left atrium and aorta, resulting in early closure of aortic valve.

Wide and Fixed Split

This is described as equal split interval between A_2 and P_2 during inspiration and expiration. It is illustrated in the diagram (Fig. 26.19C).

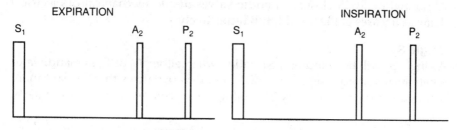

Fig. 26.19C: Wide and fixed split

Causes of Wide Fixed Splitting

1. Atrial septal defect.
2. RBBB.
3. Total anomalous pulmonary venous return.
4. Right ventricular failure.

Pathophysiology

In ASD, there is a wide splitting of second heart sound. This is because right side of heart receives more blood through the defective atrial septum, which causes delayed emptying of right ventricle and consequently delay in closure of pulmonary valve. The splitting is said to be fixed in otherwards there is no inspiratory widening. During inspiration the small extra return of blood to (right) side of the heart will not have any significant hemodynamic consequence as the right side of the heart has already received large amount of blood through ASD.

Reversed Splitting of Second Heart Sound

In this P_2 precedes A_2 and split is maximum in expiration. This is represented diagrammatically in Figure 26.19D.

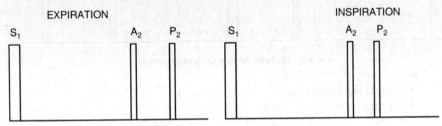

Fig. 26.19D: Reversed splitting of II HS

Associated Cardiac Conditions with Reversed Splitting
- LBBB.
- Aortic stenosis.
- Left ventricular failure.
- PDA.

Pathophysiology
Abnormal delay in closure of aortic valves due to mechanical or electrical delay as in cases of PDA and LBBB respectively.

Single S_2
A single S_2 will be heard on inspiration when either A_2 or P_2 is inaudible or when the inspiratory separation of A_2 and P_2 is so narrow that the ear cannot distinguish both components. The following are common causes of a single S_2 (Fig. 26.19E).

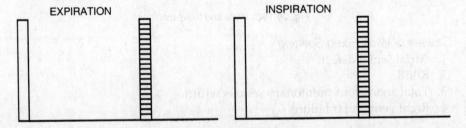

Fig. 26.19E: Single S_2

Due to Reduced Intensity of Components of Second Heart Sounds
- Pulmonary atresia
- Severe TOF, tricuspid atresia

- Truncus arteriosus
- Aortic stenosis.

P_2 Synchronous with A_2
- Atrial septal defect
- Single ventricle
- Eisenmenger's, VSD

Loud P_2—Pulmonary hypertension.

Extra-sounds

An additional or extra-sound during diastole or systole leads to one or other variety of so called triple rhythm. The various extra-sounds in systole and diastole are as follows.

Extra-sound in Diastole
1. Third heart sound (Proto diastolic gallop).
2. Fourth heart sound (Atrial gallop).
3. Summation gallop.
4. Mitral snap (Opening snap).
5. Tricuspid snap.

Extra-sounds in Systole
1. Systolic ejection clicks.
2. Systolic gallop.

Third Heart Sound

The third sound occurs in the earlier part of diastole and it coincides with rapid ventricular filling (Fig. 26.20). An audible S_3 may be present in (i) normal heart, (ii) diastolic overload states, (iii) patients who have LV dysfunction with or without overt congestive heart failure. An exaggerated S_3 is called ventricular gallop (Table 26.17).

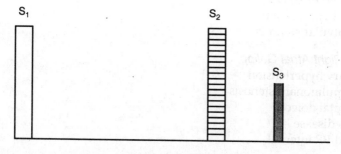

Fig. 26.20: Third heart sound

Fourth Heart Sound

The fourth sound (S_4) is a low frequency sound produced by atrial contraction and this sound is heard in late diastole. It follows the P wave by 0.14 to 0.20

Table 26.17: Third heart sound

Normal or Physiologic S₃
- Children
- Hyperkinetic states

Diastolic Overload States
- **a. Left Ventricle**
  - Mitral regurgitation
  - VSD, PDA
- **b. Right Ventricle**
  - Tricuspid regurgitation
  - Atrial septal defect

Left Ventricular Dysfunction
- Congestive heart failure
- Dilated left ventricle
- Markedly decreased ejection fraction
- Constrictive pericarditis
- Pericardial knock

sec and precedes S_1. An audible S_4 is usually abnormal and is usually indicative of increased resistance to ventricular filling. The atrial gallop sound may be caused by contraction of left or the right atrium (Fig. 26.21).

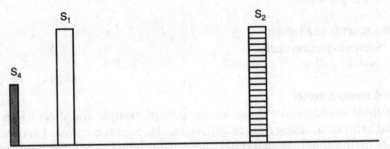

Fig. 26.21: Fourth heart sound

Causes of Left Atrial Gallop
- Systemic hypertension
- Aortic valvular stenosis.

Causes of Right Atrial Gallop
- Pulmonary hypertension
- Isolated pulmonary stenosis
- Atrial septal defect
- Ebstein's disease
- Increased PR interval.

Tips for Auscultating S₃ and S₄ (Table 26.18)

Stethoscope Technique
Have a quiet room and surroundings, routinely use left lateral position, identify LV apex impulse, use the bell with light pressure use rubber outer ring on bell.

Table 26.18: Helpful physiologic maneuvers

Alteration in venous return		Response
Increase:	Leg elevation	Increase
	Coughing	Intensity
	Sit ups	
	Abdominal compression	
	Valsalva release phase	
Decrease:	Sitting	Decrease
	Standing	Intensity
		Valsalva strain phase
Sustained hand grip (Isometric)		Increase
		Intensity

Triple Rhythm

Is described as prominent and audible third or fourth heart sound in addition to I and II heart sounds, which gives rise to a characteristic "cadence resembling the canter of a horse."

Gallop Rhythm

When triple rhythm is associated with tachycardia and other abnormalities of heart is called gallop rhythm.

Summation Gallop

Is the term used to denote the condition in which S_3 and S_4 tend to merge with each other to produce gallop sound.

Quadruple Rhythm

When 4 heart sounds namely I, II, III and IV are heard in each cardiac cycle is called quadruple rhythm.

OTHER SOUNDS

Opening Snap

The opening snap is a high pitched loud snapping or clicking diastolic sound which is best heard, just inside the apex. The diaphragm of stethoscope is more appropriate for detecting opening snap. An opening snap denotes a stenosed, but mobile mitral valve. A diagram showing relationship of heart sounds and opening snap is given below (Fig. 26.22).

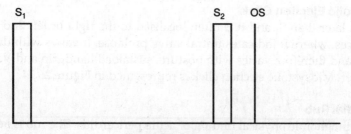

Fig. 26.22: Opening snap

Pathophysiology
Opening snap of the mitral valve appears to be due to sudden doming or tensing of stenotic anterior leaflet downwards, with a jerk thus producing a click or snapping sound.

Systolic Ejection Click
An ejection click is a high pitched sound heard best in aortic or pulmonary areas. Figure 26.23 illustrates ejection click.

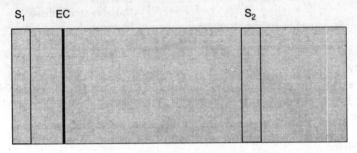

Fig. 26.23: Systolic ejection click (EC)

Presence of ejection click in aortic or pulmonary area denotes the following cardiac lesions.

Pulmonary Area
- Dilatation of pulmonary artery
- Pulmonary stenosis
- Pulmonary Hypertension
- The systolic ejection click is due to sudden doming of stenotic valve, when blood is ejected into the pulmonary artery or aorta, as in cases of PS or AS.

Aortic Area
- Aortic stenosis
- Aortic regurgitation
- Coarctation of Aorta
- Hypertension.

Midsystolic Ejection Click
It occurs later than S_1 and it is often localised to the right or left 2nd or 3rd interspaces, where it indicates mitral valve prolapse. It varies with diastolic volume and therefore varies with posture, sustained handgrip and Valsalva maneuver. Midsystolic ejection click is represented in Figure 26.24.

Pericardial Rub
It is a pathognomic physical finding of acute pericarditis. The rub is believed to be due to exudate in the pericardial sac. Characteristically rub is high pitched

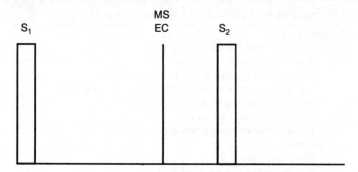

Fig. 26.24: Mid systolic ejection click

scratchy sound heard both during systole and diastole, but louder during systole. It is better heard when patient is made to sit up, leaning forward and stethoscope is held firmly on the chest.

MURMURS
These are produced by turbulence of the blood flow at or near a valve because of an abnormal communication within the heart. While describing murmurs it should be done under following headings:
1. Location.
2. Timing.
3. Conduction.
4. Pitch.
5. Amplitude (Grading).
6. Relation to respiration.
7. Relation to posture.
8. Nature of the murmur.

Grading of Murmurs
Murmurs are graded to facilitate communication with colleagues and to make long-term records. An American system of grading is as follows:

Grade I : Audible only with difficulty.
(on careful examination i.e., after tuning of ears)
Grade II : Easily heard
Grade III : Between grade II and IV
Grade IV : Murmur with thrill.
Grade V : Between IV and VI
Grade VI : Heard with stethoscope off the chest wall.

Classification of Murmurs
Murmurs are broadly divided into:
• Innocent murmurs.
• Organic murmurs.

Table 26.19: Classification of innocent murmurs

A. Systolic
   1. Vibratory murmur (Still's murmur)
   2. Pulmonary systolic murmur
   3. The peripheral pulmonary systolic murmur
   4. Supraclavicular or brachiocephalic systolic murmur
   5. Systolic mammary souffle
   6. The aortic systolic murmur
   7. The cardiorespiratory systolic murmur
B. Continuous
   1. The venous hum
   2. Continuous mammary souffle
   3. Cephalic continuous murmur

Innocent Murmurs

Definition-Murmurs that occur in the absence of either anatomic or physiologic abnormalities of the heart or circulation are called innocent, functional or physiological murmur.

The innocent murmurs are broadly classified into 7 systolic and 3 continuous murmurs. Classification of innocent murmurs is described in Table 26.19.

From this classification, following three innocent murmurs are common in pediatric practice.

Vibratory murmur Characteristics:
1. The closest acoustic analogy is like the "bizzing of a bee".
2. It is best heard between the apex and lower sternal border with the bell of sthetoscope.
3. Murmur grade ranges from 1 to 3 and occurs in midsystole.
4. Amplitude of murmur increases in the supine position and murmur intensifies during exercise, excitement or fever.
5. Most common murmur under the age of 10 years.

Pulmonary Systolic Murmur
1. It is best heard in the second left intercostal space close to the sternum and conducted upwards to the infraclavicular region.
2. Murmur is crescendo-decrescendo in configuration and occurs in midsystole.
3. Murmur is high frequency, blowing ejection systolic murmur with grade ranging from 2 to 3, best heard with diaphragm.
4. II heart sound is normally split.
5. Intensity of murmur increases during exercise, fever, or excitement.

Venous Hum
1. Most common type of innocent continuous murmur.
2. It is usually present in children and in hyperkinetic conditions such as: Anemia, thyrotoxicosis, cirrhosis, AV fistula, Postexertion, anxiety.

Characteristics
1. It is best heard in the right supraclavicular fossa but often quite loud below the clavicles.
2. Hum is a blowing continuous murmur, typically loud in diastole.
3. Murmur is abolished by following methods.
   a. Compressing the internal jugular veins.
   b. Patient turns head from the side to a midline position.
   c. Supine position.
   d. By performing Valsalva's maneuver.

Tips in auscultating Venous Hum
1. Preferable position for auscultation is sitting upright.
2. Auscultation is done using bell of stethoscope and by right hand of examiner.
3. Left hand grasps the patients chin from behind and pulls it gently to the left and upward.

Organic Murmur
Organic murmurs occur when blood flows through an abnormal valve or an abnormal orifice in the heart or between the great vessels. They are broadly classified into the following:
1. Systolic—murmur is heard between first and second heart sounds.
2. Diastole—murmur is heard between second and first sound.
3. Continuous—murmur heard continuously in both systole and diastole.

Systolic Murmurs
Systolic murmurs are classified as follows.

Ejection Systolic Murmur
Caused by forward flow of blood through a normal or diseased aortic or pulmonary valve (Table 26.20). Murmur is characterised by increasing to a peak or crescendo in midsystole and ending before the second sound. A diagrammatic representation of both aortic and pulmonary ejection systolic murmur is given in Figures 26.25A and B.

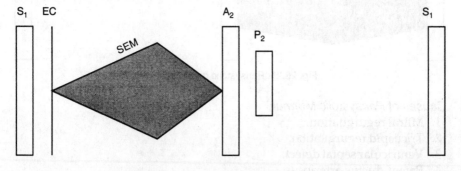

Fig. 26.25A: Aortic systolic ejection murmur (SEM)

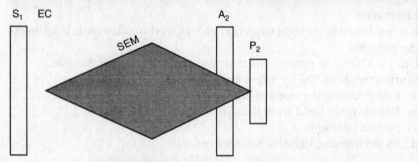

Fig. 26.25B: Pulmonary systolic ejection murmur (SEM)

Table 26.20: Causes of ejection systolic murmur

Aortic area	Pulmonary area
1. Aortic stenosis	1. Pulmonary stenosis
2. Coarctation of aorta	2. TOF
3. PDA	3. ASD
4. High output states	4. Pulmonary artery dilatation
	5. Pulmonary hypertension
	6. Innocent murmurs
	7. High output states

Pansystolic Murmur

Caused by retrograde flow of blood through an incompetent atrioventricular valve or through a ventricular septal defect. Pansystolic murmurs occupy whole of systole and continues right upto the second heart sound. In phonocardiogram recordings, murmurs appear as plateau shaped. A diagramatic representation of a murmur is given in Figure 26.26.

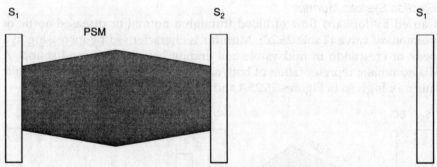

Fig. 26.26: Pansystolic murmur (PSM)

Causes of Pansystolic Murmur

1. Mitral regurgitation.
2. Tricuspid regurgitation.
3. Ventricular septal defect.
4. Patent ductus arteriosus.

Diastolic Murmur

Diastolic murmurs occur when the semilunar valves are incompetent, when the atrioventricular valves are narrowed or when they are normal, but there is an increased volume of blood flow through them. The three main types of diastolic murmurs are as follows.

Middiastolic Murmur

These are low pitched, rumbling murmurs associated with the flow of blood through the AV valves during the phase of rapid ventricular filling in diastole. The closest auditory analogue of mid diastolic rumble is "the thunder of a distant ox cart rumbling over a loose wooden bridge." The characteristic mid-diastolic murmur of mitral stenosis is low pitched rumbling murmur starting with the opening snap with a clear interval after the second heart sound.

Mid diastolic murmur is best heard when the patient is in the left lateral position. A diagramatic representation of mid diastolic murmur is given in Figure 26.27.

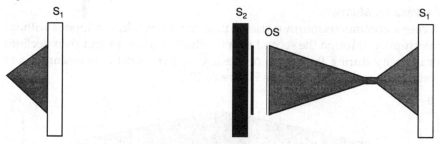

Fig. 26.27: Middiastolic murmur

Early Diastolic Murmur

This murmur is caused by regurgitation flow of blood from arterial trunk into ventricle, through an incompetent aortic or pulmonary valve. The murmur starts immediately after a second sound and attains its crescendo, almost at the start of murmur, and then declines to give rise to a decrescendo murmur. Early diastolic murmur is the most high pitched of all cardiac murmurs, best heard with the diaphragm of stethoscope and with the patient sitting up or bending forward and breath held in expiration. The early diastolic murmur of pulmonary regurgitation is known as Graham Steell murmur. A diagrammatic representation of EDM is given in Figure 26.28.

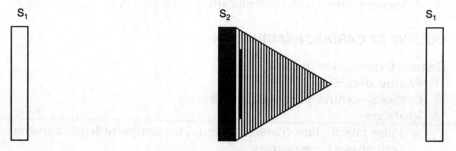

Fig. 26.28: Early diastolic murmur

Causes of early diastolic murmur
1. Aortic regurgitation.
2. Systemic hypertension.
3. Pulmonary regurgitation.
4. Pulmonary hypertension.

Atriosystolic or Presystolic Murmur

These murmurs occur when blood flows from auricle to ventricle during the phase of active atrial systole, which correspond to late diastole or presystole. It is a crescendo decrescendo murmur occuring in late diastole.

Causes of presystolic murmur
1. Mitral stenosis.
2. Tricuspid stenosis.
3. Atrial septal defect.

Continuous Murmur

A classic continuous murmur rises to peak in late systole, continuous without interruption through the second sound, which it envelops and then declines in intensity during the course of diastole. A diagramatic representation of continuous murmur is given in Figure 26.29.

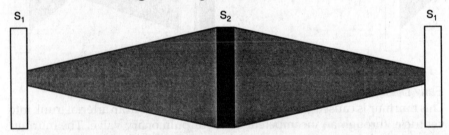

S_1 S_2 S_1

Fig. 26.29: Continuous murmur

Causes of continuous murmur
1. Patent ductus arteriosus.
2. Aorto pulmonary septal defect.
3. AV fistula or aneurysm.
4. Venous hum.
5. Pulmonary atresia with bronchial artery anastomosis.

OUTLINE OF CARDIAC EXAMINATION

General Examination in CVS
1. Posture, decubitus.
2. Cyanosis—central, peripheral, differential.
3. Vital signs:
   a. Pulse-rate, rhythm, character, volume, tension, pulse deficit, variation with phases of respiration.

    b. Respiratory rate and type of respiration.

    c. BP-upper limb, lower limb, lying down and standing.
       For pulsus paradoxus: Hill's sign.

4. Palpation of peripheral vessels: Carotid, brachial, radial, femoral, popliteal, dorsalispedis, posterior tibial.

5. Capillary filling time.

6. Growth assessment: Height, weight, head circumference, chest circumference, mid arm circumferences.

7. Clubbing-grade.

8. Signs of CCF: Increased JVP. Tender progressive hepatomegaly, pedal edema in ambulant patient, sacral edema in bed ridden patient, periorbital edema in infants, cold periphery, excessive sweating, decreased capillary filling time, pulsus alterans and basal crepitations.

9. Signs of infective endocarditis: Fever, weight loss, splenomegaly, petechiae, splinter hemorrhages, Roth's spots, Osler's nodules, Janeway lesions, change in murmur, congestive cardiac failure, meningeal signs, stroke, arthritis, hematuria, tender fingers, weakness of one side of body, prolonged treatment with high dose of penicillin.

10. Peripheral signs of AR: Water hammer pulse, Demusset's sign, Corrigan's sign, Landolfi's sign, Muller's sign, Quincke's sign, Dancing brachialis, Rosenbachin sign, Gerhardt's sign, Pistol shot femorals, Traube's sign, Durozeiz sign, Hill's sign.

11. Signs of RF: Subcutaneous nodules, erythema nodosum, arthritis, chorea, carditis.

12. Signs of carditis in rheumatic fever: Persistent tachycardia specially during sleep, bradycardia, low volume pulse, hypotension, arrhythmias, muffled first heart sound, pericardial rub, new or changing murmurs, musical murmurs, gallop rhythm, features of CCF, progressive enlargement of heart.

13. Feature suggestive of collagen vascular diseases like-SLE, JRA, etc.

14. Features of syndromes in CHD: Down syndrome, Trisomy 18,13, Turner, Marfan's syndrome, William, Holt Oram, Ellisvan Creveld, LEOPARD, etc.

15. Look for any operative scars.

CVS Proper

(Note : Four aspects of examination in inspection, palpation, percussion and auscultation).

Inspection

1. Precordial bulge
2. Apex beat

3. Pulsation

• Precordial	II left space
	III left space
	Parasternal
• Extraprecordial	Epigastric
	Suprasternal
	Right side of chest
	Back
	Over vessels and neck

4. JVP
— Pulsatile or otherwise
— Waves
— Pressure measurement
— Hepatojugular reflex
— Variation with respiration
— Variation with posture.

Palpation
1. Apex-location, nature
2. Heart sounds
3. Thrills
4. Parasternal heave-grade

Percussion
1. Right border
2. Left border
3. II left intercostal space
4. Superficial and deep cardiac dullness.

Auscultation
Auscultate in all four classical areas: mitral, aortic, pulmonary, and tricuspid area. Further ascultate in II aortic area (III left space) left lower parasternal area, neck, back and over vessels.
1. Heart sounds: Normal, abnormal, split (variation with respiration).
2. Murmurs: Location, timing, conduction, pitch, amplitude (grades), relation to respiration, relation to posture, nature.
3. Pericardial rub.
4. Extrapericardial auscultation over vessels and back.

Diagnosis of Heart Disease
Is done as per the recommendation of New York Heart Association
Etiology   : Rh, infective, congenital
Anatomy   : Enlarged heart, LA, PA, RV, PDA mitral valve deformity
Physiology : Atrial fibrillation, mitral obstruction, pulmonary hypertension,
                   Cardiac Status and prognosis:

An Algorithm for Diagnosis of CHD

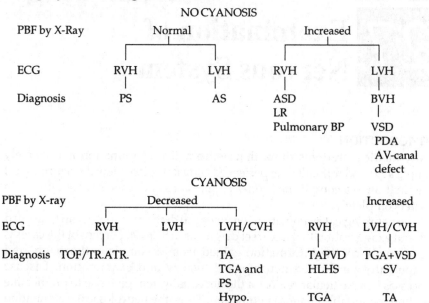

NO CYANOSIS

PBF by X-Ray	Normal		Increased	
ECG	RVH	LVH	RVH	LVH
Diagnosis	PS	AS	ASD	BVH
			LR	
			Pulmonary BP	VSD
				PDA
				AV-canal defect

CYANOSIS

PBF by X-ray	Decreased				Increased
ECG	RVH	LVH	LVH/CVH	RVH	LVH/CVH
Diagnosis	TOF/TR.ATR.		TA	TAPVD	TGA+VSD
			TGA and PS	HLHS	SV
			Hypo. Pulm Art.	TGA	TA

Syndromes with CHD

Ellisvan Creveld	—	Single Atrium, VSD
Holt Oram	—	ASD, VSD
Noonan	—	PS, ASD, Dysplastic pulmonary valve
Rubinstein Taybi	—	VSD, PDA
TAR	—	ASD, TOF
Williams	—	Supra valvar AS, Peripheral pulmonary stenosis
Vater	—	VSD, TOF, ASD, PDA
Downs	—	Endocardial cushion VSD, TOF
Trisomy 18	—	VSD, ASD, PDA
Trisomy 13	—	VSD, ASD, PDA
Turner's	—	CoA, Bicuspid Aortic valve.

(*Note*: An exhaustive list of syndromes associated with CHD is given in *Pediatric Cardiology* by Robert H Anderson, Vol. 1, Page 42-59.)

27 Examination of Nervous System

INTRODUCTION

Many medical students think that neurological examination is extremely complicated and difficult. Inexperienced clinicians often view the neurological examination as a complicated series of questions and tests that are difficult to master completely.

The neurological examination is a powerful diagnostic tool. It can be argued without exaggeration that a correct diagnosis in 85 to 90 percent of the cases is based solely on the information gained from a complete, thorough, and competently performed neurological history and examination. Disease processes in a particular region of the nervous system give rise to predictable and understandable changes in function. Thus, the neurological examination is the singularly most effective method for accurately determining the location, nature and extent of the neurologic dysfunction in a particular patient.

In this chapter, we make an attempt to present the normal neuroanatomy and physiology of the nervous system in health and a logical approach to various neurological problems in a simple way.

General Conditions and Initial Considerations

The neurological examination is time-consuming. It should never be rushed. Methodical and detailed examination of the nervous system, observing and being cognisant of relevant and so called irrelevant signs and symptoms leads on to correct diagnosis. However, a detailed neurological exam is an ordeal for the ill patient and even for a healthier child it is quite tiring. The pediatrician must take care not to fatigue the child and produce a sense of boredom. Some other facts to be borne in mind are:

1. Corrected gestational age: Especially in infants who have been born premature, the neurological responses may be according to corrected gestational age and not the chronological age.
2. Setting and serial examination: Importance must be given to the persistence of a sign on serial examination than an isolated finding.
3. Familial variation: Some diseases run in families, hence when in doubt do not forget to examine parents and other siblings.
4. Examination in handicapped: There is no single method of examiantion. The clinician must be astute enough to devise and improvise on the conventional neurological examination and make necessary modifications when examining children who are disabled and visually or hearing impaired.

5. Sensory examination and painful procedures: Sensory examination requires utmost cooperation of the patient, hence it is very difficult to put a child through an elaborate sensory examination. When necessary, a short, relevant sensory examination must be efficiently done. Care must be taken to defer frightening or painful procedures like use of ophthalmoscope etc to the last so as not to hamper further neurological examination by a terrified, uncooperative child.

Objectives of Neurological Evaluation

It is to essentially answer three questions.
1. Is there a disease involving the nervous system?
2. If yes, where is the lesion?
3. What is the nature of the lesion?

Before formulating the diagnosis, the pediatrician must remember three basic rules for CNS that go by the name of **Hughlings Jackson's Rules:**

i. No matter what the cause of lesion, symptoms will depend on the site of the lesion.

ii. Level of consciousness depends on the evolution, e.g: Lower the development affected (midbrain, pons and medulla) deeper the unconsciousness (medulla>pons>mid brain).

iii. The first function to be acquired will be the last to go, i.e. primitive reflexes disappear last.

History Taking in Neurological Patient

The single most important and informative part of the neurological evaluation is the neurologic history. A complete and accurate neurologic history alone will usually provide the knowledgeable clinician with sufficient information to think of an accurate diagnosis. In pediatric practice, the history depends most often on the mother or the care taker as very small children and infants cannot relate their complaints. Older children however may be able to tell the exact information if questioned intelligently.

There are no short cuts to taking a neurologic history. It takes practice and experience to learn how to obtain complete and accurate information from the child or his parent regarding the neurological problem. The purpose of neurological examination and other subsequent procedures serve only to narrow the differential diagnosis; but by the end of the history a reasonable idea of the diagnosis is made.

Components of a Neurological History

- Chief complaint (s)
- History of present illness
- Past medical history
- Relevant health information
- Family history
- Birth and developmental history

- Social history
- Occupational history (where relevant)
- Review of systems.

Chief Complaint

It is the first bit of information the patient or parent gives about what he feels is wrong. Naturally, it has to be in his own words, unhurried and unbiased. Some people have the habit of going on with irrelevant details while obscuring what they think is unimportant. The clinician while giving a patient hearing should get the conversation on the right track by asking a few relevant questions.

Not infrequently however, patients are seen who are seeking a second or third opinion and a diagnosis or tentative diagnosis has been already made and the informant is eager to bring it to your attention. It is prudent not to get biased by the presumably learned opinion of some one else. Always remember that your opinions or conclusions including your understanding of the complaints should be based on your own findings.

History of Present Illness (HOPI)

After the chief complaint has been described it becomes essential to develop a chronological history of events and hence ask for more details. The details of HOPI may give the first valuable clue for the diagnosis for e.g:

Onset
— Acute: (min to hrs to days) — Embolism or thrombosis
— Subacute: (days to weeks) — Infarction.
— Chronic: (months to years) — Infection, tumor, degenerative disorders

Progression
— Self limiting — Infections.
— Deterioration — Degenerative disorders
— Static — Cerebral palsy.
— Remission and exacerbation — Multiple sclerosis.

Etiology
— Genetic
— Congenital
— Infection
— Inflammation
— Prion disease
— Metabolic
— Vascular
— Neoplastic
— Degenerative

HOPI can include medical consultation for the above problems also and any investigations done thereby with results.

Past Medical History

The past history should explore:

1. Previous injuries or illnesses.
2. Previous hospitalisation and surgeries.
3. Transfusion.
4. Birth circumstances (when appropriate).

Relevant health information mainly deals with information regarding any allergies, immunisation, medications, sleep pattern, appetite, diet and recent childhood exanthems and other infectious diseases.

Family History

In cases where hereditary disorders are suspected, it is necessary to obtain a detailed family history of relatives who have severe or mild similar complaints. Consanguinity which is rare in the west is a common feature in India. If relatives with similar disease or another child with similar disease had died, the age of death and cause of death must be recorded. In cases where strong familial tendency is suspected, a three-generation pedigree chart usually helps in better understanding. Family history should also include contact with tuberculosis, family history of diabetes, hypertension and other similar or related conditions.

Social History

The living conditions, upbringing, parent child relationship, peer group relationship, educational acheivements, economic and cultural background must be enquired into. These may not give a diagnosis but may help with differential diagnosis.

Importance of asking about onset of progression of a symptom or disease: Various patterns of onset and progression in various conditions are represented graphically below. Arrow signifies point of clinical recognition (Figs 27.1A to E).

It may be noted that neurologic impairment following vascular accidents continues to remain so even after months and years (sequalae). But with toxic and infections conditions, the neurological impairment is transient or even absent after a few weeks.

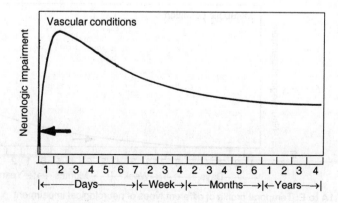

Fig. 27.1A

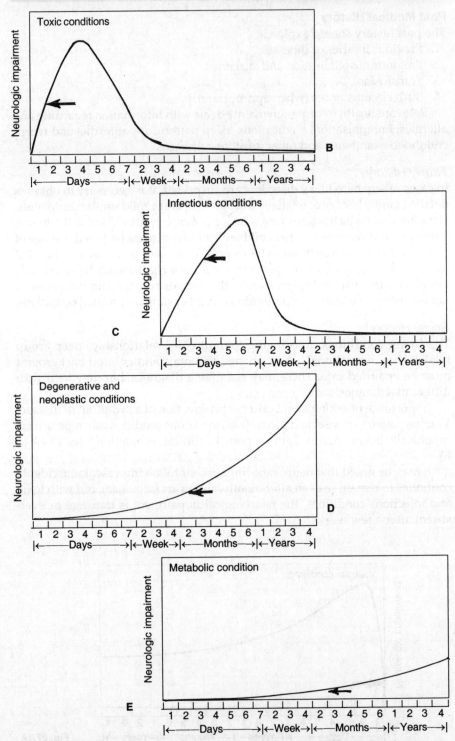

Figs 27.1A to E: Temporal profile of different types of neurological impairment

In sharp contrast, is the metabolic, neoplastic and degenerative conditions which worsen progressively over months and years.

Birth History

In pediatric neurology, birth history plays a very important role. In fact, birth history starts with antenatal history itself. The mothers status during 3 trimesters of her pregnancy, any illnesses, drug intake or exposure to radiations and toxins can affect the overall and neuro development of her unborn baby besides being the cause for various malformations, e.g. TORCH group of infections can cause a baby with small or large head with intrauterine growth restriction (IUGR) besides causing other cardiac, eye and renal anomalies, blindness, deafness and cerebral palsy in the baby.

Birth of the baby, difficult labor, use of instruments for delivery, history of birth asphyxial insult to the brain are also important in knowing the neurological status of the baby. In the postnatal period ask for early onset of convulsions, jaundice, infections and hospitalisation. The knowledge of birth history helps to decide if the disorder dealt with is congenital or acquired, static or progressive and can also help us counsel parents about the final outcome.

Developmental History

The achievement of the milestones by the child at appropriate ages must be asked for. Most parents especially mothers are keen and intelligent enough to give this information especially when compared with other sibling or other children of same age group. Developmental milestones must be evaluated in all four fields, i.e. Motor, language, adaptive and personal and social behavior. Some conditions like cerebral palsy may show predominant motor retardation, while some conditions show global development delay (Tables 27.1 to 27.3).

Regression of Attained Milestones

It is important when evaluating neurodegenerative disorders. Another important fact to be remembered is that premature babies attain development milestone according to their corrected age, not chronological age.

Table 27.1: Diagnosis of development delay (no regression)

Predominant speech delay
1. Hearing loss
2. Infantile autism

Predominant motor delay
1. Hypotonic infant
2. Ataxia
3. Hemiplegia
4. Paraplegia

Global delay
1. Chromosomal disturbances
2. Cerebral malformations
3. Intrauterine infection
4. Perinatal disorders

Table 27.2: Progressive encephalopathy onset before age two

Hypothyroidism

Aminoacidurias
1. Phenylketonuria
2. Homocystinuria
3. Histidinemia
4. Maple syrup urine disease
    a. Intermediate form
    b. Thiamine-responsive form

Disorders of lysosomal enzymes
1. Mucopolysaccharidoses
    a. Type I (Hurler)
    b. Type II (Sanfilippo)
2. Mucolipidoses
    a. Type III (I-Cell)
    b. Type IV
3. Disorders of glycoprotein degradation
    a. Mannosidosis I
    b. Fucosidoses I and II
    c. Sialidosis II (infantile form)
4. Sphingomyelin lipidosis (Nienmann-Pick type A)
5. Glucosylceramid lipidosis (Gaucher I)
6. Globoid cell leukodystrophy (Krabbe)
7. Sulfatide lipidoses (metachromatic leukodystrophy)
8. GM, gangliosidosis, I and II
9. GM gangliodisosi (Tay-Sachs, Sandhoff)

Disorders of mitochondrial enzymes
1. Subacute necrotizing encephalomyelopathy (Leigh)
2. Progressive infantile poliodystrophy (Alper)
3. Trichopoliodystrophy (Menkes)
4. Mitochondrial myopathy, encephalopathy, lactic acidosis, stroke (MELAS)

Other known enzyme deficiencies
1. Galactosemia-transferase deficiency
2. Lesch-Nyhan disease

Neurocutaneous Syndromes
1. Tuberous sclerosis
2. Neurofibromatosis
3. Chediak-Higashi syndrome

Genetic and idiopathic disorders of gray matter
1. Infantile neuroaxonal dystrophy
2. Rett syndrome
3. Infantile ceroid lipofuscinosis (Santavuori)

Genetic disorders of white matter
1. Alexander disease
2. Pelizaeus-Merzbacher disease
3. Spongy degeneration of infancy (Canaven)
4. Neonatal adrenoleukodystrophy

Progressive hydrocephalus
AIDS dementia

Table 27.3: Progressive encephalopathy: onset after age two

Disorders of lysosomal enzymes
1. Mucopolysaccharidoses types II, III and VII
2. Disorders of glycoprotein degradation
   a. Mannosidosis II
   b. Aspartyglycosaminuria
3. Disorders of glycosaminuria
4. Glucosylceramide lipidosis (Gaucher III)
5. Late-onset globoid cell leukodystroophy (Krabbe)
6. Juvenile sulfatide lipidosis

Genetic disorders of gray matter
1. Ceroid lipofuscinosis
   a. Late infantile (Bielschowsky-Jansky)
   b. Juvenile
2. Huntington' disease
3. Mitochondrial disorders
4. Xeroderma pigmentosa

Genetic disorders of white matter
1. Adrenoleukodystrophy
2. Cerebrotendinous xanthomatosis
3. Alexander disease

Infectious diseases
1. Subacute sclerosing panencephalitis
2. Chronic rubella encephalopathy
3. AIDS dementia

Occupational History

It becomes relevant in these days of child labor among the poor and under-privileged, and adolescents who take up vacational or part time jobs. The nature of the job, exposure to toxins, etc must be enquired into.

Review of Systems

Because neurologic dysfunction may result from disease or injury to other bodily functions it is essential to ask for relevant questions. The areas to be included are:
1. Skin
2. Ears, eyes, head nose and throat
3. Respiratory
4. Cardiac
5. Vascular
6. GIT
7. Renal and urinary
8. Musculoskeletal
9. Endocrine and
10. Hemopoietic.

The review of systems may reveal nothing, uncover defects or problems unrelated to the disease at present, or yield findings that might be critical in formulating a diagnosis even though they may seen nonproblematic to the patient.

Though the general principles of clinical diagnosis developed in adult neurology also apply to children, certain special problems arise to hinder the orderly sequence of thought in pediatric neurological diagnosis.

First, is that infant or young child is incapable of describing precisely his own symptoms so we must rely on the report of parents or caretaker who can never know the subjective aspects of the symptoms.

Second, the examination is hampered by the inability of a young child to co-operate in a degree that an older child or adult can. Hence, subtle approaches must be used in a child.

1. Examination should be "fun" both for the child and the examiner.
2. It may be imperative to shed the "white coat" that most children associate with painful feelings.
3. If resistance is encountered early, then it is wiser to change the approach or leave the test and reassume it later.
4. Many points may be noticed by observing a playing child; the way he manipulates his toys, etc can give vital clues about the functioning of the nervous system.
5. It may also help if the clinician joins the child in playing, something that many self conscious clinicians are averse to doing.

Equipments for Neurological Examination

1. Steel tape	Head circumferance, girth of limbs, etc
2. Stethoscope	Ascultation of head,neck, vessels, heart
3. Flash light with rubber adaptor	Pupillary reflex, pharyngeal inspection, transillumination
4. Transparent mm. ruler	Pupillary size, skin lesions size
5. Ophthalmoscope	Fundoscopy
6. Tongue blades	For depressing tongue For eliciting gag reflex For eliciting abdominal reflex
7. Key	Eliciting plantar response
8. Coffee, salt and sugar	Testing smell and taste
9. Otoscope	Auditory canal and drum
10. Tuning fork	Vibration (256 Cycles per second), Hearing
11. Cotton wisps	Corneal reflex, light touch
12. Test tubes with hot and cold water	Hot and cold sensation
13. Sterile pins	Pain sensation
14. Reflex hammer	Deep tendon reflexes
15. Coins	Steriognosis
16. BP apparatus	Routine BP, orthostatic hypotension

General Examination in Neurology

A routine physical examination including the measurement of vital data is necessary for revealing the cause of the neurological problem.

Level of consciousness of the patient gives the first indication of the sickness of the patient (dealt with subsequently). A careful head to toe examination.

Head-for lumps and bulges (for a meningioma), head circumference and anterior fontanelle.

Signs of vasomotor instability like tachycerebrale, palmar erythema, etc. must be looked for.

A thorough examination of skin and eye must be done as they are derivatives of the same germinal layer. The skin gives very vital clues for the under lying neurological disorder (Neurocutaneous syndromes).

- Cafe au-lait spots—Neurofibromatosis, Albright syndrome
- Adenoma sebaceum ⎫
- Shagreen patch ⎬ Tuberous sclerosis
- Ashleaf macule ⎭
- Heliotrope rash-Dermatomyositis
- Salmon pink maculopapular rash—evidence of collagen vascular disease or butterfly rash
- Telangiectasis—Ataxia telangiectasia
- Hemangiomas—Sturge Weber syndrome.

Also signs of tuberculosis like erythema nodosum, nonhealing ulcers, tuberculids, etc. may be seen over the skin.

A tuft of hair or a sacral dimple may be a clue to an underlying spinal abnormality such as a spina bifida. Many dysmorphic facial features may give valuable clues to various illnesses. Evidence of eye defects, cataracts, retinal angiomas, etc. also point to some underlying neurological conditions. Hence, a thorough eye examination is essential. Certain metabolic disorders have characteristic presentation as in the case of phenylketonurea, which has eczema, light colored hair, etc.

Anthropometry may reveal, short stature, Marfanoid features, etc. which give clues to neurological diagnosis. Great importance must be given to vital signs in CNS diseases. Bradycardia and high BP serve as indirect evidence of raised intracranial pressure. So also does periodic breathing. In brainstem compression syndromes, the type of respiration gives a vital evidence, irregular chaotic breathing is usually a preterminal event (dealt with in detail in Chapter on Vital Signs).

A simple observation of a child at play also gives vital clues about the kind of neurological problem.

"Skin is the part of CNS (both derived from ectoderm)
Eye is the projection of CNS and
Vascular system is the partner of CNS"

—**ML Kulkarni**

SCHEME OF EXAMINATION OF NERVOUS SYSTEM

Conventional
1. Higher mental functions.
2. Cranial nerves examination.

3. Motor system examination.
4. Coordination and gait.
5. Abnormal movements.
6. Reflexes.
7. Sensory system.
8. Autonomic nervous system.
9. Cerebellar signs.
10. Signs of meningeal irritation.
11. Signs of increased intracranial pressure.
12. Examination of skull and spine.

Extended Neurological Examination
- Developmental testing.
- Testing for newborn reflexes.

Neurological Examination in Special Situations
- The unconscious patient.
- Newborn neurological examination.

Neurologic Examination

Mental Status
Mental state examination attempts to distinguish
- Focal neurological deficit
- Diffuse neurological deficit
- Primary psychiatric illness such as depression, anxiety or hysteria presenting with somatic symptoms
- Psychiatric illness secondary to or associated with neurological disease.
  The functions assessed in mental status are
  a. Level of consciousness
  b. Attention
  c. Orientation
  d. Language function
  e. Learning and memory
  f. Cortical and cognitive function
  g. Mood and affect
  h. Thought content

Level of consciousness   There are three methods of assessment:
a. Working category-for practical purposes
b. Glasgow coma scale
c. Adelaide coma scale.

   Glasgow coma scale and Adelaide coma scale are used for progressive evaluation of an unconscions patients.

Working category   There are different terms used to describe the levels of consciousness, but the degree of alertness varies and there is no fixed demarcation.

Consciousness A state of awareness of the self and surroundings, and being responsive to various visual, auditory, tactile and thermal stimuli.

Lethargic Patient appears drowsy and may fall asleep if not stimulated, patient has difficulty in focussing or maintaining attention.

Stupor/Obtunded Patient is difficult to arouse from a somnolent state and is frequently confused when awake. Repeated stimulation is required to maintain consciousness.

Locked-in syndrome Ventral damage to the pons may rob the patient of his ability to speak or move his limbs or any muscle supplied by the lower cranial nerves. This total lack of ability to communicate may be misinterpreted as impaired awareness. However, the patients eyes are open and he can often indicate responsiveness by a vertical eye movement or a blink. EEG shows responsiveness to stimuli.

Cause is usually vascular and often fatal but occasional recovery is possible. This state must always be excluded before remarks are made over a patient who is not in coma.

Coma vigil (Akinetic mutism) Some degree of vigilance is suspected, as the patient may have open eyes which appear to follow the targets, but in truth, the patient is not alert at all.
- They do not vocalise and are doubly incontinent
- No response to noxious stimuli
- Due to bilateral frontal lobe infarction or diffuse effects of hypoxia, hypoglycemia, head surgery or hydrocephalus.
- Gross disturbance of reticular formation.
- Though superficial similarities with locked in syndrome are seen, no communication can be established with these patients.
- EEG shows no reaction to external stimuli.

Chronic vegetative state After some severe head injuries, even though no recovery of higher function occurs some patient's coma changes in that patterns of sleep and wakefulness occur. The patients may or may not be a kinetic. Their eyes open to verbal stimuli, but no communication is possible.

Respiration is well maintained, prolonged survival is possible. At postmortem, the brainstem is relatively spared, but there is extensive cortical damage.

Stupor *(Semicoma)* Patient responds only to strong, generally noxious stimuli and returns to the unconscious state when stimulation is stopped. When aroused, patient cannot interact with examiner.

Coma A state of total unresponsiveness to even deep painful stimuli. Reflex motor responses may or may not be seen.

A method commonly used to produce arousal in stuporous or comatose patients is to apply sharp pressure over a bony prominence or a cutaneous nerve and patient response is noted.

The function and part of neurological system assessed is the reticular activating system (RAS). These exert an excitatory influence on the cerebral cortex to maintain the alert state. The neurous located in the reticular formation in the midbrain and pons play a central role in this process.

Damage to this system results in a loss of nonspecific excitatory input to cortical neurons, making them less likely to respond appropriately to various stimuli.

Glasgow coma scale and Adelaide coma scale They are used for progressive assessment of an unconscious or comatose patient. It takes into consideration, three things, eye opening, best verbal response and best motor response (For details refer Chapter on Evaluation of an Emergency Situation).

Attention

A patient may be conscious, but not attentive. Attention is the ability to focus and maintain one's consciousness on a particular stimulus or task without being distracted by other stimuli. Patients who are inattentive have difficulty in concentrating on tasks and complex activities.

Attention is assessed by asking the patient to repeat short lists of objects or numbers. Inability to repeat correctly 6 number or items or more indicates a probable attention deficit. However, it must be remembered that children with poor learning and memory also do poorly in these tests.

A simple screening test is to ask the patient to spell World backwards. Attentive children can usually perform this task ; individuals with problem in maintaining attention may confuse the order of letters.

Orientation

Refers to the patient's awareness of self and certain realities of the present. We refer to these as orientation of person, place and time. Some questions asked may be:

Person : What is your name ?
What is your middle name/surname ?
How old are you ?
Who is your mother/doctor

Place : Where are we right now ?
Which city/state is this ?
Which place do you live in ?
What is your home address ?

Time : What is today's date ?
What day of the week is it ?
What time is it ?
What season is it ?
How long have you been here ? etc.

Language Function

Language is a means of communication between individuals that uses symbols to convey meaning. The symbols of a language may be pictoral in nature and serve to represent an object or an idea, or they may be sounds (phonemes) or visual images (letters) meaningless in and of themselves, that convey meaning when ordered in a particular way and presented to the ear or eye. A cortical function, language is the most sophisticated form of communication used by humans. Language disturbances profoundly affect personal interactions and cause significant functional disability.

Language disturbances, known as aphasias, must be distinguished from other problems that affect communication ability. They should be differentiated from:

- **Dysphonias**—In this, there are mechanical disturbances in speech production due to lesions of vagus nerve and vocal cords. They may sound hoarse or speak with a low volume.
- **Dysarthrias**—They typically result from cranial nerve lesions or muscle diseases and present as difficulties with resonation or articulation. They are not associated with lesions involving cortical associated neurons.

When evaluating language function, it is essential to pay attention to the following aspects.
- Spontaneous speech
- Fluency
- Comprehension
- Repetition
- Word finding and naming
- Reading and writing
- **Spontaneous speech**—A patient who demonstrates reduced or absent speech may suffer from dysarthria, aphasia, diffuse brain disease or one of a variety of psychiatric conditions. There may be poverty of thought or expression or impairment of rhythm.
- **Fluency**—Fluency in speech is word flow that is free from pauses or breaks. A simple test is to ask a patient to say words begining with a particular letter as many times as he can in 60 sec. If patient fails to produce less than 12 words-considered dysfluent.

    Care must be taken regarding the knowledge and vocabulary of the patient in that language.

    Broca's Aphasia (Motor Aphasia, Anterior Aphasia, Expressive Aphasia)

    Lesions involving left inferior frontal gyrus or areas 44 and 45 of Brodman in right handed people results in dysfluency. These patients have an articulatory struggle and use predominantely nouns and verbs. Speech lacks normal complement of preposition and grammer as a result of which it is nonfluent.
- **Stuttering** It is the difficulty in uttering the first phoneme or sound at the beginning of a conversation. The jaw and mouth may move, but no meaningful sound comes out.
- **Stammering** Repetition of phonemes at the beginning or during the course of the speech that interferes with its normal flow and rhythm.

    The causes of stammering and stuttering are not well known. They may appear spontaneously after brain injury or may be exacerbated by stress.

- **Comprehension** It refers to the ability of a patient to ascribe appropriate and correct meaning to words and sentences and can be assessed by asking a few question like—Is my sister's brother a woman or a man? etc. Patients with impaired comprehension have well articulated and prefectly fluent speech patterns, but their utterances may be out of context or devoid of appropriate content. Lesions of Wernicke's area (Posterior part of superior temporal gyrus) on the left gives this picture called wernicke's aphasia (sensory, posterior or receptive aphasia).
- **Dysarthrias** Dysarthrias are not an all or none phenomenon (Tables 27.4 and 27.5). They are divided as flaccid dysarthria due to involvement of cranial nerves and muscles of articulation and central dysarthrias or spastic dysarthrias. They both differ distinctly in voice characteristics as follows:

Table 27.4: Flaccid dysarthrias

Vocal tract muscular component	Cranial nerve affected			
	V	X	VII	XII
Laryngeal	—	Hoarse, breathy low, volume	—	—
Velopharyngeal	—	Hypernasal or nasal emission	—	—
Oral	imprecise vowels, consonants		imprecise bilateral consonants weak ptosis	imprecise vowels consonants

Table 27.5: Central dysarthrias

Central motor disorder	Vocal tract muscular component		
	Laryngeal	Velopharyngeal	Oral
1. Spasticity	Strained, strain gled, harsh low monopitch	Hypernasal	• Slow imprecise consonants
2. Rigidity	Monopitch, low volume, volume, hoarse	—	• Pseudostutter, imprecise consonants
3. Chorea	Sudden alteration in pitch and loudness	—	• Sudden alteration in vowels and consonants precision
4. Dystonia	Slow alteration in pitch, loudness, phonatony arrest	—	• Slow alternation in vowels, consonants preserved
5. Ataxia	Coarse, tremolous voice	—	• Irregular articulatory errors imprecise consonants

In children most common cause of dysarthrias is cereberal palsy.

Children with spasticity are unable to execute tongue motions, whereas children with athetoid disorders are able to execute tongue motion but unable to control extraneous motions of the tongue. Children with cerebral palsy also have mental retardation, specific language development disorder and hearing defects, all of which also contribute to speech abnormalities.

Second common cause is a cleft palate, most common anatomic defect for articulatory disorders. Most of them have hypernasal or hyponasal speech.

Those neurological disorders with primary motor unit defect or common visible anatomic defects can be logicalliy expected to produce speech and voice defects. However, some neurological syndromes and diseases are noted with unusual or abnormal voices. They are as follows (Table 27.6).

Table 27.6: Abnormal voices associated with neurological syndromes

Syndrome/Disease	Characteristic
1. 5p-syndrome (cri-du-chat)	Cat-cry
2. Bloom syndrome	Low pitched, weak growling
3. Cornelia de Lange	High pitched, hoarse
4. Dubowitz syndrome	Hoarse.
5. Happy Puppet syndrome	Paroxysms of inappropriate laughter, absent speech.
6. Hypothyroidism	Hoarse
7. Trisomy 17/18	Sea-gull like
8. Weavers syndrome	Hoarse
9. Williams syndrome	Hoarse, low pitched

- **Repetition** It is the ability to repeat single word or short lists of words without error. This is tested after fluency and comprehension. The test can be started with one word and then increased to sentences. Patients with attention deficits, learning and memory disorders may also have repetition difficulty.

  Difficulty in repetition result from lesions involving the arcuate fasciculus on the left side. Arcuate fasciculus connects Wernicke's area with Brocas area.

- **Naming and word finding** Patient is asked to name some common objects of daily use, body parts, etc. Patients with some types of aphasia may have difficulty in naming and word finding.

  Reading and writing Can be tested by giving a text to read alone without word omissions, substitutions or additions. Simple questions about the text are asked to check understanding. The patient is also given a dictation and asked to write and spell words.

  - Patients with Wernick's aphasia have difficulty in reading aloud and reading comprehension.
  - Patients with Broca's aphasia may have difficulty in reading aloud but have intact comprehension.
  - Patients who have no aphasic problems, but unable to comprehend are called *dyslexic*.
  - Agraphia refers to a disturbance of writing ability in an individual who was previously able to write.
  - Lesions are generally in the cerebral cortex and subcortical white matter of posterior temporal and anterior occipital lobes of the left hemisphere.

Test is useless in illiterate and uneducated people, and deficits means nothing to them. For people who depend on reading and writing for a living, these deficits can have a profound impact.

Overview of Language (Speech Disorders)

Process	**Abnormalities**
Hearing ————————	Deafness
Understanding	
	— Aphasia
Thought and word finding	
Voice production ————————	Dysphonea
Articulation ————————	Dysarthria

Model of Speech Understanding and Output

1. Wernicke's aphasia: Poor comprehension, fluent but often meaningless speech, no repetition
2. Broca's aphasia: Preserved comprehension, nonfluent speech, no repetiton
3. Conductive aphasia: loss of repetition with preserved comprehension and output.
4. Transcortical sensory aphasia: as in (1) but preserved repetition.
5. Transcortical motor aphasia as in (2) but repetition preserved.
6. Global aphasia-features both Wernicke's and Broca's aphasia.
7. Nominal aphasia: Lesion in angular gyrus.

Learning, Memory and Intelligence

Learning and memory depend on the integrity of the hippocampus and amygdaloid nucleus. Lesious involving these structures or their connections of the brain can cause leaining defects or amnesia.

- Immediate recall, short-term memory and long-term memory are tested.
- Visual memory and calculation are then assessed.
- Immediate recall: Narrate a small story, ask to repeat the same, with at least half the details correctly.
- Short-term memory: What did you have for breakfast, giving a short list of words or objects, ask to repeat 10-15 minutes later.
- Long-term memory: Enquire about the past with question like-When and where were you born?
  Which schools did you attend, etc.
  Necessary modifications should be done to suit the level and language of the child.

Cortical and Cognitive Function

Assessed by

- Common general knowledge questions as appropriate for the age of the child.
- Calculation ability—serial seven subtraction test and other simple sums.
- Gnosia and agnosia

Agnosia Acquired conditions characterised by inability to recognise stimuli in absence of disease involving anatomic and neural structures. Test for visual. tactile, auditory, orfactony recognition.

Visual agnosia Cannot recognise familiar objects and the lesion is in occipital visual association cortex.

Auditory agnosia Presenting the patient with sounds that familiar objects make and ask to identify present in lesions involving auditory association areas of temporal lobe.

Tactile agnosia Tested under sensory system.

PRAXIS AND APRAXIA
Praxis refers to carrying out an action. Apraxia are characterised by an inability to perform motor behavior. Specifically, apraxias are acquired disorders of learned movement present, in the absence of disease involving the "motor system" or muscle. To test for apraxia, establish first, that the sensory, motor and musculo skeletal systems are intact.

The patient must be asked to do simple tasks initially and them progress to complex tasks. Each group of muscles must be tested as apraxias may be regional eg. Buccofacial, limb, truncal, etc.

Apraxias are most frequently seen in patients with lesions involving the parietal lobe on the dominant side, although lesions in other locations of left frontal lobe may also cause apraxic disorders.

MOOD, AFFECT AND THOUGHT CONTENT
Mood and affect are components of psychological profile of the patient.

Mood refers to feelings and emotions evoked by situations, events and other occurences in daily life.

Affect refers to somatic and autonomic behaviors that are used to convey a mood or emotion.

Thought content refers to fullness and organisation of the patients thinking as reflected in conversation and behavior.

In children, these are tested only in rare and special conditions.

DELIRIUM
It is a state of confusion with disordered perceptions and decreased attention span and inappropriate response to stimuli. Some common conditions causing delirium are given herewith.

Causes of Delirium

Infections
1. Neurologic
2. Meningitis-bacterial, fungal, parasitic
   Brain abscess, cerebritis, viral encephalitis

Non-neurologic with Secondary Effects
- Exanthematous fevers
- Typhoid and typhus fevers

- Hepatic failure
- Reye's syndrome
- Influenza
- Postinfectious encephalomyelitis
- Rheumatic chorea
- Pyelonephritis
- Severe pneumonia especially pneumococcal.

Toxic

Carbon monoxide, lead and other heavy metals, organophosphates, hydrocarbons.

Vascular

- Inflammation of vessels
- Lupus erythematosus
- Polyarteritis
- Thrombosis
  - Arterial—embolic-hemolytic uremic syndrome
  - Venous sinus thrombosis
- Hemorrhage—(subarachnoid).

Medications and Drugs of Abuse

- Antihistaminics
- Atropine
- Barbiturates
- Phenothiazines
- Propranolol
- Salicylates
- Opium
- Alcohol
- Amphetamines
- Lysergic acid, etc.

Trauma

- Head surgery
- Heat stroke

Perceptual distortions Hallucinations, Illusions and Delusions:

- Hallucinations are perception of sensations in the absence of any sensory stimulus.
- Illusion on the other hand is altered perception to sensory stimulus.
- Delusions are false beliefs which cannot be corrected despite evidence to the contrary.

  These are seen in schizophrenia and psychoses, not commonly seen in children.

BEHAVIOR

Certain typical types of behavior, give a due to the underlying disease.

e.g.:
- Avoidance of eye contact and self ingrossed — Autistic behavior
- Irritable and excessive crying — Cerebral irritation due to various causes
- Self mutilating — Lesch-Nyhan syndrome

EXAMINATION OF CRANIAL NERVES

OLFACTORY NERVE

Anatomy

The peripheral neurons of the olfactory nerves are bipolar sensory cells. The distal portion of these cells, i.e. dendrites consist of ciliated processes which penetrate the mucous membrane in the olfactory region of the upper portion of the nasal cavity

These filaments are found in a small area on the medial wall of the superior nasal concha, the upper part of the septum and the roof of the nose. The central processes or neuraxes of these nerves are collected into 20 branches on each side, which form the olfactory nerves. These olfactory nerves penetrate the cribriform plate of the ethmoid bone as unmyelinated fibers and synapse in the olfactory bulb. While passing through the cibriform plate, each nerve receives tubular sheaths from the dura and pia matter. Figure 27.2 shows the distribution of olfactory nerves within the nose.

In the olfactory bulbs, the neuraxes of the olfactory nerve synapse with the dendrites of the mitral and tufted cells in the olfactory glomeruli. The neuraxes of the mitral cells (second order neurons) course posteriorly through the olfactory tract. Here, they divide into medial and lateral olfactory roots (striae). Some fibers decussate in the anterior commissure to join fibers from the opposite side.

Fibers of the medial olfactory root terminate on the medial surface of the cerbral hemisphere. (paraolfactory gyrus, subcallosal gyrus, and inferior part of the cingulate gyrus).

Fibers of the lateral olfactory root terminate in the uncus, amygdaloid nucleus, and anterior portion of the hippocampal gyrus. The hippocampi and amygdaloid nuclei on both sides are intimately related through the anterior commisure. Communications with the superior and inferior salivatory nuclei are important in reflex salivation. Figure 27.3 illustrates the main features of the olfactory pathway and its central connections.

Clinical Examination

Method of Testing

Olfactory nerve function is tested by the use of non-irritating odorants such as coffee, orange, oil of lemon, oil of cloves, oil of roses, oil of wintergreen,

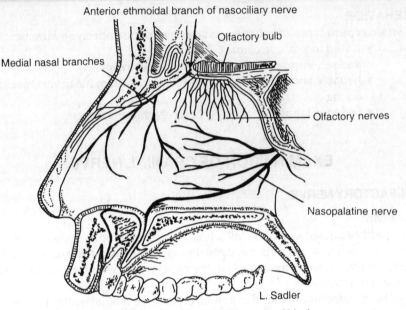

Fig. 27.2: The distribution of the olfactory nerve within the nose

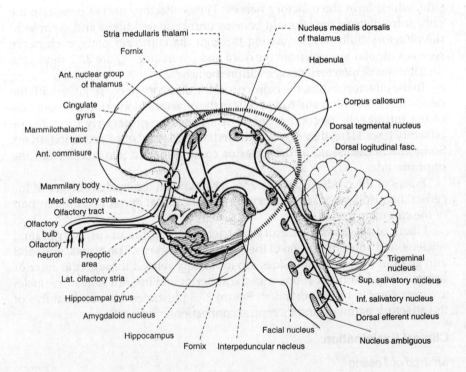

Fig. 27.3: The olfactory pathway and its central connections

eucalyptus oil. Common bedside substances such as soap, toothpaste, scents, fruits can also be used.

Avoid substances which instead of stimulating the olfactory nerve, may stimulate gustatory endorgans or the peripheral endings of the trigeminal nerve in the mucosa, e.g. chloroform may stimulate gustatory as well as olfactory endings by imparting sweet taste, pyridine may give a bitter taste, peppermint, menthol, camphor stimulate the trigeminal endings and give a feeling of coolness. Ammonia and formaldehyde also stimulate the trigeminal endings.

- Each nostril is examined separately while the other is occluded.
- With the eyes closed, the test substance should be brought near the open nostril
- Patient should be asked to inhale forcibly and indicate whether he smells something and if so, identify it.
- The process should be repeated on the other nostril and the results should be compared. After a sufficient interval, the test is repeated with two other odors. Observe the patients ability to percive, identify and name the test substance.

In infants flaring of the alae nasi in response to strong odors indicates that the sense of smell is intact.

Before evaluating loss of olfactory sensitivity, one must ascertain that the nasal passages are open. Intranasal conditions such as obstruction—allergic, atrophic rhinitis, sinusitis, polyps, may interfere with the sense of smell.

Perception of the presence of the odor indicates continuity of the peripheral nerve and its pathway.

Identification of the odor indicates intact cortical function.

A child may be able to identify the odor. The appreciation of the presence of the smell even without its recognition is sufficient evidence to rule out anosmia.

Disorders of Olfactory Function

The olfactory nerves themselves, are rarely the seat of disease, but are frequently involved in association with disease or injury of the surrounding structures. These lesions may be any where along the course of the peripheral nerve or its central pathway.

Anosmia (Anosphrasia)

Anosmia (Anosphrasia), i.e. absence of sense of smell and **Hyposmia** (impairment of olfaction) may occur in a variety of conditions.

- Trauma to the head with fracture of the ethmoid bone may cause anosmia by damaging the olfactory filaments
- Infections—meningitis
- Pernicious anemia—anosmia with perversions or loss of smell and taste
- Frontal lobe abscess or fracture of frontal or ethmoid bone
- Hydrocephalus
- Toxins—lead, calcium

- Seen in viral infections (viral hepatitis), syphilis, hypogonadism and abnormalities of zinc metabolism
- Disease of anterior cerebral artery near its origin in the circle of Willis—homolateral anosmia
- **Anosmia** It can be early sign in diagnosis and localisation of intracranial tumors, e.g. Foster Kennedy syndrome—frontal lobe tumors may cause unilateral anosmia and optic atrophy.
- **Hysterical anosmia** It is diagnosed by using irritating substances like ammonia which stimulate the trigeminal endings and volatile oils. In organic anosmia, the former will be recognised but not the latter. In hysteria neither will be recognised.

Hyperosmia

An increase in olfactory acuity seen in
- Hysteria, psychotic states
- Substance abuse
- Along with hyperacusis in migraine
- Endemic encephalitis
- Cystic fibrosis, Addison's disease, strychnine poisoning.

Parosmia (Perversion of smell)

Parosmia (Perversion of smell) and **catosmia** (presence of disaggreable odors.
- Psychic states
- Following head trauma especially uncus region
- Olfactory hallucination—presence of irritative lesion such as neoplasm or vascular lesion in the central olfactory system.

Uncinate fit Seizure preceeded by aura of a disaggreable olfactory or gustatory hallucination as a result of irritative lesion in the uncinate gyrus, hippocampus, amygdala, or temporal lobe. Olfactory stimulation can both arrest or activate such seizure. The uncinate fit is one manifestation (aura), of complex partial or temporal lobe seizure.

OPTIC NERVE

Anatomy

From the retina the fibers of the optic nerve pass backwards to form the optic chiasma. Here, fibers from the inner nasal half of each retina (representing the temporal field) decussate, while those from the outer temporal half (representing the nasal field), remain on the same side. After this chiasmal decussation, each optic tract thus consists of fibers from the outer half of the retina on the same side and from the inner half of the retina on the opposite side.

Each optic tract passes posteriorly to the lateral geniculate body of the same side (some pregeniculate fibers project to the superior colliculus). The lateral geniculate body gives rise to the optic radiation on each side.

The optic radiation passes through the post-limb of the internal capsule and projects posteriorly to the calcarine cortex of the occipital lobe. In the occipital cortex, the left half of the field of vision is represented in the right hemisphere and vice versa. The most peripheral part of the visual field is represented anteriorly in the calcarine fissure and the most medial part (macular field) is represented at the posterior part (occipital pole) (Fig. 27.4).

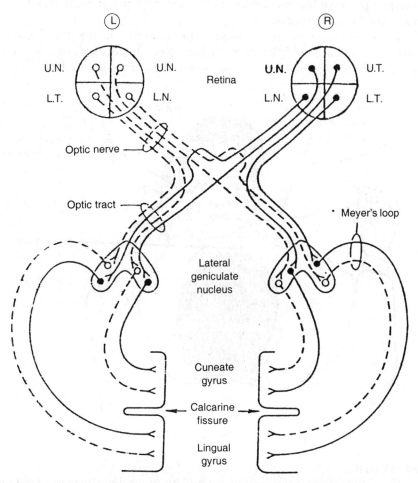

Fig. 27.4: The visual pathway. UN=upper nasal quadrant, LN=lower nasal quadrant, UT=upper temporal quadrant, LT=lower temporal quadrant

Assessment of Field of Vision

The visual fields can be assessed by several methods of varying sophistication. A simple bedside method is by comparing the extent of the patients visual field with that of the examiner.

Confrontation Test

The examiner sits opposite the patient at a distance of one meter. To test the patients right eye, ask him to cover his left eye with his left hand or the patients left eye can be covered by examiners righthand and ask to look steadily into the examiners left eye.

The examiner covers his right eye with his right hand and gazes steadily into the patients right eye. The examiner holds up his left hand in a plane midway between the patient's face and his own at full arms length to the side. The examiner keeps moving the fingers of the hand and brings it nearer untill he can just percieve the movements of the fingers. The patient is asked if he can also see the movements.

If the patient fails to see the fingers, the examiner brings them nearer. Similarly the visual field is tested in all directions, upwards, downward, left and right-using the visual field of the examiner for comparison (Fig. 27.5).

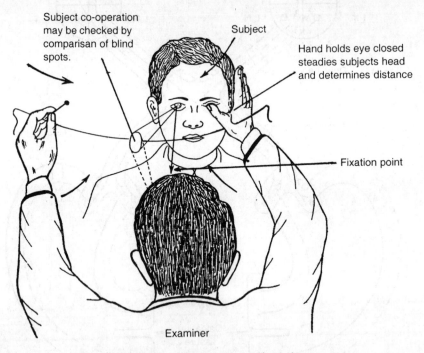

Subject co-operation may be checked by comparisan of blind spots.

Subject

Hand holds eye closed steadies subjects head and determines distance

Fixation point

Examiner

Fig. 27.5: Visual field testing by confrontation

Red Pin Test

This test outlines the central field of vision. This test is done by using a red pin head held up in the patients field in the method described above. A central area of impaired vision (central scotoma) can be recognised by this method. This method allows the patients visual field, including the size of the physiological blind spot, to be compared precisely with that of the examiner (assuming the examiner's vision is normal).

Perimetry

Visual fields can also be mapped out precisely using perimetry.

The patient is seated comfortably with his chin on a chinrest. The chinrest is adjusted in such a way that the eye being tested is oreinted at the centre of the hemispherical illuminated field. On this field, spots of light of varying size and intensity and colour are moved to detect the limits of the patients visual field.

A Bjerrums screen is used to detect objects in the centre of the visual field. Bjerrums screen is a 2 meter × 2 meter, wall mounted black screen on which test objects are presented. The patient sits at a distance of 1-2 meters with his head steady on chinrest. A white object, 1 cm in diameter is fixed to the screen at level with the patients eye. The blind spot and the peripheral visual field is then mapped out. These findings are marked on the screen and then transferred to a chart and recorded.

Visual Field Defects and their Significance

Numerous field defects are possible and the principles by which lesions are located are best illustrated by comparing a diagram of the visual pathways with principle field defects. Assessment for field defects needs cooperation of the child and depends upon the age of the child and hence field defect assessment should be conducted keeping in mind the age of the child. Diagrammatic representation of the visual pathways, the common sites of lesions are lettered and the characteristic field defects so caused are illustrated in Figure 27.6.

VISUAL ACUITY

Distant Vision

Visual acuity is measured using Snellen's test types (Fig. 27.7), a series of letters of varying sizes constructed in such a way that the top letter is visible to the normal eye at 60m, and the subsequent lines at 36, 24, 18,12,9, 6, and 5 meters respectively. Visual acuity is then recorded as per the ratio-d/D.

d—distance at which the letters are read

D—distance at which the letters should be read.

A normal person has a visual acuity of 6/6. Visual acuity of less than 1/60 is recorded as counting fingers, hand movements and perception of light.

Near Vision

Visual acuity at ordinary reading distance is assessed by using reading test types, e.g. Jaeger test chart.

The smallest print is N5. The near vision is recorded as the smallest type which the patient can read comfortably (held at a distance of 14 inches) (Fig. 27.8).

Color Vision

Color sense is tested using colored skins of wool (Holmgrens wools) or pseudoisochromatic plates (Ishihara charts). These Ishihara charts consist of multicolored dots outlining certain digits. People with defective color vision confuse cetain colors. These charts are constructed in such a way that people with abnormal color vision will read a different number on the same color plate.

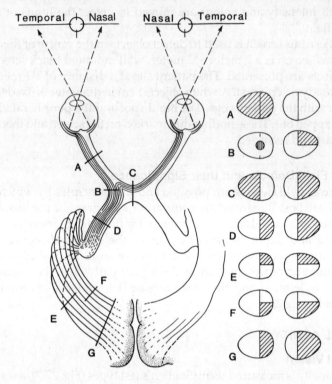

Fig. 27.6: Diagram showing the effects on the fields of vision produced by lesions at various points along the optic pathway: (A) complete blindness in left eye; (B) the usual effect is a left junction scotoma in association with a right upper quadrantanopia. The latter results from interruption of right retinal nasal fibers that project into the base of the left optic nerve (Wilbrand's knee). A left nasal hemian opia could occur from a lesion at this point but is exceedingly rare; (C) bitemporal hemianopia; (D) right homonymous hemianopia; (E and F) right superior and inferior quadrant hemianopia; and (G) right homonymous hemianopia

FUNDUS EXAMINATION

Examination of the fundus of the eye with an opthalmoscope is an important part of medical examination and often gives valuable information.

The patient should be examined in a darkroom. With practice it may be possible to examine the fundus without dilating the pupil, but for a complete examination pupils should be dilated by instilling a few drops of mydriatrics, (1% cyclopentolate or 1% tropicamide) into the conjunctival sacs.

Ask the patient to look straight ahead and to keep the eyes as still as possible. The ophthalmoscope is held a few centemetres from the patients eyes, and a suitable plus lens is used to bring the iris into focus. The ophthalmoscope is then brought as close as possible to the patient's eye and the light directed slightly towards nasal side. By doing this the optic disc can be found and the light will not fall directly on the macula (which may constrict the pupil). If the optic disc is not in focus, the strength of the lens of the ophthalmoscope should be gradually reduced untill the disk is sharply

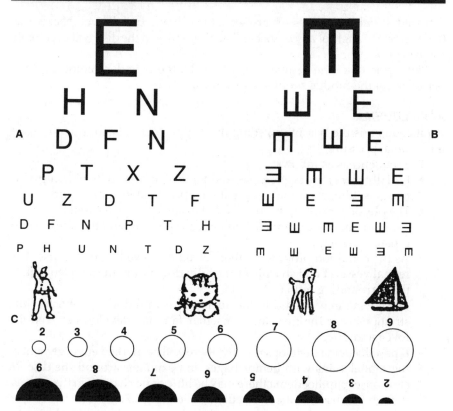

Fig. 27.7: Snellen chart—(a) letter (alphabet) chart, (b) symbol E chart, and (c) picture chart

N.5.

Boat, horse, bone, cat, cabbage, man, trousers, jewel

N.6.

Eye, ear, earth, lion, lying, road, green, dog.

N.8.

Bird, wall, silver, tower, train, gorse.

N.10.

Snail, sail, blue, jacket, clam, jockey.

N.12.

Car, crow, grey, bracket, scarlet.

N.14.

White, bank, turbot, jewel.

N.18.

Play, grain, red, goat.

N.24.

Black, frog, tree.

Fig. 27.8: Near vision chart

focussed. If only blood vessels are seen, they should be followed backwards (i.e. against the angle of any branches that are seen), and the disk will eventually come in view.

The optic disc, the retinal blood vessels, the macular region and the periphery of the fundus should be examined.

PAPILLEDEMA

Papilloedema is the passive swelling of the optic nerve head, due to raised intracranial pressure.

The sequence is as follows:
- Initially there may be increased reddness of the disk with blurring of its margins. Blurring appears first at the upper and lower margins.
- The physiological cup becomes filled in and disappears, and the retinal veins are slightly distended. Spontaneous pulsations of the retinal veins is usually absent.
- As the condition progresses, there is definite swelling of the disc. The retinal vessels bend sharply as they dip down from the swollen disk to the surrounding retina.
- The edema may extend to the adjacent area producing greyish-white striations near the disc and a macular fan may develop between the fovea and disc.
- If papilloedema develops rapidly, there will be marked engorgement of the retinal veins with hemorrhages and exudates around the disc. In slow onset papilloedema there may be little or no changes in the vessels, though the disc may be markedly swollen (Fig. 27.9).

Causes of Papilledema
1. Raised intracranial pressure due to mass lesions.
2. Raised intracranial pressure due to circulatory block
   — aqueductal stenosis
   — intraventricular tumors
   — fourth ventricle outflow block
3. Due to cerebral edema
   — posthead injury
   — postcerebral anoxia
   — benign intracranial hypertension
   — lead poisoning
   — steroid withdrawal
   — vitamin A intoxication
4. Due to raised CSF protein or altered blood products
   — postsubarachnoid hemorrhage
   — postmeningitis
   — Guillain-Barre syndrome
   — spinal cord tumors
5. The malignant phase of hypertension
6. Metabolic disorders
   — hypercapnia

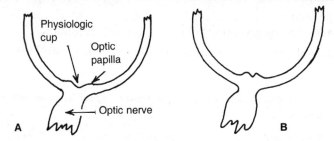

Fig. 27.9: Optic papilla in horizontal sections of the eye (a) normal optic papilla, showing slight elevation of the papillary margins and normal depth of the physiologic cup, and (b) early true papilloedema, showing elevation of the papillary margins and beginning obliteration of the physiologic cup

> — hypocalcemia
> — malignant thyrotoxic exophthalmos

7. Disorders of circulation
   — lateral sinus thrombosis
   — jugular vein thrombosis
   — superior venacaval obstruction
   — polycythemia rubra vera
   — multiple myelomatosis
   — diabetes mellitus
   — hyperlipidemia
   — vasculitis

Criteria for Diagnosis of Papilloedema

1. Elevation of the optic disk (diopters).
2. Venules   — enlargement
   — dilatation
   — tortuosity
   — absence of pulsations
3. Deflection of vessels over edge and elevated optic disc
4. Blurred disc (temporal)
5. Reddish optic disc
6. Flame shaped hemorrhages near optic disc
7. Few exudates
8. Folds and edema of retina
9. Usually bilateral
10. Advanced cases-blurring and constriction of visual fields.

Fundus Examination in Papilloedema and Optic Neuritis

Papilloedema	*Optic Neuritis*
1. Bilateral (often)	Unilateral
2. Vision-normal	Diminished
3. No pain	Pain present
4. Venous pulsations absent	Present

5. Disc elevated > 2   < 2
6. Field defect-increased blind spot   Antral scotoma.

Table 27.7 shows fundal changes in papilloedema, papillitis and optic atrophy.

Table 27.7: Appearance of fundus in papilloedema, papillitis and optic atrophy

Feature	Papilloedema	Papillitis	Optic atrophy
1. Depth	Elevated disc, physio-logical cup obliterated	Elevated disc, physio-logical cup obliterated	Shallow
2. Edge	Blurred edge	Blurred edge	Very sharp
3. Vessels	Engorged	Engorged	Narrow/few
4. Color	No venous pulse, hyperemic, hemorrhages	No venous pulse, hyperemic hemorrhages	Pallor
5. Vision	Good or enlarged blind spot	Poor vision or loss of central vision	Reduced vision

OCULOMOTOR NERVE/TROCHLEAR NERVE/ABDUCENS NERVE

Since the oculomotor, trochlear and abducens nerves all function in regulation of the eye movements, they are referred to as the ocular nerves and are examined together.

The cervical portion of the sympathetic portion of the autonomic nervous system functions with the IIIrd nerve in innervation of the eyelid and pupil, and consequently it will be considered along with the ocular nerves.

OCULOMOTOR NERVE

The IIIrd nerve arises from a nucleus in the midbrain anterior to the aqueduct of Sylvius. The nucleus is made up of:

1. A large paired lateral nuclear mass from which arise the fibers supplying the various occular nucleus [superior rectus (SR), inferior rectus (IR), medial rectus (MR), inferior oblique (IO), and levator palpebrae superioris (LPS)].
2. A median unpaired nucleus (nucleus of perlia) which is the center for convergence and accommodation
3. Edinger-Westphal nucleus, which is paired and constitutes the para-sympathetic nucleus supplying fibers to the constrictor muscle of the pupil.

The fibers from the various nuclei pass through the medial portion of the red nucleus, the substantia nigra and the cerebral peduncle and exit from the anterior surface of the midbrain. After leaving the brainstem these fibers are united to form the IIIrd nerve on each side. This nerve penetrates the dura just lateral and anterior to the post clinoid process and then passes through the upper and lateral part of the cavernous sinus.

It enters the orbit through the supraorbital fissure and separates into superior and inferior divisions. The former supplies the SR and the LPS. The latter supplies the MR, IR, and IO. It also sends a short root to the ciliary ganglion from which postganglionic fibers go as short ciliary nerves to supply the ciliary muscle and the sphincter pupillae.

TROCHCLEAR NERVE

- Smallest of the cranial nerves
- Its nuclei are situated below that of the occulomotor nerve, just anterior to the aqueduct in the grey matter of the lower midbrain.

The fibers of the trochlear nerve curve posteriorly and caudually around the aqueduct and decussate in the anterior medullary velum. It is the only cranial nerve which emerges from the posterior aspect of the brainstem. The nerve then circles around the pons and cerebral peduncle. It penetrates the dura just behind and lateral to the posterior clinoid process and passes through the cavernous sinus. It then enters the orbit through the superior orbital fissure and terminates on the SO muscle on the side opposite to the nucleus of origin.

Therefore in a nuclear lesion of the IV nerve the contralateral SO is paralysed, but in a lesion along the course of the nerve, after its decussation its ipsilateral muscle is involved.

ABDUCENS NERVE

The abducens nerve has its nucleus in the floor of the fourth ventricle within the loop formed by the facial nerve near its orgin. Fibers from the nucleus pass forward and downward and emerge in a groove between the pons and the medulla. The nerve pierces the dura opposite the dorsum sella, runs under the petrospheroidal ligament and enters the cavernous sinus. It then enters the orbit through the superior orbital fissure and supplies the lateral rectus.

Because of its long intracranial course this nerve is more frequently involved in disease processes. An increase in intracranial pressure, inflammatory exudates or hemorrhage may cause it to be pressed between the pons and the clivus. In such circumstances the VIth nerve involvement may be bilateral.

Medial Longitudinal Fasciculus (MLF)

The oculomotor, trochlear and abducens nuclei are situated one below the other in a columnar arrangement in the brainstem. They are united for coordination and conjugate action by the MLF. MLF also connects them with the nucleus of the vestibulocochlear nerve, trigeminal, facial nerve, spinal accessory, hypoglossal, the upper cervical nerves, as well as higher centers.

Due to this correlating mechanism, no isolated action of any eye muscle is ever possible, and movements of one eye are correlated with those of the other. Thus, in response to visual, auditory, sensory-vestibular stimuli, normal conjugate deviation of the eye and head ocurs. This pathway is important in auditory-ocular reflexes, vestibularocular reflex and righting reflex.

EXAMINATION OF THE PUPILS

  I. Size
 II. Shape
III. Equality
 IV. Position
  V. Pupillary reflexes   1. The light reflex.
                                     2. The accommodation reflex.
                                     3. The pain reflex.

4. The orbicularis reflex.
5 The cochlear reflex.
6 The vestibular reflex.
7. The galvanic reflex.
8. The psychic reflex.

Size

Size of pupils varies greatly with the intensity of the surrounding illumination.
In lighting of average intensity
Normally   — 3-4 mm diameter
Neonates   — pupils are small and react poorly
Adolescents— 4 mm diameter, round
Middle age — 3.5 mm diameter, regular
Old age   — 3 mm or less, irregular.

Miosis

When pupils are small (< 2 mm) they are said to be miotic. Miosis is seen in newborns, opium, organsophosphorus compound poisoning, pilocarpine, encephalitis, syringomyelia.

Mydriasis   Dilated pupils are seen in mania, atropine poisoning, damage to cervical sympathetic plexus.

PUPILLARY ABNORMALITIES (Table 27.8)

Table 27.8: Pupillary abnormalities and their causes

Reaction to light	Small pupils	Large pupils
1. Non reactive	• A-R pupil • Pontine hemorrhage • Opiates • Pilocarpine drops	• Holmes-Adie pupil • Post-traumatic-iridoplegia • Mydriatic drops • Cerebral death • Atropine poisoning • Amphetamines
2. Reactive	• Old age • Horner's syndrome	• Childhood • Anxiety • Physiological anisocoria

Pupillary Abnormalities may be due to
- Absent (Aniridia)   — Wilms tumor
- Irregular iris   — Adhesions
- Iridodialysis   — Trauma
- Coloboma   — Congenital/operative
- A-R pupil (Accommodation reflex   — Syphilis,
  present loss of light reflex miosis)   Encephalitis multiple sclerosis
- Adies pupil (Accommodation reflex   — Benign
  present, myrdiais, slow light reflex)
- Reverse ARP (loss of accommo-   — *Bilateral*-Diabetes, syphilis, basal meningitis,
  dation, light reflex present)   tumors of corpora quadrigemina.
                                                            — *Unilateral*-Diphtheria, intoxication, syphilis.

ARP: Argyll Robertson Pupil

Hippus

There is normally certain amount of alternate fluctuation in the size of pupils-pupillary unrest. When this rythmic contraction and dilatation of the pupil is present to an excessive degree it is called hippus.

Mechanism It is said to be associated with respiratory rhythm but is probably due to imbalance between the sympathetic and parasympathetic division of the autonomic nervous system. Usually seen in:
- During recovery from III nerve palsy
- During drowsiness
- Organic disease of CNS

Shape

Shape of the pupil is important in neurologic diagnosis. Normal pupil is round and regular in outline. Any irregularity, abnormality in shape, notching or serration may be significant.

Gross abnormalities in shape of pupils are usually the result of ocular disease (iritis) or eye surgery. There may be.
- Adhesion to the lens (anterior synechiae)
- A gap in the iris (congenital coloboma)

Equality

Comparison of the size of the two pupils has more significance than observation of size alone.

There may be slight difference in the size of the pupils in 15-20 percent of normal individuals. Gross inequality of pupils is called anisocoria. Sympathetic paralysis on one side will cause a smaller pupil on that side. IIIrd nerve paralysis produces dilatation of the pupil.
- Unequal pupils may be caused by iritis.
- Alternating anisocoria is seen in various CNS diseases.
- The pupil of an ambylopic/blind eye is always larger.
- In inner ear disease—ipsilateral contraction of pupil (since the pupillodilator fibers are in close proximity to the tympanic plexus in inner ear).
- Cerebral vascular accidents/head trauma—unilateral dilation and fixation of one pupil.
- Dilated fixed pupil in a comatosed patients, may give presumptive localisation of a lesion in the ipsilateral cerebral hemisphere.

Position

The pupil is usually situated in the centre of the iris. Ectopia of pupils or eccentric pupils may be the result of trauma or iritis.

Pupillary Reflexes

Light Reflex

Method The patient should be asked to look at a distant object, in order to eliminate constriction of the pupil on accommodation. A direct source of bright light is focussed into the eye being tested. Normally there is constriction of both pupils.

The response of the pupil of the eye upon which the light falls is the direct light reflex and that of the opposite eye is the consensual light reflex. This occurs due to decussation of fibers both in the optic chiasma and the Edinger-Westphal nucleus.

Constriction of the pupil is the normal response to an increase in light intensity whereas dilatation of the pupil normally occurs in response to decrease in light intensity.

Afferent pathway is through the optic nerve-pretectal nucleus—Edinger-Westphal nucleus.

Efferent fibers are carried by the occulomotor nerve through the ciliary ganglion (Fig. 27.10).
- The light reflexes must be tested in a dimly lit room.
- Patient is instructed to look straight ahead and focus at a point in the distance (to avoid constriction of the pupil that accompanies convergence).
- The examiner may place the edge of one hand against the nose and forehead to prevent light from reaching the other eye.
- The other eye should remain open during the test.
- The examiner brings the bright light of a pen torch from the side of the patients head into one eye.
- Pupillary reactions in both eyes should be examined and duly recorded.
- Normally pupils in both the eyes constrict.
- The pupillary constriction observed in the illuminated eye is referred to as the **Direct Light Reflex** and the response in the nonilluminated eye is referred to as the **Indirect, Consensual** or **Crossed-light Reflex**.
- Iridoplegia—describes a condition in which the pupil does not react to light.
- Amaurotic pupil is one that does not constrict in response to light (complete destruction of retina or optic nerve).

Swinging flashlight test
- Patient is asked to focus on a distant object in a darkened room.
- The examiner alternately shines a penlight into one eye and then the other at the rate of one cycle per second. The pupillary reaction in both eyes is observed.

  Normal response is constriction of both pupils when light is directed into each eye and slight dilatation bilaterally as the light moves across the bridge of the nose. The light-stimulated pupil constricts as a result of the direct light reflex. While the nonstimulated pupil constricts as a result of consensual light reflex.
- Paradoxic pupillary response—may be seen in patients with damage to the optic nerve but without loss of visual acuity. When light enters the normal eye, both pupils constrict. The stimulated (normal) eye due to a direct light refex and the nonstimulated (Abnormal) eye due to consensual light reflex. When the light is shifted to the abnormal eye, both pupils dilate because of a relative reduction in the intensity of light that is available to provoke the direct and indirect light reflex.

  This observation which indicates damage to the optic nerve on the side at which dilatation occurred, is referred to as an Afferent pupillary deficit

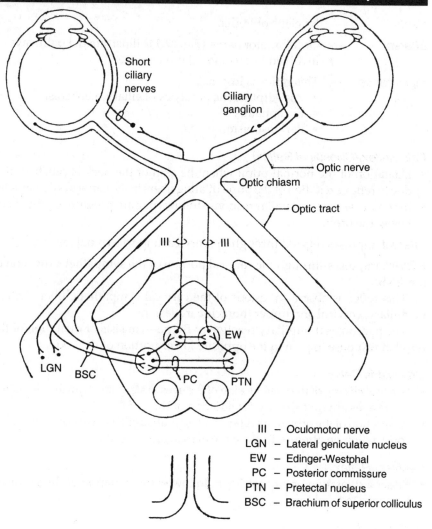

Short
ciliary
nerves

Ciliary
ganglion

Optic nerve

Optic chiasm

Optic tract

III

III

EW

LGN

BSC

PC

PTN

III — Oculomotor nerve
LGN — Lateral geniculate nucleus
EW — Edinger-Westphal
PC — Posterior commissure
PTN — Pretectal nucleus
BSC — Brachium of superior colliculus

Fig. 27.10: The neural pathways involved in the light reflexes

(Marcus Gunn pupil).
- In a patient with isolated occulomotor nerve lesion direct light reflex is absent on the affected eye but consensual light reflex is present.

Accommodation Reflex (Accommodation-convergence Synkinesis)
Is elicited by having the patient shift his gaze to some near object after having relaxed his accommodation by gazing into the distance.

This is followed by:
- Thickening of the lens
- Convergence of the eyes
- Constriction of the pupils

Afferent limb — Optic nerve
— Proproceptive fibers from Intraocular muscles.

Centre — Nucleus of Perlia.

Efferent — Occulomotor nerve (Fig. 27.11) illustrate the pathways involved in accommodation reflex.

Significance — This reflex is lost in:
- Post-diptheretic paralysis of ciliary mechanism
- Encephalitis
- Parkinsonism

Pain Reflex (Ciliospinal Reflex)
- Dilatation of the normal pupil when the skin of the neck is pinched. It is due to reflex excitation of the pupil dilating fibers in the cervical sympathetic.
- In comatose states, a similar response follows painful pressure on the cheek below the orbit.

Afferent impulses relayed through the cervical and trigeminal nerves.

Efferent impulses-through the cervical portion of the sympathetic division of the ANS.

This reflex is absent in lesions of the cervical sympathetic fibers and in medullary, cervical and upper thoracic cord lesions.

The paradoxical pupillary reaction of Byrne—consists of dilatation of the pupil in response to pain in the opposite lower portion of the body.

Orbicularis Reflex
- Forceful closing of the eyes, closing of the eyes in sleep and upward deviation of the eyes are followed by constriction of the pupils.
- A variation of the orbiculars reflex is Westphal pupillary reaction—pupillary constriction on attempt to close the eyes against resistance.

Cochlear Reflex
- Either a dilatation or a constriction followed by dilatation of the pupils in response to a loud noise.

Vestibular Reflex
- Either a dilatation or a constriction followed by dilatation of the pupils in response to stimulation of the labyrinthine system.

Galvanic Reflex
Galvanic stimulation in the region of the temple causes constriction of pupils.

Psychic Reflex
Dilatation of pupils in response to pain, fear, anxiety due to stimulation of the sympathetic division of ANS.

EXAMINING OCULAR MOVEMENT
The patient must look at a clear and definite point, such as the point of a pen or a fine point of light. The examiner then moves this point precisely and deliberately to right and left horizontally, upward and downward in the

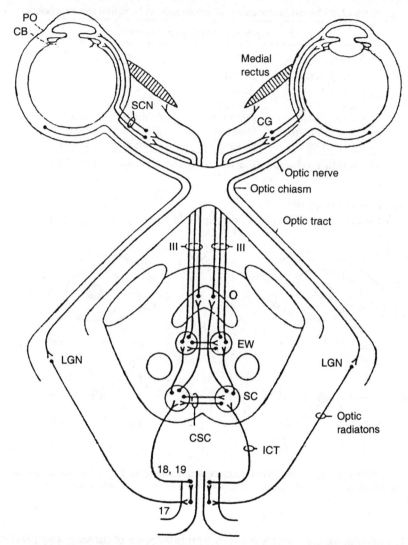

PC – Posterior commissure
CB – Ciliary body
SCN – Short ciliary nerves
O – Oculomotor nucleus (nucleus of Perlia)
III – Oculomotor nerve
EW – Edinger-Westphal
SC – Superior coiliculus

ICT – Internal corticotectal tract
CSC – Commissure of superior
       colliculus
CG – Ciliary ganglion
17 – Occipital lobe (area 17)
18, 19– Occipital lobe (area 18, 19)
LGN – Lateral geniculate nucleus

Fig. 27.11: Neural pathways involved in the accommodation reflex

midline, and vertically when the eyes are deviated to one side (Table 27.9). Do not attempt to make the eyes deviate beyond the point of comfort, and hold each deviation for at least 5 seconds. The aim is:

1. To observe lagging of one or other eye.

Table 27.9: Primary, secondary and tertiary action of different eye muscles

	Eye movements of individual muscles		
Muscle	Primary action	Secondary	Tertiary
Medial rectus	Adducts		
Lateral rectus	Abducts		
Superior rectus	Elevates	Adducts	Intorts
Inferior rectus	Depresses	Adducts	Extorts
Superior oblique	Depresses	Abducts	Intorts
Inferior Oblique	Elevates	Abducts	Extorts

Movements produced by individual extraocular muscles (Fig. 27.12).

2. To detect nystagmus.
3. In older children to analyse any diplopia the child may describe.

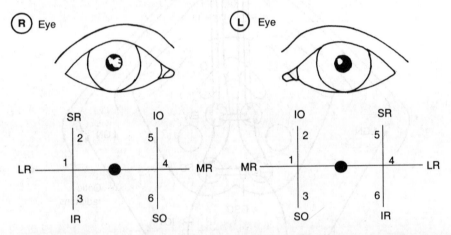

Fig. 27.12: Movement produced by individual extraocular muscles. Numbers refer to a suggested order of voluntary or following movements intended to ensure complete assessment of occular motor function. LR=latera rectus, SR=superior rectus, IR=inferior rectus, MR=medial rectus, IO=inferior oblique, SO=superior oblique

The occular muscles act together. A simplified form of considerable practical value is given below.

A. The external rectus (VIth nerve)—moves the eye horizontally outward.
B. The internal rectus (IIIrd nerve)—moves the eye horizontally inward.
C. The superior rectus (IIIrd nerve)—elevates the eye when it is turned outward.
D. The inferior oblique (IIIrd nerve)—elevates the eye when it is turned inward.
E. The inferior rectus (IIIrd nerve)—depresses the eye when it is turned outward.
F. The superior oblique (IVth nerve)—depresses the eye when it is turned inward.

The muscles paired together above act together.

Ocular Muscle Paralysis

From this scheme the following general rules can be deduced.

1. If an eye fails to move outward, there is either a VIth nerve lesion, or a local lesion of the external rectus muscle (see A above).
2. If the eye, when deviated inward, will not then move downward, there is either a IVth nerve lesion, or a local lesion of the superior oblique muscle (see F above).
3. All other defects in movement are due to IIIrd nerve lesions, a local lesion of the muscles, myasthenia gravis or an internuclear ophthalmoplegia.

In addition, however, when there is ocular muscle paralysis the unopposed pull of the normal antagonist will displace the eyeball. In paralysis of the IIIrd nerve, therefore, the eye is displaced outward, and will not move inwards or vertically. There is accompanying ptosis and pupillary dilatation, though the latter may be absent if the lesion is recovering, or is incomplete.

In VIth nerve paralysis the eye is deviated inward and will not move outward beyond the midline, but will move vertically when deviated inward.

Unfortunately, incomplete paralysis may show little visible abnormality and it is then that the diplopia produced must be investigated.

NYSTAGMUS (TALANTROPIA)

Nystagmus is slow drift in one direction with a fast correction in the opposite direction. Direction of fast phase is used to categorise nystagmus.

Types of Nystagmus

Physiological — Opticokinetic nystagmus
Peripheral — Due to vestibular involvement
Central — Central connections of vestibular or cerebellar
Retina — Due to inability to fix

Ask the patient to follow your fingers with both eyes upward, downward and sideward.

a. Pendular—Symmetrical movement at the same speed in both direction.
b. Jerk nystagmus—Fast phase in one direction and slow in other direction.
c. Note direction (one or multiple), note whether it occurs while abduction or adduction of eyes.

Peripheral nystagmus fatigus is associated with vertigo and is reduced by fixation.

1. Nystagmoid jerks—normal
2. Pendular jerks (inability to fix) e.g congenital
3. Rotary—central cause

Vertical Nystagmus (Rare)

- Indicates brainstem disease.
- Upbeat (upper brainstem lesion)-e.g: Demyelination, stroke
- Downbeat (medullary cervical junctional lesion)—e.g: Arnold-Chiari malformation, syringobulbia, demyelination.

Horizontal Nystagmus (Common)
a. Ataxic: Nystagmus of abducting eye more than adducting eye, e.g: with internuclear ophthalmoplegia as in cerebrovascular accidents (CVA).
b. Multidirectional gaze evoked—Central, cerebellar syndrome vestibular syndrome
c. Unidirectional-peripheral—Vestibular neuronitis, Minere's disease, vascular
    Central-unilateral cerebellar syndrome
    Unilateral vestibular syndrome

Rare
Opsoclonus—rapid oscillation in horizontal, rotary, vertical direction e.g: Brain stem disease, sometimes associated with neuroblastoma.
Ocular Bobbing—up and down drifting, e.g: Pontine lesion.

ANALYSIS OF DIPLOPIA

Diplopia can indicate ocular muscle weakness before it is evident to the examiner. The light rays fail to fall on exactly corresponding parts of the two retinae, and a false image is formed which is usually paler and less distinct. The rules governing the relationship of these two images are as follows:

Rule 1—Displacement of the false image may be horizontal, vertical or both
Rule 2—Separation of the images is greatest in the direction in which the weak muscle has its purest action.
Rule 3—The false image is displaced farthest in the direction in which the weak muscle should move the eye.

METHOD OF EXAMINATION

Cover one of the patient's eyes with a transparent red shield and, using a point of light, move the object to right and left horizontally, upward and downward in the midline, and vertically when the eyes are deviated to one side. In each position ask the child:
1. Whether he sees one object or two.
2. If double, do the two images lie side by side, or one above the other.
3. In which position are they farthest apart.
4. Which is the red image.

Interpretation of Results
If the images are exactly side by side, it will be only the external or internal recti that are involved. If they are one above the other, either of the obliques, or the superior and inferior recti, may be defective.

TRIGEMINAL NERVE (MIXED NERVE)

Anatomy

The sensory root takes origin from nerve cells in the trigeminal (Gasserian) ganglion and enters the lateral surface of the pons at its middle.

The fibers which conduct impulses for light touch, terminate in a large nucleus in the pons, situated lateral to the motor nucleus near the floor of the fourth ventricle, where as the fibers for pain and thermal sensation enter the (descending) bulbospinal tract, which extends as low as the second cervical segment of the cord, before ascending in the medial lemniscus.

The motor root originates from a small nucleus, medial to the main sensory nucleus, and partly from the nerve cells scattered around the cerebral aqueduct. It emerges at the side of the pons, just anterior to the sensory division, passes inferior to the trigerminal ganglion, and joins the mandibular division.

First or Ophthalmic Division
- Supplies the conjuctiva and the conjuctival surface of the upper but not of the lower lid, the lacrimal gland, the mesial part of the skin of the nose as far as its tip, the upper eyelids, the forehead, and the scalp as far as the vertex.

Second or Maxillary Division
- Supplies the cheek, the front of the temple, the lower eyelid and its conjunctival surface, the side of the nose, the upper lip, the upper teeth.
- Mucous membrane of the nose, upper part of larynx, roof the mouth, part of soft palate, the tonsils, and medial inferior part of cornea.

Third or Mandibular Division
- Supplies lower part of the face, the lower lip, the ear, the tongue and lower teeth.
- Also supplies parasympathetic fibers to the salivary glands.
- The mandibular division is joined by the motor root, which innervates the muscles of mastication (masseter, temporalis, medial pterygoid, lateral pterygoid), two muscles of the floor of the mouth-mylohyoid and anterior belly of the digastric and the tensor tympani (Fig. 27.13A) cutaneous distribution of the trigeminal nerve (Fig. 27.13B) central projections of the trigeminal nerve mediating sensation from the face.

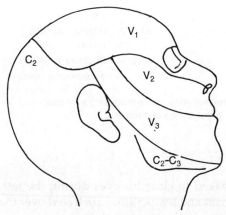

Fig. 27.13A: In cutaneous distribution of the three divisions of the trigeminal nerve. V_1=ophthalmic branch, V_2=maxillary branch, V_3=mandibular branch. Note that the skin overlying the angle of the mandible is innervated by sensory branches of cervical spinal nerves C_1 and C_3

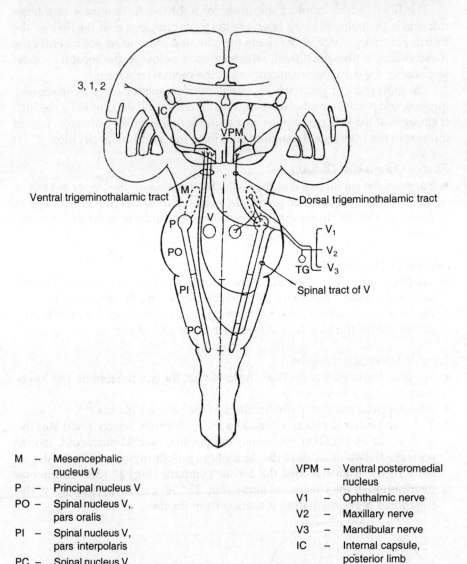

M	–	Mesencephalic nucleus V	VPM –	Ventral posteromedial nucleus
P	–	Principal nucleus V	V1 –	Ophthalmic nerve
PO	–	Spinal nucleus V, pars oralis	V2 –	Maxillary nerve
PI	–	Spinal nucleus V, pars interpolaris	V3 –	Mandibular nerve
			IC –	Internal capsule, posterior limb
PC	–	Spinal nucleus V, pars caudalis	3,1,2 –	Postcentral gyrus
V	–	Motor nucleus V	TG –	Trigeminal ganglion

Fig. 27.13B: Central projections of the trigeminal nerve mediating sensation from the face including the cornea and mouth

Clinical Examination

Sensory Component

Patient should be comfortable and asked to close his eyes during the test. Superficial skin sensations of touch, pain and temperature are tested over the areas of sensory supply of the 3 divisions of the trigeminal nerve.

For the first division (maxillary) the skin over forehead is tested. For the second division, the skin of the cheeks over the maxillary prominence is tested. For the third division (mandibular), the skin over the chin on both sides of the midline near the mental foramen is tested.

Touch   For light touch, a wisp of cotton wool or the tip of the index finger is used, ask the patient whether touch is felt and whether it feels normal. Touch can also be tested with the sharp and blunt ends of a safety pin.

Pain   Superficial pain may be tested by using a cutaneous stimuli, e.g. a pinprick. Care should be taken that the patient distinguishes between sharpness of the pinpoint and the pain it evokes. Pressure pain can be tested by pressure on deeper structures, e.g. muscles and bone.

Temperature Sense
This is examined by using test tubes containing warm and cold water. The part being tested is touched with each test tube in turn and the patient is asked whether each tube feels hot or cold.

Corneal Reflex
- This is the most sensitive test of sensory trigeminal nerve fuction.
- Patient is asked to direct his gaze to one side keeping the eyes open. The examiner then approaches the adducted eye from the lateral side with a wisp of cotton that has been twisted to a point. The examiner touches the corner over the iris just lateral to the pupil (avoid contact with conjunctiva, sclera or pupil) (Fig. 27.14).

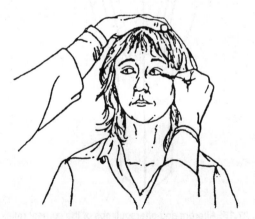

Fig. 27.14: Testing the corneal reflex

- The normal response is immediate blinking of both eyes, occasionally with movement of the head away from the stimulus.

Afferent limb   Ophthalmic division of trigeminal nerve

Efferent limb   Facial nerve (Fig. 27.15) corneal reflex pathway.

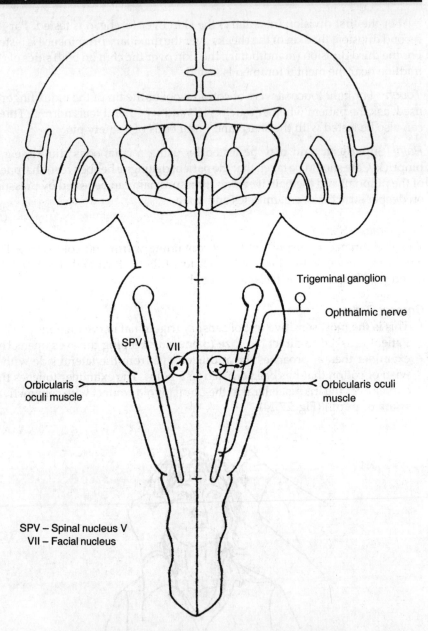

Trigeminal ganglion

Ophthalmic nerve

SPV   VII

Orbicularis
oculi muscle

Orbicularis oculi
muscle

SPV – Spinal nucleus V
VII – Facial nucleus

Fig. 27.15: Afferent and efferent limbs of the corneal reflex

- If there is damage to the ophthalmic nerve, no response will be seen in either eye if the corner of the involved side is touched. Blink response in both eyes will be observed when the cornea of the normal side is touched.
- In lesions of the facial nerve, no response is present on the involved side, when either cornea is touched. Blink response on the normal side will be present regardless of which cornea is touched.

Motor Component

To test the muscles of mastication, i.e. masseter, temporalis and medial pterygoid, patient is asked to close his mouth and clench his teeth.

The examiner palpates the contraction of the muscle on both sides. Muscle contraction should be equal and symmetrical.

The temporalis muscle can be palpated in the temporal fossa during the same maneuver.

To test the lateral pterygoid muscle, ask the patient to open his mouth and protrude the lower jaw. Deviation of the jaw to one side suggests weakness or paralysis on the ipsilateral side.

FACIAL NERVE (MIXED, MAINLY MOTOR)

Anatomy

The facial nerve is a mixed cranial nerve, serving both motor and sensory functions.

- Motor fibers innervate the muscles of facial expression including the platysma, posterior belly of the digastric, stylohyoid muscle and the stapedius muscle.
- Sensory fibers transmit taste from the anterior 2/3rd of the tongue and general sensation from the oropharyngeal musosa around palatine tonsils and a part of the skin in the external ear canal.
- Autonomic fibers innervate the lacrimal gland, submandibular and submaixillary salivary glands.

Motor Portion

The motor nucleus (largest cranial nerve motor nucleus) is in the reticular formation of the lower pons. It is made up of 2 groups of cells: the dorsal group and the ventral group.

The intracranial part of the facial nerve is made up of two distinct anatomical parts:

a. Facial nerve proper which provides motor innervation to the branchial arch derived skeletal muscles.
b. Nervus intermedius—the smaller component which is composed of sensory and autonomic fibers (Fig. 27.16A) corticonuclear projections to the facial nucleus (Fig. 27.16B) central and peripheral ganglia associated with facial nerve.
  - The facial nerve emerges from the cerebellomedullary angle and enteres the temporal bone through the internal auditory meatus. Within the temporal bone (facial canal) the motor axons course posterior medial to the middle ear structures and then inferiorly to exit the skull via the stylomastoid foramen. In the vertical part of the facial canal, it gives off a small branch to the stapedius muscle.

On exiting the stylomastoid foramen, it gives off three small branches—one to the occipital and auricular muscles and two smaller branches to the post belly of the digastric and the stylohyoid. The remaining fibers enter the

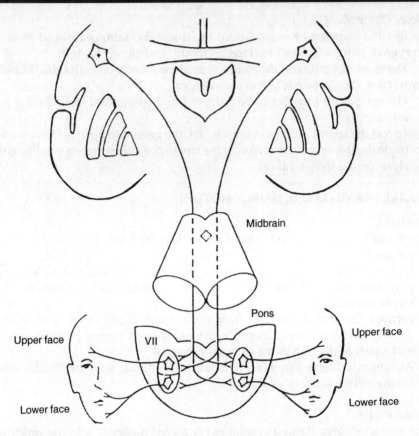

Fig. 27.16A: Corticonuclear projections to the facial nucleus

parotid gland and divide into temporofacial and cervicofacial divisions, which further divide into the terminal 5 branches, e.g. temporal, zygomatic, buccal, mandibular and cervical.

The cortical centre for the muscles of facial expression lie in the lower third of the precentral convolution. Impulses arising in the pyrimidal cells are carried through the corona radiata, genu of the internal capsule, and cerebral peduncles into the pons. Here, they decussate and in a majority supply the facial nucleus on the opposite side.

That portion of the nucleus that innervates the lower half to two-thirds of the face has, predominantly crossed, unilateral, supranuclear control, whereas the portion that supplies the upper one-third to half has bilateral control.

Sensory Portion (Nerves Intermedius)

The cell bodies of the sensory component of the facial nerve form the geniculate ganglion. The peripheral processes innervate tastebuds located ipsilaterally the Ant. 2/3rd of the tongue. Axons conveying taste course with the lingual nerve in the mouth and the chorda tympani in the middle ear. These axons ultimately join the motor axons of the facial nerve in the facial canal just above

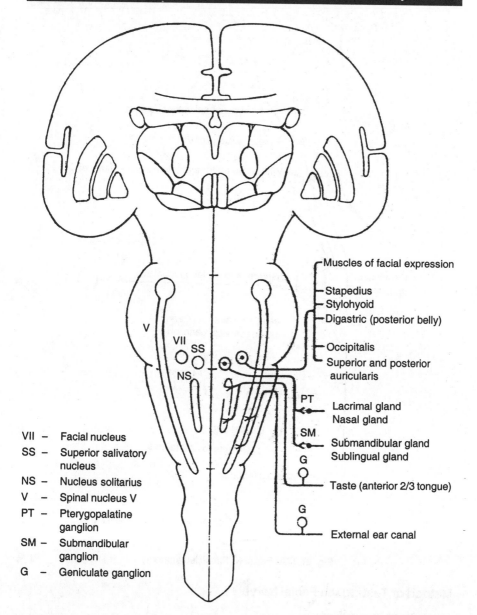

Muscles of facial expression
Stapedius
Stylohyoid
Digastric (posterior belly)
Occipitalis
Superior and posterior auricularis
Lacrimal gland
Nasal gland
Submandibular gland
Sublingual gland
Taste (anterior 2/3 tongue)
External ear canal

VII – Facial nucleus
SS – Superior salivatory nucleus
NS – Nucleus solitarius
V – Spinal nucleus V
PT – Pterygopalatine ganglion
SM – Submandibular ganglion
G – Geniculate ganglion

Fig. 27.16B: Central nuclei and peripheral ganglio associated with the facial nerve

the stylomastoid foramen. The central processes of these sensory nerves reach the brainstem as part of **nerves intermedius.** These axons then enter the tractus solitarus and terminate in the rostral part of the **nucleus solitarus.** As their nucleus also receives synaptic contacts from the neurons innervating tastebuds it is also called **gustatory nucleus** (Figs 27.17A to C) Central and peripheral course, branches of facial nerve.

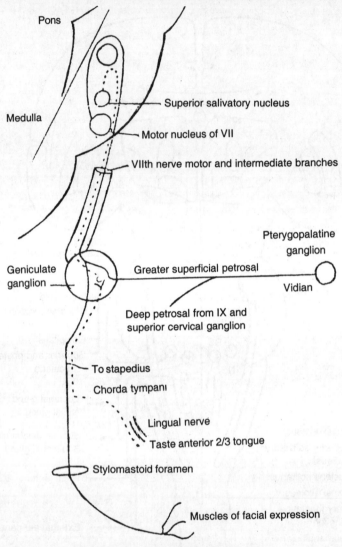

Pons

Medulla

Superior salivatory nucleus

Motor nucleus of VII

VIIth nerve motor and intermediate branches

Pterygopalatine ganglion

Geniculate ganglion

Greater superficial petrosal

Vidian

Deep petrosal from IX and superior cervical ganglion

To stapedius

Chorda tympani

Lingual nerve

Taste anterior 2/3 tongue

Stylomastoid foramen

Muscles of facial expression

Fig. 27.17A: Facial N (Simplified anatomy)

Method of Testing the Facial Nerve

Inspection/Observations

- Appearance of face—symmetry/asymmetry. Facial expressions, mobility, presence of nasolabial fold, corners of the mouth, blinking.
- The affected side of the face is expressionless.
- The nasolabial fold is less pronounced.
- The furrows of the brow may be smoothened out.
- The eye may be more widely open on the affected side than normal side.
- When the patient smiles, mouth may be drawn to the normal side.
- Drooling of saliva on the affected side.

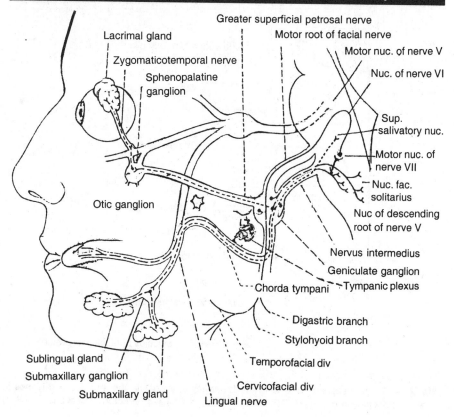

Greater superficial petrosal nerve
Lacrimal gland
Zygomaticotemporal nerve
Sphenopalatine ganglion
Motor root of facial nerve
Motor nuc. of nerve V
Nuc. of nerve VI
Sup. salivatory nuc.
Otic ganglion
Motor nuc. of nerve VII
Nuc. fac. solitarius
Nuc of descending root of nerve V
Nervus intermedius
Geniculate ganglion
Chorda tympani
Tympanic plexus
Digastric branch
Stylohyoid branch
Sublingual gland
Submaxillary ganglion
Temporofacial div
Cervicofacial div
Submaxillary gland
Lingual nerve

Fig. 27.17B: Course and branches of the facial nerve

Testing Motor Functions

1. Ask the patient to close both eyes tightly. The affected eye is either not closed, at all, or if closed, the eyelashes are not deeply burried. Closing the eyes tightly causes the corners of the mouth to be drawn up. On the paralysed side, the corner of the mouth is not drawn up. Next, try to open the eyes, while the patient attempts to close them. Normally, it is impossible to open them against the patients efforts.
2. Bells phenomenon—is a normal phenomenon in which the eyeball rolls upwards during attempted forced eye closure. It is preserved in facial palsy of LMN type.
3. Ask the patient to whistle. This is impossible.
4. Ask the child to smile or show his teeth. The mouth is drawn to the healthy side.
5. Ask the patient to inflate the mouth with air and blow out the cheeks. Tap each inflated cheek with a finger. On the affected side, air escapes easily.
6. To test the platysma ask the patient to protrude the chin and smile widely.

While testing motor functions of facial nerves the UMN and LMN innervation of the facial muscles should be considered (Fig. 27.18).

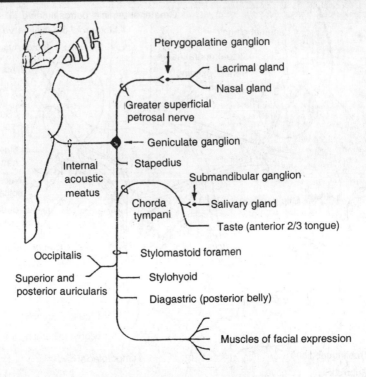

Fig. 27.17C: The peripheral course of the facial nerve, indicating the muscles and glands in nervoted (Modified from Haines, DE: Neuroanatomy: An Atlas of Structures, Sections, and Sys)

Testing Sense of Taste

Ageusia
Loss of sense of taste

Hypogeusia
Decreased sense of taste

Paraguesia
Perversions or abnormal perception of taste
- Sense of taste is tested by using strong solutions of sugar and salt, and weak solutions of citric and quinine, as tests of sweet, salt, sour, and bitter.
- These are applied to the surface of the tongue.
- Ask the child to indicate perception of the taste by pointing out to a set of cards with the tastes written on them. This should be done before the tongue is withdrawn.
- Taste may also be assessed by using a weak electrical stimulus.

Autonomic Functions
In recent lesions of the facial nerve increased lacrimation and salivation are common. This can be tested by:

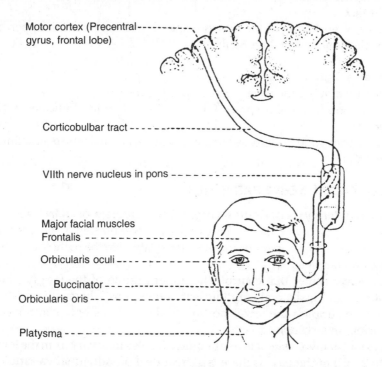

Motor cortex (Precentral
gyrus, frontal lobe)

Corticobulbar tract

VIIth nerve nucleus in pons

Major facial muscles
Frontalis

Orbicularis oculi

Buccinator

Orbicularis oris

Platysma

Fig. 27.18: UMN and LMN innervation of the facial muscles. The dotted lines indicate that the orbicularis oculi muscles receive a variable number of crossed and uncrossed axons. Therefore, the degree of weakness of the muscle varies after UMN lesions

Schirmer's test The amount of tear secretion is evaluated by hanging a litmus paper or filter paper on each lower eyelid and noting the amount of moistening on each side.

Lacrimal reflex Secretion of tears is produced, usually bilaterally, by stimulating the cornea or nasal mucosa.

Salivary reflex Flavored substances are placed on the tongue and secretion of saliva from the submaxillary duct is measured.

MOTOR REFLEXES
Certain motor reflexes of the face are affected in facial nerve lesions. These usually indicate a premature nervous system, regression to an infantile status or frontal lobe lesions.

Glabellar Reflex
- Elicited by gentle repeated percussion with a finger over the root of the nose.
- Normal response is brisk closure of the eyes during the first two or three taps. Persistent response without extinction on repeated taps is abnormal.

Snout Reflex
- Consists of purkering of the lips in response to a tap over the upper lip. This reflex is not elicited normally.

Chovostek's Sign
- Elicited by tapping the facial nerve in front of the ear
- Marked contraction and spasm following such tapping indicates hypocalcemia.

It is a response due to increased irritability of the nerve fibers to mechanical stimulation.

TYPES OF FACIAL NERVE PARALYSIS

Facial Nerve Paralysis of Central Origin (Supranuclear or UMN Type)

In central facial paralysis, there is paresis of the lower portion of the face with relative sparing of the upper portion. It is contralateral to the pathologic lesion and is rarely complete.

The nuclear center that controls the upper portion of the face has both contralateral and ipsilateral supranuclear connections whereas the nuclear centre which supplies the lower portion of the face has only contralateral supranuclear innervation.

The extent of involvement in a supranuclear palsy may vary from the lower 1/3rd to 2/3rd of the face as there is a great deal of individual variation in facial innervation.

Supranuclear lesions do not produce atrophy of the facial nuscles.

Supranuclear facial palsy is of 2 types

Volitional Palsy

In this, involvement is most marked on voluntary contraction. Paresis is apparent when the patient attempts to retract the angle of the mouth. However, on involuntary contraction such as spontaneous smiling or crying, there is preservation of function with little or no evidence of paresis.

Volitional type of central facial paresis results from involvement of
- Cortical center in the lower third of the precentral convolution that control facial movements
  or
- In the pathway between this center and motor nucleus.

Emotional Type of Central Facial Palsy

In this type of central facial palsy, impairment is marked on smiling or crying, however, patient can voluntarily retract his mouth without any difficulty. It results from—extrapyramidal, basal ganglion, thalamic or hypothalamic involvement.

In many cases of supranuclear facial palsy, there is both volitional and emotional involvement.

Peripheral Facial Palsy (Prosopoplegia)
(Nuclear, Infranuclear/ LMN Type)

In the peripheral or LMN type of facial paralysis there is:

- Flaccid paralysis of all muscles of facial expression on the involved side (ipsilateral) and paralysis is complete. In LMN type of paralysis—there is atrophy of the facial muscles.
- Affected side of face is smooth, no wrinkles on forehead.
- Eyebrow droops, eye is open, inferior lid lags
- Nose is flattened or deviated to the opposite side
- Patient is unable to raise eyebrows, frown, close the eyes, smile, cough, show his teeth, whistle, or retract the chin on the affected side.
- On attempted movement, mouth is deviated to normal side
- Food accumulates between teeth and affected cheek
- Saliva may drip from the paretic side
- There is difficulty in articulation, especially vowels which require pursing of lips
- Nasolabial folds are shallow/absent; alae nasi are sunken and do not move with respiration
- Palpebral fissure is wider than normal due to lagopthalmos (inability to close the eye)
- When the patient attempts to close the eye on the involved side, the eyeball turns upwards—Bell's phenomenon
- There is epiphora—excessive tears
- The stapedius may be paralysed—hyperacusis for low tones which appear louder and higher
- In comatose patient—function of the facial nerve is elicited by noting response to painful pressure over the supraorbital ridge.

Levator Sign of Dutemps and Cestan

Elicited by asking the patient to look down and then close the eye slowly. When present the upper lid on the paralysed side moves upwards because the levator palpebrae superioris is no longer counteracted by the orbicularis.

Negros Sign

When the patient raizes his eyes, the eyeball on the affected side deviates outwards and elevates more than the normal one-due to overaction of the superior rectus and inferior oblique.

Bergara-Waternberg Sign

It is an early and sensitive sign of both central and peripheral facial palsy. There is absence of palpable vibrations in the orbicularis oculi as the examiner attempt to open the closed eyelid against resistance.

Platysma Sign of Babinski

Failure of the platysma to contract on the affected side when the mouth is opened.

There are different types of peripheral facial paralysis, depending on the site of the lesion.

They are as follows:

Nuclear or infranuclear lesion within Pons (Tables 27.10 and 27.11)

Lesions in the pons may affect nucleus or the emerging root fibers.
- Complete ipsilateral peripheral facial nerve palsy
- Preservation of sensation and secretory function
- Due to proximity of VII Nerve nucleus with VI nerve nucleus, pontine lesions cause both ipsilateral facial paralysis and ipsilateral lateral rectus palsy.

Table 27.10: Causes of facial weakness in childhood

Congenital-structural	*Trauma-nerve compression*
Chiari malformation	Forceps pressure during delivery
Depressor anguli oris muscle abscense	Cleidocranial dysostosis
(Cardiofacial syndrome)	Histiocytosis X
Inner ear and/or facial nerve malformations	Hyperostosis cranialis interna
Mobius syndrome	Increased intracranial pressure
Syringobulbia	Petrous bone fracture from maternal sacrum
Genetic	
Facio-scapulo-humeral dystrophy	*Metabolic conditions*
Familial cranial neuropathy (recurrent)	Hyperparathyroidism
Fazio-Londe disease	Hypothyroidism
Myasthenia gravis (nonimmune mediated)	Idiopathic infantile hypercalcemia
Myotonic dystrophy	Osteopetrosis
Nemaline myopathy	
	Neoplasms
Infectious-inflammatory	Brainstem glioma
Basilar meningitis	Parotid gland tumors
Bell's palsy	
Epstein-Barr syndrome	*Vascular*
Guillain-Barre syndrome	Arterial hypertension
Miller-Fisher syndrome	Vascular syndromes of the cranial
Mycoplasma pneumoniae infection	nerves
Lyme disease (Borreliosis)	
Otitis media and mastoiditis	*Others*
Parotitis	Idiopathic cranial neuropathy
Poliomyelitis	Melkersson-Rosenthal syndrome
Ramsay Hunt syndrome *(herpes zoster)*	Multiple sclerosis
Sarcoidosis	Myasthenia gravis (immune mediated)
Trichinosis	Myathenia gravis (transient neonatal)
Tuberculosis	

Millard-Gubler syndrome Unilateral facial palsy with unilateral VI nerve palsy with contralateral hemiplegia.

Foville Syndrome Involvement of root fibers causes facial palsy with ipsilateral paralysis of conjugate gaze and contralateral corticospinal hemiplegia.

Table 27.11: Clinical localization of facial nerve lesions

Anatomic site	Facial movement	Lacrimation	Taste	Salivation	Hyperacusis
• Nucleus	Defective	Normal	Normal	Normal	Present
• Pons to internal auditory meatus	Defective	Defective	Normal	Defective	Present
• Geniculate ganglion	Defective	Defective	Defective	Defective	Present
• Ganglion to stapedius nerve	Defective	Normal	Defective	Defective	Present
• Stapedius nerve to Chorda tympani	Defective	Normal	Defective	Defective	Absent
• Below chorda tympani	Defective	Normal	Normal	Normal	Absent

Infranuclear Involvement between Pons and Facial Canal (Cerebellopontile Angle)

The facial nerve lies with the VIII Nerve in the cerebellopontile angle and internal auditory meatus. In lesions at these sites there is:
- Ipsilateral involvement of the entire face
- Tinnitus, deafness, vertigo
- Nerves intermedius is affected therefore loss of taste in the anerior 2/3rd to tongue and decreased lacrimation and salivation.

Involvement within Facial Canal

(Between internal auditory meatus and geniculate ganglion)
- Peripheral type of facial nerve palsy with involvement of nerves intermedius.
  Therefore, loss of taste and decreased lacrimation and salivation
- Hyperacusis due to palsy of nerve to stapedius
- Involvement at this site—usually uncommon

Involvement Peripheral to Geniculate Ganglion but before Departure of Nerve to Stapedius

- Unilateral complete facial palsy
- Hyperacusis
- Loss of taste, impaired secretory fuction
- Pain in the region of eardrum
- There may be herpetic eruption
- This geniculate neuralgia with herpes is called Ramsay Hunts syndrome

Involvement between Departure of Nerve to Stapedius and Departure of Chorda Tympani

- Unilateral facial palsy with loss of taste over anterior 2/3rd on tongue
- Decreased salivary secretion
- Hearing and lacrimation-not affected

Involvement within Facial Canal Distal to
Departure of Chorda Tympani (Bell's Palsy)
- Ipsilateral peripheral facial palsy alone with no other changes.

Involvement within Parotid Gland after Emergence from
Stylomastoid Foramen
- May cause partial involvement as only certain branches may be affected, therefore some muscles of facial expression may be affected.

VESTIBULOCOCHLEAR NERVE

Anatomy
The VIIIth cranial nerve is composed of two fiber systems. These are the cochlear nerve, or the nerve of hearing, and the vestibular nerve, which subserves equilbrium, coordination and orientation in space.

Vestibular Nerve
Receptors of the vestibular nerve are situated in the neuroepithelium in the cristae of the semicircular canals and the macula of the utricle and saccule, in the inner ear. Impulses are carried to the bipolar cells of the vestibular ganglion of Scarpa from which central fibers pass as the vestibular nerve. This nerve enters the medulla at its junction with the pons and fibers go to the vestibular nuclei in the medulla-lateral, medial, superior and inferior nuclei.

All four nuclei send connections to the medial longitudinal fascicullus. This pathway through connections with the nuclei of III, IV, VI and XI nerves, regulates movements of the eye, head and neck in response to stimulation of the semicircular canals. First order neurous from these nuclei go to the cerebellum through the inferior peduncle and end in the flocculomotor lobe. The nuclei also have projections to the temporal lobe (Fig. 27.19). The vestibular pathway.

COCHLEAR NERVE

Anatomy
The endorgans of the cochlear nerve are the hair cells or the auditory cells in the organ of Corti. Impulses travel to the bioplar cells of the spiral ganglion of the cohlea (cochlear ganglion). From here, central fibers emerge as the cochlear nerve. These fibers enter the brainstem at the lower border of the pons and are distributed to the dorsal and ventral cochlear nuclei

The secondary auditory tracts decussate partially and terminate in the inferior colliculus and the medial geniculate body. Fibers orginating from these pass through the internal capsule to the cortical centre for hearing in the first and second temporosphenoidal gyri (Fig. 27.20).

Examination of the Cochlear Nerve (Auditory)
- The first requirement is a quiet environment.

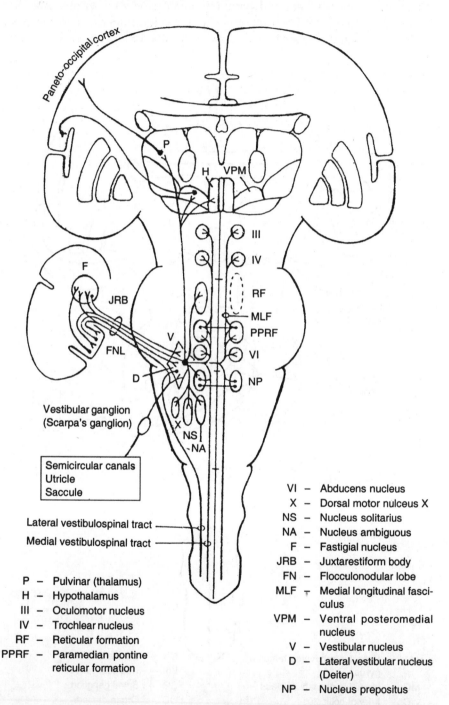

Fig. 27.19: The vestibular pathways, indicating the afferent and efferent connections of the vestibular nudei (Modified from Haines, DE: Neuroanatomy: An Atlas of Structures, Sections)

- Inspect the external ear and tympanic membrane with an otoscope. Ear should be free from obstruction such as foreign material, cerumen, ear perforation, middle ear disease, as these can alter or impair hearing ability.

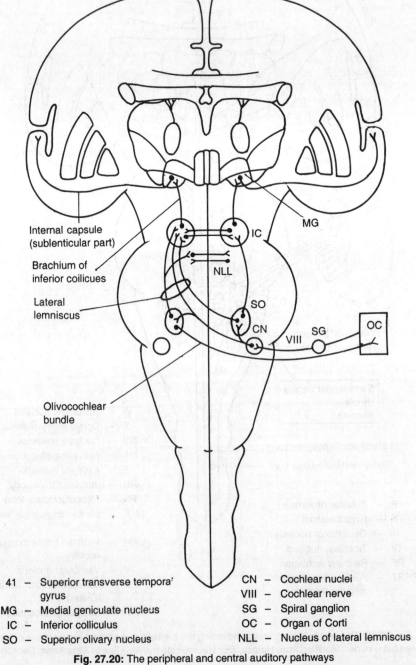

Internal capsule (sublenticular part)

Brachium of inferior coilicues

Lateral lemniscus

Olivocochlear bundle

41	–	Superior transverse temporal gyrus	
MG	–	Medial geniculate nucleus	
IC	–	Inferior colliculus	
SO	–	Superior olivary nucleus	

CN	–	Cochlear nuclei
VIII	–	Cochlear nerve
SG	–	Spiral ganglion
OC	–	Organ of Corti
NLL	–	Nucleus of lateral lemniscus

Fig. 27.20: The peripheral and central auditory pathways

- Note the distance at which the child can hear the sound produced by rubbing of fingers or ticking of a watch and compare the two sides.
- It is important to determine if deafness is due to middle ear disease (conductive) or due to auditory nerve involvemnt (Sensorineural). This is done by the Rinne's test and Weber test.

Rinne's Test

It is used to distinguish between conductive and sensorineural deafness in a patient with reduced hearing.

Performed by using a vibrating tuning fork of 256 or 512 Hz.

- The vibrating tuning fork is placed against the patients mastoid process and the patient is asked to indicate when the tone is no longer heard. At that moment the blades of the tuning fork are brought close to the external auditory meatus and the patient is asked if the tone is heard again.

In individuals with normal hearing the tone will be heard again and will continue to be heard for twice as long. This normal response is documented as AC > BC. Patients with sensorineural deafness will also hear the tone again but the duration percieved by air conduction will be decreased. In this case the test is said to be positive and is documented as AC>BC for that ear. A patient with conductive hearing loss will no longer hear the tone when the tuning fork is brought to the test auditory meatus. The Rinne's test is thus negative and is documented as BC > AC.

Weber Test

It is performed by placing the base of a vibrating tuning fork on the center of the forehead. The patient is asked to indicate on which side, if any, the tone is heard louder.

Normally the tone is heard equally on both sides. Patients with unilateral sensorineural deafness will indicate that the tone is better heard i.e., lateralised to the normal ear. (positive) Patients with unilateral conductive deafness, will indicate that the tone is louder on the diseased side i.e., lateralised to the affected ear (negative).

Fallacies with the Rinne's Test

- Lack of specificity
- Patients with profound unilateral sensorineural hearing loss or a dead ear, will report a Rinne negative when this ear is tested if the other ear has normal hearing. This is due to lack of attenuation of bone conducted sound which is heard in the non-test ear (can be solved by masking the non-test ear with a Barany noise box).

Audiometry

Audiometry is used to assess the degree of hearing loss and the likely site of pathology in the auditory pathway (Fig. 27.21).

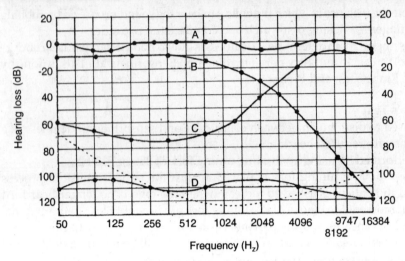

Fig. 27.21: Audiogram A–Normal curves, B–nerve deafness—loss of high tones,
C–Middle ear deafness—loss of low tones, D–Gross loss of hearing

Types of audiometry are:

Pure Tone Audiometry

In this test the threshold for pure tone sounds introduced into each ear is measured for different frequencies. Standardized sound levels are used and compared to the hearing.

In pure sensorineural hearing loss, the bone conduction thresholds mirror the air conduction thresholds, but in conductive hearing loss, the bone conduction thresholds exceed those of air (air-bone gap). This gives a measure of the degree of conductive hearing loss.

Speech Audiometry

The speech audiogram measures the patients ability to recognize and repeat lists of phonetically balanced words arranged in groups of 12, delivered at different intensities to the test ear from a tape recording. The percentage of words correctly repeated is noted at each intensity. Patients with pure conductive deafness will achieve 100 percent discrimination, but at higher intensity than normal. Patients with sensorineural deafness, are unable to achieve 100 percent discrimination at any intensity.

Impedance Audiology

In this test the impedance to the passage of sound energy is measured and is plotted graphically on a tympanogram. This is a measure of movement of the ear drum and compliance in the middle ear.

Evoked Response Audiometry

Involves a group of tests in which evoked responses in the brain are recorded following a sound applied to the ear. The averaged response is displayed on an oscilloscope as a wave form with 7 peaks.

The time taken for the impulse to peaks 1-5 (I-V latency) is measured.

Compressive lesions of the acoustic nerve will cause delay of the impulse (increased I-V latency). Similar delay is seen in patients with brainstem tumors or multiple sclerosis.

Electrocochleography (E Coch G)

It involves the insertion of a needle through the tympanic membrane, and the action potential from the cochlear nerve is measured. This test is mainly used to assess the presence of endolymphatic hydrops, e.g as in Meniere's disease.

Caloric Testing (Vestibular Function)

The patient is made to lie on a couch with the head titled at 30° (to bring the lateral semicircular canal in the vertical plane).

Patient is instructed to fix upon a point in central gaze.

The external ear canal is irrigated with water at 30°C and then 44°C for 30-40 seconds, respectively. This causes a thermal gradient across the temporal bone, which produces convection currents within the endolymph. Cold water induces nystagmus away from the ear being irrigated and warm water induces nystagmus towards the ear being irrigated. Each ear is irrigated with water at both temperatures, with a suitable delay of few minutes between each test and the induced nystagmus is timed for each of the four tests.

The evoked nystagmus may be recorded and analysed using electronystagmograpy.

Patients with nonfunctioning vestibular apparatus or complete vestibular nerve damage will not respond to caloric stimulation on that side, a condition called canal paresis.

Asymmetric response in the two eyes suggests a pontine lesion, disease involving medial longitudinal fasiculus or lesions of the extraocular nerves. A response in which both the eyes are tonically deviated to the side of the cold water irrigated ear suggests bilateral cerebral disease.

Cortical influences in the neurologically intact individual cause a rapid deviation of the eyes in the opposite direction, i.e. away from the cold irrigated side (i.e. contralateral nystagmus). If the cortical component is absent (as is coma), the fast cortically driven movement to the contralateral side is lost, but the slow vestibular driven deviation to the irrigated side will be retained (Fig. 27.22).

The ninth and tenth cranial nerves are considered together since the areas of their innervation overlap.

GLOSSOPHARYNGEAL NERVE

Functional Anatomy

This is a mixed nerve subserving both sensory and motor functions.

Motor

There are two types of motor fibers:
- Axons orginating from nerve cells in the nucleus ambiguous: These axons emerge from the brainstem immedeatly dorsal to the inferior physiological

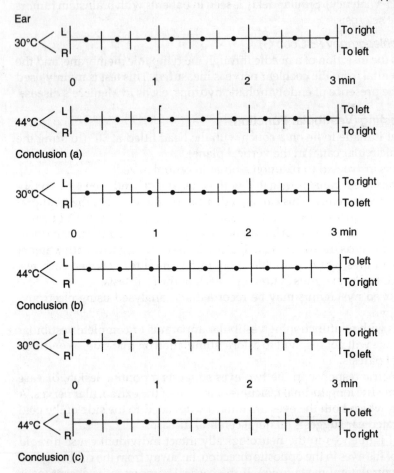

Fig. 27.22: Caloric responses. The broken line marks the time in minutes for which nystagmus on forward gaze persists after the end of irrigation. The temperature of the water is indicated on the left, the direction of the nystagmus on the right. (a) Normal response; (b) Right canal paresis in a case of acoustic neuroma; (c) Directional prepondetance to left in a case of left posterior temporal lobe tumor

olive at its rostral end. They then pass through the jugular foramen and exit the skull. These fibers provide motor innervation to the stylopharyngeus muscle (the only skeletal muscle supplied by this nerve).

- Axons originating from the nerve cells of the inferior salivatory nucleus (preganglionic parasympathetic nerve cell bodies), pass through the jugular foramen and exit the skull. These axons make synaptic contact with the neurons located in the otic ganglion. Postganglionic pararympathetic fibers from the otic ganglion innervate the parotid gland.

Sensory

The afferent fibers of the IXth nerve are also of two types: visceral and somatic. Visceral afferent fibers convey sensation from the pharyngeal mucosa, taste from the posterior one-third of the tongue and impulses from the baroreceptors in the carotid sinus. These fibes terminate in the nucleus solitarus.

Somatic afferent component is small. They convey tactile information from the external ear canal. The central processes of there axons pass through the jugular foramen and terminate in the spinal nucleus of V. Figure 27.23 shows central and peripheral ganglia associated with the glossopharyngeal nerve.

VAGUS NERVE

Functional Anatomy

The vagus nerve is a mixed cranial nerve with both sensory and motor fibers.

Sensory fibers The sensory fibers of the vagus nerve are mainly visceral in nature and transmit information from thoracic and abdominal visceral structures, chemoreceptors in the carotid body and taste receptors on the epiglottis. The cell bodies of these visceral afferent fibers are located in the nodose ganglion (immedeatly outside the jugular foramen). The central processes of the visceral afferent fibers pass through the jugular foramen and synapse in the nucleus solitarus.

The vagus nerve also carries a few somatic afferent fibers which mediate tactile sensation from the external ear canal. There axons terminate in the spinal nucleus of V.

Motor The motor component of the vagus nerve originates from two nuclei in the rostral medulla, i.e. nucleus ambigious and the dorsal motor nucleus of X.

Nucleus Ambigious

Axons arising from the nerve cell bodies in the nucleus ambigius leave the cranium through the jugular foramen.

They supply the muscles of the soft palate, the pharyngeal constrictors, and the intrinsic and extrinsic muscles of the larynx.

Dorsal Motor Nucleus of X

It contains preganglionic, parasympathetic nerve cell bodies. The axons of these cells exit the cranium through the jugular foramen and are distributed widely in the thorax and abdomen. Here, they synapse with postganglionic parasympathetic neurons which in the thorax are associated with various plexsus, e.g. pulmonary and cardiac plexus. In the abdomen they are present in the wall of the visceral structures they innervate. Figure 27.24 shows central and peripheral ganglia associated with the vagus nerve.

Clinical Examination of IX and X Nerves

The glossopharyngeal and the vagus nerves are intimately associated with each other and are similar in function. In many instances they both supply the

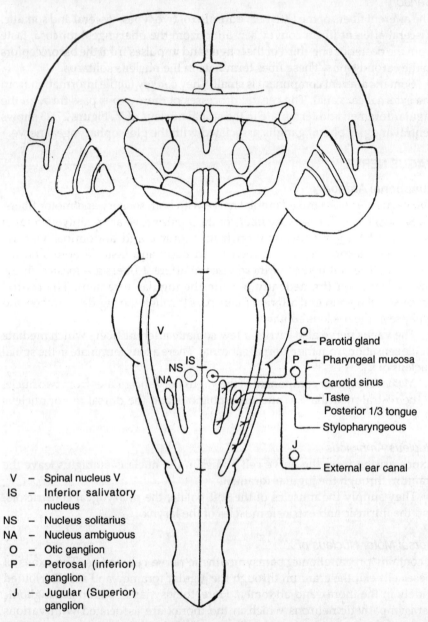

V   –   Spinal nucleus V
IS –   Inferior salivatory
        nucleus
NS –   Nucleus solitarius
NA –   Nucleus ambiguous
O   –   Otic ganglion
P   –   Petrosal (inferior)
        ganglion
J   –   Jugular (Superior)
        ganglion

O – Parotid gland
P – Pharyngeal mucosa
Carotid sinus
Taste
Posterior 1/3 tongue
Stylopharyngeous
External ear canal

Fig. 27.23: The central nuclei and peripheral ganglia association with the glossopharyngeal nerve (IX). (Modified from Haines, DE: Neuroanatomy. An Atlas of Structures, Sections and System)

same structures. They are frequently affected by the same disease processes. Often involvement of one may be difficult to differentiate from that of the other. Hence, they are evaluated together.

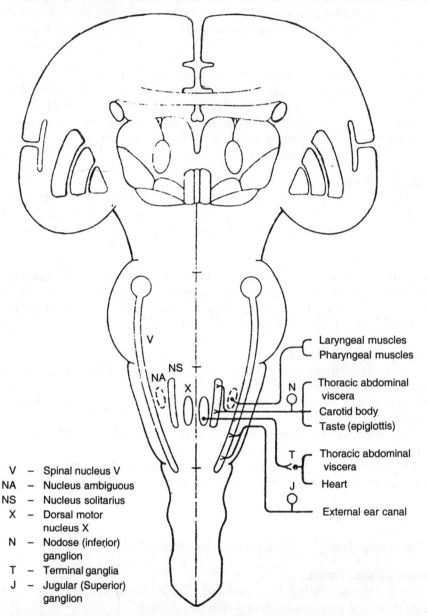

V – Spinal nucleus V
NA – Nucleus ambiguous
NS – Nucleus solitarius
X – Dorsal motor
     nucleus X
N – Nodose (inferior)
     ganglion
T – Terminal ganglia
J – Jugular (Superior)
     ganglion

Fig. 27.24: The central nuclei and peripheral ganglia associated with the vagus nerve (X)

Glossopharyngeal Nerve

The various functions of this nerve are difficult to test because these areas are also supplied by other cranial nerves and also because many of the structures it supplies, are inaccessible.

Motor Function

Motor supply is only to the stylopharyngeus muscle.

If at all any dysfunction is evident, it will be slight unilateral lowering of the palatal arch at rest (although the two sides elevate equally on effort).

Autonomic Function
Can be evaluated by noting the function of the parotid gland.

Salivary reflex	— If highly seasoned foods are placed on the tongue, flow of saliva may be seen from the Stenson's duct.
Afferent	— Carried through the glossopharyngeal.
Efferent	— Conducted from the inferior salivatory nucleus to the parotid gland.

Sensory Function
The several sensory functions of the ninth nerve are difficult to test specifically. But it is possible to test sensation in the region of tonsils, faucies, lateral and posterior pharyngeal walls, and posterior third of the dorsum of the tongue.

Reflexes
The examination of the pharyngeal and palatal reflexes form an important part of the ninth nerve examination. These reflexes are absent if there is interruption of either the afferent or efferent pathway. The pharyngeal (gag) reflex is more sensitive than the palatal (uvular) reflex.

Pharyngeal (GAG) Reflex
This reflex is elicited by applying a stimulus, such as a tongue blade or an applicator, to the posterior pharyngeal wall, tonsillar region, faucial pillars, or even the base of the tongue. The stimulus should be applied to each side of the pharynx.

If the reflex is present, there will be elevation and constriction of the pharyngeal musculature along with retraction of the tongue.

This reflex is used physiologically to initiate deglutition, exaggeration may cause the vomiting reflex. While examining a child this reflex should be tested last as it is unpleasant.

Afferent impulses — through the glossopharyngeal.
Reflex center — is in the medulla.
Efferent impulses — through the vagus nerve.

Palatal (Uvular) Reflex
It is tested by stimulating the lateral and inferior surface of the uvula or the soft palate with a tongue blade or a cotton applicator.

Normally there is elevation of the soft palate and retraction of the uvula occurring simultaneously.

Disorders of function
Lesions of the ninth nerve, especially isolated lesions are not common. The nerve is usually involved in association with the tenth, eleventh, twelfth nerve and other cranial nerves.

A lesion of the ninth nerve may be followed by a slight and transient difficulty in swallowing, especially of dry foods due to paralysis of stylopharyngeus muscle. There is no associated disturbance of speech.

Supranuclear lesions contribute to the syndrome of pseudobulbar palsy, but only if bilateral. Since the motor function of the ninth nerve is minimal, there is no clinical evidence of involvement of this nerve in pseudobulbar palsy. In nuclear lesions, such as progressive bulbar palsy, multiple sclerosis, syringobulbia, neoplasms, botulinism, there is usually associated involvement of other medullary nerves especially the Xth. In glossopharyngeal neuralgia (tic douloureux of the ninth nerve), patient experiences attacks of severe lancinating pain originating in one side of the throat and radiating along the eustachian tube to the ear.

Clinical Examination of the Vagus Nerve

Inspite of its great size and many functions, the vagus nerve is tested with difficulty and means for its examination are inadequate.

Motor Function

Motor supply is to soft palate, larynx and pharynx.

Soft palate   Observe the movements of soft palate and uvula at rest, during breathing and on phonation, usually the uvula hangs in the midline and rises in the midline on phonation.

In unilateral vagus paralysis, there is unilateral lowering and flattening of the palatal arch and the medial raphe is deviated to the normal side. On phonation uvula is retracted to the normal side.

In bilateral vagus nerve weakness, the palate cannot be elevated on phonation. On speaking air escapes into the nasal cavity and this gives speech a characteristic nasal quality.

Figure 27.25 illustrates the tests for uvular deviation.

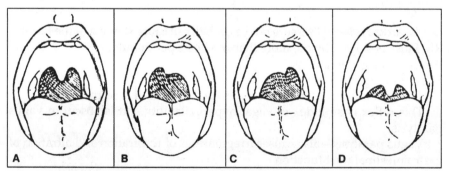

Fig. 27.25: Tests of uvular deviation (cranial nerves IX and X). (A) Normal, (B) Left IX and X palsy, (C) Right IX and X palsy, and (D) Bulbar palsy

There may be severe dysphagia for liquids and there may be regurgitation of fluids through the nasal cavity.

Palatal reflex   In unilateral vagus paralysis, the palatal reflex is lost on the involved side.

In bilateral vagus weakness, the palatal reflex is lost bilaterally.

Pharynx Functions of pharynx are tested by observing contraction of the pharyngeal muscles on phonation-In unilateral paralysis, the Vernet's videau phenomenon many be seen, i.e. curtain movement of the pharyngeal wall to the normal side.
- By testing the pharyngeal reflex
- Noting character of patients speech.
- Difficulty in swallowing liquids and solids especially for solids.
- Coughing may be impaired and there may be decrease in the cough reflex.

Larynx Examination of the larynx includes.
- Noting the character and quality of the voice
- Abnormalities of articulation
- Difficulty with respiration
- Impairment of cough
- Examination of the vocal cords by laryngoscopy.

Normally the vocal cords are abducted during inspiration and adducted on phonation and coughing. Note the position of the vocal cords at rest and movement on phonation and inspiration. In unilateral laryngeal paralysis, voice is hoarse and the vocal cords take up a position between adduction and abduction. In bilateral paralysis, phonation and coughing are impossible and there may be inspiratory stridor. In bilateral adductor palsy, voice is reduced to a whisper.

Autonomic Functions
Of the vagus nerve are difficult to test clinically.

It is the most important parasympathetic nerve of the body.

Vagal paralysis can cause tachycardia and stimulation can cause bradycardia.

Oculocardiac reflex Pressure on the eyeball can cause slowing of the HR and RR. Pulse is slowed by not more than 5-8 beats per minute.
Afferent—trigeminal nerve
Efferent—vagus nerve.

This reflex is inconstant, unstandardised and influenced by emotion.

This reflex is an index of vagal hyperirritability and is absent in vagus paralysis.

Vagus paralysis—also causes irregularities of respiration and altration of gastrointestinal tract function.

Level of Vagus Nerve Involvement
It may be supranuclear, nuclear or infranuclear. Supranuclear involvement is significant when bilateral as in pseudobulbar palsy-dysphagia and dysarthria are due to bilateral supranuclear involvement. Extrapyramidal supranuclear involvement may cause difficulty in swallowing, talking and anomalies of respiratory rhythm.

Nuclear involvement may occur in bulbar poliomyelitis, GB syndrome, botulism, neoplasms vascular lesions.

In slowly progressive lessions as in progressive bulbar palsy, there may be fasciculations of palatal, pharyngeal and laryngeal muscles.

In medullary compression due to trauma, raised intracranial pressure, edema-projectile vomiting and marked variations in HR, RR, and BP.

Infranuclear involvement may follow lesions.

- At the base of the brain-meningitis, basal hemorrhage, aneurysms, skull fractures.
- In the jugular foramen-(along with IX, XI, XII)
- Along the course of the nerve
- Diabetes, toxic, deficiency states affecting the peripheral nerve.
- Diptheritic involvement.
- Individual branches of the vagus nerve may be involved in disease processes in neck, mediastinum, thorax, abdomen.

SPINAL ACCESSORY NERVE

Purely motor nerve that innervates the trapezius and Sternocleidomastoid muscles.

Anatomy

Although considered a cranial nerve, the cells of its origin, are in the upper cervical segments of the spinal cord.

The axons from these cells emerge laterally from the spinal cord and enter the cranium through the foramen magnum. In the cranium, these axons lie in close proximity to axons originating in the nucleus ambiguous which supply the muscles of larynx and pharynx. The fibers then course towards the jugular foramen and exit the skull along with the IX and X cranial nerves. In the neck it supplies the sternocleidomastoid and the trapezius muscles.

Figure 27.26 shows the central and periphral connections of the spinal accessory nerve.

Clinical Examination

This nerve is examined by testing the actions of the 2 muscles.

Inspection of the neck and shoulders for atrophy and fasciculations followed by palpation of both the muscles.

Testing the Sternocleidomastoid

Contraction of this muscle turns the face to the opposite side.

Patient is asked to turn the head to the opposite side against resistance while the examiner palpates the contralateral sternocleidomastoid muscle. This is repeated on the opposite side. Muscle power is noted and compared on both sides (Fig. 27.27).

Testing the Trapezius

Contraction of the trapezius causes upward rotation of the scapula and is involved in shoulder elevation. Patient is asked to elevate or shrug the shoulders against resistance. Muscle power is noted and compared. When the

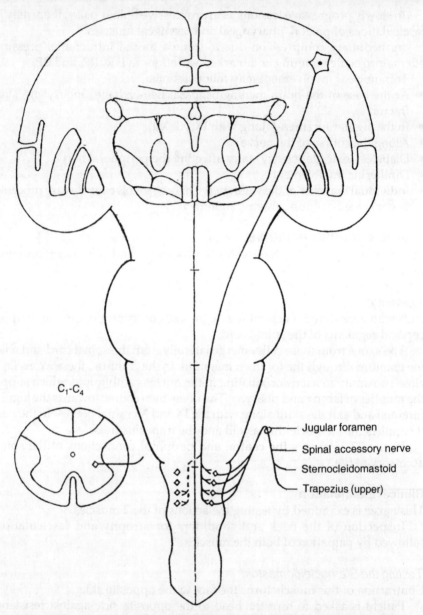

C₁-C₄

Jugular foramen

Spinal accessory nerve

Sternocleidomastoid

Trapezius (upper)

Fig. 27.26: The central peripheral connections of the spinal accessory nerve (XI)

arm is extended anterior to the horizontal, there may be winging of the scapula on the affected side (although less marked than in paralysis of seratius anterior).

CRANIAL NERVE: HYPOGLOSSAL NERVE

Anatomy

The hypoglossal nerve is a purely motor nerve which supplies the muscles of the tongue and the depressors of the hyoid bone.

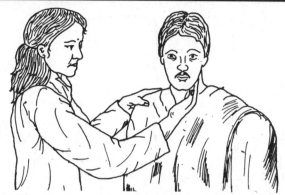

Fig. 27.27: Testing the strength of the sternocleidomastoid muscle (cranial nerve XI)

This nerve arises from the hypoglossal nucleus in the medulla in the lower part of the floor of the fourth ventricle. It emerges from the medulla between the anterior pyramid and the olive. It then travels through the hypoglossal canal and then exits the skull. Through the various branches, it supplies the intrinsic muscles of the tongue, as well as hyoglossus, styloglossus and genioglossus.

The intrinsic muscles of the tongue are concerned with alteration of the shape of the tongue, i.e. narrowing, elongating, shortening and broadening. These movements are required for speech, swallowing and mastication.

The extrinsic muscles, draw the tougue forward (genioglossus), depress the tongue (hyoglossus and chondroglossus) and draw the tongue upwards and backwards (styloglossus).

Figure 27.28 shows the central and peripheral connections of the hypoglossal nerve.

Clinical Examination

Inspection: of the tongue resting in the floor of the mouth. Carefully examine the position, mass, atrophy and contour of the tongue. Note any abnormal movements such as fasciculations or tremors. Inspect the position of the tongue at rest and protrusion for paralysis as illustrated in Figure 27.29.

Fasciculations

They are small contractions like movements that are evident when the tongue is at rest. They may not be as evident when the tongue is protruded, e.g. Spinal muscular atrophy.

Tremors

They are accentuated on protrusion of the tongue. They usually disappear when the tongue is at rest whereas fasciculations persist. Coarse tremors are seen in parkinsonism. All tremors may be accentuated by protrusion of the tongue or by talking.

In chorea, there may be irregular, jerky movement of the tongue and patient is unable to keep the tongue protruded.

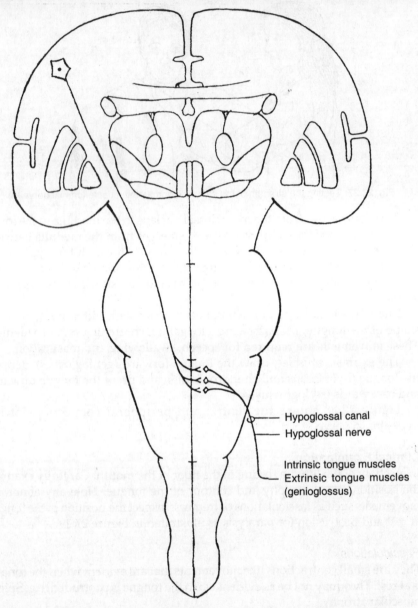

Hypoglossal canal
Hypoglossal nerve

Intrinsic tongue muscles
Extrinsic tongue muscles
(genioglossus)

Fig. 27.28: The central and peripheral connections of the hypoglassal nerve (XII)

Athetoid
Dystonic movements, habit spasms and tics may involve the tongue.

Palpation of the tongue should be done to assess and confirm unilateral atrophy. When atrophy is present there is loss of muscle substance, first apparent at the tip and borders of the tongue. The tongue is wrinkled, furrowed, and the mucous membrane on the affected side is thrown into folds.

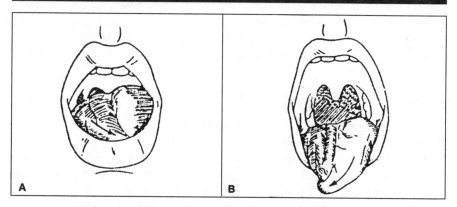

Fig. 27.29: Hypoglossal nerve (cranial nerve XII). (A) Right XII paralysis, tongue at rest, and (B) Right XII paralysis, tongue protruding

Movements of the Tongue

Patient is asked to protrude the tongue and move it in and out; side to side, up and down—both slowly and rapidly.

Ask the patient to press the tip of the tongue against the cheek, while the strength of this pressure is tested by the examiners finger placed outside the cheek.

Morphologic Changes of the tongue may have diagnostic significance.
- Ankyloglossia (tongue tie) may simulate paresis.
- Macroglossia is seen in Down's syndrome and cretinism.
- Tongue hypertrophy is seen in parkinsonism and other dyskinesias where the tongue is constantly protruded.

SPEECH

Patients with hypoglossal nerve lesions have difficulty uttering lingual words. A simple test is to ask the patient to say "la, la, la " or "tee, tee, tee" or "dee dee dee". These sounds will be poorly pronounced as normal enunciation requires pushing the tongue against the hard palate.

These patients may also have difficulty with manipulation of food in the mouth and swallowing (dysphagia).

Patients with bilateral lesions of the hypoglossal nerve may have difficulty with respiration as the tongue tends to fall backwards into the oropharynx.

Types of Paralysis

Glossoplegia (paralysis of the tongue) may be due to supranuclear, nuclear or infranuclear lesions.

In Supranuclear Lesions

Of the hypoglossal nerve, there is paresis with deviation of the tongue but no atrophy. Since the genioglossus, the principal protractor of the tongue has crossed supranuclear innervation, the tongue protrudes towards the paralysed side, but to the side opposite the cerebral lesion.

In Nuclear and Infranuclear Lesions

There is atrophy of the involved side of the tongue in addition to paralysis and deviation. The deviation is towards the paralysed side which is also the side of the lesion.

EXAMINATION OF MOTOR SYSTEM

Brief Review of Neuroanatomy Related to Examination of Motor System

The motor systems are composed of functionally organized groups of neurons that regulate muscle activity necessary for the maintenance of posture and the purposeful and coordinated perturbations of posture we refer to as movement. From a clinical perspective, the motor system makes it possible for individuals to express their wants, needs, feelings, experiences, and general state of health and wellbeing. Motor system dysfunction not only can make it difficult for people to carry out activities of daily living efficiently and effectively but, in more extreme cases, may deprive them of the ability to satisfy basic needs or even to communicate their wants and needs to others. The clinician therefore must be able to recognize motor disturbances, understand their meaning and significance, and take corrective measures when possible or necessary.

To organize an approach to the examination of the motor systems, the motor systems can be divided into **peripheral** and **central components**. The peripheral components consist of alpha and gamma motor neurons, their axons, the skeletal muscles they innervate, and the neuromuscular junction. The central components consist of functionally organized groups of neurons in the forebrain, brainstem, and cerebellum, which are known to influence the activity of alpha and gamma motor neurons.

The following brief summary of the organization of the peripheral and central components of the motor systems will acquaint or reacquaint with fundamental concepts that form the basis for specific tests of motor function and will help the clinican to interpret the result of these tests.

Peripheral Components

The peripheral components of the motor systems are composed of muscles of various types and the neurons that innervate them. Physiologically and functionally, two distinct types of muscles can be divided extrafusal muscles and intrafusal muscles. Extrafusal muscles cross one or more joints and therefore are directly involved in the control of posture and the production of movement. Extrafusal muscles are innervated by alpha motor neurons, so named because they transmit nerve impulses at velocities that define the alpha range (80 to 120 meters per second). Intrafusal muscles are small, striated muscles located in the polar regions of the muscle spindle. Contraction of intrafusal muscle fibers increase tension in the muscle spindle but do not result in movement. Muscle spindles are innervated by gamma motor neurons, so named because they transmit nerve impulses more slowly, at velocities that define the gamma range (15 to 30 meters per second).

An important concept regarding the peripheral components of the motor system is the motor unit defined as consisting of an alpha motor neuron, its axon and collateral branches, and all of the skeletal muscle fibers it axon and collateral branches, and all of the skeletal muscle fibers it innervates. Motor units in muscles used for fine, skilled movements such as speech, eye control, or manipulation tasks with the hands tend to be small, meaning that the ratio of alpha motor neurons to the number of skeletal muscle fibers they innervate is low. In contrast, motor units in muscles used predominantly for postural and locomotor activities, such as the paraspinal and limb-girdle muscles, tend to be considerably larger, with a single alpha motor neuron providing motor innervation to many skeletal muscle fibers.

Alpha motor neurons are frequently referred to as lower motor neurons; with their axons and collateral branches, they constitute the final common pathway by which nerve impulses reach skeletal muscles to cause them to contract. The final common pathway, therefore, is the final link in the chain of neurons that control posture and movement.

Central Components

The central components of the motor systems are functionally more numerous and organizationally more complicated than are the peripheral components. Two distinct types of central nervous system neurons that influence motor behavior can be described: upper motor neurons and neurons composing functional systems that influence upper motor neurons. With regard to the latter, this discussion will be limited to the neurons and neuronal pathways commonly associated with the cerebellum and basal nuclei.

Upper Motor Neurons (Cortical)

Clinically, the term upper motor neuron is generally used to refer to nerve cells located in the primary motor regions of the cerebral cortex. These cells are located in the posterior part of the frontal lobe (areas 4, 6 and 8) and in the anterior part of the parietal lobe (areas 3, 1, 2 and 5). In the neurologic examination, cortical upper motor neurons can be divided into two groups: those that influence alpha and gamma motor neurons located in cranial nerve motor nuclei and those that influence alpha and gamma motor neurons located in the ventral horn of the spinal cord. Axons of the former compose the corti-conuclear (corticobulbar) tracts. Axons of the later compose the corticospinal system, which course through the brainstem to influence lower motor neurons in the spinal cord. The motor system examination focuses primarily on motor functions mediated by spinal motor neurons.

Corticospinal upper motor neurons are organized somatotopically in the primary motor cortices of the posterior frontal and anterior parietal lobes. Corticospinal neurons that influence lower motor neurons located at lumbar and sacral spinal levels are found along the medial surface of the hemisphere, in the sagittal sulcus, whereas those that affect lower motor neuron of cervical and upper thoracic levels are located on the dorsal and dorsolateral surfaces of the hemisphere. The axons of these cells course through the subcortical white matter (corona radiata) immediately deep to the cortical areas from which they arise (Fig. 27.30). At the level of the thalamus, they lie in the posterior

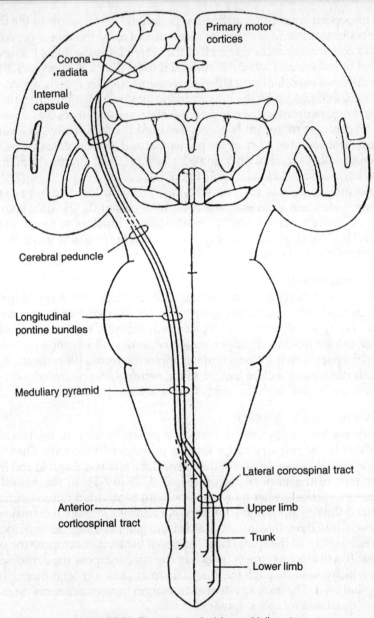

Fig. 27.30: The corticospinal (pyramidal) system

limb of the internal capsule; at the level of the midbrain, they lie in the middle portion of the cerebral peduncle. Corticospinal fibers retain their somatotopic organization in both the internal capsule and the cerebral peduncle. The fibers pass through the pontine nuclei, and at the level of the medulla oblongata, they lie on its ventral surface, forming the medullary pyramid. The majority of these axons cross the midline in the pyramidal decussation. In the spinal cord, corticospinal axons that crossed the midline in the pyramidal decussation constitute the lateral corticospinal tract, and those that remained uncrossed form the anterior ventral corticospinal tract. Within the spinal gray matter, these axons make either direct or indirect synaptic contact with the dendrites of alpha motor neurons and, to a lesser degree, with those of gamma motor neurons.

Corticospinal axons have frequently been referred to as part of the pyramidal system, a name reflecting the fact that the axons are located within the medullary pyramid. The term corticospinal system is sometimes also used to refer to these fibers.

Clinically Important Anatomic Facts

First, about 85 to 90 percent of the approximately 1 million axons that form each medullary pyramid decussate at caudal medullary levels to achieve a position in the contralateral half of the spinal cord. These axons occupy a position in the dorsal part of the lateral funiculus and are organized somatotopically so that those axons that will terminate at more caudal levels (Fig. 27.30). Collectively, these axons constitute the lateral corticospinal tract, which extends the full length of the spinal cord. Axons that do not cross the midline in the pyramidal decussation maintain their ventral position within the spinal cord and are located in the ventral funiculus of the spinal cord, where they constitute the anterior (ventral) corticospinal tract. But do not seem to be somatotopically organized within the ventral funiculus.

The relative position of the lateral and anterior corticospinal tracts within the spinal white matter suggests that they may preferentially influence specific lower motor neuron pools within the ventral horn. The lateral corticospinal tract axons influence predominantly limb-related lower motor neurons, whereas anterior corticospinal tract axons seem to exert their effects on neurons innervating axial muscle groups. Moreover, lateral corticospinal tract axons that terminate at spinal levels forming the brachial plexus seem to exert a greater influence on lower motor neurons that innervate the finger flexors and wrist extensors than on other functionally related groups of lower motor neurons.

Second, axons composing the lateral corticospinal tract are not equally distributed to all levels of the spinal cord. Estimates indicate that approximately 55 percent of the axons forming the lateral corticospinal tract terminate at spinal levels contributing to the brachial plexus (C-5 through T-1), with an additional 25 percent ending in spinal segments of origin of the lumbosacral plexus (L-2 through S-2). Lateral corticospinal tract axons terminate within the spinal gray matter on the ipsilateral side.

In contrast, the axons of the anterior corticospinal tract seem to be distributed fairly evenly to all spinal segments. Moreover, unlike lateral corticospinal axons, as many as 50 percent of the axons of the anterior corticospinal tract may recross the midline in the anterior white commissure of the spinal cord to make synaptic contact with alpha motor neurons in the medial portion of the ventral horn on the contralateral side. This observation suggests that axial muscles, which are innervated by lower motor neurons in the medial portion of the ventral horn, receive synaptic input from both cerebral hemispheres, whereas limb muscles (particularly distal limb muscles) are influenced exclusively by the contralateral cerebral cortex.

A third clinically important fact regarding corticospinal axons concerns those that decussate at the level of the caudal medulla in the pyramidal decussation. Axons that terminate at more rostral levels of the spinal cord decussate more rostrally in the pyramidal decussation, while those destined for more caudal spinal levels cross more caudally in the pyramidal decussation (Fig. 27.30). This observation may be valuable when interpreting motor findings produced by small, localized lesions in the ventral part of the caudal medulla.

Upper Motor Neurons (Brainstem)

In addition to the cerebral cortex, certain brainstem nuclei also contain upper motor neurons. Chief among these nuclei are the red nucleus, the vestibular nuclei, the nuclei of the superior colliculus, and nuclei of the mesencephalic tegmentum.

Red Nucleus

The red nucleus is the origin of axons that cross the midline at caudal mesencephalic levels and lie in the lateral part of brainstem reticular formation. In the spinal cord, these axons lie intermingled with those of the lateral corticospinal tract and, like lateral corticospinal tract axons, terminate in motor nuclei located largely in the lateral part of the ventral horn (Fig. 27.31). The majority of the axons of the rubrospinal tract end at the level of the cervical enlargement, although the tract has been shown to extend caudally to upper sacral levels. The red nucleus influences upper limb flexor muscle groups predominantly, although effects on other upper limb muscle groups cannot be ruled out. It is unlikely that rubrospinal tract axons exert any significant influence on lower motor neurons that innervate axial muscles.

Vestibular Nuclei

The vestibular nuclei are the origin of two descending tracts that influence spinal lower motor neurons. The lateral vestibulospinal tract originates from the lateral vestibular nucleus (Deiter's nucleus) and lies in the ventral part of the ipsilateal lateral funiculus (Fig. 27.31). The tract extends the full length of the spinal cord, suggesting that it influences motor neurons innervating both upper and lower limb muscles. The location of these axons within the spinal white matter suggests further that their influence is exerted predominantly on extensor muscle groups of the upper and lower limbs. The inferior and medial vestibular nuclei are the origin of axons that lie medially in the caudal brainstem, intermixed with the axons of the medial longitudinal fasciculus. In the spinal cord, these axons form the medial vestibulospinal tract and are found in the ventral funiculus of the spinal cord. The medial vestibulospinal tract contains axons originating from both the ipsilateral and contralateral vestibular nuclei. The position of these axons in the ventral funiculus of the

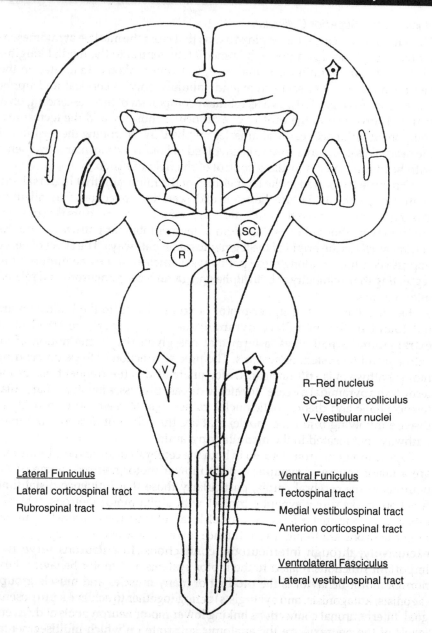

R–Red nucleus
SC–Superior colliculus
V–Vestibular nuclei

Lateral Funiculus
Lateral corticospinal tract
Rubrospinal tract

Ventral Funiculus
Tectospinal tract
Medial vestibulospinal tract
Anterion corticospinal tract

Ventrolateral Fasciculus
Lateral vestibulospinal tract

Fig. 27.31: The origin, course, and location within the spinal cord of major upper motor neuron pathways

spinal cord suggests that they preferentially influence axial muscle groups, particularly extensor muscles of the neck and trunk. The vestibulospinal pathways exert excitatory effects on extensor muscles of the limbs, particularly limb-girdle muscles, and on extensor muscles of the neck and trunk.

Nuclei of the Superior Colliculus

The superior colliculus, the origin of axons that cross the midline at midmesen-cephalic levels occupy a position immediately ventral to the medial longitu-dinal fasciculus. Within the spinal cord, tectospinal axons are located in the ventral funiculus and seem to extend caudally only to cervical and upper thoracic levels (Fig. 27.31). The tectobulbar component of this descending fiber system is involved in the control of extraocular muscles, and the tectospinal component influences cervical muscles involved in controlling the position of the head. This pathway seems to be involved in linking extraocular movements with head movements to allow control of the field of vision.

Other nuclei located in the tegmentum of the midbrain (that is, dorsal and ventral tegmental nuclei) are the origin of descending projections that infleunce lower motor neurons in the brainstem and spinal cord. The dorsal tegmental nuclei may be thought of as the origin of tegmentobulbar pathways, and the ventral nuclei as the origin of the tegmentospinal pathways. The effect of nerve impulse conduction along these pathways is unclear; it may be important in regulating the excitability of both alpha and gamma motor neurons and related interneurons.

Because the axons of upper motor neurons located in the brainstem are not found in the medullary pyramid, they are properly referred to as extrapyramidal pathways, a term that has given rise to the notion of an extrapyramidal system or systems. The precise function of these descending motor pathways is still unclear. Unfortunate also is the frequent use of the term "extrapyramidal disease" to refer to disease processes involving particular telencephalic and diencephalic nuclei, rather than to refer more correctly to disease involving brainstem nuclei that are the origin of descending motor pathways not located in the medullary pyramid.

Upper motor neurons located in both the cerebral cortex and the brainstem are a major source of synaptic input to lower motor neurons. Some of the neurons in the cerebral cortex, particularly those that influence distal limb function, make direct synaptic contact with alpha motor neurons, whereas others exert indirect effects by way of local interneurons. Brainstem upper motor neurons are thought to influence lower motor neurons largely, if not exclusively, through interneuronal connections. Interneurons serve two important functions related to the motor systems and motor behavior. First normal motor behavior is the product of many muscles and muscle groups (agonists, antagonists, and synergists) acting together to achieve a purposeful goal. Interneuronal connections linking lower motor neuron pools at different levels of the neuraxis are the anatomic substrate on which multisegmental motor neurons act and is therefore as important as excitation for normal motor behavior. These important inhibitory functions are considered to be mediated by specific groups of local interneurons.

Several specialized regions of the brain, which, by virtue of their fiber connections, influence the activity of the upper motor neurons just described. Three functionally and clinically distinct sources of input to upper motor neurons are considered:

1. The association cortex
2. The basal nuclei
3. The cerebellum

Only a brief review is presented here. This brief synopsis is intended to make the tests of motor function described later in the chapter and their interpretation seem reasonable and appropriate.

Association Cortex

The cerebral cortex is functionally diverse collection of nerve cells. One way of ordering our thinking is to distinguish between primary cortical areas (sensory and motor) and association areas of the cortex. Primary sensory cortices receive input from specific thalamic nuclei, or in the case of smell, from the olfactory bulb. Primary motor cortices, by definition, contain neurons that contribute axons to the corticospinal and corticobulbar (corticonuclear) tracts. The remaining areas of the cerebral cortex are referred to as association cortices. The association cortices can be further divided into sensory association cortex and motor associations cortex.

The primary sensory cortices project heavily to related sensory association cortices, where some interpretation of the sensory experience takes place. Sensory association cortices, in turn, project to other association cortices within the same hemisphere and, through the corpus callosum and other commissural connections, to association cortices in the contralateal hemisphere. Many sensory association areas project in turn to the primary motor and motor association cortices, thereby providing cortical upper motor neurons with information transmitted to and processed by brain areas associated with the sensory systems.

The prefrontal areas of the frontal lobe are rich source of input to the primary motor cortices, particularly to those areas lying anterior to upper motor neurons and is important not only in the control of simple voluntary movements but also in the regulation and expression of emotionally charged motor behaviors. Thus, upper motor neurons located in the primary motor cortices can be influenced by a wide variety of cortical areas, each of which may be influenced by a wide variety of cortical areas, each of which may be involved in very different aspects of brain function. Damage to association areas of the cerebral cortex or to the axons that interconnect these areas with the motor cortex typically presents as apraxias and agnosias. Other signs and symptoms not associated with motor function may also be produced by lesions that affect the motor and sensory association cortices.

Basal Nuclei

The basal nuclei are a group of subcortical structures located deep within each cerebral hemisphere. They consist of the striatum (caudate and putamen), the globus pallidus, and the amygdaloid nucleus. Input to the basal nuclei originates largely from the cerebral cortex and is directed mainly to the striatum. The striatum also receives synaptic input from the substantia nigra. Striatal efferent neurons terminate largely in the globus pallidus. The globus pallidus is the major output nucleus of the basal nuclei and is the origin of fibers that influence upper motor neurons in both the brainstem (red nucleus and dorsal and ventral tegmental nuclei) and cerebral cortex (corticospinal and corticobulbar neurons, influences through the ventral anterior and ventral lateral nuclei of the thalamus. The globus pallidus is strongly influenced by neurons located in the subthalamic nucleus. Although the exact role of the basal nuclei and their associated nuclei in the control of posture and movement remains unclear, specific deficits associated with disease or injury involving several of these nuclei are well-characterized.

A simple but useful, idea regarding the function of the basal nuclei is to consider them important in determining which upper motor neurons need to be activated (or inhibited) to produce a desired motor behavior. This idea is based on clinical observations suggesting that motor deficits associated with disease involving the basal nuclei are characterized by the inappropriate receuitment of motor units (too many or too few) for the intended behavioral task. In some cases, movements are difficult to initiate, and in others, unintended or unneeded movements are present. Not infrequently, both types of problems are evident in the same patient.

Cerebellum

The cerebellum receives input from the vestibular apparatus, muscle spindles located throughout the body, the inferior olivary nuclei, and the cerebral cortex by way of the pontine nuclei. Like the basal nuclei, the output of the cerebellum is directed toward upper motor neurons in the brainstem and cerebral cortex. Brainstem upper motor neurons influenced by the cerebellum are located chiefly in the red nucleus and the vestibular nuclei. Cortical upper motor neurons are those that give rise to the corticospinal and corticobulbar tracts. Cerebellar influences on cortical upper motor neurons, like those of the basal nuclei, are mediated by way of projections through the ventral lateral nucleus of the thalamus. The cerebellum is important in determining when upper motor neurons need to be activated (or inhibited) to produce a desired movement. Motor deficits associated with diseases of the cerebellum are characterized by an inappropriate sequencing in the activation and deactivation of upper motor neurons and, consequently, of lower motor neurons. Patients with cerebellar disease appear to have difficulty adjusting the amplitude, direction, and velocity of their intended movements.

In summary, lower motor neurons and their axons represent the final common pathway that leads to muscle contraction. Lower motor neurons are influenced by upper motor neurons located in both the cerebral cortex and brainstem. Upper motor neuron influences are mediated largely by way of local interneurons, which can exert either excitatory or inhibitory effects on lower motor neuron pools. Upper motor neurons, in turn, are influenced by a wide range of brain areas, including association areas of the cerebral cortex, the basal nuclei, and the cerebellum. Ultimately, the function of the motor systems is to excite or inhibit selected lower motor neuron pools required to carry out a particular motor behavior, and to do so in the proper sequence. The signs and symptoms produced by lesions affecting particular components of the motor system reflect an inability to properly carry out these two important physiologic processes.

FUNCTIONAL COMPONENTS OF MOTOR SYSTEM INCLUDES (IN BRIEF)
A. Upper motor neurons (UMN)
B. Internuclear neurons-in between upper and lower motor neurons
C. Lower motor neurons (LMN)

Upper Motor Neurons
The primary motor projection cortex is located in the anterior wall of the central sulcus and the adjacent portion of the precentral gyrus, corresponding to the distribution of the Betz cells (giant pyramidal cells). These cells control the movement of the opposite side of the body. The motor cortex has the body represented in an upside down fashion except that face and individual muscles are represented separately. Motor action from the cerebral cortex comes down in two ways:
1. Directly down to cranial nerve nuclei or anterior horn cells (corticobulbar and corticospinal pyramidal tracts).
2. First to basal ganglia and then to lower motor neurones (anterior horn cells). This is extrapyramidal system.

UMN is the nerve cells of the motor cortex with its processes which pass through the internal capsule, to the brainstem and spinal cord. In the brain stem they end around the cranial nerve nuclei and in the spinal cord they end around the spinal motor nuclei in ventral gray horn of the spinal cord. Ninety-five percent cross over, 5 percent are ipsilateral. In cranial nerves, control is almost always unilateral except 12th and facial nerve which have bilateral innervation.

Extrapyramidal system consists of cortical portion, striatal portion (basal ganglia, thalamus and subthalamus, corpus striatum) tegmental (rednucleus and connections) concerned with postural adjustments, autonomic integration. Lesion of extrapyramidal system at any level diminishes or abolishes voluntary movements and replaces them with involuntary movements. There are dyskinesia and rigidity along with autonomic disturbances.

LMN is the final common pathway from anterior horn cell of spinal cord to peripheral nerve to motor end plates of the muscle.

Main Clinical Features of Motor Disorders
I. **LMN syndrome**
   • Weakness
   • Decreased muscle tone
   • Absent tendon reflexes
   • Muscle wasting, often severe
   • Fascultation in affected muscles
   • Distribution of weakness and wasting consistent with lesion in spinal segment, nerve root or peripheral nerve.

II. UMN syndrome

- Weakness in corticospinal distribution, shoulder abduction and finger movements, hip flexion and toe dorsiflexion
- Spastic increase in muscle tone
- Increased tendon reflexes
- Extensor plantar response
- Little or no atrophy

III. Extrapyramidal syndrome

- Plastic or spastic increase in muscle tone
- Abnormal postures
- Involuntary movements and tremors
- Normal or increased tendon reflexes
- Plantar responses normal or extensors.

Motor System

It is tested under the following headings.

- A. Bulk (Nutrition)
- B. Tone
- C. Power
- D. Coordination and gait
- E. Abnormal movements
- F. Reflexes

Nutrition

The bulk of muscles of both upper and lower limbs is looked for on inspection by careful comparison between two sides and by actual measurement at identical points on both limbs. A difference of > 0.5 cm is considered significant. Sometimes there is generalised wasting. Some other findings seen are.

Atrophy When muscle mass is diminished in size, and the limb loses its normal contour. It may result from LMN lesions, muscular dystrophies, disuse atrophy, peroneal atrophy. Atrophy is proximal in myopathies and distal in neuron disease.

Hypertrophy There is increase in size of the muscle. It may be due to developmental defect or may result from increased occupational use and myotonia congenita.

Pseudohypertrophy There is no increase of muscular element but hypertrophy is due to increase of fibrous and other elements. Seen in pseudohypertrophic muscular dystrophy (DMD, etc).

Tone

Muscle tone (tonus) is a state of continuous mild contraction of the muscle dependent upon the integrity of the CNS, peripheral nerves and properties of the muscle itself. Alternatively tone is defined as the degree of tension present in a muscle at rest.

To test the tone, the child must be relaxed and comfortable and lying supine with the head and neck in neutral position.

Tone is tested by

a. Inspection of the muscle
b. Palpation of the muscle
c. Passive movements of the joints (Resistance to passive movements)
d. By shaking the limb

a. *Inspection* The atonic limbs assume a posture of limpness and lies externally rotated. If both lower limbs are hyptonic they will be in "pitched frog" position.

Hypertonic muscles stands out prominently and depending on the muscles involved, limb will have different postures, e.g. decorticate, decerebrate etc.

b. *Palpation* Atonic muscle on palpation is soft and flabby and hypertonic muscle is rigid and spastic.

Passive movements of the joints Normal muscle has a certain amount of resilience and when passively stretched by a joint movement, a certain amount of involuntary resistance is encountered.

Method

Upperlimbs

Arms Take the hand as if to shake it and hold the forearm, first pronate and supinate the forearm, then roll the hand around at the wrist. Hold the forearm at the elbow and move the arm through the full range of flexion and extension at the elbow (Fig. 27.32).

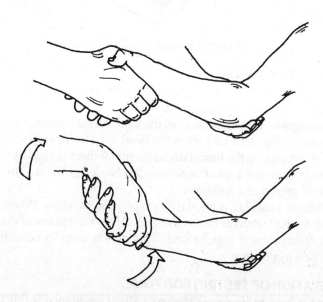

Fig. 27.32: Testing tone in upper limbs

A simple test would be to raise both arms and let them passively fall comparing on 2 sides.

Test the tone by passively moving all the joints in their possible movements.

Lower limbs Tests for assessment of tone in the lower limbs is often usually done in knee and ankle joints. However, the tone should be tested by passively moving all the joints (Proximal and distal) in their possible movements.

At hip With the patient lying with legs straight, roll the knee from side to side. This also induces relaxation (Fig. 27.33).

At knee Put the hand behind the knee and lift it rapidly, watch the heel. Hold the knee and ankle. Flex and extend the knee.

At ankle Hold the ankle and flex and dorsiflex the foot.

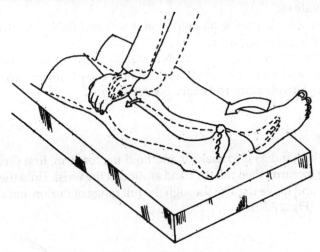

Fig. 27.33: Roll the knee for testing the tone

Testing Tone in Neck Muscles

a. Place both hands under the occipital region and gently raise the head forwards until the chin rests on the chest.

b. Bring the supine child to the edge of the table or bed with shoulders resting on the edge of the table and allow the head to be independent of support. In case of hypotonia, the head falls suddenly. If there is rigidity the head is pulled back due to spasm of neck muscles. Neck rigidity due to any cause is a sign of meningeal irritation.

c. Neck drop or head lag is an early sign of polio myelitis. When a child is lifted off the bed with his hands the neck follows the plane of the trunk, in early poliomyelitis it lags behind. This also is seen in conditions with generalised hypotonia.

INTERPRETATION OF TESTING FOR TONE

Normal tone is said to be present when a slight resistance is felt through a whole range of movement.

Decreased Tone

Loss of resistance through movement. Heel does not lift off the bed when knee is lifted quickly. Decreased tone is noted in all LMN disorders, shock period of UMN lesion (few minutes to weeks), in certain brain lesions, and systemic disorders(PEM, Rickets, etc).

Marked loss of tone is called flaccidity.

Causes of Hypotonia

Combined Central and Peripheral Nervous System Disease

1. Adrenoleucodystrophy
2. Cerebellothalamospinal degeneration
3. Infantile neuroaxonal dystrophy
4. Metachromatic leucodystrophy
5. Krabbe's disease
6. Prader Willi syndrome
7. Zelleweger syndrome

Upper Motor Unit Disease

1. Any acute cerebral insult: CVA, HIE,
2. Infections like (viral, bacterial, fungal, parasitic)
3. Chromosomal anomalies: Down's syndrome, Prader Willi's
4. Congenital motor disease: Atonic or Ataxic cerebral palsy.
5. Incontinentia pigmenti.
6. Metabolic diseases: Carnitine deficiency, gangliosidosis, hypercalcemia, hyperglycinemia, hypocalcemia, Niemann-Pick disease, organic acidemias, renal tubular acidosis.
7. Toxicity: Bilirubin, magnesium, phenobarbitol phenytoin, sedative drugs.
8. Trauma: Brain, spinal cord injury.

Lower Motor Unit System Disease

1. Arthrogryposis multiplexa congenita
2. Carnitine deficiency
3. Connective tissue disease — Ehler-Danlos syndrome
4. Anterior horn cell — Spinal muscular atrophy
   — Poliomyelitis
5. Peripheral nerve — Familial dysautonomia
   — Guillain-Barré syndrome
   — Polyneuropathies
6. Neuromuscular junction — Botulism
   — Myasthenia gravis syndrome
7. Muscle — Congenital myopathies
   — Glycogen storage disease
   — Hypothyroidism
   — Polymyositis

Increased Tone

Resistance increases suddenly (the catch), heel leaves easily when knee is lifted (spasticity).

- Increased through whole range of movement, as if bending a lead pipe (lead pipe rigidity), i.e. increased tone both in flexors and extensors throughout the movement.
- Regular intermittent break in tone throughout the whole range of movement (cog wheel rigidity) (Table 27.12). In pyramidal lesion flexor muscle in upper limbs, extensor muscles in lower limbs will show increased tone. Spasticity is exaggeration of stretch reflexes and expresses itself as: (a) diminished voluntary movements, (b) Increased resistance to passive movement, (c) Increased reflexes and clonus. Development of spasticity is selective and involves the extensors of the legs and flexors in the arms. Loss of movement is proportional to the degree of spasticity.

The following types of hypertonicity are seen:

Clasp Knife (spasticity)	— Sign of upper motor neuron type of lesion.
Cog-wheel rigidity	— Intermittent action of agonists and antagonists-valuable sign of extrapyramidal involvement.
Lead pipe rigidity	— Characteristic of extrapyramidal but may also be seen in extreme spasticity of UMN type.
Decerebrate rigidity	— All limbs extended, arms pronated, fists closed and feet plantar flexed. Lesions of brainstem (Fig. 27.34).

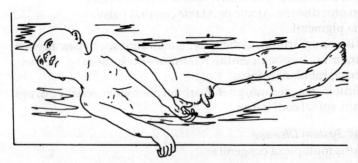

Fig. 27.34: Decerebrate rigidity

Decorticate positioning — Upperlimbs are flexed, lower limbs extended, seen in extensive lesions at the level of basal nuclei or between basal nuclei and cortex (Fig. 27.35).

Other conditions and signs presenting with alteration in tone:

Paratonia or gegenhalten: The patient apparently opposes your attempts to move the limb and is usually seen in bilateral frontal lobe damage.

Myotonia: Slow relaxation following action. Make a fist and release suddenly-myotonic hand unfolds slowly, found in dystrophia myotonica.

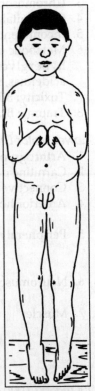

Fig. 27.35: Decorticate posture

Table 27.12: Clinical differentiation of spasticity and rigidity

Spasticity (A component of the pyramidal syndromes)	Rigidity (A component of the extrapyramidal syndromes)
Clasp-knife phenomenon, in hemiplegic, quadriplegic, monoplegic, or paraplegic distribution	Lead-pipe phenomenon, often with cog wheeling and tremor at rest. Usually in all four extremities but may have a "hemi" distribution.
The examiner elicits the claspknife phenomenon, a catch-and yield sensation, by a quick jerk of the resting extremity	The examiner elicits the lead-pipe resistance of rigidity by making a relatively slow movement of the patient's resting extremity
Clonus and hyperreflexia	No clonus; reflexes not necessarily altered
Extensor toe sign	Normal plantar reflexes
Tends to predominate in one set of muscles such as flexors of the upper extremity and the extensors of the knee and plantar reflexors of the ankle	Tends to affect antagonistic pairs of muscles equally
EMG shows no activity with the muscle at complete rest	EMG tends to show electrical activity with the muscle as relaxed as the patient can make it

Dystonia: Patient maintains posture at extremes of movement with contraction of agonist and antagonist.

Percussion myotonia: It may be demonstrated when a muscle dimples following percussion with a patellar hammer. Most commonly sought in abductor pollicis brevis and tongue.

Tripod sign: Child is asked to sit up from recumbent position. He does so, slowly, raises his back in one stiff column and balances by keeping his hands on the bed behind his back the knees are drawn up simultaneously.

Kiss the knee: A child is asked to sit up and kiss his knee. He is unable to do so as there is spasm of back muscles, and head and neck.

Both the above signs are signs of acute poliomyelitis(Non-paralytic) and indicate spinal muscular rigidity.

Adductor sign: Extreme pain on trying to adduct the thighs of a child. The tendon of adductor stands out taut near the pubic attachment.

Scarf sign: In extreme hypotonia, it is almost possible to wrap the whole arm around the neck as if it were a scarf.

TESTING FOR MUSCLE POWER
Power is strength of muscle to perform movement.
Important points to be kept in mind while testing the muscle power.
- It should be steady exertion by both the child and doctor
- Force applied to resist the movement should be gentle especially in hypertonic muscle as it may produce painful cramps.

- Strength of the muscle will commensurate with age and built of the child. Power applied to resist should be proportionate accordingly.
- Power should be tested on the, supposed to be normal side in the same muscle first.
- Degree of weakness should be noted (Grading power).
- Constancy of muscle weakness should be noted any improvement on encouragement or rest ?
- Last but most important, is there any coexistent painful condition ? e.g. injury, inflammation or mechanical defect, contracture of muscle, ankylosis of joint which impair the movement.

Muscle power testing is carried out in groups of muscles as given below. It is graded as:

5— Normal power, movement against gravity and resistance.

4— Muscle though able to make normal movement is overcome by resistance.

3— Movement against gravity but not against additional resistance.

2— Movement with gravity eliminated; normal movement is possible only under some particular positions.

1— Visible or palpable flicker of contraction but no movement.

0— Total paralysis.

Types of Muscular Weakness

Weakness due to Pyramidal Tract Lesions

This tends to be a weakness that is incomplete except in the acute stages, or in the presence of a grossly destructive lesion. It affects particular movements rather than particular muscles, and is most marked in the abductors and extensors of the upper limb, and the flexors of the lower limb. Normally it is associated with increase of tone and exaggerated reflexes. Distribution is more distal than proximal, particularly in the upper limbs, where hand movements are affected earliest.

Weakness due to Extrapyramidal Lesions

This is more of a hindrance of movement due to equal resistance from agonists and antagonists, than to true loss of muscle power. It is generalized throughout the limb and associated with rigidity and often with resultant suppression of the reflexes.

Weakness due to Lower Motor Neuron Lesions

This is usually very marked, but, except in extensive polyneuropathies, is limited to the muscles having that segmental supply. If of long standing, it is associated with marked wasting and loss of those tendon reflexes in which the affected muscles play a part. A lesion at anterior horn or anterior root level picks out those muscles whose sole or maximal supply is from that segment, and these muscles may show fasciculation. At peripheral nerve level it affects all the muscles supplied by that nerve. In a polyneuropthy, this type of weakness is often maximal peripherally in the arms and legs, and usually symmetrical.

Weakness due to Muscular Lesions

This can range from weakness of one muscle, such as after a local injury, to weakness of every muscle, such as in some cases of polymyositis. This type of weakness is either very localized, or very widespread but patchy. The muscles affected correspond either to the supply of a particular spinal segment or a particular peripheral nerve. There is often individual muscle wasting, pseudo-hypertrophy, or tenderness. The related reflexes are lost.

REVIEW OF FACTORS RELATED TO WEAKNESS

Symptoms of Neuromuscular Disease

Slow motor development
Easy fatigability
Frequent falls
Abnormal gait
    Waddle
    Toe-walking
    Steppage
Specific disability
    Arm elevation
    Hand grip
    Rising from floor
    Climbing stairs

Signs of Neuromuscular Disease

Observation
    Functional ability
    Atrophy and hypertrophy
    Fasciculations
Palpation
    Tenderness
    Muscle texture
Examination
    Strength
    Tendon reflexes
    Myotonia
    Joint contractures

Causes of Acute Generalized Weakness

Infectious disorders
    Enterovirus infections
    Guillain-Barre syndrome
Neuromuscular blockade
    Tick paralysis
    Myasthenia gravis
    Botulism

      Periodic paralysis
           Hypokalemic
           Hyperkalemic
           Normokalemic
           Acute intermittent porphyria

Causes of Progressive Proximal Weakness

1. Spinal cord disorders
2. Juvenile spinal muscular atrophy
   a. Autosomal recessive
   b. Autosomal dominant
   c. Hexosaminidase A deficiency
3. Limb-girdle myasthenia
   a. Familial
   b. Sporadic
4. Muscular dystrophies
   a. Duchenne/Becker
   b. Limb-girdle
   c. Facioscapulohumeral syndrome
5. Inflammatory myopathies
   a. Dermatomyositis
   b. Polymyositis
6. Metabolic myopathies
   a. Acid maltase deficiency
   b. Other carbohydrate myopathies
      1. Myophosphorylase deficiency
      2. Debrancher enzyme deficiency
   c. Muscle carnitine deficiency
   d. Mitochondrial myopathies
7. Endocrine myopathies
   a. Thyroid
   b. Parathyroid
   c. Adrenal cortex

Causes of Progressive Distal Weakness (Table 27.13)

Spinal Cord Disorders
Spinal Muscular Atrophy
Hereditary Motor Sensory Neuropathy (HMSN)
1. HMSN I   :   Charcot-Marie tooth
2. HMSN II   :   Neuronal Charcot-Marie tooth
3. HMSN III   :   Dejerine-Sottas
4. HMSN IV   :   Refsum
Other Genetic Neuropathies
1. Sulfatide lipidoses: Metachromatic leukodystrophy
2. Other leukodystrophies
3. Disorders of pyruvate metabolism
4. Familial amyloid neuropathy

Neuropathies with Systemic Diseases
1. Drugs
2. Toxins
3. Uremia
4. Systemic vasculitis

Idiopathic Neuropathy
1. Chronic demyelinating neuropathy
2. Chronic axonal neuropathy

Myopathies
1. Myotonic dystrophy
2. Hereditary distal myopathies

Scapulo (humeral) peroneal
1. Neuronopathy
2. Emery-Dreifuss syndrome
3. With dementia

Table 27.13: Differentiating points of the muscular dystrophies

Type of Dystrophy	Genetic Type	Age at Onset (Years)	Age at Disability (Years)	Pattern of Weakness
Duchenne	X-linked	0.5	10-15	Proximal
Becker	X-linked	5-15	15-25	Proximal
Limb-girdle	X-linked	10-30	20-40	Proximal
Facioscapulohumeral	Autosomal dominant	10-30	30-50	Proximal arm, face
Myotonic	Autosomal	10-30	30-50	Distal limbs, face
Scapuloperoneal	Autosomal dominant	20-30	30-50	Proximal arm and
	Autosomal recessive	0-10	5-15	distal leg
Emery-Dreifuss	X-linked	5-15	25-50	Proximal arm and distal leg

WEAKNESS MAY BE MONOPLEGIC, HEMIPLEGIC, PARAPLEGIC OR QUADRIPLEGIC

Acute Monoplegia

Plexopathy/Neuropathy
1. Acute neuritis
   a. Idiopathic plexitis
   b. Osteomyelitis, plexitis
   c. Tetanus toxoid (?) plexitis
   d. Poliomyelitis
2. Hereditary
   a. Hereditary brachial neuritis
   b. Hereditary recurrent pressure palsy
3. Injury
   a. Traction injuries
   b. Pressure injuries
   c. Lacerations

4. Stroke
5. Complex migraine
6. "Hemiparetic" seizures

Acute Hemiplegia
Cerebraovascular disease
Epilepsy
Migraine
Diabetes mellitus
Infection
Trauma

Progressive Hemiplegia
Arteriovenous malformation
Brain abscess
Cerebral hemisphere tumor
Demyelinating diseases
Adrenoleukodystrophy
Late onset globoid leukodystrophy
Multiple sclerosis

Spinal Paraplegia

Congenital
1. Dysraphic states
   a. Myelomeningocele
   b. Tethered spinal cord
2. Syringomyelia
3. Arteriovenous malfmormations
4. Atlanto-axial dislocation

Tumors
1. Ependymoma
2. Astrocytoma
3. Neuroblastoma
4. Other

Acute Transverse Myelitis
1. Idiopathic
2. Devic syndrome
3. Encephalomyelitis

Infections
1. Diskitis
2. Polyradiculoneuropathy
3. Epidural abscess
4. Tuberculous osteomyelitis

Trauma in Newborn
1. Transection
2. Infarction

Trauma in Childhood
1. Concussion
2. Fracture dislocation
3. Epidural hematoma

Familial Spastic Paraplegia

Quadriplegia

Spastic Quadriplegia
Causes:
1. **Cortical Lesion:**
   A. Cerebral palsy.
   B. Decerebrate state due to anoxia, hydrocephalus, diffuse sclerosis, pineal tumors, etc.
   C. Congenital disorders e.g., microcephaly.
2. **Brainstem Lesion:**
   A. Vertebrobasilar insufficiency
   B. Brainstem space occupying lesions.
   C. Infections, e.g. bulbar poliomyelitis.
   D. Degeneration conditions: syringobulbia, motor neurone disease, etc.
   E. Demyelinating disease, e.g. disseminated sclerosis.
3. **High Cervical Cord Lesion:**
   A. Fracture dislocation of cervical spine
   B. Craniovertebral anomaly.
   C. Cervical spondylosis
   D. Hematomyelia.
   E. Cervical cord tumors.

Flaccid Quadriplegia
Causes:
1. **Polyneuropathy**
   A. Acute infective polyneuritis
   B. Porphyria
   C. Diphtheria
   D. Botulism
   E. Triorthocresyl phosphate (TOCP)
   F. Infectious mononucleosis
   G. Infective hepatitis.
2. **Muscle diseases**
   A. Acute myasthenia gravis
   B. Periodic paralysis
   C. Polymyositis

3. **Anterior horn cell disease:** Poliomyelitis
4. **Brainstem lesions with neuronal shock.**

Summary of Assessment of Muscle Weakness

1. UMN lesion or LMN lesion
2. Pyramidal or extrapyramidal
3. LMN — Anterior horn cell: Patchy, fasciculations
   Nerve root type: Patchy, fasciculations, root pain, girdle pain
   Peripheral nerve: Along the distribution of the nerve
   Myoneural junction type: Character depends on disease, e.g. myasthenia gravis
   Muscle: Character depends on disease, e.g. DMD
4. Note whether the weakness is
   a. Proximal or distal
   b. Symmetrical or asymmetrical
   c. Flexors or extensors
   d. Any particular muscle
   e. Ascending or descending
   f. Acute or chronic, periodic
   g. Static or progressive
   h. Grading of muscle power
   i. Weakness of muscles or movements
   j. Associated features—tone, wasting, reflexes.

Muscle Power Testing in the ARMS

In the arms, an UMN or pyramidal weakness predominantly affects finger extension, elbow extension and shoulder abduction. Elbow flexion and grip are relatively preserved.

Innervation of the upper limb is mainly by three nerves.

- Radial nerve and branches supply all extensors in the arm.
- Ulnar nerve supplies all intrinsic muscles of the hand except
  L — Lateral two lumbicals
  O — Opponens pollicis
  A — Abductor pollicis brevis
  F — Flexor pollicis brevis
The above are supplied by median nerve.

Pronator Test

It is a simple screening test. Ask the patient to hold arms out in front with palms facing upwards and to close eyes tightly and watch position of arms.

- -One arms pronates and drifts down—weakness on that side.
- Both arms drift downwards in bilateral weakness
- Arm rises—cerebellar disease
- Fingers continuously move up and down—deficit of joint position sense.

TESTING INDIVIDUAL ACTIONS AT VARIOUS JOINTS

Shoulder Abduction

Ask patient to lift out both elbows to the side and push up against resistance (Fig. 27.36).

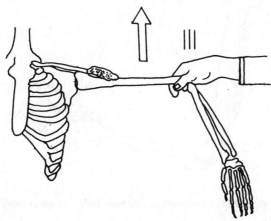

Fig. 27.36: Testing should be abduction (Adapted from Fuller)

Muscle : Deltoid
Nerve : Axillary nerve
Root value : C_5

Elbow Flexion

Hold the patient's elbow and wrist and supinate. Ask patient to pull his hands towards his face against resistance (Fig. 27.37).

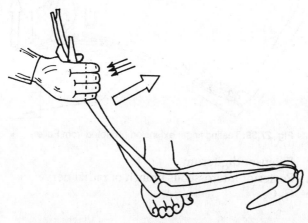

Fig. 27.37: Testing elbow flexion (Adapted from Fuller)

Muscle : Biceps brachii
Nerve : Musculocutanous
Root : C_5, C_6.
If pronated, brachioradialis comes into action.

Elbow Extension

Hold patients elbow and wrist. Ask to extend the elbow (Fig. 27.38).

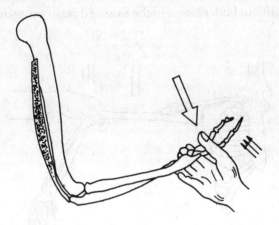

Fig. 27.38: Testing elbow extension (Adapted from Fuller)

Muscle : Triceps
Nerve : Radial nerve
Root : $C_6 C_7 C_8$

Finger Extension

Fix the patient's hand. Ask patient to keep fingers straight and press against extended fingers (Fig. 27.39).

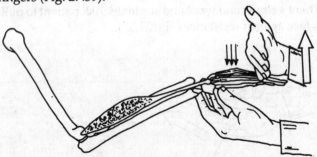

Fig. 27.39: Testing finger extension (Adapted from Fuller)

Muscle : Extensor digitorum
Nerve : Posterior interosseous branch of radial nerve
Root : $C_7 C_8$.

Finger Flexion

Close your finger on the patients finger, palm to palm. Ask patient to grip your fingers and attempt to open patients grip (Fig. 27.40).

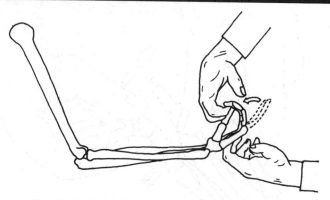

Fig. 27.40: Testing finger flexion (Adapted from Fuller)

Muscle : Flexor digitorum profundus and superficialis
Nerve   : Median and ulnar
Root   : C_8.

Finger Abduction

Ask the patient to spread his fingers out. Hold the middle and other fingers together and ask to spread the index finger (Fig. 27.41).

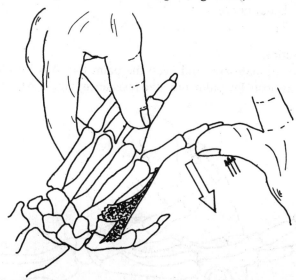

Fig. 27.41: Testing finger abduction (Adapted from Fuller)

Muscle : Dorsal interosseous
Nerve   : Ulnar nerve
Root   : T_1

Finger Adduction

Ask patient to bring his fingers together. Make sure the fingers are striaght. Fix the middle, ring and little finger. Ask the child to attempt to abduct the index finger (Fig. 27.42).

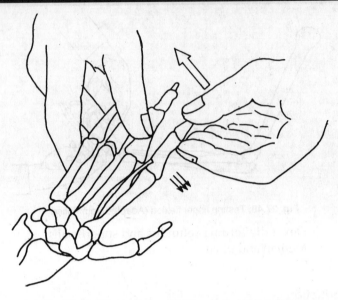

Fig. 27.42: Testing finger adduction (Adapted from Fuller)

Muscle   : Second palmar interossi
Nerve   : Ulnar nerve.
Root   : T_1

Thumb Abduction

Ask patient to supinate arm and keep the palm flat. Ask him to bring the thumb towards nose. Fix palm and give resistance (Fig. 27.43).

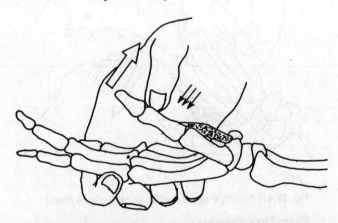

Fig. 27.43: Testing thumb abduction (Adapted from Fuller)

Muscle   : Abductor pollicis brevis
Nerve   : Median nerve
Root   : T_1

The other muscles tested in case of abnormalities are:

Serratus Anterior

Stand behind the patient in front of a wall. Ask the patient to push the wall with arms straight with hands at shoulder level. Look at scapula. Muscle weakness causes winging (Fig. 27.44).

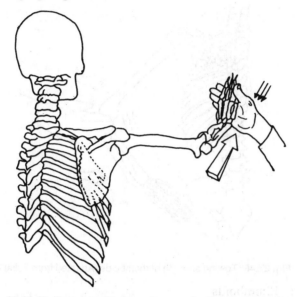

Fig. 27.44: Testing strength of serratus anterior (Adapted from Fuller)

Nerve   :   Long thoracic nerve
Root   : $C_5\, C_6\, C_7$.

Trapezius

Go behind the patient and compare the line and curve of the trapezii, making certain that he is sitting symmetrically upright. Then ask him to raise his shoulders towards his ears. Now try to depress the shoulders forcibly. Even the most feeble patient is normally able to resist the maneuver (Fig. 27.45).

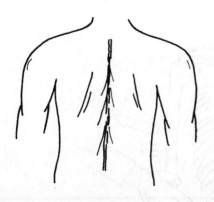

Fig. 27.45: Testing the strength of trapezius, ask the patient to raise his shoulders toward his ears

Muscle :   Trapezius
Nerve   :   Spinal accessory nerve

Rhomboids

Ask the patient to put his hands on his hips. Hold his elbow and ask him to bring elbow backward (Fig. 27.46).

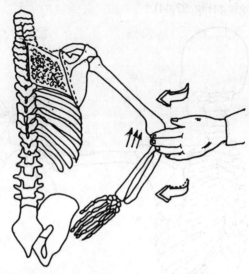

Fig. 27.46: Testing strength of rhomboids (Adapted from Fuller)

Muscle   :   Rhomboids
Nerve   :   Nerve to rhomboids
Root   : $C_4 C_5$.

Supraspinatus

Stand behind the patient. Ask him to lift his arm from the side against resistance (Fig. 27.47).

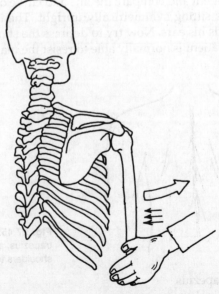

Fig. 27.47: Testing strength of supraspinatus (Adapted from Fuller)

Nerve   : Suprascapular nerve
Root   : C_5

Infraspinatus
Stand behind the patient hold his elbow against his side with the elbow flexed, asking him to move his hand out to the side and resist this movement at the wrist (Fig. 27.48).

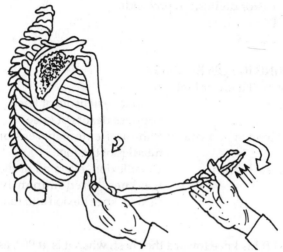

Fig. 27.48: Testing strength of infraspinatus (Adapted from Fuller)

Nerve   : Suprascapular nerve
Root   : $C_5\,C_6$.

Brachioradialis
Hold the patients forearm and wrist with forearm semipronated. Ask patient to pull hands to his face (Fig. 27.49).

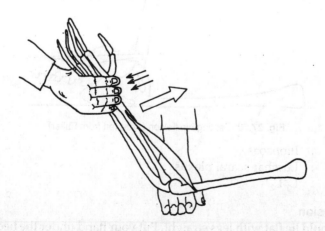

Fig. 27.49: Testing strength of brachioradialis (Adapted from Fuller)

Muscle   : Brachioradialis
Nerve   : Radial nerve
Root   : C_6

Long Flexors of Little or Ring Finger
Ask the patient to grip your fingers. Attempt to extend the distal inter-
phalangeal joint of the little and ring finger.
Muscle   : Flexor digitorium profundus
Nerve   : Ulnar nerve
Root   : C_8.

POWER TESTING IN LOWER LIMBS
Nerves supplying the lower limbs are:

Femoral nerve	: Supplies extensors of knee
Sciatic nerve	: Supplies flexors of knee
Posterior tibial branch of sciatic	: Plantar flexion, inversion and small muscles of the foot.
Common peroneal branch	: Dorsiflexion, eversion of the ankle UMN weakness predominantly affects hip flexion, knee flexion and foot dorsiflexion.

Hip Flexion
Ask patient to lift his knee toward the chest, when it is at 90°, ask him to pull
it up as hard as he can against resistance (Fig. 27.50).

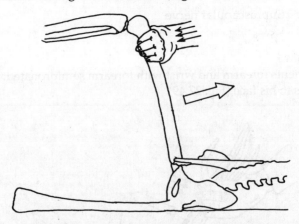

Fig. 27.50: Testing hip flexion (Adapted from Fuller)

Muscle   : Iliopsoas
Nerve   : Lumbar scaral plexus
Root   : $L_1 L_2$.

Hip Extension
Patient should lie flat with legs straight. Put your hand under the heel and ask
to push it down (Fig. 27.51).

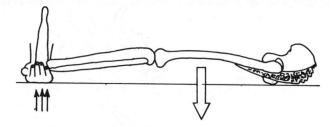

Fig. 27.51: Testing hip extension (Adapted from Fuller)

Muscle   :   Gluteus maximus
Nerve   :   Inferior gluteal nerve
Root   : $L_5 S_1$.

Hip Abductors

Fix one ankle, ask the patient to push the other leg out at the side and resist this movement by holding the other ankle (Fig. 27.52).

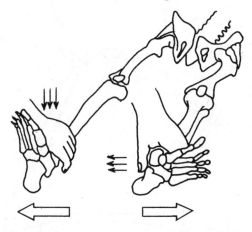

Fig. 27.52: Testing strength of hip abductors (Adapted from Fuller)

Muscle   :   Gluteus medius and minimus
Nerve   :   Superior gluteal nerve
Root   : $L_4 L_5$

Hip Adductors

Ask patient to keep ankles together. Fix one ankle and try and pull the other ankle out (Fig. 27.53).

Muscle   :   Adductors
Nerve   :   Obturator nerve
Root   : $L_4 L_5$.

Knee Extension

Ask patient to bend the knee till 90°, then ask to straighten leg against resistance (Fig. 27.54).

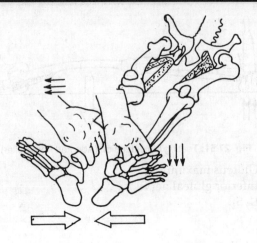

Fig. 27.53: Testing strength of right hip adductors (Adapted from Fuller)

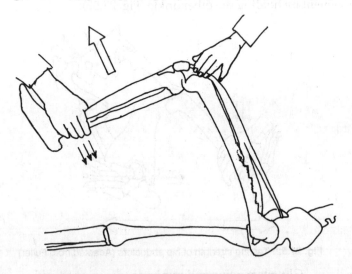

Fig. 27.54: Testing knee extension (Adapted from Fuller)

Muscle : Quadriceps femoris
Nerve : Femoral nerve
Root : $L_3 L_4$

Knee Flexion

Ask the patient to bend his knee and bring his heel toward his bottom. When the knee is at 90°, try to straighten out the leg, holding the knee, watch hamstrings (Fig. 27.55).

Muscles : Hamstrings
Nerve : Sciatic nerve
Root : $L_5 S_1$.

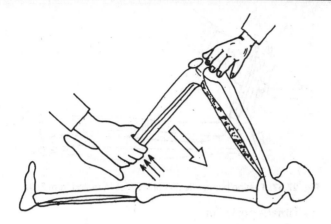

Fig. 27.55: Testing knee flexion (Adapted from Fuller)

Foot Dorsiflexion

Ask the patient to move the ankle back and try to bring toes towards his head. When ankle is past 90°, try to overcome this movement; watch the anterior compartment (Fig. 27.56).

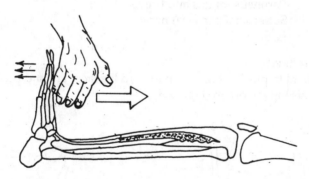

Fig. 27.56: Testing dorsiflexion of the foot (Adapted from Fuller)

Muscle	:	Tibialis anterior
Nerve	:	Deep peroneal nerve
Root	:	L_4 L_5.

Plantar Flexion of Foot

Ask the patient to point his toes away from his head, with his leg striaght. Try to over come this (Fig. 27.57).

Muscle	:	Gastrocnemius
Nerve	:	Posterior tibial nerve
Root	:	S_1.

Foot Inversion

With the ankle at 90° ask the patient to turn his foot inwards against resistance (Fig. 27.58).

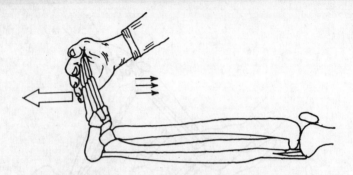

Fig. 27.57: Testing plantar flexion of the foot (Adapted from Fuller)

Muscle : Tibialis posterior
Nerve : Tibial nerve
Root : $L_4 L_5$.

Foot Eversion

Ask the patient to turn his foot out to the side. Try and then bring the foot to the midline (Fig. 27.59).

Muscle : Peroneus longus and brevis
Nerve : Superficial peroneal nerve
Root : $L_5 S_1$.

Big Toe Extension

Ask the patient to pull his big toe up toward his face. Try and push the distal phalanx of his big toe down (Fig. 27.60).

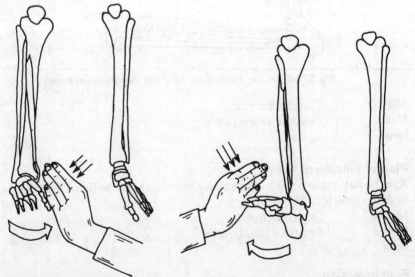

Fig. 27.58: Testing inversion of the foot (Adapted from Fuller)

Fig. 27.59: Testing eversion of the foot (i) (Adapted from Fuller)

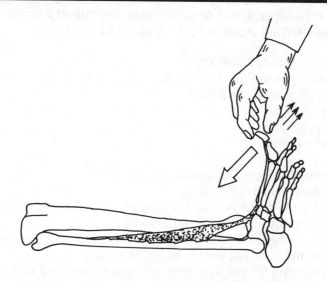

Fig. 27.60: Testing eversion of the foot (ii) (Adapted from Fuller)

Muscle : Extensor digitorum longus
Nerve : Deep peroneal
Root : L_5.

Extension of the Toes

Ask the patient to bring his toes towards the head. Press against the proximal part of his toes and watch the muscle (Fig. 27.61).

Muscle : Extensor digitorum brevis
Nerve : Deep peroneal
Root : $L_5 s_1$.

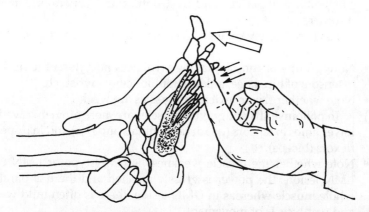

Fig. 27.61: Testing extension of the toes (Adapted from Fuller)

MUSCLE POWER TESTING IN INDIVIDUAL CIRCUMSTANCES
(SOME IMPORTANT POINTS FOR CONSIDERATION)

Muscle Power Testing in Poliomyelitis
The patient is put in the following three positions to bring in or eliminate gravity in different muscle groups.
1. Supine position
2. Prone position
3. Lateral position

Muscle Power Testing in Unconscious or
Uncooperative Patient or in Infants
1. By noting the position of limb, e.g. weak lower limb is rotated laterally with lateral side of thigh touching the bed.
2. By allowing the limbs to drop from similar position and noting the manner in which they fall. The weaker limb falls rapidly.
3. By stimulating the parts of limb with sharp object and noting the force with which the limb is withdrawn.

Testing Power when Minimal Weakness is Anticipated
1. For lower limbs
   - Ask the patient to stand on one leg
   - Hop on one leg
   - In supine position lift both lower limbs and hold them in air and see which one falls earlier.
2. For upper limbs ask the patient to hold both upper limbs in front of trunk and hold them in air, watch which one falls earlier.
   - Next note whether the weakness is symmetrial or asymmetrical.
        Symmetrical weakness is an important feature of GB syndrome and congenital myopathies and dystrophies and generalised metabolic disorder.
        Asymmetrical weakness is seen in paralytic poliomyelitis, peripheral nerve lesions.
   - Note groups of muscle having weakness at different joint. Flexors, extensors of hip, knee, ankle, shoulder elbow wrist, etc.
   - Note whether flexor/extensor muscles are weak.
        In poliomyelitis antigravity muscles are more often involved, i.e. in lower limbs extensors (quadriceps, tibials anterior) and in upper limbs flexors (biceps).
   - Note whether the muscle weakness is UMN type or LMN type. In LMN lesions the power is grossly affected and there is paralysis of whole muscle whereas in UMN lesion, there is often mild weakness and paralysis is of movement.
   - Note also which individual muscle is paralysed by doing specific test described for each muscle.
   - Do not forget to assess muscle power in chest muscles and abdominal muscles.

This is done by "splinting techniques." If diaphragm is paralysed splinting of chest causes severe respiratory distress. In chest wall muscle paralysis (intercostal muscles) splinting of abdomen causes respiratory distress.

- Assess power of neck muscle. In weakness of neck muscles there will be head drop.
- Assess involvement of bulbar muscles.
- Combing, throwing is used to assess proximal muscle power of upper limbs.
- Climbing, sitting from standing and getting up from sitting position is used to assess proximal muscles of lower limbs.
- Tip toe walking is used to assess extensor muscles of lower limb (Quadriceps and tibialis anterior).
- Heel walking is used to assess flexor muscles of lower limb (Hamstring and calf muscles).

Table 27.14: The power at different joints can be assessed in the following manner
(Normal and good power only is considered)

Upper extremities joint	Normal and good
Shoulder Flexion to 90 degrees (Fig. 27.62)	Sitting with arm at side, elbow slightly flexed. Stabilize scapula. Patient flexes arm to 90 degrees (palm down). Resistance is given above elbow.
Shoulder extension (Fig. 27.63)	Face lying with arm inwardly rotated. Stabilize scapula. Patient extends arm through range of motion. Resistance is given above elbow.
Shoulder abduction to 90 degrees (Fig. 27.64)	Sitting with arm at side in midposition between inward and outward rotation. Elbow flexed a few degrees. Stabilize scapula. Patient abducts arm to 90 degrees without outward ratation at shoulder joint (palm down). Resistance is given above elbow joint.
Shoulder horizontal abduction (Fig. 27.65)	Face lying with shoulder abducted to 90 degrees, upper arm resting on table and lower arm hanging vertically ove edge. Stabilize scapula. Patient raises upper arm through range of motion. Resistance is given above elbow. Motion takes place primarily at glenohumeral joint and not between scapula and thorax.
Elbow flexion (Fig. 27.66)	Sitting with arm at side and forearm supinated. Stabilize upper arm. Patient flexes elbow through range of motion. Resistance is given proximal to wrist joint.
Elbow extension (Fig. 27.67)	Facelying with shoulder abducted to 90 degrees and forearm hanging vertically over edge of table. Stabilize upper arm.

Contd...

Contd...

Upper extremities joint	Normal and good
	Patient extends elbow through range of motion. Resistance is given above wrist joint in plane of forearm motion.
Wrist flexion (Fig. 27.68)	Sitting with forearm resting on table. Muscles of thumb and fingers relaxed.
	Stabilize forearm.
	Patient flexes wrist.
	To test flexor carpi radialis, resistance is given at base of second metacarpal bone in direction of extension and ulnar deviation (Illustrated).
	To test flexor carpi ulnaris, resistance is given at base of fifth metacarpal bone in direction of extension and radial deviation.
Wrist extension (Fig. 27.69)	Sitting with forearm resting on table. Muscles of fingers and thumb relaxed.
	Stabilize forearm.
	Patient extends wrist
	To test extensor carpi radialis longus and brevis, resistance is given on dorsal surface of second and third metacarpal bones in direction of flexion and ulnar deviation.
	To test extensor carpi ulnaris, resistance is given on dorsal surface of fifth metacarpal bone in direction of flexion and radial deviation.
LOWER EXTREMITIES	
Hip extension (Fig. 27.70)	Face lying with legs extended.
	Stabilize pelvis.
	Patient extends hip through range of motion.
	Resistance is given above knee joint.
Hip flexion (Fig. 27.71)	Sitting with legs over edges of table.
	Stabilize pelvis.
	Patient flexes hip through last part of range of motion.
	Resistance is given above knee joint.
Hip abduction (Fig. 27.72)	Side lying with leg slightly extended beyond midline. Lower knee flexed for balance.
	Stabilize pelvis.
	Patient abducts leg through range of motion.
	Resistance is given above knee joint.
Hip adduction (Fig. 27.73)	Side lying with leg resting on table and upper leg supported in approximately 25 degrees of abduction.
	Patient adducts leg until it contacts upper leg.
	Resistance is given above knee joint.
Knee Extension (Fig. 27.74)	Back lying with leg to be tested over end of table.
	Opposite leg flexed at knee and hip, with foot resting on table (for pelvic stabilization).
	Stabilize thigh above knee joint.
	Patient extends knee through range of motion.
	Resistance is given above ankle joint (Pad should be used under knee).

Contd...

Contd...

Upper extremities joint	*Normal and good*
Knee flexion (Fig. 27.75)	Face lying with legs straight. Stabilize pelvis. Patient flexes knee. Grasping above ankle, therapist outwardly rotates leg and resists flexion to test biceps femoris.
Foot dorsiflexion (Fig. 27.76)	Back lying with heel over edge of table. Stabilize lower leg. Patient dorsiflex and inverts foot, keeping toes relaxed. Resistance is given on medial dorsal aspect of foot. **Note:** Patient should be cautioned to keep big toe relaxed to avoid substitution by extensor hallucis longus.
Ankle plantar flexion (Fig. 27.77)	Standing on leg to be tested. Knee straight. For Normal grade, patient raises heel from floor through range of motion of plantar flexion. Patient can complete motion four or five times in good form.

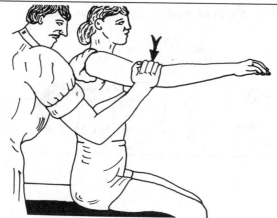

Fig. 27.62: Shoulder flexion to 90 degrees

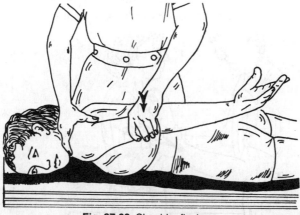

Fig. 27.63: Shoulder flexion

COORDINATION

A coordinated combination of a series of motor actions is needed to produce a smooth and accurate movement. This requires integration of sensory feed back

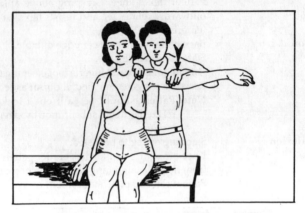

Fig. 27.64: Shoulder abduction to 90 degrees

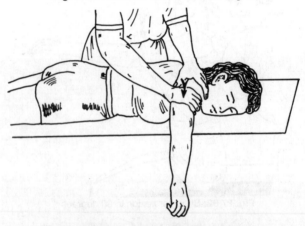

Fig. 27.65: Shoulder horizontal abduction

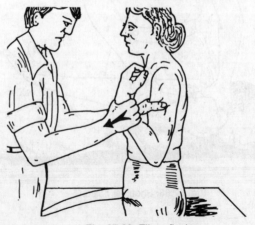

Fig. 27.66: Elbow flexion

and motor output. This integration occurs mainly in the cerebellum. Loss of joint position sense can produce some incoordination which worsens when

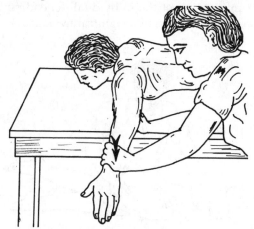

Fig. 27.67: Elbow extension

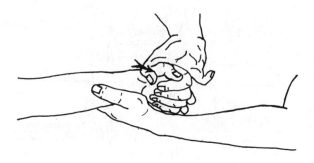

Fig. 27.68: Wrist flexion

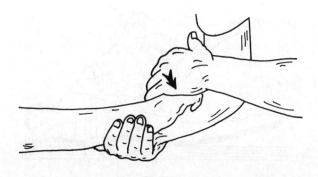

Fig. 27.69: Wrist extension

the eyes are closed. Fine coordination is not fully developed until 4-6 years of age. Hence, methods of testing coordination must be adapted to the level of neuro muscular maturation of the individual depending on the post natal age. Coordination cannot be tested if signifcant weakness is present.

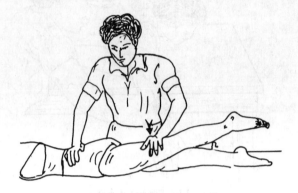

Fig. 27.70: Hip extension

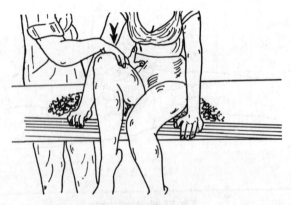

Fig. 27.71: Hip flexion

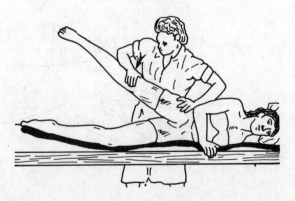

Fig. 27.72: Hip abduction

Testing

Testing coordination in older children and adults can be done by standard neurological methods, whereas, in infants and young children testing of coordination is mainly achieved by observational skills.

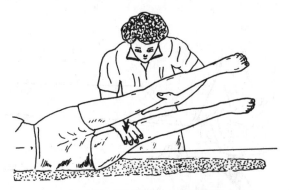

Fig. 27.73: Hip adduction

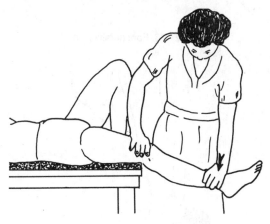

Fig. 27.74: Knee extension

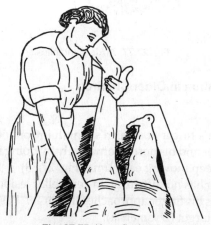

Fig. 27.75: Knee flexion

In infants and young children day to day activities give more valuable information. They should be observed while they are playing. The way they handle things, the way they pickup objects, the way they walk should be observed because, these actions need coordinated movements, a gross analysis can be done.

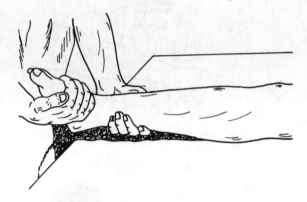

Fig. 27.76: Foot dorsiflexion

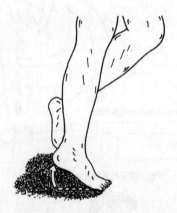

Fig. 27.77: Ankle plantar flexion

Testing Coordination in Older Children

Finger Nose Test

Hold the examiner's finger at an arm's length infront of the patient. Ask him to touch your finger and his nose alternatively by doing it progressively faster. The finger must keep moving each time (Fig. 27.78).

Normal person has no difficulty. In cerebellar lesion, patient develops an intention tremor as his finger approaches the target. Past pointing is present if he overshoots his target (Dysmetria).

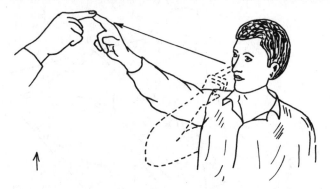

Fig. 27.78: Testing finger-nose test

Repetitive Movements

Ask patient to perform some repetitive movements like supinate and pronate rapidly, etc. In cerebellar lesion there is incordination and the patient is unable to do so or has irregularity or slowness of movement (dysdiadokokinesia) (Fig. 27.79).

A subtler and superior method is thigh slapping test. Test each hand separatly. Ask the patient to slap his thigh, alternating first with the palm and then with the back of the hand, as rapidly and rhythmically as possible making an audible sound (demonstrate initially how to do) (Fig. 27.80). The dysrhythmia of the ataxic hand can be seen as well as heard.

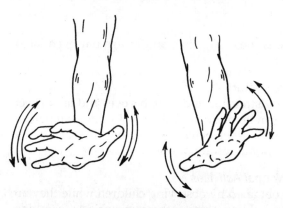

Fig. 27.79: Pronation-supination test for dystaxia-dysmetria of the hands. Notice the even excursions of the normal right hand, and the uneven excursions of the ataxic left hand

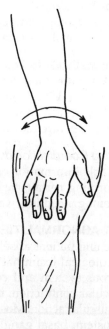

Fig. 27.80: Thigh-slapping test for dystaxia-dysmetria. The cerebellar patient slaps irregularly, and turns the hand too little in alternately slapping, the front and the back of the hand on the thigh touch too much

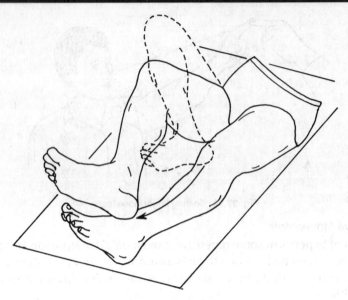

Fig. 27.81: The heel-shin test

Heel-shin Test
The patient is asked to touch the heel of the leg along the shin of the other repeatedly. In cerebellar lesion there will be disorganised movement with the heel falling off the anterior part of the shin, knee falling from side to side (Fig. 27.81).

Tandem Walking
Walking along a straight line is most sensitive, and brings out even latent ataxia especially truncal ataxia.

Other Methods to Test Coordination
1. Ask patient to hold arms outstretched and close his eyes and tell to keep in this position, push the arm up or down suddenly. In a normal person, they rapidly return to normal. In cerebellar disease, they oscillate several times before returning to normal resting position.

Testing Coordination during Normal Activities
Valuable information can be obtained by observing children while they are performing certain tasks, e.g. holding objects, throwing objects, combing, buttoning, needling, walking, eating, writing, picking up objects, etc.

GAIT ABNORMALITIES
Watching patient arise, stand and walk forms the most important aspect of neurological examination. A normal gait requires integrity of peripheral nervous system and central nerves system, good proprioception, vision, muscular contraction, reciprocal limb actions, righting reflexes, coordination of muscular action. Most disorders of muscles, nerves, spinal cord, cerebellum, brainstem, basal ganglia and cerebrum cause disturbance of gait that are characteristic.

Types of Gaits

Developmental Gaits
1. Reflex stepping of neonate.
2. Cruising—infant takes steps when steadied by parent.
3. Toddler's gait—broad base, short jerky irregular step, semiflexed posture of arms and frequent falls.
4. Mature gait—Norrow based, heel-toe strike contrabody movement and reciprocal swings of arms.

Neuromuscular Gaits
1. Club foot gait
   a. With tibial torsion-in toed or pigeon toed gait
2. Lordotic wadling gait (pride of pregnancy gait) (duck like gait)
   Causes:-   DMD, CDH (bilateral), polymyosities,
               Engelman's syndrome
               Myelodysplasia, slipped femoral
               epiphysis (bil), achondroplasia
3. Toe drop or foot drop gait (high stepping)
   High steps are taken due to foot drop to avoid tripping of toes, walks cautiously watching the flour.

   Symmetrical   Distal peripheral neuropathy (toxic metabolic, heridofamilial, Charcot-Marie Tooth's progressive peroneal atrophy).

   Heel drop gait   tibial nerve palsy

   Flail foot gait   complete sciatic nerve palsy
4. Toe walking: Normal toddler, spastic diplegia, autistic or retarded child, DMD, sometimes familial.

Sensory Gaits
   Painfull sole or hyperesthetic gait—patient bears as little weight on the painful side as possible.
   Radicular pain gait or antalgic gait—due to slipped disc pain radiating along the leg.
   Nocturnal flipping hand gait—carpel tunnel syndrome
   Flipping hand gait—autism, mental retardation
   Tabetic, dorsal column or sensory ataxic gait—foot is placed on the ground with a thud (stamping gait)
   Blind persons gait—slow, deliberate, searching steps

Cerebellar Ataxic Gaits (Staggering or Reeling Gait)
Patient walks like a drunken man. Unsteady uncoordinated and cannot walk in straight line or around a chair.

Spastic Gait
Hemiplegic gait (circumduction gait) patient circumducts a leg dragging the toe, placing the ball down without a heel strike, with the ipsilateral arm held in partial flexion.

Paraplegic Gait
Spastic diplegic gait (Scissor gait, due to excess adductor tone at hip joint. *Crouch gait*—with knees flexed while walking)
    Spastic ataxic gait (Cerebral palsy, spinocerebellar degeneration).

Basal Ganglion Gait

Shuffling gait—Short steps, does not lift the feet from the floor, has the march a petits pas (the march of small steps)

Parkinsonian gait—Walks slowly with short steps, lacks arm swing, turns enblock like a statue.

Festinating gait—Small short steps as if chasing one's own center of gravity.

Choreiform gait—Choreiform movements increase during walking.

Spastic athetoid gait—Athetosis with spasticity.

Equinovarus dystonic gait—Intermittent inturning of the foot that causes difficulty in walking, e.g. dystonia .

Dromedary gait—Like camel (exhibiting rise and fall of trunk), e.g. dystonia musculorum deformans.

Cerebral Gait (Apraxic gait)

Dancing bear gait   Stepping on the same spot as if trying to free the feet from thick, sticky mud, e.g. bilateral cerebral lesion like Alzheimer's disease.

Psychiatric Gaits

Astasia abasia (astasia = not standing; abasia = not walking) in hysteria.
    Hysterical inability to stand and walk. The patient is ataxic and sways from the hip rather than ankles. It increases on attention and patient does not hurt himself.

Gait as an Expression of Biological Sexual Orientation (Sexual Orientation of Brain)

Male gait   Pelvis movements less, armswing straight

Female gait   Pelvis movements more, increased carrying angle

Male homosexuals gait Dainty steps, swishy hips, exaggerated wrist movements.

Lesbian's gait   Aggressive

INVOLUNTARY MOVEMENT

Examination

Involuntary movements are those patterns of muscle contractions which cannot be stopped at person's will or on observer's command. They are due to structural or biochemical lesion in the basal ganglion, reticular formation and cerebellum.

These are best appreciated only on seeing affected patients. Armed with right vocabulary, most common abnormal movements can be described. There is frequently a considerable overlap between various syndromes and several types of abnormal movements are often seen in the same patient, for example, tremor and dystonia in a parkinsonian patient on treatment.

Three aspects are looked into in evaluating for a movement disorder (abnormal or involuntary movement).

1. Positive phenomenon: Abnormal positions maintained, additional movements seen.
2. Latent phenomenon: Abnormal phenomenon that can be revealed by using various maneuvers, e.g. rigidity on testing tone and abnormal postures brought on writing (writer's cramp).
3. Negative phenomenon: The inability to do things, for example, a slowness in initiating actions (bradykinesia).

To Evaluate Latent Phenomenon

On walking; the following may occur or increase
- Rest tremor
- Dystonic posturing
- Chorea

Finger nose testing may reveal
- Action tremor
- Intention tremor
- Myoclonus may exacerbate
- Choreic movements.

Repetitive movements—slowed or break up easily—bradykinesia.

Writing becomes progressively slower and the patient may hold the pen in an unusual way (writer's cramp).

Describe

1. Pattern of movement—Jerky, twisting, repetitive, flinging.
2. Distribution
3. Rate
4. Amplitude
5. Force
6. Factors increasing
7. Factors decreasing
8. Relation to sleep
9. Relation to emotion
10. Onset and progression
11. Associated feature

ABNORMAL MOVEMENTS

Types

Fibrillation

Spontaneous random contraction of denervated muscle fiber detected by EMG, seen clinically in spinal muscular atrophy in the tongue.

Fasciculation

Twitching of a small part of a muscle due to random discharges of LMN.
Benign fasculation are common in normal person, e.g.
Eyelids and during exhaustion and fatigue.

Pathological: AHC Damage-Polio, SMA (I) Nerve root irritation often associated with atrophy, hyporeflexia and weakness.

Tremor

Rhythmic, regular oscillations of a body part

Types:

1. Resting tremors (3-5 cycles per second [CPS]) often seen in parkinsonism, has low amplitude and regular frequency of 5 CPS, disappear during intentional movement and increases during emotional stress.

   There are two descriptive types   a. Pillrolling

                                                    b. Drum beating

2. Parkinsonism tremors are often associated with leadpipe or cogwheel rigidity, over all bradykinesia, akathesia (an irresistible need to move).

3. Intentional (ataxic tremor) regular tremor of low or moderate amplitude that appear during intentional movement (Finger nose test).

4. Positional or postural tremor: Occurs in maintaining a certain posture, e.g. holding head up or out stretching of hand. These are seen in cerebellar lesion or in their pathways. A combination of resting tremor, intention tremor, postural tremor constitutes "rubral tremor" due to a lesion in Dentato rubral or dentothalamic tract.

5. Tremors of anxiety, hypoglycemia and hyperthyroidism are fine and fast (10CPS)

Clinical Evaluation of Tremors

1. Distribution (Hand, jaws, tongue, head, trunk, legs)
2. Rate (3-12 CPS)

   Physiological-10 CPS

   Parkinsonism-5 CPS
3. Amplitude (fine, coarse)
4. Relation to movement— Intentional (cerebellar)

                                      Posture—postural

                                      Rest (Resting—parkinsonism)

                                      End point tremor (Finger-nose test—cerebellum)
5. Relation to sleep and emotion—All disappear in sleep and increased during emotions
6. Response to drugs
7. Associated symptoms

Chorea (Like English twist dance !)

Sudden

Jerky

Nonrepetitive

Resembling fragments of normal movements

Most prominent in extremities, however seen in tongue, face

Exaggerated by emotion and action

Quasipurposive movement

Disappear during sleep

Common causes: Rheumatic chorea
Drug induced
TB meningitis
Encephalitis,
Chorea gravidarum

Rare causes: Wilson's disease
Huntington's chorea
Typhoid,
Diphtheria
Leukodystrophies
Hallovarden Spartz syndrome
Carbon monoxide poisoning

Rheumatic chorea is often associated with:

a. Hypotonia
b. Pendular jerks
c. Flexor plantars
d. Brisk superfical reflexes
e. Milk maid's grip
f. Facial grimace
g. Bad handwriting
h. Dinner fork deformity of hand
i. Explosive speech, dysarthria
j. Jack in box tongue
k. Choreic hand
l. Other features of rheumatic disease like arthritis, carditis, subcutaneous nodules.

CHOREA

Differential Diagnosis

Congenital
Cerebral palsy

Degenerative
Canavan's spongy degeneration

Genetic
- Ataxia telangiectasia
- Bassen-Kornweiz disease
- Benign familial chorea
- Dystonia musculorum deformans
- Fabry's disease
- Familial paroxysmal choreoathetosis
- Friedreich's ataxia
- Glutaric acedemia
- Huntington's chorea

- Incontinentia pigmenti
- Lesch Nyhan syndrome
- Phenylketonuria
- Porphyria
- Sturge-Weber disease
- Tardive dyskinesia
- Wilson's disease

Infectious

- Diphtheria
- Encephalitis
- Neurosyphilis
- Pertussis
- Post streptococcal
- Typhoid fever

Metabolic and Endocrine

- Addison's disease
- Beriberi
- Cerebral lipidoses
- Hypocalcemia
- Hypoglycemia
- Hypomagnesemia
- Hyponatremia
- Hypoparathyroidism
- Kernicterus
- Polycythemia
- Thyrotoxicosis
- Vitamin B_{12} deficiency in infants
- Wilson's disease

Neoplastic

- Brain tumors

Toxic

- Carbon monoxide
- Isoniazid
- Lithium
- Mercury
- Phenothiazines
- Reserpine
- Scopolamine

Traumatic

Burns in children

Unknown and Miscellaneous
- Hyperkinetic syndrome
- Intranuclear hyaline inclusion
- Parietal chorea

Vascular
- Henoch-Schönlein purpura
- Cerebral infarction
- Lupus erythematosus
- Posthemiplegic chorea

  In Pediatric clinical practice the most common cause for chorea is Syndenham's chorea and hence it is described in detail:

Sydenham's Chorea
Characteristic features of choreiform movements
1. Involuntary movements
2. Sudden, jerky
3. Nonrepetitive
4. Occurring at distal joints
5. Quasipurposive
6. Disappear during sleep
7. Exaggerated by emotions and presence of people are other features seen in Sydenham's chorea.
8. Associated movements
9. Emotional lability
10. Muscular hypotonia
11. Pendular jerks (or depressed or absent deep tendon reflexes)
12. Brisk superficial reflexes especially abdominal reflexes.
13. Signs in chorea:
    a. Hand:
        - Choreic hand (Dinner fork deformity).
          Subluxation of hand with extended fingers.
        - Pronator sign—when upper limbs are held above head, there will be pronation of forearms, flexion of wrists and hyperextension of MCP & IP joints.
        - Milk maid's grip—alternate loosening of grip on the examiners finge.
        - Clumsy hand writing.
    b. Oral:
        - Explosive speech
        - Dysarthria
        - Jack in box—sudden protrusion of the tongue when asked to protrude the tongue.
        - Adder tongue—alternate protrusion and retraction of tongue.
14. Examine for other features of rheumatic fever:
    Carditis
    Subcutaneous nodules, arthritis.

15. Clinical types of Sydenham's chorea:
    a. Hemichorea
    b. Manic chorea: Emotional disturbance is more
    c. Paralytic chorea: Due to excessive hypotonia
    d. Chorea gravidarum: Seen in pregnancy

Treatment:
A. Three-drug regime:
   1. Diazepam   — 0.3 mg/kg body wt/day ⎫
   2. Phenobarbitone — 3-8 mg/kg body wt/day ⎬ 4-6 weeks
   3. Chlorpromazine — 2 mg/kg body wt/day ⎭
B. Sodium valporate — 20 mg/kg body wt/day for 10-14 days
C. Inj. procaine penicillin 4 L IM daily for 10 days followed by injecting benzathine penicillin 12 lacs IM once every 3 weeks for life long.
D. Attend to nutrition
E. Avoid injuries

Daily Follow-up of Patients with Chorea
1. For abnormal movements
   • Hand writing
   • Coordination in use of hands
2. For cardiac involvement
   • Sleeping pulse rate
   • Intensity of first heart sound (muffling)
   • Appearance of murmurs
3. State of nutrition
4. Injury prevention

Long-Term Follow-up and Prognosis
1. Cardiac involvement in 1/3 cases after 10 years
2. Recurrence of chorea in 1/3 cases
3. Tics
4. Cognitive function defects.

ATHETOSIS (Like Bharatnatyam !)
Slow twisting movements of the periphery—mostly fingers and wrists.

Differential Diagnosis of Diseases Causing Athetosis

Degenerative/Familial Diseases
• Hallervorden-Spatz disease
• Progressive pallidal atrophy
• Tuberous sclerosis
• Wilsons' disease
• Pelizeaus-Merzbacher disease

Toxic Causes
• Hyperbilirubinemia
• Kernicterus

- Sepsis
- Sulfonamides
- Hepatitis
- Carbon monoxide poisoning
- Lithium
- Barbiturates

Metabolic Diseases
- Birth Anoxia
- Lesch-Nyhan syndrome
- Tay-Sach's disease
- Phenylketonuria

Vascular Diseases
- Residual infantile hemiplegia
- Emboli

Infections
- Measles
- Pertussis
- Diphtheria
- Tuberculosis
- Encephalitis

Trauma
- Birth trauma

Neoplasm
- Rare cause of hemiathetosis

DYSTONIA (Like Break Dance !)
Prolonged slow alternating contraction and relaxation of agonists and antagonists often occurring in proximal joints and cause abnormal posturing of limbs (twisting) for a prolonged period of time (like scoliosis, contractures of joints).

Sometimes they are focal, e.g. spasmodic torticolis, writer's cramp.

Differential Diagnosis
1. Congenital and developmental
   - Benign dystonia of infancy
   - Cerebral palsy (dystonic form)
   - Dyspeptic dystonia with hiatus hernia
   - Paroxysmal torticollis in infancy.
2. Degenerative disorders:
   - Ataxia telangiectasia
   - Dystonia musculorum deformans

- Focal dystonias
- Hallervorden-Spatz syndrome
- Hemidystonia
- Idiopathic torsion dystonias
- Leber disease
- Myoclonic dystonia
- Subacute necrotising encephalomyelopathy
- Dystonia—parkinsonian syndrome
3. Infectious disease:
   - Viral encephalitis
4. Metabolic conditions:
   - GM_1 ganglosidosis
   - GM_2 gangliosidosis
   - Glutamic acidemia
   - Mitochondrial encephalomyelopathies
   - Phenylketonuria
   - Wilson's disease
5. Reaction to medications
   - Bethanechol
   - Carbamazepine
   - Phenothiazine
   - Reserpine
6. Psychogenic—Munchausen syndrome
7. Sleep abnormalities—Paraoxysmal sleep dystonia

HEMIBALLISMUS (Like Russian Ballet !)

Violent flinging movements of one-half of the body. (Ballista means to throw as in ballistics).

Lesion is in subthalamic nuclei

Causes: Tubercular meningitis

Encepahalitis

Vascular accident in the region of subthalamic nuclei

TIC: Spontaneous stereotyped muscle contraction often involving face. They can be momentarily stopped by volition. They are often associated with obsessive-compulsion personality traits.

CHILDHOOD TICS

Etiological Classification

Idiopathic
- Acute simple transient tic (<1yr)
- Persistent simple or multiple tic of childhood (Remits by adult life)
- Chronic simple or multiple motor tics (Persists throughout life)
- Gilles de La Tourette syndrome

Secondary tics
- Postencephalitis
- Sydenham chorea
- Head trauma
- Carbon monoxide poisoning
- Post-stroke
- Acanthocytosis
- Drugs—levodopa, phenytoin, carbamazepine, etc.
- Mental retardation syndromes and chromosomal anomalies.

OTHER TYPES OF ABNORMAL MOVEMENTS

Oculogyric Crisis
Spontaneous upward deviation of eyes and head, seen with resting tremor and lead pipe rigidity.
Causes: Phenothiazine drugs.

Tardive Dyskinesia (Meige's Syndrome)
A therapy resistant hyperkinesia usualy with predominant face, lip and tongue movement, that appear after prolonged ingestion of psychotropic medications.

Akathisia
An irresistible need for movement characterised by irresistible, restless movements and shifting of postures often seen in parkinsonism.

Myoclonic Jerks
Sudden shock like spontaneous contraction of a muscle or a group of muscles causing startle like phenomena. These are due to sudden discharge from reticular activating sites of brainstem (Tables 27.15 and 27.16).

Physiological
Hypnogagic and hypnopompic jerks (before falling asleep and during waking).

Pathological
Infantile myoclonus, SSPE, encephalitis, tuberous sclerosis, etc. may be flexor, extensor or mixed. Salam seizures, where in, head and trunk suddenly bend, and are characterstic of infantile spasm (West's syndrome).
   Myoclonus may be static or progressive. Static myoclonus is usually benign. Progressive myoclonus usually indicates the presence of a metabolic, hereditary or infectious process.
   Myoclonus may be grouped by the following general categories.
1. Genetic: Essential myoclonus, progressive myoclonus, progressive myoclonus epilepsy (e.g. Lafora disease), and storage conditions (e.g. lipidosis).
2. Seizure disorders: Idiopathic epilepsy and infantile spasms.
3. Brain injury: Anoxia, toxins and metabolic disorders.
4. Viral infections.
5. Miscellaneous: Opsoclonus, nocturnal myoclonus and palatal myoclonus.

Table 27.15: Myoclonic jerks may be rythmic v/s arrhythmic

Classification	Bodypart	Rhythm	Stress response	Sleep response	Sensory response	Motor response
Arrhythmic	Varies often fluctuates	Irregular and variable	Increase	Absent	Increase	Increase
Rhythmic	Segmental	Regular	Unchanged	Present	Unchanged	Unchanged

MYOCLONUS

Arrhythmic

Table 27.16: Myoclonus arrhythmic jerks

Reticular reflex myoclonus	Cortical reflex myoclonus
Primarily affects proximal muscles	• Primarily affect distal muscles
Generalized myoclonic response to sensory stimuli	• Sensory stimuli evoke myoclonus that is limited to distal muscles
Specific EEG abnormalities, related but not synchronous with movements	• EEG abnormalities usually synchronous with the myoclonic jerks
Sensory-evoked potentials of normal voltage	• Sensory-evoked potentials of high voltage
Brainstem activation caudo rostral	• Brainstem activation is rostrocaudal

Historic data, including any familial incidence of movement disorders, are essenital. Exposure to anoxia, toxins, or trauma should be ascertained. The examination should determine whether myoclonus is focal or generalised.

Classification of Myoclonus

Segmental
1. *Brainstem*
   a. Eye
   b. Palate
   c. Jaw
   d. Face
   e. Neck and tongue
2. *Toxic*
   a. Limb
   b. Trunk
   c. Diaphragm
3. *Etiology*
   a. Vascular
   b. Infections
   c. Demyelinating
   d. Neoplastic
   e. Traumatic
   f. Unknown.

Generalised (Subcortical, Brainstem or Spinal Cord Involvement, Table 27.17)

Acute and subacute
1. Encephalomyelitis (including polio)
2. Toxic and infections
   a. Other infection
      i. Tetanus
      ii. Nonspecific
   b. Strychnine
   c. Other (including drugs)
3. Anoxia
4. Metabolic (Uremia, hepatic insufficiency)
5. Degenerative (inclusion body encephalitis)

Table 27.17: Selected causes of myoclonus

Congenital	Neuronal ceroid-lipofuscinosis
Aicardi syndrome	Pyridoxine dependency
Cerebral agenesis	Tay-Sachs disease
Holoprosencephaly	Uremia
Porencephaly	Wilson's disease
Syringomyelia	
	Unknown
Toxic	Myoclonic encephalopathy of infancy
Antihistamines	(with or without neuroblastoma)
Lead intoxication	
Minamata disease	**Degenerative**
Pentylenetetrazol	Familial progressive myoclonic epilepsy
Tranquilizers	Infantile myoclonic spasms
	Incontinentia pigmenti
Trauma	Lafora body disease
Anoxia	Multiple sclerosis
Intracerebral hemorrhage	Progressive degeneration of gray matter
Subdural hematoma	(Alpers disease)
	Ramsay-Hunt syndrome
Vascular	Sturge-Weber syndrome
Thrombosis: cortex,	Sudanophilic leukodystrophy
cerebellum, brainstem, and spinal cord	Tuberous sclerosis
	Unverricht-Lundborg disease
Metabolic and endocrinologic	
Aminoacidopathies	**Infectious**
Hyperglycinemia	Acute and chronic encephalitis
Maple syrup disease	Herpes zoster meningoencephalitis
Phenylketonuria	Malaria
Hallervorden-Spatz syndrome	Polio
Hepatic failure	Postencephalitic syndrome
Hypoglycemia	Postimmunization syndrome
Hypoxia	Smallpox
Kwashiorkor	Subacute sclerosing parencephalitis
Menke's disease	Tuberculous meningitis

Contd...

Chronic
1. Progressive myoclonus epilepsy (Lafora bodies, lipidoses, Ramsay-Hunt syndrome).
2. Nonprogressive intermittent myoclonus with epilepsy.
3. Essential myoclonus (paramyoclonus multiplex).
4. Nocturnal myoclonus.

Any approach to the problem of a child with myoclonus must be the result of a systematic appraisal for known associated conditions.

REFLEXES

A tendon reflex results from the stimulation of a stretch sensitive gamma efferent which, via a single synapse, stimulates a motor nerve leading to a muscle contraction.

Root values can be recalled counting from ankle upward (Fig. 27.82).

Simplified diagram of the arc for the tendon reflex is illustrated in Figure 27.83.

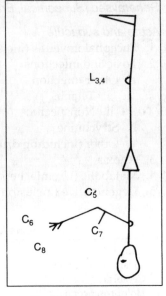

Fig. 27.82: Root values of reflexes

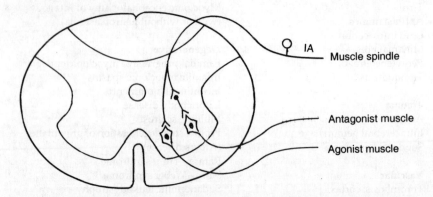

Fig. 27.83: The afferent and efferent limbs of the muscle stretch reflex

Graded as follows:
0 –		No response
1 +	:	Sluggish or diminished
2 +	:	Active or expected response
3 +	:	Brisk
4 +	:	Brisk with clonus

Approach to Deep Tendon Reflexes
1. To find the optimal stimulus by varying the position of the limb which will give the best results.

2. Always use whole length of patellar hammer and let it swing with swinging movements of the hammer at the wrist (Fig. 27.84).
3. Correct plane of tendon to elicit reflexes.
4. Re-enforcement method
5. Certain positions-
   Ex: For ankle jerk-put the child on mothers shoulder and come back and elicit the reflex
6. If there is significant tone
   Deep tendon reflexes may not be elicited so reduce the tone by moving the limbs.
7. Isolated exaggerated reflex is of no significance.
8. Upto 2 years-normal plantar may be extensor.
9. Equivocal response, i.e. only extensor or only fanning seen in pyramidal lesion.

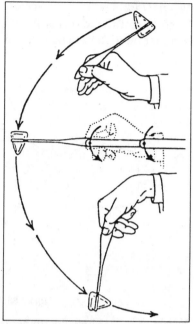

Fig. 27.84: Technique for striking a blow with a reflex hammer. Notice the loose, double pivot action at the wrist and fingers

Jaw Jerk

With the patient's jaw sagging loosely open the mouth, place your finger across the jaw and strike a crisp blow and watch the movement of the jaw (Fig. 27.85).

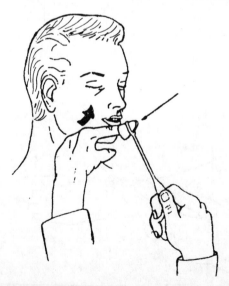

Fig. 27.85: Jaw reflex. With the patient's jaw sagging loosely open, the jaw and strikes it acrisp blow, the thin arrow shows the direction of the percussion hammer blow, the thick arrow shows the response

Biceps Jerk

Place patient's hand on his abdomen. Place your index finger on tendon. Swing hammer on to it. Watch biceps muscle (Fig. 27.86).

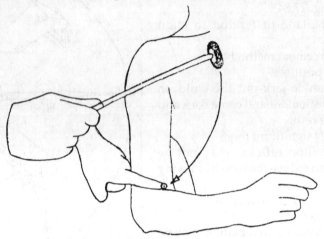

Fig. 27.86: Testing the biceps reflex

Nerve : Musculocutaneous, root value C5 C6

Supinator Reflex (Misnomer; muscle involved is brachioradialis)

Arm flexed on the abdomen, finger on the radial tuberosity. Hit the finger with the hammer and watch the brachioradialis muscle (Fig. 27.87).

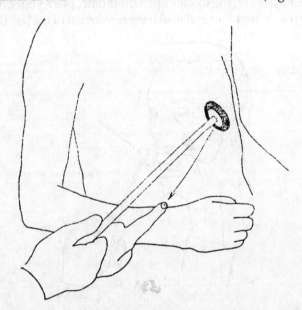

Fig. 27.87: Testing the supinator reflex

Nerve : Radial nerve, root value C6 (C5).

Triceps Jerk

Draw the arm across the chest, holding the wrist and elbow at 90°. Strike the triceps tendon directly with patellar hammer. Watch the muscle (Fig. 27.88).

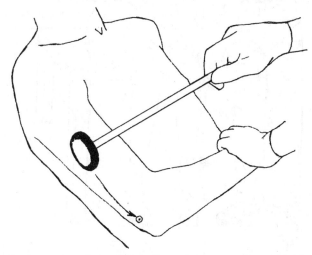

Fig. 27.88: Testing the triceps reflex

Nerve   :   Radial nerve, root value: C7.

Knee Jerk (Quadriceps Femoris Reflex)

Place the arm below the knee so that the knee is at 90°. Strike below the patella; watch the quadriceps (Figs 27.89A to C).

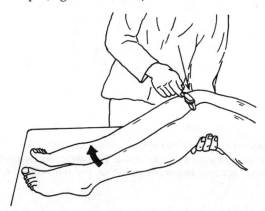

Fig. 27.89A: Quadriceps femoris reflex, patient supine. The ex-bends the patient slight tension on the patellar tendon. The blow then will deform the tendon and transmit a stretch to the muscle

Nerve   :   Femoral, root value: L3-L4.

Patellar Clonus

With the leg straight, grip the patella and briskly bring it downwards, a rhythmic contraction is noted. It is always abnormal, indicates UMN type of lesion (increased stretch).

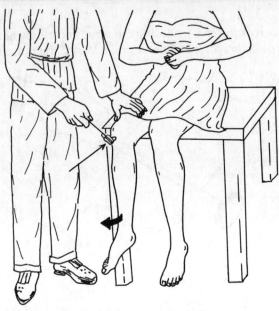

Fig. 27.89B: Pull method (of jendrassik) for reinforcing the quadriceps reflex. The patient locks the hands and pulls apart hard while the ex-strikes the tendon

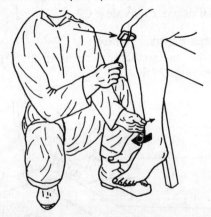

Fig. 27.89C: Counterpressure method for reinforcing the quadriceps reflex. The ex-applies slight thumb pressure (small arrow) against the patient's tibia. The patient counteracts the thumb pressure by slight tension in the quadriceps femoris muscle. Then the ex-strikes the quadriceps tendon

Ankle Reflex

Hold foot at 90° with medial malleolus facing the ceiling. The knee should be flexed and lying to the side, strike achilles tendon and watch calf muscles (Fig. 27.90A).

Nerve   :   Tibial, root value S1 S2.

Alternatives Methods of Testing Ankle Jerk
1. Legs straight, place your hand on ball of the foot, strike your hand, watch muscles of the calf (Fig. 27.90B).

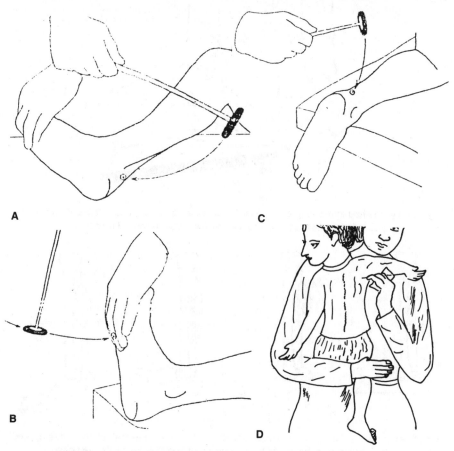

Figs 27.90A to D: (A to C) The ankle reflex and (D) Position for eliciting ankle jerk in infants

2. Ask patient to kneel on a chair so that ankles hang loosely over the edge. Strike achilles tendon directly (Fig. 27.90C).
3. In infants, the ankle jerk can be elicited with the infant on mother's shoulders (Fig. 27.90D).

Ankle Clonus
Dorsiflex the ankle briskly. Maintain the foot in that position, rhythmic contraction > 3 beats is abnormal (Figs 27.91A and B).

Reinforcement
If any reflex is not obtainable directly, then ask the patient to do some reinforcement like linking hands across the chest and pull them apart as you try for reflex. In children, crying is a very good reinforcement (Fig. 27.92).

OTHER ALLIED REFLEXES

Hoffmann Reflex
The terminal phalanx of the patient's middle finger is flicked downward between the examiner's finger and thumb. In states of hyperreflexia, organic

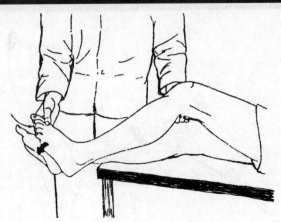

Fig. 27.91A: Method for eliciting ankle clonus. The ex-jerks upward and a little outward on the patient's foot (thin arrow). The thick arrow is the downward response

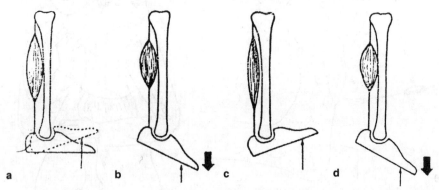

Fig. 27.91B: Mechanism of ankle clonus. The thin arrow represents the light pressure applied by the examiner to the ball of the patient's foot, the thick arrow the response

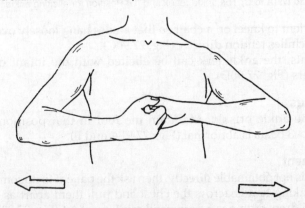

Fig. 27.92: Reinforcement

or emotional, the tips of the other fingers flex and the thumb flexes and adducts. If this finding is on one side only, it can sometimes be an early sign of unilateral pyramidal tract disease (Fig. 27.93).

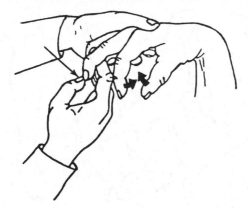

Fig. 27.93: Finger flexion reflex (Hoffman's method). With a thumb, the ex-flexes the distal phalanx of the finger, while pressing up with the index finger. Then the ex-releases the phalanx abruptly, allowing it to up shaprly. The abrupt release and resultant extension of the phalanx stretches the flexor muscles, causing fingers and thumb to flex. The patient's MSRs must be very brisk for this method to work

Wartenberg's Sign

The patient supinates his hand, slightly flexing the fingers. The examiner pronates his hand and links his similarly flexed fingers with the patient's. Both then flex their fingers further against each other's resistance. Normally, the thumb extends, though the terminal phalanx may flex slightly. In pyramidal tract lesions, the thumb adducts and flexes strongly. Unfortunately this is not a constant sign but if present on one side only, it can indicate an early state of pyramidal tract disease (Fig. 27.94).

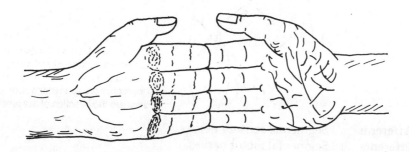

Fig. 27.94: Wartenberg's sign. Normal result. Note thumb extension of the patient

Rossolimo's Reflex

The patient lies supine with the leg extended and the foot partially dorsi-flexed. The ball of the foot is then struck with the hammer and in hypertonic states there is a brisk contraction of all toes. The same reflex can be obtained by flicking the toes in an upward direction. Its significance is the same as the finger flexion reflex in the upper limb (Fig. 27.95).

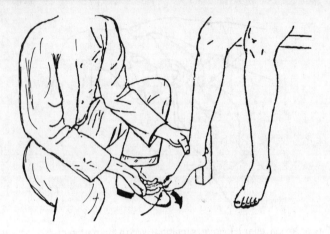

Fig. 27.95: Toe flexion reflex (Rossolimo's method).
The maneuver is identical with the finger flexion method

SUPERFICIAL REFLEXES

Abdominal Reflex

Using a blunt stick, lightly scratch the abdominal wall as indicated in figure. The abdominal wall on the same side must contract (Fig. 27.96).

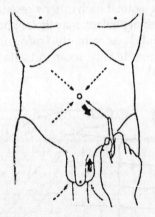

Fig. 27.96: Method for eliciting the superficial abdominal and cremasteric reflexes. The thin arrows are the direction of the examiner's stroke. The thick are the direction of the response

Afferents	:	Segmental sensory nerves.
Efferents	:	Segmental motor nerves.
Roots	:	Above umbilicus: T_8-T_9.
		Below umbilicus T_{10}-T_{11}.

Absent reflex seen in:
- Obesity
- Previous abdominal operations.
- Frequent pregnancy
- Pyramidal tract involvement above that level
- Peripheral nerve abnormality.

Plantar Response (Babinski's sign)

Explain procedure to the patient. Gently draw a blunt stimulus along the lateral border of the sole along the foot pad. Watch the big toe and remainder of the foot. Figures 27.97A and B shows the reflex arc of the plantar reflex.

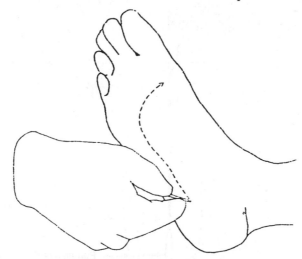

Fig. 27.97A: Testing the plantar response

Responses

- All toes flex flexor response—Negative Babinski's sign—Normal
- Great toe extends, other toes spread-extensor plantar response-**Babinski's sign-positive**
- No movement-No response
- Big toe extends, other toes extend, ankle flexes-withdrawal response-repeat gently or try alternate methods

    Few important points for practical consideration

- Scratching the lateral side of sole with key is the best method for eliciting plantar response. In infants toe nail may be used to give stimuli (Fig. 27.97C).

    See the initial response. Stop as soon as you get the response.

- In younger children asymmetry is more important.
- Plantar response can be normally extensor upto 18-24 months.
- Repeated stimulation causes exhaution of the reflex.
- Plantar response should not be mistaken for plantar grasp which is normally present in infants upto 7 months. In plantar grasp the stimulus is given at the ball of toes on medial side, where as to elicit plantar response noxious stimulus is applied to lateral side of sole.
- The length, strength and speed of stimulus are all important in eliciting plantar response.

Positive Babinski Sign

Indicates UMN lesion. It may be normally seen till the age of 2 years when myelination has not taken place. Too much weight cannot be placed on this

the
Pre
her
sm.
occ

Inf
ile

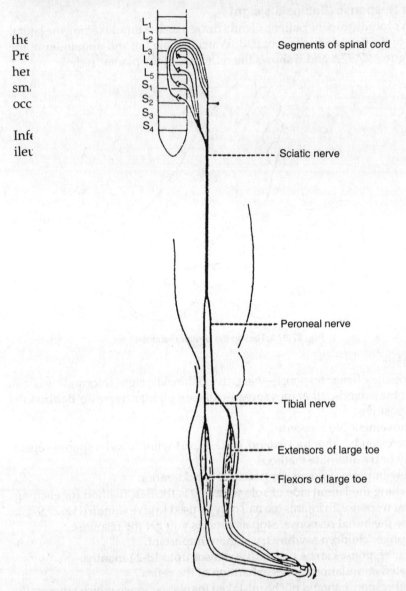

Segments of spinal cord

L₁
L₂
L₃
L₄
L₅
S₁
S₂
S₃
S₄

Sciatic nerve

Peroneal nerve

Tibial nerve

Extensors of large toe

Flexors of large toe

Fig. 27.97B: Reflex arc for the plantar reflexes. For simplicity, the diagram shows the flexor hallucis brevis in the cali rather than in the foot

sign in isolation. A negative sign may be seen if profound weakness is seen in the muscles leading to inability to extend the toe or if there is a sensory abnormality interfering with the afferent part of the reflex.

Alternative Methods
To elicit same response see Figures 27.98A to G and Table 27.18.

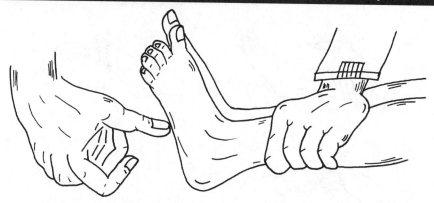

Fig. 27.97C: Plantar reflex by nail scratch (extensor response). Best method in infants

Table 27.18:

Descriptive name	Eponym	Maneuver
A. Plantar toe reflex	Babinski	• Move an object along the lateral aspect of the sole
B. None	Chaddock	• Move an object along the lateral side of the foot.
C. Achilles-toe reflex	Schaeffer	• Squeeze hard on the Achilles tendon.
D. Shin-toe reflex	Oppenheim	• Press your knuckles on the patient's shin and move them down.
E. Calf–toe reflex	Gordon	• Squeeze the calf muscles momentarily.
F. Pinprick–toe reflex	Bing	• Make multiple light pinpricks on the dorsolateral surface of the foot.
G. Toe pull reflex	Gonda, Stransky	• Pull the 4th toe outward for a brief time and release suddenly.

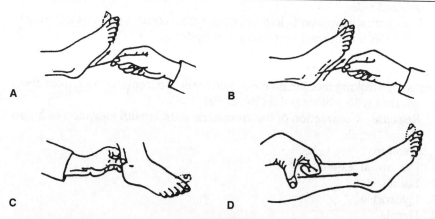

Figs 27.98A to D

Conjunctival and Corneal Reflex

Afferent	:	Ophthalmic division of trigeminal nerve
Reflex center	:	Pons

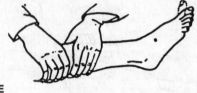
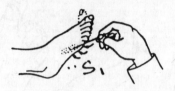

E   F

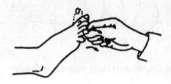

G   **Figs 27.98A to G:** Methods for eliciting the extensor toe sign

Efferent   :   Facial nerve
Method   :   The examiner touches the cornea or conjunctiva from the
                   side with a wisp of cotton. In response to this stimulus there
                   is closing of the same eye (direct) and opposite eye (Con-
                   sensual response) (See examination of trigeminal nerve).

Significance
1. In unilateral trigeminal nerve lesion, resulting in corneal and conjunctival
   anesthesia, stimulation of these structures fails to produce direct or consensual response but stimulation of opposite side results in production of
   both of these.
2. In unilateral facial palsy with weakness of orbicularis occuli, when either
   cornea is stimulated response occurs only on the normal side, not on
   affected side.
3. Conjuctival response is less important than corneal response. It may be
   absent in few normal persons and in hysteria.

Cremasteric Reflex (L1)
Elicited by stroking the skin on the upper, inner aspect of the thigh from above
downwards with a blunt point (Fig. 27.96).
   Response   Contraction of the cremastric muscle with elevation of homolateral testicle.
   Absent in:
1. Pyramidal lesions
2. Local lesion
3. Hydrocele
4. ̄ Hernia

Bulbocavernous Reflex (S2-S4)
Elicted by pressing the glans penis
   Response   Contraction of the bulbocavernous muscle, felt at the junction
   of the penis and the scrotum

Absent in:
1. Pyramidal lesion
2. Reflex arc lesion

Anal Reflex (S4-S5)

Elicited by stroking or pricking the skin or mucous membrane in the perianal region.

    Response   Contraction of the external anal sphincter

    Absent in:
1. Pyramidal lesion
2. Lesion of local reflex arc of S4-S5.

DEVELOPMENTAL REFLEXES

Primitive reflexes are essential in normal development. Response to these reflexes prepares the child for progressive development, such as rolling over, sitting, crawling, standing, etc. In normal development, these primitive spinal and brainstem reflexes gradually diminish in order that higher patterns of righting and equilibrium reactions may become manifested (Table 27.19). When inhibitory control of higher centers is disrupted or delayed, primitive patterns dominate to the exclusion of higher, integrated sensorimeter activities. Certain neurologic dysfunctions are believed to result from specific CNS lesions. Such lesions release primitive, abnormal reflexes from inhibition normally exerted by higher centers. These more primitive reflexes result in abnormalities manifested by phylogenetically older postures and movements and abnormal muscle tone.

    There are three levels of reflexive development.

Table 27.19: Normal sequential development

Levels of CNS maturation	Correspondence levels of Reflexive development	Resulting levels of motor development
Spinal and/or Brain Stem Midbrain	Apedal Primitive reflexes Quadrupedal Righting reactions	Prone-lying Supine-lying Crawling Sitting
Cortical	Bipedal Equilibrium reactions	Standing Walking

Apedal

Predominance of primitive spinal and brainstem reflexes with motor development of a prone or supine-lying child.

Quadrupedal

Predominance of midbrain development with righting reactions and motor development that of a child who can right himself, turn over, assume crawling and sitting positions.

Bipedal

At cortical level of development reveals equilibrium reactions with motor development that of a child who can assume the standing position and ambulate.

Spinal reflexes are mediated by areas of the CNS Deiters' nucleus which is in the lower third of the pons (Tables 27.20 and 27.21). Spinal reflexes are "phasic" or movement reflexes which coordinate muscles of the extremities in patterns of either total flexion or extension. Positive or negative reactions to spinal reflex testing may be present in the normal child within the first two months of life. Positive reactions persisting beyond two months of age may be indicative of delayed maturation of the CNS negative reactions are normal. Complete domination by these primitive spinal reflexes results in an apedal (prone, supine-lying) child.

Table 27.20: List of developmental reflexes

Mediated at	Reflexes
1. Spinal cord level	Flexor withdrawal
	Extensor thirst
	Crossed extensor
2. Brainstem level	Asymmetrical tonic neck
	Symmetrical tonic neck,
	Tonic labyrinthine (prone and supine)
	Positive supporting reaction
	Negative supporting reaction
3. Midbrain level	Neck righting
	Body righting
	Labyrinthine righting (prone and supine)
	Optical righting (Prone and supine)
4. Cortical	(Various balancing reflexes)
	Four foot kneeling
	Sitting
	Kneel standing
	Hopping
	See-saw
	Simian position
5. ? Semicircular canals	Moro reflex
? Labyrinths	Landau reflex
? Neck proprioceptors	Protective extensor thurst
(Automatic movement reactions)	(Parachute reflex)

Brainstem reflexes are mediated by areas from Deiters' nucleus to the red nucleus which sits at the most caudal level of the basal ganglia. Brainstem reflexes are "static" postural reflexes and effect changes in distribution of muscle tone throughout the body, either in response to a change of the position of head and body in space (by stimulation of the labyrinths), or in the head in relation to the body (by stimulation of proprioceptors of the neck muscles. Positive or negative reactions to brain stem reflex testing may be present in the normal child within the first four to six months of life. Positive reactions persisting beyond six months of age may be indicative of delayed motor maturation of the CNS. Negative reactions are normal. Complete domination by these primitive brainstem reflexes results in an apedal (prone, supine-lying) child.

Table 27.21: Development reflexes

Reflexes	Test position	Test stimulus	Negative reaction	Positive reaction
SPINAL CORD LEVEL				
Flexor Withdrawal	Patient supine Head in mid-position Legs extended.	Stimulate sole of foot.	Controlled maintenance of stimulated leg in extension or volitional with-drawal from irritating stimulus	Uncontrolled flexion response of stimulated leg. (Do not confuse with response to tickling).
(Positive reaction is normal upto two months of age. Positive reaction after two months of age may be one indication of delayed reflexive maturation.)				
Extensor Thrust	Patient supine. Head in mid-position. One leg extended, opposite leg flexed.	Stimulate sole of foot of flexed leg.	Controlled maintenance of leg in flexion.	Uncontrolled extension of stimulated leg. (Do not confuse with response to tickling).
(Positive reaction is normal upto two months of age. Positive reaction after two months of age may be one indication of delayed reflexive maturation.)				
Crossed Extension	Patient supine. Head in mid-position One leg flexed, opposite leg extended.	Flex the extended leg	On flexion of the extended leg, the opposite leg will remain flexed	On flexion of the extended leg, the opposite, or initially flexed, leg will extend.
(Positive reaction is normal upto two months of age. Positive reaction after two months of age may be one indication of delayed reflexive maturation.)				
BRAINSTEM LEVEL				
Asymmetrical Tonic Neck	Patient supine Head in mid-position Arms and legs extended.	Turn head to one side.	No reaction of limbs on either side.	Extension of arm and leg on face side, or increase in extensor tone; flexion of arm and leg on skull side, or increase in flexor tone. ("Like Fencing Position")
(Positive reaction is normal upto four to six months of age. An obligatory ASTN reflex is pathologic at any age. Positive reactions after six months may be one indication of delayed reflexive maturation.)				

Contd...

Table 27.21 contd...

Reflexes	Test position	Test stimulus	Negative reaction	Positive reaction
Symmetrical Tonic Neck 1	Patient in quadruped position or over tester's knees	Ventroflex the head.	No change in tone of arms or legs.	Arms flex or flexor tone dominates; legs extended or extensor tone dominates. ("Like dog drinking water")
(Positive reaction is normal upto four to six months of age. An obligatory ASTN reflex is pathologic at any age. Positive reactions after six months may be one indication of delayed reflexive maturation).				
Symmetrical Tonic Neck 2	Patient in quadruped position or over tester's knees	Dorsiflex the head	No change in tone of arms or legs.	Arms extend or extensor tone dominates; legs flex or flexor tone dominates. ("Like howling dog")
(Positive reaction is normal upto four to six months of age. An obligatory ASTN reflex is pathologic at any age. Positive reactions after six months may be one indication of delayed reflexive maturation).				
Positive Supporting Reaction	Hold patient in standing position.	Bounce several times on soles of feet.	No increase of tone (Legs volitionally flex)	Increase of extensor tone in legs. Plantar flexion of feets, genu recurvatum may occur
(Positive reaction is normal from 3 to 8 months of age. Positive reaction after eight months of age may be one indication of delayed reflexive maturation.)				
Negative Supporting Reaction	Bring patient to standing position	Weight-bearing position	Release of extensor tone from positive supporting allows platigrade feet and flexion of legs.	No release of extensor tone, positive supporting persists.
(Normal reaction is sufficient release of extensor tone to allow flexion for reciprocation. Abnormal reaction is continuation of positive supporting reflex beyond eight months of age. A reaction of excessive flexion on weight bearing is abnormal beyond four months of age).				

Contd...

Table 27.21 contd...

Reflexes	Test position	Test stimulus	Negative reaction	Positive reaction
MIDBRAIN LEVEL				
Neck Righting	Patient supine. Head in mid position Arms and legs extended	Rotate head to one side, actively or passively	Body will not rotate	Body rotates as a whole in the same direction as the head.
	(Positive reaction is normal from birth to six months of age. Positive reaction beyond six months of age may be one indication of delayed reflexive maturation. Negative reaction over one month of age is one indication of delayed reflexive maturation.)			
Body Righting Acting on the Body	Patient supine Head in mid position Arms and legs extended	Rotate head to one side, actively or passively	Body rotates as a whole (neck righting) and not segmentaly	Segmental rotation of trunk between shoulders and pelvis, e.g. head turns then shoulders, finally the pelvis.
	(Positive reaction emerges about six months of age and continues to eighteen months of age. Negative reaction over six months of age may be one indication of delayed reflexive maturation.)			
Labyrinthine Righting Acting on the Head 1	Hold blindfolded patient in space. Prone position.	Prone position in space *per se.*	Head does not raise automatically to the normal position	Head raises to normal position, face vertical, mouth horizontal
	(Positive reaction is normal about one to two months of age and continues throughout life. Negative reaction after two months of age may be one indication of delayed reflexive maturation.)			
Labyrinthine Righting Acting on the Head 2	Hold blindfolded patient in space. Supine position.	Supine position in space *per se.*	Head does not raise automatically to the normal position.	Head raises to normal position, face vertical, mouth horizontal
	(Positive reaction is normal about six months of age and continues throughout life. Negative reaction after six months of age may be one indication of delayed reflexive maturation.)			

Contd...

Table 27.21 contd...

Reflexes	Test position	Test stimulus	Negative reaction	Positive reaction
Optical Righting 1	Hold patient in space. Prone position	Prone position in space *per se*.	Head does not raise automatically to the normal position	Head raises to normal position, face vertical, mouth horizontal
(Positive reaction normally appears soon after labyrinthine righting acting on the head (1-2 months) and continues throughout life. (Optical righting reactions in all positions are valid only if the labyrinthine righting is not present). Negative reaction after this time may be one indication of delayed maturation.)				
Optical Righting 2	Hold patient in space. Supine position	Supine position in space *per se*.	Head does not raise automatically to the normal position.	Head raises to normal position, face vertical, mouth horizontal.
(Positive reaction is normal about six months of age and continues throughout life. Negative reaction after six months of age may be one indication of delayed reflexive maturation.)				
CORTICAL LEVEL (Mainly balancing reflexes and few of them are described)				
Sitting	Patient seated on chair.	Pull or tilt patient to one side.	Head and thorax do not right themselves; no equilibrium or protective reactions (It is possible to have positive reactions in some body parts but not in others).	Righting of head and thorax, abduction-extension of arm and leg on raised sied (equilibrium reaction), and protective reactions on lowered side.
(Positive reactions are normal about ten to twelve months of age and continue throughout life. Negative reactions after twelve months of age may be one indication of delayed reflexive maturation.)				
Hopping 1	Patient in standing position. Hold by upper arms.	Move to the left or to the right side.	Head and thorax do not right themselves; no hopping steps to maintain balance.	Righting of head and thorax, hopping steps sideways to maintain equilibrium.
(Positive reactions normal about fifteen to eighteen months of age and continue throughout life. Negative reactions after eighteen months of age may be one indication of delayed reflexive maturation.)				

Contd...

Table 27.21 contd...

Reflexes	Test position	Test stimulus	Negative reaction	Positive reaction
Hopping 2	Patient in standing position. Hold by upper arms	Move forward	Head and thorax do not right themselves; no hopping steps to maintain balance.	Righting of head and thorax, hopping steps sideways to maintain equilibrium.
	(Positive reactions normal about fifteen to eighteen months of age and continue throughout life. Negative reactions after eighteen months of age may be one indication of delayed reflexive maturation.)			
Dorsiflexion	Patient in standing position. Hold under axillae	Tilt patient backwards.	Head and thorax do not right themselves; no dorsiflexion of feet.	Righting of head and thorax, feet dorsiflex
	(Positive reactions normal about fifteen to eighteen months of age and continue throughout life. Negative reactions after eighteen months of age may be one indication of delayed reflexive maturation.)			
See-saw	(Patient must be able to maintain standing balance) Patient in standing position. On same side, hold by hand and foot, flex hip and knee.	Pull arm forward gently and slightly to lateral side.	Head and thorax do not right themselves; Inability to maintain standing balance	Righting of head and thorax; slight abduction and full extension of manually flexed knee to maintain equilibrium.
	(Positive reaction normal about fifteen months of age and continue throughout life. Negative reactions after fifteen months of age may be one indication of delayed reflexive maturation.)			
Simian Position	Patient in squat-sitting position	Tilt to one side.	Head and thorax do not right themselves; inability to assume or maintain position, lack of equilibrium or protective reactions.	Righting of head and thorax, abduction-extension of arm and leg on raised side (equilibrium reaction), and protective on the lowered side.
	(Positive reactions normal about fifteen to eighteen months of age and continue throughout life. Negative reactions after eighteen months of age may be one indication of delayed reflexive maturation.)			

Contd...

Table 27.21 contd...

Reflexes	Test position	Test stimulus	Negative reaction	Positive reaction
? Semicircular canals **? Stretch receptors** **In the neck** **Moro Reflex**	Patient in semi-reclined position.	Drop head backward	Minimal or no startle response	Abduction, extension (or flexion, external rotation of arms; extension and abduction of the fingers.
(Positive reaction is normal from birth to four months of age. Positive reaction after four months of age may be one indication of delayed reflexive maturation).				
Landau Reflex	Patient held in space, supporting thorax. Prone position.	Head raised, actively or passively.	Spine and legs remain in flexed position.	Spine and legs extend. (When head is ventroflexed, spine and legs flex.)
(Positive reaction is normal from six months to two and one half years of age. Positive reaction after two and one half years of age may be one indication of delayed reflexive maturation. Negative reaction is normal from birth to six months of age and from 30 months through out life.)				
Protective Extensor Thrust (Parachute Reflex)	Patient prone. Arms extended over-head.	Suspend patient in air by ankles or pelvis and move head suddenly towards floor.	Arms do not protect head, but show primitive reflex reaction, such as, ATNR or STNR.	Immediate extension of arms with abduction and extension of fingers to protect the head.
(Positive reaction is normal about six months of age and remains throughout life. Negative reaction after six months of age may be one indication of delayed reflexive maturation.)				

Righting reactions are integrated at the midbrain level above the red nucleus, not including the cortex. Righting reactions interact with each other and work toward establishment of normal head and body relationship in space as well as in relation to each other. These are the first such reactions to develop after birth and reach maximal concerted effect about age ten to twelve months. As cortical control increases, they are gradually modified and inhibited and disappear towards the end of the fifth year. Their combined actions enable the child to roll over, sit up, get on his hands and knees, and make him a quadrupedal child.

Equilibrium reactions are mediated by the efficient interaction of cortex, basal ganglia and cerebellum. Maturation of equilibrium reactions brings the individual to the human bipedal stage of motor development. They occur when muscle tone is normalized and provides body adaptation in response to change of center of gravity in the body. They emerge from six months on. Positive reaction at any one level indicates the next higher level of motor activity is possible.

Automatic movement reactions are a group of reflexes observed in infants and young children which are not strictly righting reflexes, but which are reactions produced by changes in the position of the head and involve either the semicircular canals, or labyrinths, or neck proprioceptors. Like righting reflexes, they appear at certain stages of development and their persistence, or absence, can be observed in patients under pathological conditions.

The development of a child can also be assessed by observing and examining the child by 180° flip examination.

Salient features:

- Gross motor assessment should be performed on a firm surface
- In supine posture observe the-posture (decerebrate, decorticate, opisthotonus, pithed frog, scissoring)
  — Sucking
  — Rooting
  — Glabellar tap
  — Moro reflex
  — Flexor withdrawal
  — Extensor thurst
  — Crossed extensor
  — Asymmetric tonic neck reflex
  — Tonic labyrinthine (supine)
  — Neck righting
  — Body righting
  — Labyrinthine righting (supine)
  — Plantar grasp
  — Palmar grasp

While the child is being drawn into sitting position, by traction note the degree of head control.

Grasp reflex can also be assessed when the child is being pulled to sit. In sitting position look for the curvature and arching of the back and lateral tilt.

Ventral suspension	—	Landau reflex
	—	Parachute reflex
	—	Galants reflex
Vertical position	—	Placing
	—	Stepping
	—	Hopping
	—	DeLange's sign
	—	See-saw
Prone position	—	Symmetrical tonic neck reflex (Over the examiners knees)
	—	Tonic labyrinthine (prone)
	—	Labrinthine righting (prone)
	—	Optical righting (prone)

In prone position observe for the head lift and note for the arm support.

EXAMINATION OF SENSORY SYSTEM

Brief Review of Sensory System Neuroanatomy

The sensory systems are composed of both neural and non-neural structures that function to provide us with an awareness of the environment in which we live. Normal sensory function can be thought of as being composed of four distinct processes: sensory transduction, impulse transmission, perception, and sensory interpretation.

Functional Anatomy

Sensory transduction is the process where by stimuli or energy applied to the body results in the generation of action potentials in peripheral nerves. Sensory transduction is achieved either by specialized receptors located in visceral and somatic structures, or directly in peripheral nerve fibers without specialized receptors, which are sensitive to changes in the microenvironment in which they are located. Sensory receptors transduce or convert a particular form of energy into nerve impulses, which are transmitted toward the central nervous system (CNS).

Impulse transmission is the process whereby information about the environment in the form of action potentials is brought to the CNS and distributed to regions where, among other functions, perception and interpretation occur. Afferent nerve cells with cell bodies located in dorsal root ganglia and cranial nerve sensory ganglia transmit nerve impulses from the periphery to the CNS. Within the CNS, several ascending pathways are involved in distributing nerve impulses to specific areas of the brain important perception and interpretation. Perception is the phenomenon of experiencing the environment and change in it. Specific nuclei of the dorsal thalamus and gyri of the cerebral hemispheres are thought to be involved in sensory perception. In humans, the primary sensory cortex is the postcentral gyrus of the parietal lobe.

Sensory interpretation is a process in which meaning and significane are assigned to the perceived attributes of an event or object in the environment.

It results in recognition of the vent or object and is based on some previous experience with it. Sensory interpretation is a higher cortical function and invovles areas of the cerebral cortex commonly referred to as association cortices. The recognition or interpretation of tactile stimuli involves the association cortex of the parietal lobe.

The anatomic and functional organization of the sensory systems focusing on somatic sensory functions mediated by spinal nerves and pathways, functions that are routinely evaluated in the sensory part of the neurologic examination are briefly reviewed.

The transmission of nerve impulses from the receptor in the periphery to the CNS occurs along the axons of afferent nerve cells derived from the neural crest. The peripheral processes of spinal afferent neurons combine to form segmental spinal nerves, which may intermingle further in plexuses. (i.e. brachial or lumbosacral) to form specific peripheral nerves. Dorsal root ganglion cells and their peripheral processes vary in size. The more thickly myelinated afferent fibers transmit nerve impulses to the spinal cord more rapidly than do the thinly myelinated and nonmyelinated fibers.

Transmission of nerve impulses from the dorsal root ganglion to the spinal cord occurs along axons that form the dorsal roots. As each root approaches the spinal cord, it further divides into a series of longitudinally oriented rootlets that penetrate the pial surface in the region of the dorsolateral fissure. The axons within each rootlet segregate in such a way that the more thickly myelinated fibers enter the cord slightly medial to the more thinly myelinated and unmyelinated axons (Fig. 27.99).

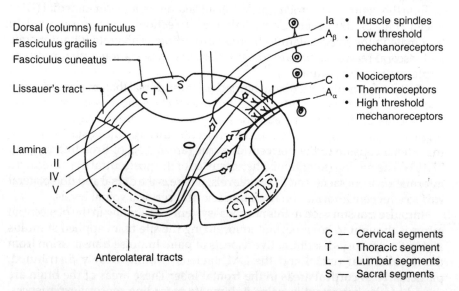

Fig. 27.99: The spinal cord termination sites of different classes of primary afferent nerve

Most of the axons entering the spinal cord via the dorsal root terminate in the ipsilateral dorsal horn. In general, low-threshold, rapidly adapting, encapsulated receptors tend to be associated with thickly myelinated afferent fibers, whereas high-threshold, slowly adapting, unencapsulated receptors, including nociceptors and thermoreceptors, tend to be associated with thinly myelinated and unmyelinated afferent nerve fibers. These general concepts serve as the bases for selecting particular stimuli for use in the sensory portion of the neurologic examiantion.

Within the spinal cord, nerve impulses are transmitted to more rostral levels of the neuraxis by way of two major ascending pathways, the anterolateral system (ALS) and the dorsal column-medial lemniscus system (DC-ML). The anatomic organization and function of each of these ascending systems is briefly reviewed.

Anterolateral System (ALS)

The ALS is composed of several ascending tracts that occupy a position in the anterolateral white matter of the spinal cord. These fibers originate in cells on the contralateral side of the spinal cord, in the dorsal, intermediate, and ventral horns. The axons cross the midline in the anterior white commissure before accumulating in the anterolateral white matter. The axons that form the anterolateral tracts are somatotopically organized. Those that subserve sacral and lumbar segments are dorsolateral to those that subserve sacral and lumbar segments are dorsolateral to those that subserve thoracic and cervical levels. A somatotopic organization is retained throughout the brainstem. The most important of the ascending pathways that make up the ALS are the spino-thalamic, spinoreticular, and spinotectal tracts. Spinothalamic tract, as the name implies, terminates in particular nuclei of the dorsal thalamus. These nuclei include the ventral posterolateral (VPL), intralaminar, and dorsomedial (DM) nuclei (Fig. 27.100). Some spinothalamic projections are also reported to terminate in the hypothalamus, thereby providing a substrate for autonomic and visceral reactions that are sometimes seen in association with noxious or unpleasant sensory stimuli.

Thalamocortical projections from each of these dorsal thalamic nuclei differ and are thought to be important in different aspects of the sensory experience. Nerve cells in the VPL nucleus are somatotopically organized and are the origin of a somatotopically organized projection through the posterior limb of the intenal capsule to the postcentral gyrus (areas 3,1,2 of Broadmann) (Fig. 27.101). The medial (interhemispheric) surfce of the postcentral gyrus receives information from sacral and lumbar levels, whereas the dorsal and dorsolateral surfaces receive information from thoracic and cervical spinal levels.

Impulse transmission in this neuronal system terminating in the postcentral gyrus is thought to be important in localizing the site of an applied stimulus and in the sensory-discriminative aspects of pain. Impulse transmission from the intralaminar nuclei and the DM nucleus is more widely distributed, particularly to cortical areas in the frontal lobe. These areas of the brain are thought to be important in value judgments regarding sensory experiences, complex reactions to sensory stimulation, and in motivational and affective responses to noxious or painful experiences. Spinoreticular projections coursing through the anterolateral tracts and spinal lemniscus terminate in nuclei scattered throughout the reticular formation of the brainstem (Fig. 27.100).

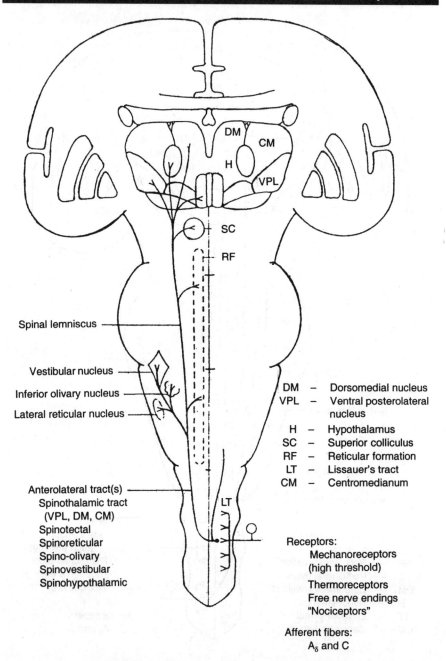

DM – Dorsomedial nucleus
VPL – Ventral posterolateral
nucleus
H – Hypothalamus
SC – Superior colliculus
RF – Reticular formation
LT – Lissauer's tract
CM – Centromedianum

Spinal lemniscus

Vestibular nucleus

Inferior olivary nucleus

Lateral reticular nucleus

Anterolateral tract(s)
Spinothalamic tract
(VPL, DM, CM)
Spinotectal
Spinoreticular
Spino-olivary
Spinovestibular
Spinohypothalamic

Receptors:
Mechanoreceptors
(high threshold)

Thermoreceptors
Free nerve endings
"Nociceptors"

Afferent fibers:
A_δ and C

Fig. 27.100: Brainstem and forebrain nuclei that receive afferent
input from axons of the anterolateral system

These nuclei in turn participate in a number of functions, three of which are pertinent to our understanding of normal neurologic function and the neurologic examination.

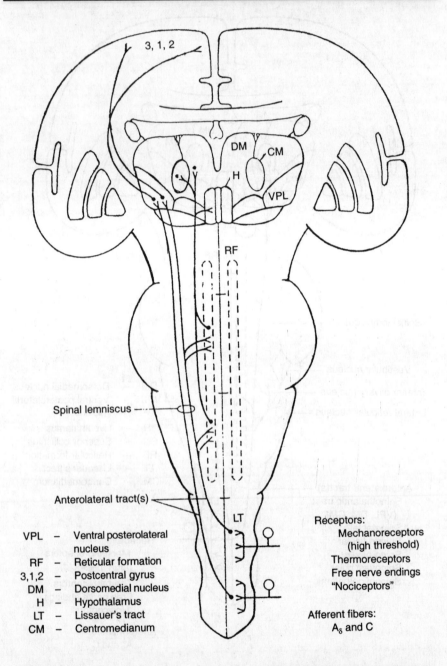

Fig. 27.101: The course and termination of major components of the anterolateral system

First, ascending projections originating in the brainstem reticular formation exert an excitatory effect on the cerebral cortex, mediated through the thalamus. Activity in this ascending reticular activating system (ARAS) is essential to maintenance of the conscious state. As activity in the ARAS is depressed, so is level of consicousness. When we apply noxious sensory stimuli in an effort to arouse a comatose or stuporous patient, we are increasing neural activity in spinoreticular, reticulothalamic, and thalamocortical pathways in an effort to raise the level of consciousness.

Second, descending projections from the brainstem reticular formation to autonomic and somatic motor neurons in the spinal cord activate defense systems to protect the individual from continuing exteroceptive insult. In this sense, spinoreticular projections activate moderately complex, automatic behaviors that are part of self-protective defensive mechanisms.

Third, descending projections from specific nuclear regions of the brainstem reticular formation exert an inhibitory influence on the very ascending tract cells that excited them in the first place.

The final pathway to consider in this brief review of the ALS is the spino-tectal tract. The axons of this tract lie intermixed with those of the spinothalamic and spinoreticular tracts in the spinal crod and brainstem. At the level of the midbrain, spinotectal axons terminate in the deeper layers of the superior colliculus (Fig. 27.100). Nerve cells of the superior colliculus that receive spinal input are the origin of axons that descend through the brainstem and enter the spinal cord as the tectospinal tract. Tectal projections to the brainstem (tectobulbar) are distributed to the extraocular nuclei. The pathway helps mediate eye movements to bring a stimulated area of skin into the visual field. In the spinal cord, tectospinal fibers terminate on interneurons and lower motor neurons that innervate muscles that support the neck and move the head. Activity in this pathway also helps to bring stimulated areas into view by producing appropriate movements of the head. The spinotectal component of the ALS can therefore be viewed as the ascending portion of a neural system that can be used to orient the position of the eyes in the skull and the head on the trunk in response to stimulation of the skin.

Dorsal Column-Medial Lemniscus System

The dorsal column-medial lemniscus system is a phylogenetically newer ascending pathway. The dorsal columns (dorsal funiculi) are composed of two smaller fasciculi: the fasciculus gracilis and the more laterally located fasciculus cuneatus (Fig. 27.99). The fasciculus gracilis is composed of the central processes of large dorsal root ganglion cells subserving sacral, lumbar and lower thoracic spinal segments of the ipsilateral side. The cell bodies of axons forming the fasciculus cuneatus are located in dorsal root ganglia associated with upper thoracic and cervical levels of the spinal cord (Fig. 27.102). The dorsal columns are somatotopically organized, with fibers subserving sacral segments being most medial and those transmitting impulses from cervical levels being most lateral (Fig. 27.99).

The axons in the fasciculus gracilis and cuneatus terminate at the level of the caudal medulla oblongata, in the nucleus gracilis and nucleus cuneatus, respectively. Nerve cells in these two nuclei are the origin of axons that cross the midline in a rostroventral trajectory and assume a position in the medulla immediately dorsal to the medullary pyramid. The crossed axons of these nuclei form a somatotopically organized bundle of fibers referred to as the medial lemniscus (Fig. 27.102). The fibers of the thalamus. From the VPL

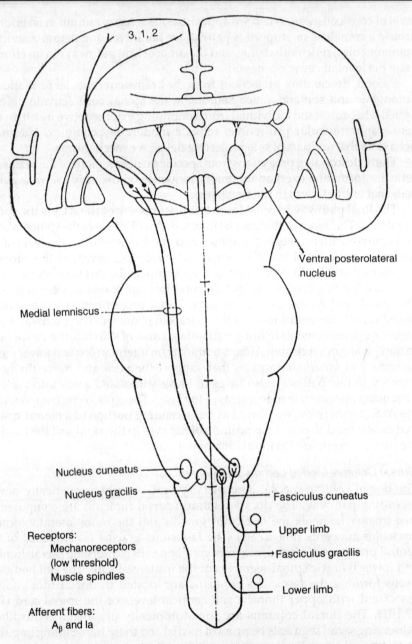

Receptors:
Mechanoreceptors
(low threshold)
Muscle spindles

Afferent fibers:
A_β and Ia

Fig. 27.102: The course and termination of axons of the dorsal column-medial lemniscus system 3, 1, 2 = Postcentral gyrus

nucleus, nerve impulses are transmitted to the postcentral gyrus (areas 3,1,2) by way of thalamocortical projections occupying the posterior limb of the internal capsule. The dorsal column-medial lemniscus system is somatotopically organized throughout its course, making it ideally suited for localizing stimuli applied to discrete regions of the body.

The disease or injuries involving these specific cortical, nuclear, and white matter areas produce definable perceptual deficits involving somatotopically appropriate areas of the body.

Sensory interpretation is a process whereby recognition or meaning is attributed to perceived stimuli. With regard to cutaneous sensory stimuli, this process includes several related functions, including the ability to identify a stimulus based on its tactile characteristics. Identifying objects by touch (stereognosis), recognizing number or letters written on the skin (graphesthesia), and differentiating between different weights (barognosis) are cortical functions involving sensory association cortices of the parietal lobe. Patients with focal disease involving these cortices alone present with fascinating deficits of recognition even though they are able to perceive tactile stimuli.

The anatomic organization of different components of the peripheral nervous system must be understood to correctly identify and localize disease processe affecting these structures. An adequate knowledge of peripheral neuroanatomy also is essential. The reader must become familiar with the cutaneous distribution of both segmentally derived sensory fibers (dermatomes) and postplexus peripheral nerves. Figures 27.103 and 27.104, illustrate regions of the body innervated by particular segmental or peripheral nerves.

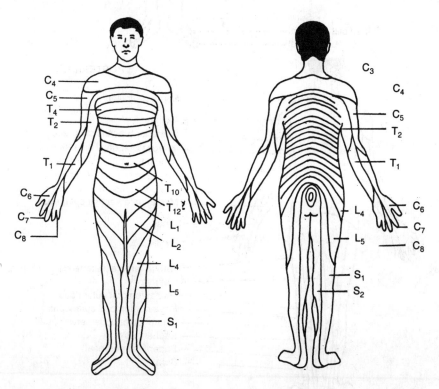

Fig. 27.103: The sensory dermatomes

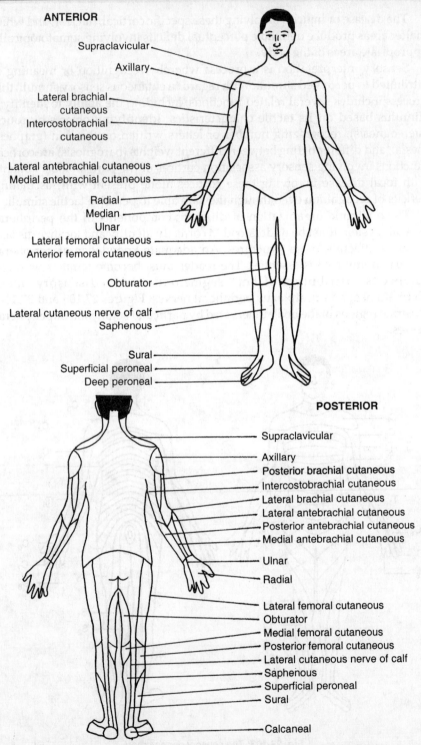

ANTERIOR

Supraclavicular
Axillary
Lateral brachial cutaneous
Intercostobrachial cutaneous
Lateral antebrachial cutaneous
Medial antebrachial cutaneous
Radial
Median
Ulnar
Lateral femoral cutaneous
Anterior femoral cutaneous
Obturator
Lateral cutaneous nerve of calf
Saphenous
Sural
Superficial peroneal
Deep peroneal

POSTERIOR

Supraclavicular
Axillary
Posterior brachial cutaneous
Intercostobrachial cutaneous
Lateral brachial cutaneous
Lateral antebrachial cutaneous
Posterior antebrachial cutaneous
Medial antebrachial cutaneous
Ulnar
Radial
Lateral femoral cutaneous
Obturator
Medial femoral cutaneous
Posterior femoral cutaneous
Lateral cutaneous nerve of calf
Saphenous
Superficial peroneal
Sural
Calcaneal

Fig. 27.104: The sensory distribution of peripheral cutaneous nerves

SENSORY FUNCTION

Both primary and cortical discriminatory sensations are evaluated by having the patient identify each sensory stimuli. Each sensation is tested in each major peripheral nerve. Routinely evaluated sites are hands, lower arms, abdomen, feet and lower legs. Sensory discrimination of face is with cranial nerves.

Each sensation is tested with patients eyes closed.

- Use minimal stimulation initially and gradually go on increasing until patient becomes aware of it.
- Stronger stimulus is needed over the back, buttocks and heavily cornified areas where the level of sensitivity is lower in other sensitive areas.
- Test contralateral areas and ask patient to compare with each sensation, there should be:
  - Minimal differences side to side
  - Correct interpretation of sensation
  - Discrimination of side of body tested
  - Location of the stimulus

Primary Sensation (Table 27.22)

Touch

Tested with cotton wool or the head of a pin on all parts of the body. Patient keeps eyes closed and he is asked to indicate the site where he has been touched.

Table 27.22: Clinical tests of sensory function

Functional systems	Clinical tests
Anterolateral systems	Pin prick
	Thermal sense
	Deep pain
Dorsal column-Medical lemniscus	Light touch
	Vibratory sense
	Position sense
Cortical sensory function	Traced figure identification
	Object idenfitication
	Double simultaneous stimulation

The following sensations should be tested:

Pain

Tested with a pin prick on all parts of the body, any area where it is not felt adequately is noted. The test may be modified by alternating sharp and blunt edge of a sterile needle. Care must be taken not to allow summation effect- give a gap of at least 2 sec between 2 stimuli. The patient may be asked to identify as sharp or dull pain.

Pressure (Deep pain)

Squeezing the trapezius, calf or biceps muscle, patient should experience discomfort.

Temperature
Only when pain sensation is not intact, temperature is tested. Roll test tubes of hot or cold water alternately against the skin, in an unpredicted pattern to evaluate temperature sensation. Ask the patient to indicate which temperature is perceived and where it is felt.

Vibration
Place the stem of a vibrating tuning fork against several bony prominences starting distally. The sternum, wrist, finger joints, shin, ankle and elbow and toes, all may be tested. A buzzing or tingling sensation should be felt. Ask the patient to tell you where the vibration is felt.

Position of Joints
Hold the joint to be tested (great toe) or finger by the lateral aspects to avoid giving a clue about the direction it was moved. Begin with the joint in neutral position, raise or lower the digit, and ask the patient to tell you which way it was moved. Return it to neutral position before moving it in another direction. Repeat procedure so that great toe and finger of hand are tested. The range of movements should be around 10 degrees (Fig. 27.105).

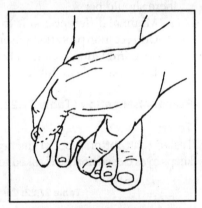

Fig. 27.105: Method of separating the digits to test position sense in the fourth toe. The ex-grasps the toe on the sides and randomly moves it up and down

Cortical Sensory Functions
Cortical or discriminatory sensory function tests cognitive ability to interpret sensations associated with coordination abilities. Inability to perform these should make you suspect a lesion in the sensory cortex or the posterior column of spinal cord. The patient's eyes are closed during these procedures.

Stereognosis
Hand the patient familiar objects (key, coin) to identify by touch and manipulation. Tactile agnosia, an inability to recongise objects by touch, suggests a parietal lobe lesion.

Two-Point Discrimination
Use two sterile needles and alternately touch the patients skin with one or two points simultaneously at various locations over the patients body. Find the distance at which the patient can no longer distinguish two points. The minimal distances of discriminating two-points varies in various locations tested.

Extinction Phenomenon
Simultaneously touch the cheek, hand or other area on each side of the body with a sterile needle. Ask the patient how many stimuli there are and where they are. Both the sensations must be felt.

Graphesthesia
With a blunt pen, draw a letter or a number on the palm or any other body location. Repeat the procedure each time using a different figure. The letter or number should be easily recognised.

Point Localisation
Touch an area on the patient's skin and withdraw the stimulus. Ask the patient to point to the area touched. There should be no difficulty in localising the stimulus. Usually tested simultaneously with superficial tactile sensation.

Procedures for Testing Integrity of Individual Spinal Tracts

Spinal tracts	Neurologic tests
Ascending tracts	
Lateral spinothalamic	— Superficial pain
	— Temperature
Anterior spinothalamic	— Superficial touch
	— Deep pressure
Posterior column	— Vibration
	— Deep pressure
	— Stereognosis
	— Two-point discrimination
	— Point localisation

Signs and Symptoms Associated with Various forms of Myelopathy

1. **Complete transection** : Bilateral weakness,
   Fig. 27.106A
   Bilateral loss of all modalities below level of lesion, DTR's may be decreased initially (spinal shock), but then bilateral increase with bilateral extensor plantar response. Neurogenic bladder present

2. **Hemisection** : Ipsilateral weakness
   Fig. 27.106B
   Below level of lesion
   Ipsilateral vibration and position sensory loss
   Contralateral pain and temperature loss
   At level of lesion
   All sensory loss ipsilaterally
   Increased DTR's and extensor plantars (Ipsilateral)

3. **Posterior columns** : No weakness, often associated with corticospinal tract involvement.
   Fig. 27.106C
   Postion and vibration loss
   DTR's normal (or may be increased or decreased depending on the disease)
   Neurogenic bladder usually present, may be absent

4. **Corticospinal** : Unilateral or bilateral weakness
   Fig. 27.106D
   No sensory loss
   DTR's (Similar to complete transection)
   Neurogenic bladder present

5. **Anterior two-thirds**   : Bilateral weakness
   Fig. 27.106E   Upper motor neuron—below level of lesion
                               Lower motor neuron—at level of lesion
                               Position and vibration spared, may have sacral
                               sparing
                               DTR's (similar to complete transection)
                               Neurogenic bladder present

6. **Central core**   : Weakness may be lower motor neuron type at
   Fig. 27.106F   the level, in late stages-upper motor neuron signs
                               Pain and temperature absent with position and
                               vibration spared at the level of lesion. If lesion
                               enlarges, there may be loss of sensation with
                               sacral sparing
                               DTR's decreased at the level of lesion—early in
                               the disease, without Babinski's sign.
                               Late in the disease, features may be that of
                               complete transection
                               Neurogenic bladder may be absent/present

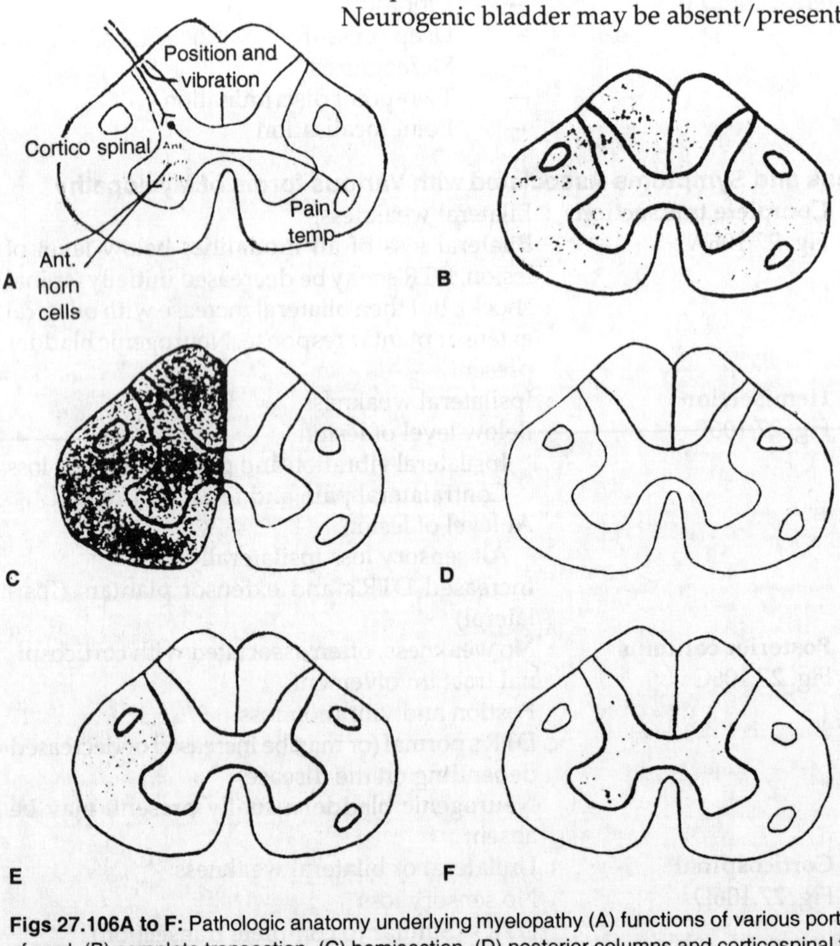

Figs 27.106A to F: Pathologic anatomy underlying myelopathy (A) functions of various portions of cord, (B) complete transection, (C) hemisection, (D) posterior columns and corticospinal tract (funicular myelopathy), (E) anterior two-thirds, and (F) core

Sensory Changes in Various Diseases

Polyneuropathy
- Symmetrical glove and stocking anesthesia
- Distal parts more affected, all modalities of sensations involved.
- Calf tenderness is present.

Cauda Equina and Conus Lesions
Loss of all modalities of sensations involving especially lower sacral segments leading to perianal anesthesia.

Multiple Root Involvement
Varying degrees of impairment of cutaneous sensations in the distribution of nerve roots, pain is more affected than touch.

Brainstem Syndrome
- Loss of touch, pain and temperature on same side of face and opposite side of the body due to involvement of trigeminal tract or nucleus and lateral spinothalamic tract.

Thalamic Syndrome
- Loss of all modalities of sensation on opposite side of the body.
- Spontaneous and disabling pain.

Partial Lobe Syndrome
- Primary modalities of sensation affected in deep seated parietal lobe lesions.
- Loss of tactile localisation, discrimination, asteriognosis.

Hysterical
- Complete hemianesthesia with reduced hearing, vision, taste and smell.
- Sharply defined sensory loss-not along any nerve.
- Position sense is never affected.

AUTONOMIC NERVOUS SYSTEM
Comprises of the sympathetic and parasympathetic system.

Sympathetic System Stimulation Causes
- Tachycardia
- Dilatation of bronchi
- Release of adrenaline/noradrenaline (maintains BP)
- Decreases bowel motility
- Inhibition of micturition (Relaxes detrusor, stimulates internal urethral sphincter).
- Increases sweating
- Increases dilatation of pupils

Outflow : T_1-L_2.

Parasympathetic System Stimulation Causes
- Bradycardia
- Constriction of bronchi

- Increase in salivation and lacrimation
- Increase in bowel motility
- Erections
- Initiation of micturition
- Constriction of pupils.

Outflow: Cranial nerves III, VII, IX, and X and S_2-S_4

Examination

- Check pulse rate in lying and standing posture
- Check blood pressure in supine and erect posture
- Look at the color of the skin and note any flushing check for tachy cerebrale and sweating.
- Feel the skin temperature
- Look for bladder and bowel involvement.

Always ask for drug intake. Many drugs interfere with autonomic function like beta blockers and anticholenergic drugs.

Bladder Function

The bladder has two chief sources of nerve supply

a. Autonomic nervous system—Serves with impulses of involuntary nature.
b. Cerebrospinopudendal—Subserves volitional control pathway.

Autonomic Nervous System

Comprises of the sympathetic and parasympathetic system.

Sympathetic supply is from the grey matter of the L_{1-4}: These fibers after passing through the celiac and superior mesenteric ganglia form the presacral nerve. At the level of S_1 vertebrae the presacral nerve divides into two hypogastric nerves which after synapsing at the hypogastric ganglion supply the fibers to the urinary bladder (Fig. 27.107).

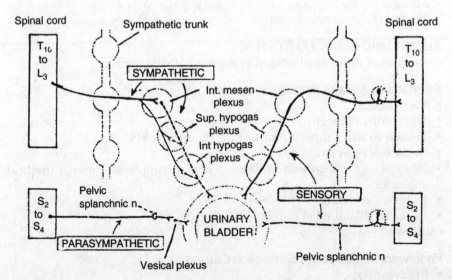

Fig. 27.107: Scheme to show the innervation of the urinary bladder

Stimulation of the sympathetic system causes relaxation of detrusor and contraction of the sphincter (internal) and stops micturition.

Parasympathetic nerve supply is from the sacral 2-4 segments, pass through the pelvic nerves (nervi ergentes) which terminate in the hypogastric ganglia. The postganglionic fibers innervate the detrusor, trigone and the internal sphincter. Stimulation of the parasympathetic system causes contraction of the detrusor and relaxation of the internal sphinecter causing the bladder to empty.

Cortical fibers control micturition, voluntarily through the pudendal nerve that supples the external sphincter.

Afferent supply of the bladder:

The afferent fibers take two pathways

a. Along the sympathetic into the dorsal nerve roots of L_1- L_2 and lower thoracic segments.
b. Along the sacral autonomic into the sacral dorsal nerve roots.
    They subserve the following functions;
    i. They indicate the degree of distentsion of the bladder.
    ii. Convey pain sensibility.

The centre for integration of these impulses is at the cortex at the top of the motor area on the medial aspect of the hemisphere.

Physiology of Micturition

As the bladder fills, its internal pressure slowly rises. Contraction waves appear which stimulate the pressure receptors in the muscle coat and send afferent impulses up the spinal cord and to the brain which give rise to a "desire to micturate." If it is inconvenient to micturate, then impulses from the cortex via the sympathetic nerves cause elongation of bladder muscles by relaxation of the detrusor and constriction of the internal urethral sphincter. The pressure in the bladder falls and the "desire to micturate" temporarily passes off. Adults have better voluntary control of bladder than children.

On the other hand, the bladder can be voluntarily emptied in response to the desire to micturate. The impulses from the cortex, then travel down the sacral segments along nerviergentes to relax the internal sphincter and contract the detrusor. Simultaneous relaxation of the external sphincter also occurs and the bladder is emptied. Causes and features of different types of bladder anomalies are given in Table 27.23.

EXAMINATION OF CEREBELLUM

Classic Findings of Cerebellar Dysfunction
- Hypotonia
- Nystagmus
- Staggering gait
- Titubation

Other Symptoms and Signs in Cerebellar Dysfunction
- Action tremor
- Asthenia

Table 27.23: Causes and clinical features of various types of bladder anomalies

Type	Lesion	Causes	Bladder sensation	Emptying	Capacity	Tone	Cystometrogram
1. Uninhibited	Loss of cortical inhibitory control	* Meningitis * Brain tumor * Multiple sclerosis	Preserved	Complete but Uninhibited	Reduced	Normal	uninhibited vesical contraction Normotonic curve
2. Automatic (Reflex Neurogenic)	Complete lesion involving both ascending and descending pathways in spinal cord above S2	* Transverse myelitis * Spinal cord injury * Cord compression	Lost	Bladder gets emptied as soon as its gets filled but emptying is poor	Reduced	Increased	Uninhibited vesical contraction Hypertonic curve
3. Autonomous	Lesion involving Sacral spinal centres (S2,3,4) syndrome	* Meningo-myelocele * Caudaequina * Conus medullaris lesion	Lost	Constant dribbling	Usually decreased (variable)	Usually increased	Flat hypotonic curve with no vesical contraction
4. Motor denervated	Efferent fibers from lower motor neuron S2,3,4	—	Preserved	Distended bladder severe pain	Increased decompensated	Decreased decompensated	Painful overflow incontinence
5. Sensory denervation (rare)	Afferent pathway, posterior column	* Diabetes * Syphilis * Disc prolapse	Lost	Distended but no pain	Increased	Decreased (Hypotonic)	Hypotonic curve Painless overflow incontinence

- Ataxia
- Decompensation of movements
- Dysdiadochokinesia
- Dysmetria
- Dyssynergia
- Impaired rebound
- Pendular deep tendon reflexes

Examination of Arms and Hands
- Finger to nose test
- Finger to finger to nose test
- Rapid alternating movements (hands, fingers, tongue)
- Rebound
- Tone evaluation

Examination of Gait
- Foot tapping
- Heel to shin maneuver
- Heel to toe walking
- Hopping in place (one foot)
- Romberg's sign
- Tandem walk
- Walking in a circle

Cerebellar Signs
1. Head tilt
2. Ataxic gait
3. Heel to toe walking
4. Fall in centrifugal direction during turning
5. Head nodding (Titubation)
6. Intention tremor (Dysmetria)
7. Dysdiadokokinesia
8. Finger-nose-finger test
9. Heel to shin test
10. Dysarthria—scanning speech
11. Nystagmus
12. Saccadic eye movements
13. Ocular dysmetria
14. Skew deviation
15. Hypotonia
16. Hyporeflexia/pendular knee jerk
17. Cerebellar fits
18. Truncal ataxia

Localisation Value
1. Hypotonia — Ipsilateral hemisphere
2. Dysmetria — Hemisphere

3. Ocular dysmetria   — Mid vermis
4. Truncal ataxia   — Posterior vermis and basillar structures
5. Gait ataxia   — Anterior vermis
6. Dysarthria   — Mid vermis

Tests for Cerebellar Dysfunction

Abnormality	Method of examiantion
Gait dystaxia (broad basal stance and broad based gait)	Free walking for broad based gait and tandum walking
Nystagmus	Inspect and have patient follow your finger through fields of gaze.
Arm dystaxia and irregular alternating movements	Finger-to-nose; pronation-supination test; thigh slapping test
Overshooting	Wrist-slapping test and arm pulling test
Leg dystaxia (other than gait)	Heel-to-knee test; shin tapping test
Hypotonia	Inspection for rag doll postures and rag doll gait; passive movement of extremities; pendular knee reflexes.
Nystagmus, skew deviation	Watch eyes, ask patient to follow your finger
Slurred speech (dysarthric) and scanning speech	Talk to patient
Ataxic gait	Test gait

Cerebellar syndromes

1. Cerebellar hemisphere syndrome (mainly posterior and variable anterior) — Dysarthria, arm overshooting, hypotonia, dystaxia of arm, gait, trunk and leg.
   Nystagmus, is bidirectional, coarser to side of lesion, fast component to side of gaze

2. Rostral vermis syndrome (Anterior lobe) — Hypotonia, gait, trunk and leg dystaxia (arm variable), no nystagmus and truncal ataxia, no dysarthria

3. Caudal vermis syndrome (Flocconodular and posterior lobe) — Gait, truncal ataxia
   Nystagmus, variable hypotonia

4. Pancerebellar syndrome (All lobes) — All features mentioned above

ATAXIA

One of the main presentation of cerebellar disease is ataxia.

Findings often Associated with Ataxia

1. Chronic otitis media/sinusitis   — Ataxia telangiectasia
2. Cataracts and Aniridia   — Sjögren's syndrome

3. Conjunctival telangectasia,   — Ataxia telangiectasia
   Bronchiectasis, malignancy
4. Cherry red spot   — Taysach's disease
5. Retinitis   — Refsum disease, Sjogren Larsen,
                                   Basson- Kernweig syndrome
6. Cardiomyopathy and stroke   — Friedreich's, Moya-moya
                                   Homocystinuria
7. Hyperpnea   — Joubert syndrome
8. Apnea, sighing   — Leigh's
9. Malabsorption   — Vit E deficiency
10. Acrodermatitis   — Zinc deficiency
11. Icthyosis   — Sjögren Larsen
12. Pellagra   — Hartnup disease
13. Alopecia   — Biotinidase deficiency
14. Diabetes mellitus   — Friedreich's ataxia
15. Unusual odour   — MSUD, Chediak-Higashi.

Causes of Ataxia

Congenital
- Agenesis of cerebellum
- Hemiagenesis
- Vermis aplasia with dysraphic malformation
- Dandy Walker malformation
- Hypoplasia
- Microgyria
- Congenital cerebellar atrophy
     Granular layer
     Purkinje layer
     Treatable causes of inherited ataxia are given in Table 27.24.

Familial, Degenerative and Metabolic Ataxia

0-6 months
- Marinesco-Sjogren   — Dementia, cataract
- Joubert   — Hyperpnea, retardation
- Gillespie syndrome — Aniridia, mental retardation
- Behr's syndrome   — Optic atrophy, spasticity, MR

6 months-6 years
- Ataxia telangiectasia   — Recurrent infections, telangiectasia
- Spastic ataxia   — Spastic paraplegia, dementia
- Olivo pontocerebellar atrophy   — Seizure, blindness, ophthalmoplegia.
- Tay-Sach's   — Cherry red spot
- Neuronal ceroid lipofuscinosis   — Optic atrophy, spastic dimentia
- Chediak-Higashi   — Recurrent infections, partial albinism
- SSPE   — Dementia, ophthalmoplegia, neuro-
                                     pathy
- Sandhoff   — Dementia, myotonic epilepsy

Table 27.24: Treatable causes of inherited ataxia

Disorder abnormality	Metabolic features	Clinical	Treatment
1. Bassen-Kornweig syndrome	Abetalipoproteinenia	Acanthocytosis, retinitis pigmentosa, fat malabsorption	Vit E
2. Hartnup disease	Tryptophan malabsorption	Pellagra rash, intermittent ataxia	Niacin
3. Familial-periodic ataxia	Unknown	Episodic attacks worse with pregnancy or OC pills	Acetazolamide
4. Mitochondrial complex defects	Complexes I, III, IV	Encephalomyelopathy	? Riboflavin
5. Multiple carboxylase deficiency	Biotinidase deficiency	Alopecia, rec infection, variable organic acidemia	Biotin
6. Pyruvate dehydrogenase deficiency	Block in EM and Kreb cycle	Lactic acidosis, ataxia	Ketogenic diet,
7. Refsum disease	Phytanic acid hydrolase	Retinitis pigmentosa, Cardiomyopathy, neuropathy, ichthyosis	Dietary restriction of phytanic acid
8. Urea cycle defects	Urea cycle	Hyperammonemia	Protein restriction, arginine, Alpha-ketoacids.

6-16 years
- Friedreich's ataxia
- Adrenoleucodystrophy
- Metachromatic leucodystrophy
- Abetalipoproteinemia
- Bassen-Kornwitz
- Pelizeaus-Meizbacher disease
- Refsum disease
- Rett syndrome

Intermittent ataxia
- Hartnup disease — Pellagra
- MSUD (Variant) — Odor, encephalopathy
- Hyperammonemia — Encephalopathy
- Acute intermittent porphyria — Abdominal pain
- Holocarboxylase defeciency — Recurrent infection, alopecia
- Acordermatitis enteropathica — Rash.

Endocrinological Causes
- Acquired hypothyroidism
- Cretinism

Infectious or Postinfectious
- Acute cerebellar ataxia
- Cerebellar abscess

- Diphtheria
- Echovirus
- Fischer syndrome
- Infectious mononucleosis (EBV infection)
- Infectious polyneuropathy
- Japanese-B- encephalitis
- Mumps encephalitis
- Pertussis, polio, typhoid, varicella
- Postbacterial meningitis

Neoplastic
- Frontal lobe tumors
- Hemispheric cerebellar tumors
- Midline cerebellar defects (tumors)
- Neuroblastoma
- Pontine gliomas
- Spinal cord tumors

Traumatic
- Acute cerebellar edema
- Acute frontal lobe edema

Toxic

Endogenous : Neuroblastoma

Exogenous : Alcohol, clonazepam, phenobarbetone
phenytoin, primidone, lead encephalopathy

Vascular

Angioblastoma of cerebellum

Basilar migraine

Cerebellar embolism/thrombosis/hemorrhage

Posterior cerebellar artery disease

Von-Hippel-Lindu disease

SIGNS OF MENINGEAL IRRITATION

First of All: Care must be taken, not to perform these tests in a patient with cervical instability-e.g. trauma or in patients with rheumatoid arthritis for the fear of precipitating spinal injury or atlanto axial dislocation, respectively.

Neck Stiffness (Nuchal Rigidity)

The patient lying supine on a flat surface.

Place your hand behind the patient's head and

- Gently rotate the head as if patient was indicating "no"-feel for the stiffness or resistance to movement (Fig. 27.108).
- Gently lift the head off the bed; try to make the patient's chin touch the sternum feel for the tone in the neck.
- Watch the legs for hip and knee flexion.

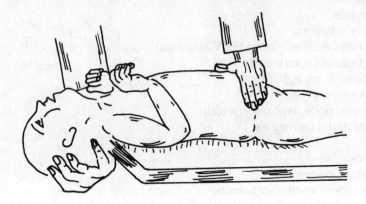

Fig. 27.108: Examination for neck rigidity

- In older child neck rigidity may be tested as illustrated in Figure 27.109.

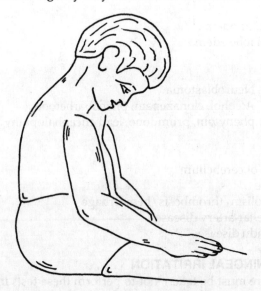

Fig. 27.109: Neck rigidity in older child. Child asked to touch chin to front of chest without opening mouth

Normally

The neck moves easily in both planes, with the chin easily reaching the chest on neck flexion.

Neck Rigidity

It occurs on movement: indication meningeal irritation

Common causes

- Meningitis (bacterial/viral)
- Subarachnoid hemorrhage

- Any cause of raised ICP
- Severe cervical spondylosis
- Cervical lymphadenopathy
- Severe pharyngitis/retropharyngeal abscess.
- Phenothiazine reaction
- Kernicterus
- Strychnine poisoning

Kernig's Sign

Patient lying supine, the leg is flexed at the hip with the knee flexed and then the knee is extended. Resistance to this movement is an indication of meningeal irritation (Fig. 27.110). If unilateral, it indicates radiculopathy.

Kernig's sign is absent in the non-CNS causes of neck stiffness.

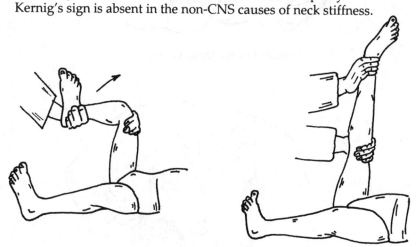

Fig. 27.110: Kernig's sign

Brudzinski's Signs
  a. Leg sign
  b. Neck sign
  c. Symphysis sign

Leg Sign
Maneuver is done as for Kernig's sign, the leg on the other side also flexes at the hip if there is meningeal irritation (Fig. 27.111).

Neck Sign
Hip and knee flexion in response to neck flexion, indicates meningeal irritation (Fig. 27.112).

Symphysis Sign
Pressure over pubic symphysis causes flexion of both lower limbs.

Straight Leg Raising Test (Test for Radicular Entrapment)
With the patient lying flat on the bed, lift the leg, holding the heel. Note the angle attained and any difference between 2 sides (Fig. 27.113A).

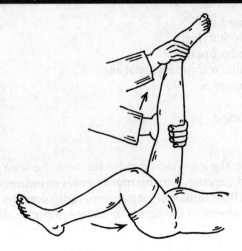

Fig. 27.111: Brudzinski's sign (leg)

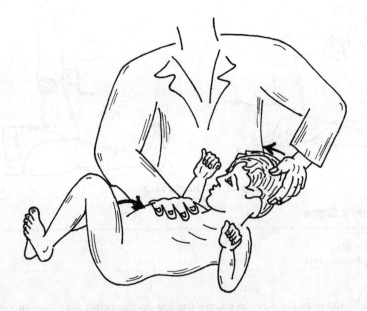

Fig. 27.112: Brudzinski's sign (neck)

Normal >90°; less in older patients
Limitation with pain in the back = nerve root entrapment

Lasegue's Sign

Once the leg is raised to a particular level in the straight leg raising test, and the patient gets pain, the foot is dorsiflexed. If the pain worsens, it is due to sciatica (Fig. 27.113B).

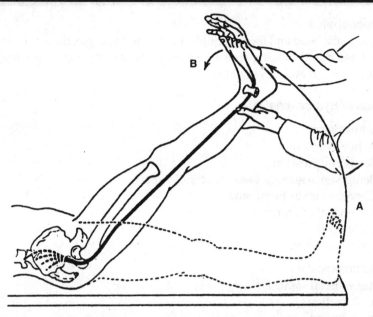

Fig. 27.113: Straight-knee leg-raising test (A) the-ex elevates the leg, (B) the ex then dorsiflexes the foot. Both maneuvers stretch the sciatic nerve and elicit pain if the nerve roots are inflamed, compressed, or imprisoned by a mechanical lesion

SCHEME OF CNS EXAMINATION: SUMMARY
a. General physical examination in CNS
b. Scheme of neurological examination

General Physical Examination
1. General Appearance
2. Level of Consciousness
3. Head — Shape (Brachy, dolicho, oxy, plagiocephaly)

        size — plot on standard curve, micro, macro, swelling, symmetry

        Fontanel — size (plot on curves), bulge, tenseness, pulsation, depression

        Sutures
        Macewan's sign
        Ascultating of head for bruit
        Transillumination of head

Causes of Large Head

1. *Hydrocephalus* Excessive volume of cerebrospinal fluid in the skull

2. *Megalencephaly* Enlargement of the brain.

3. *Thickening of the skull*

Hydrocephalus

Hydrocepalic head and face resemble an inverted triangle, the forehead being large, bossed and bulging forward over the orbits, the eyes being displaced slightly forward and downward.

Causes of Hydrocephalus

Communicating
1. Achondroplasia
2. Basilar impression
3. Benign enlargement of subarachnoid space
4. Choroid plexus papilloma
5. Meningeal malignancy
6. Meningitis
7. Posthemorrhagic

Noncommunicating
1. Aqueductal stenosis
   a. Infectious
   b. X-linked
2. Chiari malformation
3. Dandy-Walker malformation
4. Klippel-Feil syndrome
5. Mass lesions
   a. Abscess
   b. Hematoma
   c. Tumors and neurocutaneous disorders
   d. Vein of Galen malformation

Hydranencephaly
1. Holoprosencephaly
2. Massive hydrocephalus
3. Porencephaly

Megalencephaly

Anatomic Megalencephaly
1. Genetic megalencephaly
2. Megalencephaly with neurologic abnormality
3. Megalencephaly with achondroplasia
4. Megalencephaly with gigantism (Sotos syndrome)
5. Neurocutaneous disorders
   a. Hypomelanosis of Ito
   b. Incontinentia pigmenti
   c. Linear nevus sebaceous syndrome
   d. Neurofibromatosis
   e. Tuberous sclerosis

Metabolic Megalencephaly
1. Alexander disease
2. Canavan disease
3. Galactosemia—transferase deficiency
4. Gangliosidosis
5. Globoid leukodystrophy
6. Maple syrup urine disease
7. Metachromatic leukodystrophy
8. Mucopolysaccharidoses

Conditions with a Thickened Skull Causing Macrocephaly
1. Anemia
2. Cleidocranial dysostosis
3. Craniometaphyseal dysplasia of Pyle
4. Epiphyseal dysplasia
5. Hyperphosphatemia
6. Leontiasis ossea
7. Orodigitofacial dysostosis
8. Osteogenesis imperfecta
9. Osteopetrosis
10. Pycnodysostosis
11. Rickets
12. Russel dwarf

Microcephaly
Premature fusion of sutures, fontanelle closed, orbits flat, protruding eyes.

Conditions Causing Microcephaly

Primary Microcephaly
1. Microcephaly vera (genetic)
2. Chromosomal disorders
3. Defective neurulation
   a. Anencephaly
   b. Encephalocele
4. Defective prosencephalization
   a. Holoprosencephaly (arhinencephaly)
   b. Agenesis of the corpus callosum
5. Defective cellular migration

Secondary Microcephaly
1. Intrauterine disorders
   a. Infection
   b. Toxins
   c. Vascular
2. Perinatal brain injuries
   a. Hypoxic-ischemic encephalopathy
   b. Intracranial hemorrhage

    c. Meningitis and encephalitis
    d. Stroke
  3. Postnatal systemic diseases
    a. Chronic cardiopulmonary disease
    b. Chronic renal disease
    c. Malnutrition

Terms that Describe Head Shapes

Acrocephaly	— High, tower-like head with vertical forehead
Brachycephaly	— Broad head with recessed lower forehead
Oxycephaly	— Pointed head
Plagiocephaly	— Flattening of one side of head
Scaphocephaly	— An abnormally long and narrow head (dolicocephaly)
Trignocephaly	— Triangular-shaped head with a prominent vertical ridge in the midforehead

Disorders Associated with Craniostenosis

1. Ataxia telangiectasia
2. Familial hypophosphatemia
3. Hyperthyroidism
4. Idiopathic hypercalcemia
5. Mucopolysaccharidoses
6. Polycythemia vera
7. Rickets   a. Renal rickets
                 b. Vitamin D deficient
                 c. Vitamin D resistant
8. Sickle cell disease
9. Thalassemia major

Spine and Peripheral Nerves

Deformity—Kyphoscoliosis
Pot's spine
Epidural abscess
Metastasis
Meningomyelocel
Spina bifida oculta (tuft of hair lipoma, hemangioma sinus, etc.)
Localising cord lesions from spinal lesions
    Cervical-add 1
    1-6th-add 2
    7-10th-add 3
    10th thoracic overlies L1 and L2
    11th thoracic overlies L3 and L4
    12th thoracic overlies L5 and S1
    1st lumbar all sacral and coccygeal

Salient features and related physical findings

a. Spine bifida : Paraplegia
Trophic ulcers,
Bladders symptoms

b. Spina bifida Oculta (Tuft of hair, : Paraplegia
pigmentation, dimple, lipoma, Trophic ulcers
hemangioma, at the site) Bladder symptoms

c. Scoliosis : Friedreich's ataxia

d. Gibbus : TB, secondaries in spine
mucopolysaccharidosis

e. Tenderness : TB spine, secondaries, tumors

f. Diastometamyelia : Paraplegia

g. Short neck, low hair line : Cranio-vertebral anomalies

Peripheral Nerves

Thickening of Nerves : Hereditary neuropathy
Leprosy
Neurofibromata

Face

Typical facies (Myopathic, DMD, facial palsy, etc)
Dysmorphism (Down's syndrome)
    (Nose, mouth, chin, etc)
Ectodermal dysplasia, teeth

Eyes

Slant, dystopia canthorum, epicanthic folds
Hypo and hypertelorism
Corneal opacity, buphthalmos, cataract,
Pupillary changes, KF ring.
Anisocoria, coreatasia, corectopia, ptosis, enophthalmos, exophthalmos,
    macrocornea,
Microcornea.

Skin

Anemia, cyanosis, jaundice, neurocutneous markers (Cafe-au-lait spots, incontinenti pigmenti, tuberous sclerosis, facial hemangioma) rashes of collagen vascular diseases and childhood infections. Trophic changes, callosities, telangiectasia, petechiae, nodule, ulcer and pigmentation changes.

- Signs of vasomotor instability — Tachycerebrate, shock
- Allergic reaction dermatographia
- Scleroderma — Muscle wasting, weakness, dys-
    phagia, dysarthria.
- Neurofibromatosis — Neurofibroma, cafe-au-lait spots,
- Tuberous sclerosis — Ash leaf spots, shagreen patch,
    adenoma sebaceum
- Herpes zoster — Segmental level of lesions

- Herpes simplex — Encephalitis
- Common exanthema — Encephalitis
- Rash of systemic vasculitis, drugs
- Rash of pellagra — Hartnup disease
- Light sensitive eruptions — Porphyria, SLE
- Erythema nodosum — TB
- Scars, burns — Syringomyelia, leprosy
- Ulcers (orogenital) — Behcet's syndrome
- Butterfly rash — SLE
- Cutaneous angiomata

Facial naevi	:	Sturge-Weber disease
Spinal segmental nevi	:	Disorders of neural crest Syringomyelia Spinal astrocytoma
Midline pink nevi	:	Congenital craniospinal abnormalities
Spider nevi	:	Hepatic cirrhosis Pregnancy
Familial hemorrhagic telangiectasia	:	Telangiectases on spinal arachnoid and skin

Ear

Discharge, mastoid abnormalities, auricular abnormalities, temporomandibular joint abnormalities.

Vital Signs

Pulse.

Respiratory rate, type of respiration

Blood pressure

Peripheral Vessels, Cardia and Lungs

- Very slow pulse rate : Increased intracranial pressure
  Vasovagal seizures
  Complete heart block (Strokes Adams attacks)
- Very fast pulse rate : Nervousness
  Systemic infections
  Thyrotoxicosis
  Paraxysmal tachycardia
  Severe hemorrhage.
- Heart sounds : Cardiac murmurs—significant in chorea
  MS+AR—cerebral emboli, infective endocarditis
  AS—fainting attack
  CHD—cerebral abscess
  MVP—embolism

Signs of Increased Intracranial Pressure

Bounding pulse

Increased systolic BP

Increased head size in infants
Bulging AF in infant
Papilloedema
Macewan's sign
Unilateral pupillary dilatation

Lymphadenopathy, Hepatosplenomegaly and Abdominal Masses

Handedness

Meningeal Signs
Curled up posture, photophobia, tripod signs, neck rigidity, Kernig's sign, Brudzinski's sign (Leg and Neck).

Higher Mental Functions
1. Level of consciousness
2. Glasgow coma scale
3. General behavior and appearance (normal, hyperactive, agitated, quiet, etc).
4. Orientation in person, space, time
5. Attention span
6. Memory—instantaneous, immediate, recent, past, remote
7. Emotional status
8. Delusion, illusion, hallucinations
9. Language
   • Spontaneous speech
     Dysphonia
     Dysarthria
     Dysphasia
     Dysprosody (difficulty with melody, rhythm, accent, pitch and intonations)
   • Fluency
   • Comprehension
   • Repetition
     • Naming and word finding
     • Reading and writing
10. Intellectual capacity
     Cognitive and cortical functions
     Fundamentals of knowledge
     Calculative knowledge
     Gnosia
     • Visual
     • Auditory
     • Finger
     Praxia
     • Buccofacial
     • Limb

- Trunk
- Constriction

Mood

Thought content

Developmental Screening

Developmental quotient

Mental retardation grading

Special Senses

Vision

Hearing

Cranial Nerves

I Smell

II Optic

- Visual acuity

Reading

Object handling, following objects

Snellen's charts (Letter, E-chart, Figure chart)

Blink responses

Finger counting, hand movements

Opticokinetic nystagmus

PL, PR

- Visual fields

Confrontation test, perimetry

- Fundoscopic examination-disk, vessels, optic cup, macula, color size.

III, IV and VI

Palpebral fissure (Ptosis)

Pupils

Ocular movements

Tracking • Abduction
  - Abduction with elevation
  - Abduction with depression
  - Adduction
    - Adduction with elevation
    - Adduction with depression

Volitional—(Same as above)
  - Light reflex (Direct and indirect)
  - Accommodation reflex

V Sensory

Corneal reflex

Ophthalmic maxillary and mandibular nerves

Rooting reflex in infants
Motor—Strength (masseter, temporali's, pterigoids)

VII Sensory—(Taste)
Motor—Facial muscles
- Frontalis
- Orbicularis oculi
- Zygomaticus
- Buccinator
- Orbicularis oris
- Platysma

VIII Cochlear
- Whispered voice
- Watch test
- Rinne's test (AC: BC)
- Weber's test (Lateralising to)

Vestibular
- Gaze nystagmus
- Past pointing
- Caloric test

IX and X Movments of Uvula and Softpalate
Gag reflex,
Voice
Enunciation

XI (Spinal Accessory)
Sternocleidomastoid and trapezius

XII Atrophy, Fibrillation, Deviation on Protrusion and Enunciation

Motor System
1. Abnormal postures — Decerebrate
   Decorticate
   Hemiplegic
   Pithed frog
   Opisthotonus
   Curled up posture
   Tonic neck reflex
2. Nutrition-measurement of girth at symmetrical points
3. Muscle power — Grading
   — Daily activities (Walking, sitting, standing, climbing)
   — Proximal or distal weakness
   — Symmetric or asymmetric

      — Flexor or extensor
      — Groups of muscles at different joints
        (flexors, extensors, adductors, abductors and rotators)

4. Muscle tone (by resistance and passive movements, by feel, posture, by shaking, excessive mobility at joint)
5. Coordination
(finger nose test, finger finger nose test, heel knee test, hand movements, walking, dysdiadochokinesis, hand writing, gait, rebound phenomenon.
6. Abnormal movements

Reflexes
    Deep
    Superficial
    Somatic

Deep
    Jaw, biceps, triceps, supinator, knee, ankle
    Clonus—ankle, patellar, finger clonus

Superficial
    Corneal, conjunctival, abdominal, cremastric and
    Plantar, bulbocavernous
    Glabellar tap reflex
    Hoffman sign
    Other tests for eliciting pyramid lesions

Somatic
    Bladder, bowel

Sensory
    Cortical   — Graphesthesia
                    — Stereognosis
                    — 2-point discrimination
    Posterior column — Light touch
                    — Vibration
                    — Position
    Lateral column   — Temperature
                    — Deep pain
                    — Pin prick

Cerebellar Signs
    Hypotonia
    Nystagmus
    Skew deviation
    Incoordination

Ataxic gait
Truncal ataxia
Pendular muscles stretch reflexes

Autonomic Nervous System
Sphincter disturbances
Vital signs
Salivation, lacrimation and sweating
Tachycerebrate, palmar erythema.

GAIT
Spastic, stamping (post column), high stepping, ataxic, festinent... waddling, scissor, limping, astasia abasia

Developmental Reflexes
180° Flip examiantion

Final Inference
Note at historical level   Onset
Progression of the disease

After History and Detailed Examination Decide
1. What are the parts of nervous system involved
2. Location of the lesion
3. What is the lesion
4. Differential diagnosis

READY RECKONER OF EXAMINATION OF NERVOUS SYSTEM

Cranial Nerves and Their Function
  I. Sensory—Smell perception and interpretation
  II. Sensory—Visual acuity, field of vision, color vision
  III. Motor—Elevate eyelid, most extraocular muscles except lateral rectus and superior oblique.
  Parasympathetic—Pupillary constriction, change of lens shape.
  IV. Motor—Downward and inward eye movement
  V. Motor—Jaw opening, clenching, chewing and mastication sensory-sensation to cornea, iris, lacrimal gland, conjunctiva, eyelid, forehead, nasal and oral mucose, teeth, tongue, facial skin.
  VI. Motor—Lateral eye movement
  VII. Motor—Muscles of facial expression, platysma, stapedius.
  sensory—Taste, sensation to pharynx
  Parasympathetic—Salivation, tears
  VIII. Hearing and Equilibrium
  IX. Motor—Swallowing, phonation
  Sensory—Nasopharynx, gag, taste
  Parasympathetic—Salivary gland, carotid reflex

Table 27.25: Localization of neurological lesions

Anatomical regions	Signs of lesion	Tests to detect the lesion
a. Above the foramen magnum.	*i. Signs are contralateral unless specified otherwise* *ii. One or more sign may be absent in any individual case* *iii. Losses may be total or partial*	
1. Frontal lobe	headache motor seizures, focal, jacksonian or generalized • hemiplegia or monoplegia (usually with central facial palsy and often palatal or lingual weakness) • disorientation in time, space and person • confusion and mental changes • expressive aphasia • motor apraxia • Witzel Sucht's syndrome, (excessive jocularity, response to questions with silly answers)	Grasp and after grasp reflexes sucking reflex present even after the age of its normal disappearance in infancy **Tests for cerebral lesion** • orientation in time, space ane person • attention span • memory • affect • ability to interpret proverbial phrases • ability to follow simple and or complex commands • serial seven • arithematic • spelling • reading • writing • alteration in personality • Feeding • speech (perception, nominal, syntactic, expressive aphasia) • Two-point discrimination • vibratory and position sense • stereognosis • ability to differentiate right from left • muscle power
2. Parietal lobe	• headache • Jacksonian sensory seizures • loss of vibratory and position sense • loss of two-point sensibility • graph anesthesia • astereognosis	

Contd...

Contd...

Anatomical regions	Signs of lesion	Tests to detect the lesion
3. Temporal lobe	• headache • unicinate fits–unusual taste, smells, hallucinations, *de javu* (feeling of having already seen a place or person, never seen before, deja etende (comments never heard before are incorrectly regarded as repetition of previous conversation) *ja mais vu* (there is a feeling of unfamiliarity with a situation that one has already experienced) • auditory perceptive aphasia • homonymous hemianopsia or quadanopsia • somnambulism • clouding of consciousness	
4. Occipital lobe	• visual aura (flashes of light, blindness) • homonymous hemanopsia, frequently with macular sparing or incongruity occasionally there is quadrantic hemianopia • there may be failure to appreciate colour, form and movement • word blindness and 'mind blindness'	• visual fields
5. Parieto-occipital lobe	• difficulty in performing simple arithematic • viual perceptive aphasia • nominal aphasia • difficulty in differentiating one finger from another • Gerstaman's syndrome, unable to differentiate right from left	
6. Pyramidal tract	• upper motor neurone involvement of one or more cranial nerves, V, VII, X, XI, XII • hemiplegia, quadriplegia • muscle spasticity	• loss of superficial and cremasteric reflexes • pathological reflexes elicited, i.e., Babinskis, Oppenheim, Chaddok, Hoffman, Tromner, Gordon, Rossolimo and Marie-Foix

Contd...

Contd...

Anatomical regions	Signs of lesion	Tests to detect the lesion
		• physiological reflexes
	• spastic neurogenic bladder	• muscle power
	• exaggerated physiological reflexes	• patellar and ankle clonus
7. Medial lemniscus	• numbness and tingling	• vibratory sense
	• loss of vibratory sense	• sense of position
		• finger nose test (eyes closed)
	• loss of deep touch and position sense	• stereognosis
		• two-point sensibility
	• dysmetria	• ataxic gait
	• ataxia accentuated by closing the eyes	• Romberg's sign
		• graphesthesia
8. Thalamus	• hemianesthesia, followed by	• proprioceptive sensations
	• excessive sensibility to thermal and painful stimuli	• extroceptive sensations (touch, pain and temperature)
	• the pains are greatly aggravated by emotional stress and fatigue	
	• spontaneous pains	
	• misinterpretation of other stimuli (e.g., light touch, or tickling may give unpleasant sensation)	
	• may be ataxia	
	• choreiform movements from simultaneous involvement of corpus striatum	
	• hemiparesis with simultaneous involvement of internal capsule	
9. Spinothalamic tracts	• loss of pain and temperature sense	• sensations of pain and temperature (hot and cold test)
	• loss of superficial touch (rare)	• tests for sacral sparing
10. Superior cerebellar ped- uncle or brachium con-	• in coordinated movements of limbs	• tests for coordination
	• hypotonia	• muscle tone

Contd...

Contd...

Anatomical regions	Signs of lesion	Tests to detect the lesion
juctivum (ipsilateral changes)	• dysdiadochokinesia • dyssynergia • dysmetria often with intesion tremors • decreased deep tendon reflexes (rarely) • head tilt and posturing (rarely)	• tendon reflexes
11. Extrapyramidal tract	• emotional instability (uncontrollable bursts of laughter or bouts of weeping) • involuntary tremors at rest (disappear during sleep) • clownish and short stepping gait • chorea • athetosis • mask like facies • monotonous speech • muscular rigidity (cogwheel or plastic) • fixed head and trunk • propulsion and retropulsion	• facial expression • Myerson's eye signs • affect • speech • muscle tone • gait • propulsion and retropulsion tests • spontaneous movements • check for Kayser-Fleischer ring
12. Cerebellar hemisphere (ipsilateral changes)	• syllabic or staccato speech • reeling, broad based gait • intension tremors • nystagmus • incoordinated movement of limbs • hypotonia • decreased tendon reflexes • dysadiadochokinesia • dyssynergia • head tilt and posturing (occasionally)	• gait • muscle tone • physiological reflexes • nystagmus (horizontal rotary) • speech test (sound repetition) • rock test, • finger nose test (look for intention tremors) • supination and pronation test • patting test • rebound test

Contd...

Contd...

Anatomical regions	Signs of lesion	Tests to detect the lesion
13. Vermis of cerebellum	• trunk ataxia • rocking forward and backward in Romberg position • difficult in standing erect, falls backwards or forwards	• heel-to-knee test • ability to button clothes • ability to circle chair, clockwise and anticlockwise • leg swinging test of Wartenberg
14. Vestibular system	• dissociated (ataxic) nystagmus • disconjugate deviation of eyes • vertical nystagmus	• vertigo • nystagmus • general symptoms (tachycardia, nausea, vomiting, lowered blood pressure) • Caloric test
15. The cerebellopontine angle	• cerebellar signs (ibid) • muscle power and tone medulla (upper motor neurone signs on the opposite side of the body, rarely amounting to definite paralysis. • sings of cranial nerve involvement (on the same side as the lesion) V, VII and VIII cranial nerves	• signs of pressure on pons and • V, VII and VIII cranial nerves as described subsequently
16. Cranial nerves	i. Signs are ipsilateral ii. Losses may be total or partial iii. One or more signs may not be present in any individual case iv. After excluding raised intracranial tension, CSF should be done	
Olfactory nerve Cranial I (sensory)	• abnormally acute sense of smell (hyperosmia) • loss of sense of smell (anosmia) • perverted sense of small (parosmia)	• testing smell (each nostril separately) with non-irritating volatile substance like, clove oil camphor, turpentine, peppermint

Contd...

Contd...

Anatomical regions	Signs of lesion	Tests to detect the lesion
	• loss of sense of taste, only the primary sensations of taste (sweet, bitter, salt and sour) remain	• testing taste
Optic nerve Cranial II (sensory)	i. The nerve	
	• papilloedema	• visual acuity
	• papillitis	
	• optic atrophy (primary and secondary), central and paracentral scotomata	• visual fields • fundus examination
	• peripheral constriction of visual field	• color vision
	• loss of visual acuity, unilateral blindness	
	ii. Optic chiasma	
	• bitemporal hemianopia or quadranopsia	
	• altitudinopsia (usually bilateral) a defect of upper lower half of the visual field	
	• optic atrophy	
	• paracentral scotomata (rarely)	
	iii. Optic tract	
	• contralateral homonymous hemianopsia (without macular sparing)	
	• Wernicke's hemianopic pupillary response	
	iv. Optic radiations	
	• contralateral homonymous hemianopsia	
	• quadrianopsia (unilateral or bilateral)	
	v. Occipital lobe.	
	Contralateral homonymous hemianopsia, (often with out macular sparing)	

Contd...

Contd...

Anatomical regions	Signs of lesion	Tests to detect the lesion
III. Oculomotor nerve	i. Nerve	**Tests for III, IV and VIth nerves**
	• ptosis, may be associated with compensatory wrinkling of the forehead on the same side	• size of the palpebral fissure
	• lateral deviation of eye (exotropia)	• finger following for ocular movements
	• paralysis of medial, upward and downward gaze	• accomodation
	• concensual light reflex	• light reflex
	• inability to elevate eye when turned medially	
	• dilated fixed pupil (does not react to light, accommodation or concensual stimulation)	
	• loss of visual acuity	
	• diplopia and dizziness	
	• external strabismus with downward deviation	
	• limitation of ocular movements	
	• nystagmus	
	• tilting of head to compensate for diplopia	
	• hippus (alternate dilatation and constriction of pupil under uniform illumination) seen in chorea (rheumatic)	
	• ossilopsia (optical illusion of movement of fixated objects)	
	ii. Third nerve nucleus	
	• paresis of individual orbital muscles, such as superior and inferior oblique, peripheral lesion of the nerve give complete paralysis)	• in nuclear lesion when head is kept immoible and gaze fixed on an object, eyes may follow the movement of object, or when the patient is unable to follow the
	• conjugate deviation (both eyes turned to same side)	
	• paralysis of convergence (loss of accommodation)	
	• nystagmus	

Contd...

Contd...

Anatomical regions	Signs of lesion	Tests to detect the lesion
	iii. supranuclear lesions (of frontal and occipital lobes) <ul><li>paralysis of conjugate gaze to the eyes opposite side with deviation of the eyes to the side of the lesion</li><li>individual ocular muscles not affected, hence no squint and diplopia</li><li>reverse in the irritative processes, due to over-action of affected muscles</li><li>muscles controlling a particular movement paralysed</li></ul>	moving object with his eyes he fixes the gaze on object and head rotates passively, or gaze may remain fixed on object and eyes take upm position of deviation
IV Trochlear nerve (motor) contralateral signs if lesion is nuclear	<ul><li>head tilts away from the side of lesion</li><li>nystagmus</li><li>cannot look down (hence difficulty in descending stairs</li><li>diplopia</li></ul>	<ul><li>prism tests for ability of internal and external rectus muscle to coalesce</li><li>diplopia testing with red glass or Maddox rod</li></ul>
VI Abducens nerve (motor)	<ul><li>medial deviation of eye (esotropia)</li><li>squint</li><li>paralysis of lateral gaze</li></ul>	
Internuclear paralysis lesion of brainstem, interrupting connections between VI nerve nuclei	<ul><li>ophthalmoplegia internuclearis i.e., dissociation of movements of two eyes on looking laterally, On moving the eyes away from the side of lesion, ipsilateral eye fails to move beyond the position of central fixation. Opposite eye has partial outward movement plus nystagmus, (ataxic nystagmus)</li></ul>	test movements of eyeball
III, IV, VI nuclear lesion	<ul><li>is rare (in bulbular paralysis and progressive muscular atrophy, all the three nuclei are involved together.)</li><li>Chronic progressive complete ophthalmoplegia</li></ul>	

Contd...

Contd...

Anatomical regions	Signs of lesion	Tests to detect the lesion
V. Trigeminal nerve (mixed nerve)	• loss of sensation of all modalities over forehead to bregma and overarm face excluding angle of jaw • loss of sensation of all modalities in oral cavity except taste • dissociate anesthesia i.e., loss of pain but not touch (involvement of spinal tract of Vth nerve, e.g. in syringobulbia) • close the jaw tightly and palpate masseter • paralysis of muscles of mastication with deviation of the jaw to the affected side • Trismus (lock jaw) due to spasm of the muscles of mastication, in rabies, tetany, tetanus, epilepsy and hysteria • weak bite • nerve tenderness at areas of emergence of divisions of nerve • trigger zones of pain • attacks of sharp cutting pain, marked if Gasserian ganglion or peripheral branches are involved. • loss of reflexes like jaw jerk, sneez, conjunctival and corneal. Jaw jerk exaggerated in supranuclear palsy • impaired hearing due to paralysis of tensor tympani • trophic and secretory disturbances causing anosmia (due to dryness of nose, moisture is necessary to smell), ulceration of face, loss of teeth	• Sensations of forehead, face and oral cavity, including taste • corneal reflex • jaw jerk • sneeze reflex • ability to chew • trigger zones of neuralgia
VII. Facial nerve (mixed nerve mainly motor)	i. Unilateral paralysis a. emotional facial weakness, i.e. deviation of mouth to normal side on smiling. Deviation disappears on	

Contd...

Contd...

Anatomical regions	Signs of lesion	Tests to detect the lesion
	voluntary movements (1) lesions of opposite thalamus and (2) connections of thalamus with frontal lobe.)	
	b. Upper motor neurone facial weakness (lesion at any point between the opposite cortex and facial nucleus in pons). The upper face is spared because they have bilateral innervation and are controlled by both cerebral cortices	• loss of ability to show teeth and smile • unable to whistle • no loss of taste • salivation not affected • reflexes retained • emotional response • ipsilateral hemiplegia or monoplegia
	• on showing teeth, angle of mouth deviates to healthy side with • deepening of nasolabial folds on that side • eyes can be closed normally • paralysis is of spastic type	
	c. Lower motor neurone facial weakness (final common pathways between the nucleus and the muscle is interrupted, cutting off all stimuli to both upper and lower facial muscles lesion is on the same side) • ironing out of the nasolabial fold • widening of palpebral fissure • inability to elevate eyebrows • loss of ability to show teeth • loss of ability to smile • loss of ability to whistle • weak corneal reflex • loss of taste on anterior 2/3 of tongue • fasciculations of facial muscles	• symmetry of face at rest and during voluntary facial movement • ability to close the eyes tightly • ability to wrinkle the forehead

Contd...

Contd...

Anatomical regions	Signs of lesion	Tests to detect the lesion
	• blepharospasm	• ability to show teeth
	eyelids the eyeball on the effected side is seen to turn upwards)	• ability to smile
	• excape of fluids on drinking—because angle of mouth is drooping	• sense of taste
	• difficulty in articulation—due to paralysis	• corneal reflex
	To localize the exact site of lesion keep in view following considerations.	• if a child does not smile, ask her to whistle. This often results in successful smile, though whistle may be unsuccessful
	i. with lesion in pons, hemiplegia is on the opposite side.	
	ii. when lesion is between the brainstem and departure of chorda tympani in the middle ear, salivation, taste and tear production is affected, with distortion of sounds due to palsy of stapedius muscle.	
	iii. In lesions of cerebello-pontine angle, V and VIIth nerves are also involved.	
	iv. When lesion is in the middle ear after the branching of superficial petrosal branch, but before branching off of chorda tympani; secretion of tears is normal, taste and salivation affected.	
	v. In lesions of nucleus of the facial nerve in facial canal, beyond departure of chorda tympani, there is only weakness of facial muscles.	
	vi. Lesion of the nerve in parotid gland or in the muscles themselves; only some of the facial muscles are paralysed.	

Contd...

Contd...

Anatomical regions	Signs of lesion	Tests to detect the lesion
	d. Bilateral facial nerve paralysis	
	i. bilateral emotional facial palsy	• watch facial expression at rest and on voluntary facial movement
	• mask like face	• "hot potato speech" (as though speaking with hot potato in mouth)
	• complete lack of normal play of expression	
	• there is diminished blinking, but when occurs is normal	• sense of taste
	• There is transformation when the patient smiles	• ability to smile
		• ability to whistle
	ii. bilateral upper motor neurone paralysis	
	• mask like expression of face not marked	
	• blinking little affected	
	• mouth appears well during ordinary conversation, but cannot be moved on command	
	iii. bilateral lower motor neurone palsy.	
	• flattening of all normal folds	
	• corners of the mouth sag	
	• all attempts at voluntary movement fail	
	• on an attempt to close eyes or blink, whites of eyes are seen	
	• talks as if there is extensive ulceration in the mouth.	

In long-standing facial paralysis, there may be aberrant re-innervation any attempt at facial expression results in inappropriate facial expression for emotions, which surprises the audience and is embarrassing to the patient.
Primary muscular disorders mimicking facial palsy are, myasthenia gravis, muscular dystrophy and dystrophia myotonia.

VIII Accoustic nerve cochlear nerve, vestibular nerve (composite sensory nerve)	A. Cochlear nerve (for hearing)	• otoscopic examination
	• nerve deafness, loss of ability to hear wrist watch or whispered voice	• hearing acuity, watch test, whisper test, audiogram
	• tinnitus	• Webers test
		• Rinne's test

Contd...

Contd...

Anatomical regions	Signs of lesion	Tests to detect the lesion
	• hearing scotomas (deafness to certain pitches and noises)	• Bing's test
	ii. supranuclear lesions (lesion of superior temporal gyrus of dominant cerebral hemisphere)	
	• auditory hallucinations	
	• sensory aphasia or word deafness (can) hear but unable to understand the word)	
	B. Vestibular nerve	• rotation test
	• vertigo	• caloric test
	• horizontal nystagmus, slow component usually to the side of lesion	• past pointing test
		• Romberg's sign
IX. Glossopharyngeal (mixed nerve)	• loss of sensation in oropharynx	• pharyngeal or gag reflex
	• gag reflex absent	• Vernet *re deau* phenomenon (constriction of pharyngeal wall when saying 'Ah')
	• slight dysphagia normal	• carotid sinus reflex, (pressure over the carotid sinus produces slowing of the heart and fall in blood pressure)
	• deviation of uvula to affected side	
	• loss of sensation pharynx, tonsils, fauces and posterior 1/3 of tongue	
	• loss of constriction of posterior pharyngeal wall when saying, "Ah"	
	• increased salivation (involvement of tympanic plexus in middle ear lesion)	
	• rarely nystagmus of uvula	
	• sometimes tachycardia (disturbance or carotid sinus reflex)	
X. Vagus nerve (mixed nerve)	bilateral nuclear lesion (medullary) or bilateral motor neurone lesion (voluntary movements impaired but reflex movements remain) no move ment of palate and pharynx	• palate and uvula, position and movement
		• ability to say, A,E,I,O,U
		• ability to swallow
		• gag reflex

Contd...

Contd...

Anatomical regions	Signs of lesion	Tests to detect the lesion
	• dysphagia • nasal regurgitation of fluids • nasal speech • spasticity of tongue • exaggerated jaw jerk • difficulty in phonation • palatal nystagmus (constant rythmic vertical oscilla-tions of the palate) • pharyngeal (gag) reflex absent • voice hoarse and deep, utterances of high notes impos-sible	• laryngoscopy
XI. Accessory nerve (motor)	• sternomastoid weakness (unilateral or bilateral) weak-ness in turning head to opposite side • trapezius weakness, weakness in elevation of shoulders	• ability to turn head from side to side • ability to shrug the shoulders • sternomastoid muscle

XII. Hypoglossal nerve	a. unilateral lower motor neurone lesion
	  • tongue weak and atrophied on the affected side
	  • on protrusion deviates to paralysed side
	  • tremors and fasciculations
	b. bilateral lower motor neurone lesion
	  • global atrophy of tongue
	  • with little or no movement
	c. nuclear or medullary lesion (flaccid paralysis)
	  • fasciculations, sensory disturbances, loss of deep sensations, e.g. pain and temperature sense, involv-ing half of the face or body. This will be bilateral in midline lesions
		• ability to protude the tongue in straight line
		• move the tongue from side to side and lick each cheek with it
		• any atrophy or tremors

Contd...

Contd...

Anatomical regions	Signs of lesion	Tests to detect the lesion
	• If lesion is bilateral, tongue is completely paralysed with dysphagia, dysarthria and difficulty in chewing food	
	d. cortical lesions	
	• dysarthria	
	• ataxia of tongue	
	e. striatum lesions (e.g. in chorea) irregular rhythmic movements of tongue	
	f. supranuclear (spastic paralysis)	
	• contralateral hemiplegia and paralysis of tongue	
	• on protrusion tongue deviates opposite to the side of lesion	
	• no atrophy or fibrillation	
	• contralateral hemiplegia and ipsilateral paralysis of tongue (lesion of pyramid near the decussation)	
	g. bilateral upper motor neurone lesion	
	• weak and	
	• bunched up tongue	
	• sluggishness of all voluntary movements	
	• no deviation of tongue but cannot move rapidly from side to side on protrusion	
	h. pseudobulbar palsy is bilateral upper motor neurone paralysis affecting the VII, IX, X and XIIgh cranial nerves	
	i. Bulbar palsy lower motor neurone paralysis affecting the VII, IX, X and XII cranial nerves	
b. Involvement below the foreman magnum	i. signs are ipsilateral unless otherwise specified.	
	ii. one or more signs under each structure may be absent in individual cases.	

Contd...

Contd...

Anatomical regions	Signs of lesion	Tests to detect the lesion
	iii. Losses may be total or partial.	
	iv. X-ray of vertebral column indicated.	
	v. CSF examination after exclusion of raised intracranial tension, should be done.	
1. Anterior motor horn or root	• flaccid muscles • weakness confined to individual muscles • loss of deep tendon reflexes • muscular atrophy • loss of anal reflex • flaccid neurogenic bladder (if S 2, 3 or 4 is involved) • vasomotor changes (if lateral horn is involved)	• muscle tone • muscle power • reflexes
2. Lateral column	• increased deep tendon reflexes • ankle, patellar, wrist, clonus • Babinski, Oppenheim, Chaddock, Tromner, reflexes • loss of superficial abdominal and cremasteric reflexes • muscular weakness (diffuse but distal muscle involvement) more marked • loss of involuntary movement • muscle spasticity • spastic gait • spastic neurogenic bladder (can be flaccid in acute lesions)	• deep tendon reflexes (physiological reflexes) • clonus • abnormal reflexes (pathological reflexes) • superficial reflexes • muscle tone • muscular power • gait
3. Spinocerebellar tract	• usually there are no signs unless there is associated involvement of cerebellum	
4. Lateral spinothalamic tract (contralateral changes)	• loss of temperature sensation	• sensations of pain and temperature • loss of temperature sensation

Contd...

Contd....

Anatomical regions	Signs of lesion	Tests to detect the lesion
5. Ventral spinothalamic tract (contralateral changes)	• loss of superficial touch (rarely)	• sensation of touch
6. Ventral commissure (bilateral changes)	• Loss of pain • loss of temperature	• sense of pain and temperature sensation's-hot and cold test • gait • Romberg sign • sensation of touch, position sense and vibration • tendon reflexes • finger nose test (eyes closed) • two-point sensibility • stereognosis • graphesthesia
7. Posterior column	• ataxia • Romberg's sign • numbness and tingling and position senses • loss of deep touch • dysmetria • loss of deep tendon reflexes • flaccid neurogenic bladder • loss of vibratory sense • radicular pains • broad based ataxic gait, accentuated by closing the eyes	
8. Sensory roots	• flaccid muscles • numbness and tingling • loss of vibratory and position sense • segmental loss of touch, pain and temperature • absent tendon reflexes without atrophy • trophic changes • flaccid neurogenic bladder (if S2, 3 or 4 involved)	• sensations of touch, pain, position and vibration • deep sensations of testicle and Achilles tendon • gait • muscle tone • physiological reflexes • rectal and bladder tone and control
9. Peripheral nerves	• high stepage gait • weakness • paresthesia • tenderness of nerves and muscles	• test for all sensory modalities • muscle size and tone • muscle power • physiological reflexes

Contd....

Contd...

Anatomical regions	Signs of lesion	Tests to detect the lesion
	• glove and stocking anesthesia (non-segmental combined sensory loss) • loss of vibratory and position sense • absent deep tendon reflexes • muscular atrophy • trophic and vasomotor changes • fibrillations and reaction of degeneration	• check trophic changes vasomotor changes • muscle and nerve tenderness
10. Sympathetic ganglion	• Horner's syndrome • anhidrosis • vasomotor changes (dermatographia) • hypertension	• palpaberal fissures • pupils • pulse • blood pressure • intestinal mobility • mecholyl test "seat function" • cocaine test
11. Myoneural junction	• inability to chew • inability to count • inability to blink eyes without fatigueing	• tests of muscle power
12. Muscles	• waddling gait • muscular weakness (proximal more than distal) • muscular atrophy (occasionally hypertrophy and pseudomuscular hypertrophy) • tendon reflexes diminished but retained for long time • no fasciculations or reaction of degeneration	• gait • muscle bulk • Tests of muscle power • myotonic reflex (delayed relaxation of hand grip)
13. Pseudotumor cerebri (benign intracranial hypertension)	• headache • papilloedema • no neurological manifestations	• only positive test is fundus eamination **Causes are:** i. following ear infection

Contd...

Contd...

Anatomical regions	Signs of lesion	Tests to detect the lesion
		ii. associated with thrombi in superior longitudinal or lateral sinus
		iii. hypovitaminosis A
		iv. hypervitaminosis A
		v. use of tetracycline
		vi. cortiosteroids
		vii. endocrine disorders
Raised intracranial tension		
A. prior to fusion of skull suures	a. Constant signs	• fundus examination
	• hydrocephalus; head enlarged in all diameters, most marked at vertex and least at the base	• Macewin's sign (percussion on skull gives characteristic hollow, craked pot note)
	• suture open and widened	• neurological examination
	• anterior fontanelle widely open and full	• X-ray skull
	• face triangular and small contrasting markedly with large rounded forward projecting forehead.	
	• setting sun, appearance of the eyeballs (downward pressure of the orbital plate of frontal bone on the eyeballs)	
	• distended subcutaneous veins of scalp	
	• scanty hair on scalp	
	• exaggerated deep tendon reflexes	
	• bradycardia	
	• respiration slow and shallow	
	• respiratory arrhythmias (Cheyne Stokes breathing)	
	• arrest of growth	
	b. variable signs	
	• convulsions	
	• mental retardation	
	• spastic paralysis of the limbs	

Contd...

Contd...

Anatomical regions	Signs of lesion	Tests to detect the lesion
	• nystagmus • deafness • headache and vomiting • papilloedema and optic atrophy	
B. Post-skull sutural union	• headache • vomiting • convulsions • slow cerebration and apathy • periods of somnolence • exaggerated deep tendon reflexes • extensor plantar response • paresis of lower limbs first and later extending to upper limbs • no sensory loss • visual impairement • diplopia, to begin with intermittent • convergent squint • papilloedema • giddiness, (feeling of faintness and general unsteadiness especially on stooping) • vertigo • deafness • cranial nerve paralysis • incoordination of movements • bradycardia • respiration slow and shallow • respiratory arrhythmia • anosmia	• fundus • neurological examination • X-ray skull

(Adapted from BK Sohi (Eds) *Pediatric Clinical Methods*, Ist Edition; 1993: CBS Publishers and Distributors, Delhi).

    X. Phonation, swallowing, sensation behind ears, heart, lung, GIT, (other abodminal viscera).
   XI. Motor—Head turn, shrugging of shoulders.
  XII. Motor—Tongue movements, articulation, swallowing.

Cranial Nerve Testing

       I. Smell
      II. Visual acuity, color, field of vision.
III, IV, VI. Ocular movements, eyelid drooping, pupillary reflex, accommodation reflex.
      V. Corneal reflex, sensation, muscles of mastication
    VII. Inspect facial movements and test taste
  VIII. Hearing, Rinne's, Weber's test
    IX. Taste (bitter, sour), gag relfex, swallowing
     X. Gag, swallowing, voice, nasal regurgitation
    XI. Trapezius and sternomastoid function
   XII. Speech
          Tongue strength

Indirect Cranial Nerves Examination

Newborn and Infants

Cr. II, III, IV and VI	Optical blink reflex
	Follow objects
	Dolls eye maneuver
Cr N V	Rooting and sucking reflex, chewing and biting.
Cr N VII	Crying, smiling, wrinkles of forehead, nasolabial fold
Cr VIII	Acoustic blink reflex
	Dolls eye maneuver (for vestibular problem and eye muscle problem)
Cr. IX	Swallowing and gag
Cr. XII	Sucking and swallowing
	Pinch infants nose, mouth will open and tip of tongue will rise in a midline position.

For Young Children

      II. Snellen E or picture chart, visual field
III, IV, VI. Follow objects
      V. Chewing, sensation over face, corneal reflex
    VII. Shows teeth, crying smiling
   VIII. Turn to sound, audiometry
IX and X. Gag reflex
XI and XII. Protrudes tongue, shrugs shoulders and raise arms

SOFT NEUROLOGICAL SIGNS

These are defined as particular forms of deviant performance on a motor or a sensory test in the neurological examination that is abnormal for that age.

Significant caution must be exercised in the interpretation of the soft neurologic signs. Testing for soft neurologic signs is cumbersome. It involves observation of a series of timed motor tasks and also a comparison with those of normal children of the same age and sex (Table 27.26).

Table 27.26: Observation of motor tasks for soft sign finding

Activity	Soft sign finding	Latest expected age for disappearance
1. Walking (Gait)	Stifflegged with foot tapping quality, unusal posturing of the limbs	3 years
2. Heel walking	Difficulty in remaining on heels for 10 ft distance	7 years
3. Tiptoe walking	Difficulty in remaining on toes for a 10 feet distance	7 years
4. Tandem gait	Difficulty in walking heel to toe unusual posturing of arms	7 years
5. One foot standing	Unable to remain on one foot longer than 5-10 sec	5 years
6. Hopping in one place	Unable to rhythmically hop on each foot	6 years
7. Motor stance (arms ext. infront, feet together, eyes closed)	Drifting of arms, mild writhing movement of fingers	3 years
8. Visual tracking	Difficulty in following the object with eyes when the head is still, nystagmus	5 years
9. Rapid thumb to finger test	Rapidly touching thumb to finger in sequence is uncoordinated; unable to suppress mirror movement in contralateral hand	8 years
10. Rapid alternating movements of hands	Irregular speed and rhythm with pronation and supination of hands	10 years
11. Finger nose test	Unable to repeatedly touch finger and nose	7 years
12. Rt- Lt-discrimination	Unable to identify Rt and Lt sides of ones own body	5 years
13. Two-point discrimination	Difficulty in localising and discriminating when touched in one or two places	6 years
14. Graphesthesia	Unable to identify geometric shapes you draw on child's open palm	8 years
15. Stereognosis	Unable to identify common objects placed in the hand	5 years

Interpretation

Soft neurological signs may be present in an intellectually normal child, but the presence of 2 or more such signs in a child points to a neurologic dysfunction. It may be cerebral palsy or even attention deficit disorder. Therefore, rather than jumping to a conclusion, it is better to monitor the child closely.

Types

- Mirror movements
- Head bobbing/Foot tapping

- Dysdiadokokinesia
- Finger agnosia
- Stimulus extinction
- Choreiform movements
- Lateral dominance
- Verbal dyspraxia
- Strabismus

These may be evaluated and elicited by a few activities.

Table 27.27: Structures of brainstem and their functions

Medulla	Higher control of respiration, vasomotor function
Cr. N IX to XII	Higher respiration centre. Reflexes of swallowing, coughing, vomiting, sneezing and hiccup, cough, relay station for ascending and descending spinal tract that cross in medulla.
Pons	Reflexes of pupillary action and eye movements regulates
Cr.N V-VIII	respiration, houses portion of respiratory center control. Voluntary muscle through pyramidal tract.
Mid Brain	Reflex center for eye and head movement
Cr. N III-IV	Auditory relay pathway Corticospinal tract pathway
Diencephalon	Relay impulses between cerebrum, cerebellum, pons and
Cr. N I and II	medulla, conveys all
Thalamus	Sensory impulse except olfaction to and from cerebrum before reaching associated sensory area. Integrates impulse between motor cortex and cerebellum, influence voluntary movements and motor response, cortical level of consciousness, consciousness perception of sensation and abstract feelings.
Epithalamus	Houses pineal body. Sexual development and behavior.
Hypothalamus	Major processing center of internal stimuli for ANS temperature control, water osmolality, feeding behavior and neuroendocrinal control.
Pituitary	Hormonal contral of growth, lactation and metabolism.

Testing Spinal Tracts

Ascending

Lateral spinothalamic	—	Superficial pain
	—	Temperature
Anterior spinothalamic	—	Superficial touch
	—	Deep pressure
Posterior column	—	Vibration
	—	Deep pressure
	—	Position
	—	Stereognosis
	—	Point location
	—	Two-point discrimination
Anterior and dorsal spinocerebellar	—	Proprioceptive

Table 27.28: Motor clinical syndromes of neurological deficits

I. **Lower motor neuron** (Includes ant. horncell, nerve root, peripheral nerve, myoneural junction)	• Paralysis of individual muscle or sets of muscle in root or peripheral nerve distribution • Atrophy of denervation early • Hypotonia • Hypo or absent DTR • Fasciculation and fibrillation (AHC disease or nerve root irritation) • Sup. reflexes absent • Sensory changes if peripheral nerves or nerve roots involved.
II. **Upper motor neuron** Cortical motor neurons to Cr. N. nuclei or AHC in spinal cord	• Paralysis of movements in hemi, quadri, para or monoplegic distribution • Disuse atrophy late and slight. • Brisk DTR and clonus common • Extensor plantar response. • Clasp knife spasticity • Tone in upper limb flexors, extensors of knee and flexors of ankle more • Absent abdominal or cremastic response.
III. **Basal motor nuclei of extra-pyramidal system** (Basal ganglia) Includes: • Cerebrum: Caudate-putamen (Striatum) Globus pallidus (Pallidus) • Diencephalon: Somatomotor relay nuclei of thalamus (anterior and lateral ventral nucleus) Subthalamic nucleus, zona incerta • Mid brain: Reticular formation, Red nucleus substantia nigra	• Rigidity (lead pipe or cogweel) • Hypokineia • Involuntary movements—tremors, patterned hyperkinesia (Chorea athetosis, dystonia)
IV Cerebellar (Cerebellar hemis-phere (mainly post. lobe) Rostral vermis (Ant. lobe) Caudal vermis and (Flocco-nodular and post. lobe) pancerebellar syndrome)	Gait dystaxia—broad based, ataxic gait, difficult tandem gait Nystagmus Arm dystaxia and irregular alternating movement (Finger nose test, pronation and supination test) Overshooting (Wrist slapping arm pulling test) Leg dystaxia (heel knee test) Hypotonia (Pendular knee jerk)

Descending

Lateral and anterior pyramidal	Rapid rhythm with alternating movements Voluntary movement Deep tendon reflexes Plantar reflex

Medial and lateral   Posture, gait, Romberg's
reticulospinal   Instinctual reaction

Primitive Reflexes Routinely Tested

1. Rooting
2. Sucking
3. Swallowing
4. Plantar grasp
5. Palmar grasp
6. Placing
7. Stepping
8. Moro's
9. Trunk incurvation
10. Tonic neck reflex (Fencing)

Less Commonly Evaluated Primitive Reflexes

Glabellar
Galant (Trunk Incurvation)
Landau
Parachute
Neck righting
Symmetrical tonic neck reflex
Delange's sign

Root Values of Commonly Tested Superficial and Deep Tendon Reflexes (Figure in the Bracket, Most Important Root)

Superficial Reflexes   :   Upper abdominal T7, 8 and 9
                                Lower abdominal T10-T11
                                Cremasteric T12 (L1) L2
                                Plantar L4 L5 (S1) and S2
Deep Tendon Reflexes   :   Biceps C5-C6
                                Brachioradialis C5-C6
                                Triceps C6 (C7) C8
                                Patellar L2 (L3) (L4)
                                Ankle (S1) S2

Table 27.29: Differentiating points of UMN and LMN lesions

UMN lesion	LMN lesion
Spasticity	Flaccidity
No atropy	Atrophy
Loss of power of function	Loss of power of individual muscle
DTR increased	DTR decreased or zero
Superficial reflex absent	Sup reflex absent
Plantars upgoing	Plantars down going or absent
No fasciculation	Fasciculation may be present

Cardiovascular Accidents in Reference to the Artery Involved, the Area Supplied and the Clinical Presentation

Table 27.30

Artery	Area supplied	Clinical syndrome
1. Int. carotid art	Cerebral hemisphere diencephalon	Unilateral blindness Severe contralateral hemiplegia Hemianesthesia, profound aphasia
2. MCA	Cerebrum communication language space, sensation and voluntary movement	Alteration in communication cognitive, mobility and sensation
3. ACA	Medial surface and upper convexity of frontal and parietal lobe and medial surface of hemisphere which includes motor and sensory cortex limbs than upper serving legs	Emotional liability confusion Urinary incontinence, impaired mobility with sensation greater in lower limbs than upper limbs
4. PCA	Medial and inf. temp. lobe, medial occipital lobe, thalamus, post. hypothalmus and visual receptive area	Hemianesthesia Hemiplegia, homonymous hemianopia Receptive aphasia Cortical blindness
5. Vertebral or basilar	Brainstem and cerebellum	T1A
	a. (Incomplete occlusion)	Unilateral and bilateral weakness of limbs diplopia, nausea, vomiting, tinnitus dysphasia, dysarthria
	b. Anterior portion of pons	Locked instate (No movement exept eyelids, sensation and consciousness preserved)
	c. Complete occlusion and hemorrhage	Coma miotic pupil decerebration Respiration and circulation abnormality, Death
6. Posterior inferior cerebellar art	Lateral and post medulla	Wallenberg syndrome, dysphasia and dysphonia ipsilateral anesthesia of face and cornea for pain and temp (touch preserved), ipsilateral Horner syndrome, contralateral loss of pain and temperature in trunk and extremities, ipsilateral decompensation of movement
7. Ant. inf. and sup. cerebellar artery-	Supplies cerebellum	Difficulty in, articulation, swallowing, movement of limbs and nystagmus
8. Ant spinal art	Ant spinal cord	Flaccid paralysis below level of lesion, loss of pain, touch and temperature. Proprioception retained
9. Post spinal art	Post spinal cord	Sensory loss specially proprioception, vibration, touch and pressure. Movements present.

MCA=Middle cerebral artery; ACA=Anterior cerebral artery; PCA=Posterior cerebral artery; TIA=Transient ischaemic attack.

Table 27.31: Patterns of sensory loss in some individual conditions

1.	Single peripheral N	— All or selected modality of sensation loss along the distribution of nerve lost sensation is less than anatomic distribution of nerve because of overlap
2.	Polyneuropathy	— Glove and stocking distribution All modalities slow change
3.	Transection of spinal cord (complete)	— All forms of sensation are lost below the level of lesion
4.	Brown-Sequard syndrome	— Ipsilateral motor and proprioceptive and contralateral loss and pain and temp

Table 27.32: Corticospinal (Pyramidal) tract lesions at different levels and their clinical manifestations

1.	Cortical lesions	Often produce monoplegia on the contralateral side. To produce hemiplegia the lesion should be massive.
2.	Corona radiata	Lesions produce monoplegia on the contralateral side. To produce hemiplegia lesion should be massive.
3.	Internal capsule	Dense hemiplegia on the other side usually with UMN type of VII nerve palsy on the hemiplegic side.
4.	Midbrain	Ipsilateral III nerve palsy and contralateral hemplegia (Webers syndrome).
5.	Pons	Ipsilateral VI and VII nerve palsy. Contralateral hemiplegia (Millard-Gubler syndrome)
6.	Medulla	Bilateral pyramidal signs, Lower cranial nerve palsy IX, X, XI, XII.
7.	Cervical spinal cord	Quadriplegia
8.	Thoracic spinal cord	Ipsilateral monoplegia

Clinical Variation of UMN (Pyramidal) Syndrome

Classic Hemiplegic Distribution
From cortex to caudal level of the pons causes weakness on contralateral side. The arm is weaker than the leg and the finger movements are weakest of all.

Double Hemiplegia
Here, the lesion interrupts both pyramidal tracts rostral to the medulla. All four limbs and bilateral lower part of face are involved.

Pseudobulbar Palsy
Bilateral interruption of corticobulbar components of the pyramidal tract at cerebral or brainstem level. This causes weakness of oropharyngeal muscles with dysphagia, dysarthria and spastic dysphonia. Emotional movements are preserved.

Spastic Diplegia
Bilateral pre and perinatal cerebral lesion causing bilateral pyramidal syndrome with legs more involved than arms and bulbar muscles relatively spared. Involuntary movements like athetosis are common.

Locked in Syndrome

Bilateral interruption of the pyramidal tracts in the basis pontis or cerebral peduncles cause UMN paralysis of all volitional movements except vertical eye movements. Patient will be conscious. Patient may only respond by up and down movements of eyes.

Quadriplegia (Tetra Plegia)

Bilateral interruption of pyramidal tracts in the caudal medullar or cervical region paralyses volitional movements of trunk and all 4 limbs with loss of volitional bladder and bowel control and volitional control of breathing. It spares corticobulbar fibers to face and bulbar muscles.

Paraplegia

Bilateral interruption of pyramidal tract caudal to cervical region causes UMN paralysis of legs and loss of bladder and bowel control.

Monoplegia

A small lesion in motor cortex and internal capsule causes contralateral weakness of one arm or leg. A lesion in thoracic cord causes monoplegia on the ipsilateral side.

Extensor plantar may be absent in cerebral or spinal shock or a lesion in spinal reflex arch—peroneal nerve injury, long afferent impulse, etc.

Differential Diagnosis of Neurological Symptoms

Table 27.33: Differentiating points between extramedullary and intramedullary spinal tumors

Extramedullary	Intramedullary
1. Root pains and local spinal tenderness are common	Rare
2. Paresthesia rare and often late	Common and early
3. Muscle spasms common	Rare
4. Bladder and Bowel disturbances occur late	Early
5. Hemisection of cord or Brown-Sequard syndrome may occur (ipsilateral motor and proprioceptive and contralateral loss of pain and temp)	Rare
6. Spasticity and other pyramidal signs prominent	Less common
7. No sensory dissociation	Dissociation of sensation is common, i.e. there is loss of sensations of pain and temperature, while touch in preserved.
8. Muscle atrophy uncommon	Common
9. Trophic change uncommon	Common
10. CSF changes due to spinal block are common	Rare

LIMP: In practice it is essential to evaluate if a child is limping due to a neurological or non-nurological cause. List of conditions causing limp.

Table 27.34: Neurological and non-neurological conditions causing limp

Neurological causes	Non-neurological
CNS	**OSSEOUS**
Cerebrovascular accident	Potts disease, osteomyelitis
Meningitis, encephalitis	Legg perthes disease, Osgood-Schlatter
Acute infantile hemiplegia	disease, paraspinal abscess
Acute cerebellar ataxia	Rickets, Blount's disease
Malingering, drug toxicity	Intervertebral disc problem, Caffey's disease.
Peripheral nerves	Articular
GB syndrome	Transient synovitis
Acute polio, transverse myelitis, periodic	SLE and other collagen
paralysis	vascular diseases, JRA,
Tick paralyses	Acute rheumatic fever, HS purpura, inflam-
Soft tissue	matory bowel disorder
Strain, sprain, hematoma, callous, ingrown	Serum sickness
toenail, myositis, viral	Hemophilia
Trichinosis	Hepatitis
Cellulitis	Dislocated hip
Infection	Brucellosis
Scurry	
Bakers cyst.	

Paralysis and Sensory Deficit Immediately after Spinal Cord Transection

Transection at Medullocervical junction or C1-C3
- Complete apnea
- Complete quadriplegia
- Complete anesthesia distal to lesion
- Patient dies if not ventilated
- If lesion is distal to T1, sensorimotor deficit affects only trunk and legs

During Spinal Shock
- Flaccid paralysis of muscles
- Flaccid bladder and bowel paralysis with incontinence
- All deep tendon reflexes and superficial reflexes lost
- Earliest to reappear is anal spincter tone
  In the next stage
      Increased deep tendon reflexes
      Spasticity
      Extensor plantars
      Reflex emptying of bladder and bowel
  In slow cord compression spastic paraplegia occur from the starting.
  Some twitching, sweating and reflex elimination of urine and feces can occur.

Abdominal Reflex/Cremastric Reflex (Various Conditions)
1. Normally absent in small infants and appear with maturation.
2. Abdominal reflexes may be absent in obese patients.

3. Abdominal reflexes disappear after acute UMN lesions and later they may recover.
4. If the brain lesion occurs early these reflexes regularly return, as in cerebral palsy.
   Anal reflex is the first to return after spinal shock.

Paroxysmal Disorders of Infancy
Apnea and Breathholding
1. Cyanotic
2. Pallid

Table 27.35: Causes of lethargy and coma

Epilepsy	c. Urea cycle disorder, heterozygote
1. Postictal state	d. Glycogen storage disorders
2. Status epilepticus	e. Systemic carnitine deficiency
Hypoxia-Ischemia	2. Renal disease
1. Cardiac arrest	a. Uremic encephalopathy
2. Cardiac arrhythmia	b. Hypertensive encephalopathy
3. Congestive heart failure	c. Dialysis encephalopathy
4. Near drowning	d. Complications of immunosuppression
5. Neonatal	3. Hepatic disease
6. Hypotension	4. Disorders of osmolality
a. Autonomic dysfunction	a. Hypernatremia
b. Dehydration	b. Hyperglycemia
c. Hemorrhage	c. Hyponatremia
d. Pulmonary embolism	d. Hypoglycemia
Increased Intracranial Pressure	5. Endocrine disorders
1. Cerebral abscess	a. Adrenal insufficiency
2. Cerebral edema	b. Hypoparathyroidism
3. Cerebral tumor	c. Thyroid disorders
4. Herniation syndromes	6. Other metabolic disorders
5. Hydrocephalus	a. Burn encephalopathy
6. Intracranial hemorrhage	b. Parenteral hyperalimentation
a. Spontaneous	c. Hypomagnesemia
b. Traumatic	d. Vitamin B complex deficiency
Infectious Disorders	**Toxic**
1. Infections of the brain	1. Prescription drugs
a. Bacterial meningitis	2. Substance abuse
b. Fungal meningitis	3. Toxina
c. Viral encephalitis	**Trauma**
d. Reye syndrome	1. Concussion
2. Postinfectious encephalomyelitis	2. Contusion
3. Postimmunization encephalopathy	3. Intracranial hemorrhage
4. Systemic infections	a. Epidural hematoma
a. Fever	b. Subdural hematoma
b. Sepsis-toxic shock	c. Intracerebral hemorrhage
c. Shock-encephalopathy syndrome	4. Neonatal
Metabolic and Systemic Disorders	
1. Inborn errors of metabolism	1. Hypertensive encephalopathy
a. Neonatal presentation	2. Intracranial hemorrhage-nontraumatic
b. Disorders of pyruvate meta-	3. Systemic lupus erythematosis
bolism	4. Vasculitis

Seizures
1. Febrile seizures
   a. Simple febrile
   b. Epilepsy
   c. Infectious
2. Afebrile seizures
   a. Generalized tonic-clonic seizures
   b. Epilepsy
   c. Infectious
3. Myoclonic seizures
   a. Infantile spasms
   b. Benign myoclonic epilepsy
   c. Severe myoclonic epilepsy
   d. Lennox-Gastaut syndrome

Migraine
1. Benign paroxysmal vertigo
2. Paroxysmal torticollis
3. Cyclic vomiting

Sources of Headache
Intracranial
   Cerebral and dural arteries
   Large veins and venous sinuses
Extracranial
   Extracranial arteries
   Periosteum/sinuses
   Muscles attached to skull
   Cervical roots
   Cranial nerves

Diagnostic Features of Headache
   Length of illness
   Frequency and duration
Location
Quality
Time of day
Associated features
Factors that precipitate
Factors that relieve

Migraine Equivalents
Acute confusional migraine
Transient global amnesia
Basilar migraine
Benign paroxysmal vertigo

Hemiplegic migraine
Paroxysmal torticollis
Ophthalmoplegic migraine
Cyclic vomiting

Presenting Features of Increased Intracranial Pressure
Large head
Bulging fontanelle
Failure to thrive
Setting-sun sign
Shrill cry
Diplopia
Headache
Mental changes
Nausea and vomiting
Papilledema

Herniation Syndromes

Unilateral (Uncal) Transtentorial Herniation
1. Decreasing states of consciousness
2. Respiratory irregularity
3. Dilated and fixed pupil
4. Homonymous hemianopia
5. Increased blood pressure, slow pulse
6. Decerebrate rigidity

Bilateral (Central) Transtentorial Herniation
1. States of decreasing consciousness
2. Pupillary constriction or dilation
3. Impaired upward gaze
4. Irregular respiration
5. Decerebrate or decorticate rigidity

Cerebellar (Downward) Herniation
1. Neck stiffness or head tilt
2. States of decreasing consciousness
3. Impaired upward gaze
4. Irregular respirations
5. Lower cranial nerve palsies

Secondary Pseudotumor Cerebri

Drugs
1. Corticosteroid withdrawal
2. Nalidixic acid
3. Oral contraceptives

4. Tetracycline
5. Vitamin A

Systemic Disorders
1. Guillain-Barre syndrome
2. Iron deficiency anemia
3. Leukemia
4. Polycythemia vera
5. Protein malnutrition
6. Systemic lupus erythematosus

Head Trauma
Infections
1. Otitis media
2. Sinusitis

Metabolic
1. Adrenal insufficiency
2. Diabetic ketoacidosis (treatment)
3. Galctosemia
4. Hyperadrenalism
5. Hyperthyroidism
6. Hypoparathyroidism
7. Menarche
8. Pregnancy

Disturbances of Sensation

Hereditary Sensory and Autonomic Neopathy (HSAN)
1. HSAN I   :   Autosomal dominant
2. HSAN II   :   Autosomal recessive
3. HSAN III   :   Familial dysautonomia
4. HSAN IV   :   With anhydrosis
5. HSAN   :   X-linked
6. HSAN   :   With spastic paraplegia
7. Familial amyloid neuropathy

Brachial Neuritis
1. Neuralgic amyotrophy
2. Recurrent familial brachial neuropathy
3. Sympathetic reflex dystrophy

Lumbar Disk Herniation

Syringomyelia

Foramen Magnum Tumors

Thalamic Syndromes

Congenital Insensitivity (Indifference) to Pain
1. Mental retardation
2. Lesch-Nyhan syndrome
3. With normal nervous system

Neural Crest Syndrome (Table 27.36)

Table 27.36: Clinical symptomes of neural crest syndrome corresponding to different tissues

Tissues	Clinical symptoms
Spinal ganglia	Absence of pain
Sympathetic ganglia	Anhydrosis
Pia-arachnoid	Dural thickening
Induction of enamel	Enamel aplasia
Skin pigment	Blondde hair, fair skin
Forebrain cells	Mental retardation

Table 27.37: Metabolic screening in progressive ataxias

Disease	Abnormality
	Blood
Adrenoleukodystrophy	Very-long-chain fatty acids
Ataxia-telangectasia	IgA, LgE, alpha-fetoprotein
Abetalipoproteinemia	Lipoproteins, cholesterol
Hypobetalipoproteinemia	Lipoproteins, cholesterol
Mitochondrial disorders	Lactate, glucose-lactate tolerance
Sulfatide lipidosis	Arysulfatase-A
	Urine
Hartnup disease	Amino acids
Maple syrup urine disease	Amino acids
	Fibroblasts
GM2 gangliosidosis	Hexosaminidase
Refsum disease	Phytanic acid
Carnitine acetyltransferase deficiency	Carnitine acetyltransferase
	Bone Marrow
Neurovisceral storage	Sea-blue histiocytes

Causes of Stroke

Idiopathic Infarction

Moya Moya disease

Cartoid Disorders
1. Trauma
2. Infection
3. Fibromuscular dysplasia

Heart Disease
1. Congenital
2. Rheumatic
3. Mitral valve prolapse

Sickle Cell Anemia

Lipoprotein Disorders

Cancer
1. Disseminated intravascular coagulation
2. L-asparginase-induced thrombosis
3. Methotrexate-induced infarction
4. Metastatic neuroblastoma

Venous Thrombosis

Intracerebral hemorrhage
1. Neonatal
2. Arteriovenous malformations

Homocystinuria

Table 27.38: Evaluation of cerebral infarction

	Evaluation	*Condition*
Blood	CBC, ESR culture anti-DNA, lipid profile lactic acid	Bacterial endocarditis Hyperlipidemia Leukemia Lupus erythematosus MELAS Polycythemia Sickle cell anemia
Urine	Nitroprusside reaction Urinalysis	Homocystinuria Nephritis Nephrosis
Heart	EKG Echocardiogram	Bacterial endocarditis Congenital heart disease Mitral valve prolapse Rheumatic heart disease
Brain	Arteriography	Arterial dissection Arterial thrombosis Arteriovenous malformation Fibromuscular hypoplasia Moya moya disease, vasculitis

Differential Diagnosis of Intracranial Hemorrhage
1. Arteriovenous malformations
2. Blood dyscrasias
   - DIC
   - ITP
   - Leukaemia
3. Brain tumor

Table 27.39: Differential diagnosis of intracerebral hemorrhage

Arteriovenous malformation
Blood dyscrasias

1. Disseminated intravascular coagulation
2. Idiopathic thrombocytopenic purpura
3. Leukemia

Brain tumors
Hemorrhagic infarction

1. Cerebral emboli
2. Sagittal sinus thrombosis
3. Sickle cell anemia
4. Systemic lupus erythematosus

Hypersensitivity vasculitis

Table 27.40: Slowly progressive disorders sometimes misdiagnosed as cerebral palsy

Condition	
Polyneuropathy	1. Metachromatic leukodystrophy
	2. GM gangliosidosis II
	3. Infantile neuroaxonal dystrophy
	4. Hereditary motor and sensory neuropathies
Ataxia	1. Ataxia-telangiectasia
	2. Friedreich's ataxia
	3. A beta lipoproteinemia
Spasticity—chorea	1. Lesch-Nyhan syndrome
	2. Pelizaeus-Merzbacher disease
	3. Rett syndrome
	4. Familial spastic paraplegia
	5. Sea-blue histiocytosis

4. Hemorrhagic infarction
   - Cerebralemboli
   - Sagittal sinus thrombosis
   - Sickle cell anemia
   - SLE
5. Hypersensitivity vasculitis

Differential Diagnosis of Chorea as Presenting or Prominent Symptom

Genetic Disorders
1. A beta lipoproteinemia
2. Ataxia-telangiectasia
3. Benign familial chorea
4. Fahr disease
5. Familial paroxysmal choreoathetosis
6. Hallervorden-Spatz disease
7. Hepatolenticular degeneration (Wilson disease)
8. Huntington disease
9. Infantile bilateral striatal necrosis
10. Lesch-Nyhan syndrome
11. Machado-Joseph disease

Drug-induced Movement Disorders
1. Anticonvulsants
2. Antiemetics
3. Oral contraceptives
4. Psychotropic agents
5. Stimulants

Systemic Disorders
1. Hyperthyroidism
2. Lupus erythematosus
3. Pregnancy (chorea gravidarum)
4. Sydenham (rheumatic) chorea

Tumors of Cerebral Hemisphere

Conditions that may Include Choreothetosis

Cerebral Palsy
1. Congenital malformations
2. Kernicterus
3. Perinatal asphyxia
4. Unknown causes

Genetic Disorders
1. Ceroid lipofuscinosis
2. Dystonia musculorum deformans
3. Incontinentia pigmenti
4. Phenylketonuria
5. Porphyria
6. Pelizaeus-Merzbacher disease
7. Rett syndrome

Infectious Diseases
1. Bacterial meningitis
2. Viral encephalitis

Metabolic Encephalopathies
1. Addison's disease
2. Burn encephalopathy
3. Hypocalcemia
4. Hypernatremia
5. Hypoparathyroidism
6. Vitamin B deficiency

Vascular-Poststroke

Differential Diagnosis of Torticollis and Head Tilt
- Benign paroxysmal torticollis
- Cervical cord tumors
- Cervical cord syringomyelia
- Cervicomedullary malformations

- Diplopia
- Dystonia
- Familial paroxysmal choreoathetosis
- Juvenile rheumatoid arthritis
- Posterior fossa tumors
- Sandifer syndrome
- Spasmus nutans
- Sternocleidomastoid injuries
- Tic and Tourette syndrome

Differential Diagnosis of Acquired Ophthalmoplegia

Brainstem

1. *Tumor*
   a. Brainstem glioma
   b. Craniopharyngioma
   c. Pineal region tumors
   d. Lymphoma
   e. Leukemia
   f. Metastases

2. *Vascular*
   a. Migraine
   b. Infarction
   c. Hemorrhage
   d. Vasculitis
   e. Arteriovenous malformation

3. *Multiple sclerosis*

4. *Brainstem encephalitis*

5. *Intoxication*

6. *Subacute necrotizing's encephalopathy*

Nerve

1. Increased intracranial pressure
2. Postinfectious
   a. Idiopathic (postviral)
   b. Polyarticuloneuropathy
   c. Miller-Fisher syndrome
3. Infections
   a. Orbital cellulitis
   b. Diphtheria
   c. Gradenigo's syndrome
   d. Meningitis
4. Familial recurrent neuropathies
5. Trauma
   a. Orbital
   b. Head
6. Vascular
   a. Migraine

    b. Aneurysm
    c. Cavernous sinus thrombosis
    d. Cartoid cavernous fistula
7. Tumor
    a. Orbital tumors
    b. Cavernous hemangioma
    c. Sellar and parasellar tumors
    d. Sphenoid sinus tumors
8. Inflammatory
    a. Tolosa-Hunt syndrome
    b. Orbital pseudotumor
    c. Sarcoidosis

Neuromuscular Transmission
1. Myasthenia gravis
2. Botulism

Myopathies
1. Fiber type disproportion myopathies
2. Mitochondrial myopathies
3. Oculopharyngeal dystrophy
4. Vitamin E deficiency
5. Thyrotoxicosis

Acute Unilateral Ophthalmoplegia
1. Increased intracranial pressure
2. Idiopathic (postviral)
3. Migraine
4. Myasthenia gravis
5. Orbital tumors
6. Gradenigo syndrome
7. Aneurysm
8. Brain tumors
    a. Brainstem glioma
    b. Parasellar tumors
    c. Tumors of pineal region
9. Multiple sclerosis
10. Brainstem stroke
11. Recurrent familial
12. Inflammatory
    a. Tolosa-Hunt syndrome
    b. Orbital pseudotumor
13 Trauma
    a. Orbital
    b. Head

Causes of Acute Loss of Vision

Demyelinating Optic Neuropathy
1. Idiopathic optic neuritis

2. Neuromyelitis optica
3. Multiple sclerosis

Ischemic Optic Neuropathy
1. Retinal migraine
2. Retinal artery obstruction
   a. Embolism
   b. hemoglobinopathy
   c. Coagulopathy

Cortical Blindness
1. Migraine
2. Posttraumatic transient cerebral blindness
3. Benign occipital epilepsy
4. Anoxic encephalopathy
5. Occipital metastatic disease

Trauma
1. Posttraumatic transient cerebral blindness
2. Retinal injuries
3. Indirect optic neuropathy
4. Carotid dissection

Pseudotumor Cerebri

Toxic Optic Neuropathy

Measles Retinitis

Pituitary Apoplexy

Hysteria

Causes of Progressive Loss of Vision

Disorders of the lens
1. Cataract
2. Dislocation of the lens

Hereditary Optic Atrophy
1. Leber optic neuropathy
2. Dominant optic neuropathy
3. Juvenile diabetes mellitus—optic atrophy

Compressive Optic Neuropathies
1. Aneurysm
2. Arteriovenous malformations
3. Craniopharyngioma
4. Hypothalamic and optic tumors
5. Pituitory adenoma
6. Pseudotumor cerebri

Orbital Tumors

Retinal degenerations
1. Abnormal lipid metabolism
   a. A beta lipoproteinemia
   b. Hypobetalipoproteinemia
   c. Neuronal ceroid lipofuscinosis
   d. Niemann-Pick's disease
   e. Refsum disease
2. Abnormal carbohydrate metabolism
   a. Mucopolysaccharidosis
   b. Primary hyperoxaluria
3. Aminoacidopathies
   a. Cystinosis
   b. Cystinuria
4. Other syndromes of unknown etiology
   a. Cockayne syndrome
   b. Laurence-Moon-Biedle syndrome

Corneal Clouding in Childhood
1. Cerebrohepatorenal syndrome
2. Congenital lues
3. Fabry disease (ceramid trihexosidosis)
4. Familial high-density lipoprotein deficiency (Tangier disease)
5. Generalized gangliosidosis GM
6. Juvenile metachromatic dystrophy
7. Marinesco-Sjogren disease
8. Mucolipidosis
9. Pelizaeus-Merzbacher disease

Definitions

Amblyopia	Defective visual acuity after correction of refractive error, customarily reserved for visual loss associated with strabismus.
Amaurosis	Partial or total loss of vision
Cortical blindness	Visual loss due to cerebral disease uncomplicated by abnormalities of the orbit or anterior visual pathways.
Obscurations	Transitory episodes of visual loss of blurring
Photopsias	Abnormal visual sensations (hallucinations) such as flashing lights.
Scotoma	A visual field defect. Central scotoma involves the point of fixation and indicates macular or optic nerve disease. Ceco-central scotoma involves the blind spot and suggests optic nerve disease. Arcuate scotoma follows the pattern of the retinal fiber bundless and indicates retinal or optic nerve disease.

Table 27.41: Classic brainstem syndromes

Syndromes	Findings	Structures
Lateral medullary syndrome; also known as Wallenberg's syndrome, posterior inferior cerebellar artery (PICA) syndrome, lateral medullary plate	Voice change from ipsilateral vocal cord paralysis Ipsilateral decreased gag response Ipsilateral loos of pain and temperature sensation on face Ipsilateral Horner's syndrome Ipsilateral cerebellar findings Contralateral loos of pain and temperature sensation of body Vertigo, nystagmus, vomiting	Nucleus ambiguous or roots of X Nucleus solitarius or roots of IX Descending tract and nucleus of V Descending sympathetic tract Inferior cerebellar penducle Lateral spinothalamic tract Vestibular nuclei
Inferior lateral pontine syndrome; also known as Foville's syndrome, anterior inferior cerebellar artery syndrome	Ipsilateral lower motor neuron facial weakness and loss of taste sensation on anterior-two-thirds of tongue Ipsilateral deafness Ipsilateral loss of pain and temperature sensation on face Ipsilateral loss of horizontal conjugate gaze Ipsilateral Horner's syndrome Contralateral loss of pain and temperature sensation of body	VII VIII Descending V Pontine paramedial reticular formation Descending sympathetic Lateral spinothalamic
Superior lateral pontine syndrome; also known as superior cerebellar artery syndrome	Ipsilateral ataxia and intention tremor of arm and leg Ipsilateral Horner's syndrome Contralateral loss of pain and temperature sensation on face and body	Superior cerebellar peduncle Descending sympathetic Lateral spinothalamic and ventral ascending V
Posterior cerebral artery syndrome	Loss of sensation on contralateral body with concomitant pain Hemiballismus Field defect Material specific memory defect Global amnesia	Thalamus Subthalamus Occipital lobe Unilateral medial temporal lobe Bilateral medial temporal lobe or ischemia of one temporal lobe with the other previously damaged.
Medial medullary syndrome; also known as Dejerine's syndrome, anterior spinal artery syndrome, alternating inferior hemiplegia	Ipsilateral flaccid tongue weakness Contralateral hemiplegia Sometimes contralateral loss of position and vibration sensation	XII Pyramidal tract Medial lemniscus

Contd...

Contd...

Medial pontine syndrome; also known as Millard-Gubler syndrome, medial penetrating pontine arteries, alternating middle hemiplegia	Ipsilateral lateral rectus palsy	VI nerve
	Contralateral hemiplegia with face usually involved	Corticospinal and corticobulbar tracts
	Sometimes contralateral loss of position and vibration sensation	Medial lemniscus
	Sometimes loss of adduction of ipsilateral eye during conjugate gaze	MLF
Medial midbrain syndrome; also known as Weber's syndrome, medial penetrating midbrain artery, superior alternating hemiplegia	Ipsilateral complete III nerve palsy	III rootlets
	Contralateral hemiplegia	Corticospinal and corticobulbar tracts
Paramedial midbrain syndrome	Ipsilateral complete third nerve palsy, so that the eye is down and out, the lid has ptosis, and the pupil is dilated and not responsive to light	Roots of III
	Contralateral ataxia and intension tremor of arm	Red nucleus and decussation of superior cerebellar peduncle after its crossover
	Sometimes contralateral loss of position and vibration sensation	Medial lemniscus
	Sometimes contralateral loss of pain and temperature sensation	Lateral spinothalamic tract and ventral secondary ascending tract of V

Table 27.42: Differential diagnosis of upper motor neuron weakness

Symptom	Hemispheric	Brainstem	Cord
Weakness	(1) Almost always unilateral; (2) usually will affect upper and lower extremities; (3) with midline lesion, there may be bilateral lower-extremity weakness	May be unilateral or bilateral	(1) Usually bilateral; (2) if unilateral, pain and temperature may be decreased in opposite extremity; (3) lower extremities more frequently affected than upper extremities; (4) motor level with increased DTR's below level, absent DTR's at level; (5) may have atrophy at level
Cranial nerve defects	May have: II—hemianopsia; III, IV, VI—eye deviates toward lesion and away from hemiparesis; pupils normal except in carotid disease; V—corneal reflex decrease;VII—lower facial weakness; XI—head deviation toward lesion; X, XII—palate and tongue may deviate transiently	May have: III, IV, VI-nerve paresis; eyes deviate toward hemiparesis; pupil abnormalities; V-motor weakness and decreased sensation; VII-upper and lower face weakness; VIII-vertigo and deafness; IX-decreased sensation and absent gag; difficulty swallowing	None
Sensory defects	May have (1) hemianesthesia (2) disorders of cortical sensation (i.e, astereognosis, agraphasthesia, position sense abnormality)	May have (1) hemianesthesis; (2) loss of pain and temperature with intact vibration and position, intact pain and temperature	May have (1) position and vibration absent on one extremity, pain and temperature on other extremity, (2) sensory level on trunk, (3) absence of pain and temperature unilaterally or bilaterally with intact position and vibration, (4) opposite of No. 3, (5) cape like distribution.
Bladder dysfunction	Usually absent; may be present with bilateral disease	Usually absent; may be present with bilateral disease	Usually present
Cerebellar defects	Absent	May be present	Absent
Behavior disturbances	Aphasia, agnosia, apraxia, agraphia, alexia, etc.	Absent	Absent

28 Evaluation of the Musculoskeletal System

INTRODUCTION

The very word orthopedics means *straight child* but unfortunately many pediatricians feel uncomfortable when it comes to examination of bones and joints of children. In this chapter a step-by-step approach is presented for evaluation of musculoskeletal system.

AGE

Infancy

1. Arthrogryposis multiplex congenita (Birth)
2. Congenital syphilis (Few weeks to months after birth)
3. Scurvy (usually 6-24 months)
4. CTEV (Birth)

Childhood

1. Rheumatic fever (> 3 yr)
2. Rheumatoid arthritis (> 14 yr)
3. Kawasaki disease (Less than or equal to 5 yr)
4. ALL (Peak incidence around 4 yr)
5. Perthe's disease (2-12 yr)

Adolescence

1. Slipped capital femoral epiphysis (SCFE)
2. SLE
3. Spondylarthropathies (Ankylosing spondylitis, Reiter's disease, reactive arthritis)
4. HSP (> 2 yr)
5. Osteosarcoma
6. Ewing's sarcoma

Any Age

1. Osteomyelitis
2. Septic arthritis
3. Trauma (Fracture)

SEX

In general, most diseases occur with equal frequency in both sexes. However, certain diseases are more common in males and some in females (Table 28.1).

Table 28.1: Diseases common in males and females

Males	Females
1. Hemophilia with hemarthrosis	1. SLE
2. Perthe's disease	2. Developmental dysplasia of hip (DDH)
3. Ewing's sarcoma	
4. Osteosarcoma	
5. Henoch-Schonlein purpura	
6. Spondylarthropathies	
7. Growing pains	

Chief Complaints

Diseases of skeletal system manifest mainly in the form of the following:

Pain

This is the main complaint of a patient with arthritis. However, pain is conspicuous by its absence, in Charcot's joint (e.g. Secondary to syringomyelia), Clutton's joint (e.g. Secondary to congenital syphilis), enquiry must be made mainly about the following points:

a. *Onset*

Acute	— e.g. Septic arthritis, trauma, rheumatic arthritis.
Insidious	— e.g. Collagen vascular disease.
Following trauma	— Fracture, dislocation. In osteosarcoma trauma and ensuing pain brings attention of patients towards the swelling.

b. *Character*

Dull aching	— e.g. Chronic arthritis (TB, RA)
Throbbing	— e.g. Septic arthritis.

c. *Site* — Pain may be felt in the *muscle* (myositis) or affected *joint* (arthritis) or it may be a *referred pain* from the other joint (e.g.-Hip disease—pain can be felt in the knee; caries of cervical spine-pain referred to occiput; intervertebral disc lesion-pain felt around the chest wall). Pain usually remains localised to one particular joint, but in certain diseases, it shows fleeting nature (e.g. Rheumatic fever, disseminated gonococcal infection, rat bite fever, etc.).

d. *Relieving and aggravating factors* — In general, pain following fracture or arthritis is *relieved by rest* and increased by movement. However, *constant pain* indicates joint effusion, hemarthrosis or joint dislocation.

In rheumatoid arthritis pain and stiffness are more in the early morning and decrease as the day advances.

In tuberculous joint, when the articular cartilages are destroyed, the pain increases during sleep. Because, when the patient is awake during the day, there is a protective muscular spasm which immobilises the joint. During sleep, the muscles relax and allow friction between the eroded articular surfaces, giving rise to *"night-cry."*

   Dramatic relief of pain with aspirin indicates rheumatic arthritis.

Joints Involved

Major joints	— Rheumatic fever, JRA, hemophilia, pyogenic arthritis.
Small joints	— Rheumatoid arthritis, gout.
Unusual joints	— Temporomandibular joint
	(Pain during chewing, ear pain) — JRA
	— Cricoarytenoid joint (hoarse voice) — JRA
	— Sternoclavicular (chest pain) — JRA
	— Sacroiliac—Ankylosing spondylitis
	— Great toe—Gout
	— Atlanto-occipital—Rheumatoid arthritis.

Number of joints involved

Monoarticular	— Pyogenic, TB, hemophilia, leukemia.
Pauciarticular	— JRA, hemophilia
Polyarticular	— Rheumatic fever, JRA.

Abnormal Movement

Following abnormalities can be noted

Reduced movement	Painful reduction in movement, with a limp (Antalgic gait)—arthritis.
Absent movement (Pseudoparalysis) e.g.	Scurvy Congenital syphilis Acute lymphoblastic leukemia (ALL) Hemarthrosis, septic arthritis
Increased range of movement e.g.	Marfan syndrome Homocystinuria Congenital contractural arachnodactyly Ehlers-Danlos syndrome Stickler's syndrome
Movement in abnormal direction	Fracture
Abnormal gait e.g.	Painful limp (Antalgic gait) Arthritis Perthes' disease SCFE. Waddling gait with lumbar lordosis — DDH

Involuntary movements	They could be convulsion, jitteriness, fasciculations, choreoathetosis, dystonia, ballism.
Myotonia is indicated by	Choking episodes, dysphagia, garbled speech, difficulty in defecation, prolonged eye closure following sneezing, inability to relax a grip (e.g. while shaking hands), inability to relax smile (*Cheshire cat smile*).

Change in the Skeletal Contour
a. Abnormal shape of foot   e.g. CTEV
b. Short stature   e.g. Skeletal dysplasias (like achondroplasia)
c. Long stature   e.g. Marfan syndrome
d. Swelling   e.g. joint effusion, osteosarcoma, Ewing's sarcoma
e. Multiple fracture with malunion   e.g. Osteogenesis imperfecta.

Miscellaneous
a. Fracture following trivial trauma (pathological #)
   e.g.   Osteogenesis imperfecta,
                                     Osteopetrosis,
                                     Solitary bone cyst,
                                     Osteosarcoma
                                     Chronic osteomyelitis.
b. Joint locking   — loose bodies in the joint
c. Weakness, wasting, fatigue — muscular weakness.

Past History
One should enquire about the previous history of:
- Trauma—previous trauma is sometimes responsible for subsequent osteoarthritis.
- Tuberculosis
- Osteomyelitis
- Surgery on bones/joints
- Chronic illness (e.g. chronic renal failure produces osteoporosis)

Family History
The following history should be elicited in musculoskeletal disorders.
- History of congenital abnormalities of hip (DDH)/foot(CTEV)
- History of scoliosis
- History of arthritis : RA, ankylosing spondylosis, gout
- History of bleeding tendency in males : Hemophilia
- History of genetic disorders : Osteogenesis imperfecta, rickets.

If the family history is suggestive of musculoskeletal disorders, it is very important to draw a 3 generation pedigree.

Birth and Developmental History
Following history is important:
- Reduced fetal movements indicates—congenital myopathies.
- Prematurity, perinatal asphyxia, need for special ventilatory support—congenital myopathies.
- Abnormal presentation, large for gestation, birth injuries—fracture, nerve damage.
- Cryptorchidism, poor suck, weak cry, reduced activity—congenital myopathies.
- Delayed motor milestones, floppy baby—myopathy, cerebral palsy.

Examination of Musculoskeletal System

Equipments
- Skin marking pencil
- Tape measure
- Reflex hammer
- Goniometer
- Stethoscope.

The examination begins as the child enters the examination room. One should note how the child walks, sits, rises from sitting position, takes off shirt, buttons the shirt and responds to other directions given during the examination. One should inspect anterior, posterior and lateral aspects of the patient's posture, ability to stand erect, the symmetry and body parts and alignment of extremeties. One should also note any lordosis, kyphosis or scoliosis.

One should also observe the extremities for overall size, shape (any gross deformity); skin folds, swelling in relation to bones/joints.

One should always compare the two sides after placing the extremities in symmetrical position.

EXAMINATION
Examination is done as follows:
1. Gait
2. General physical examination
3. Local examination   — Examination of muscles
                        — Examination of bones and joints
4. Functional assessment
5. Systemic examination.

Gait
Gait is defined as propulsive movement of body, characterised by *"stance phase"* and *"swing phase"*. Gait is formally tested by exposing the lower limbs (by taking off the clothes) and asking the child to walk bare footed, on a flat surface. The child should be asked to walk away from the examiner, to turn round a given point and then to come towards him again. The child is also made to

walk on his toes (tests plantar flexion) and heels (tests dorsiflexion) and stand on one leg (tests gluteus medius).

Normal Gait

One complete walk cycle consists of a stance phase (when foot is on the ground, supporting as well as propelling the body forward) and a swing phase (when the foot is advanced forward without ground contact). Each leg alternately goes through stance and swing phase rhythmically, carrying the body forward. There is a simultaneous swinging of the arms so as to maintain support.

Normal gait at different stages,

1. 1 year child — Wide based stance, short steps, elbows flexed. No reciprocal arm movement. Foot stroke occurs with inital heel stroke
2. 2-year-old child — Increased velocity and step length
   — Decreased cadence
3. After 3 years — Towards adult pattern
4. 7 years — Adult pattern

Abnormal Gait

A child who bears weight for longer duration on one side than the other, during walking has a painful limp (*Antalgic gait*).

If he walks with the hip markedly flexed, holding his thigh while walking and bears weight at the tip of the toes for as brief a time as possible, he probably has pain in the hip. If he walks on the outside of the foot, there is probably pain in the metatarsophalangeal joint of great toe. If a child lifts the whole foot at once without a smooth heel-off-toe-off cycle, it indicates a painful foot/stiff knee.

In-toe and out-toe gait (Fig. 28.1) This is determined by asking the child to walk straight. The long axis of the foot is compared with the direction in which the child is walking. If the foot is directed inwardly it is called in-toe gait (commonly due to internal femoral torsion and internal tibial torsion). If the foot is directed outwardly, it is called out-toe gait (commonly due to external tibial and femoral torsion).

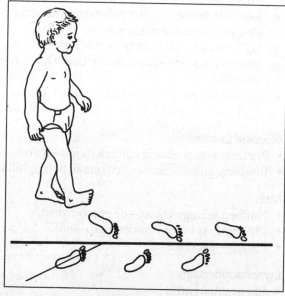

Fig. 28.1: In-toe gait

For other types of gait, refer to '*neurological examination*', in this book.

General Physical Examination

Following points give clue to the underlying diagnosis:

Fever

Arthritis, osteomyelitis, leukemia.

Toxicity

Septic arthritis, acute osteomyelitis, leukemia.

Inadequacy of Peripheral Perfusion

Peripheral perfusion to an extremity should be determined by checking the peripheral pulses and capillary refill. Poor peripheral perfusion could indicate compartment syndrome (For example, following supracondylar fracture of humerus) or shock (due to fracture of long bones with internal bleeding or septicemia secondary to septic arthritis or osteomyelitis).

Cutaneous Lesions

a. *Rheumatic arthritis*—erythema marginatum-rare.
b. *Rheumatoid arthritis*—small, evanescent, macular rash, often with central pallor, mainly found on the trunk and proximal extremities, usually appearing during febrile periods.
c. *Lyme arthritis*—erythema chronicum migrans (ECM) rashes are erythematous, and itchy, seen in the intertriginous areas, gradually expand in all directions.
d. *Henoch-Schonlein purpura*—petechiae/palpable purpura, associated with urticaria-angioedema, seen in crops, mainly over the buttocks and lower extremities.
e. *Kawasaki disease*—rash is polymorphous and primarily truncal, dry fissured lips, periungual desquamation.
f. *SLE*—malar rash with butterfly distribution.
g. *Draining sinuses*—fixed to the underlying bone indicates chronic osteomyelitis.
h. *Dermatomyositis*—heliotrophic rash, Gottron's papules
i. *Tight skin*—scleroderma, Mixed connetive tissue disorder (MCTD)

Mucosal Lesions

- Bilateral non purulent conjunctivitis—Kawasaki disease.
- Bleeding gums—Scurvy, leukemia, hemophilia.

Nails

- Nailbed telangiectasia—dermatomyositis,
- Clubbing, splinter hemorrhages—SBE
- Pitting—psoriasis

Lymphadenopathy

- Rheumatoid arthritis
- SLE
- Kawasaki disease (usually cervical LN)

- ALL
- Serum sickness.

Eyes

- *Blue sclera* — indicates osteogenesis imperfecta.
- *Iridocyclitis* — indicates JRA
- *Phlycten* — indicates tuberculosis
- *Cataract* — indicates long-term steroids consumption (JRA, SLE, etc.)
- *Retinopathy* — indicates long-term chloroquine consumption (JRA)

LOCAL EXAMINATION

Examination of Muscles

Examination of muscles is done under the following headings:

Inspection

Certain important inspectory findings give clue to underlying diseases; e.g.

Congenital absence of a muscle may be isolated

e.g.—P. major

Associated with a syndrome   e.g.—Absence of

P. major — absent nipple, breast and anterior axillary fold (Poland syndrome)

P. major — associated with leukemia

Temporalis — associated myotonia

Depressor angulioris — CHD

Muscle wasting It may be due to.

- *Non-neuromuscular diseases*—Here, strength is well preserved in relation to the degree of muscular wasting.

  Example: Quadriceps wasting following arthritis of knee (localised wasting), tuberculosis, malignancy, marasmus (generalised wasting).

- *Neuromuscular disease.*

  LMN paralysis—More pronounced wasting.

  UMN paralysis and myopathy—Less pronounced wasting.

Muscle hypertrophy It may be

- *Pseudohypertrophy*—Associated with decrease in power.

  e.g. DMD-Calf muscle hypertrophy.

  True hypertrophy—With no loss of power.

  e.g. Athletes, healthy adolescents, congenital adrenal hyperplasia (with virilisation).

Involuntary movements It may be in the form of chorea, athetosis, ballismus, dystonia, tremors, tics, convulsions, jitteriness, fasciculations.

Palpation

All muscles should be palpated for tone, tenderness, induration, etc. (Table 28.2).

Following points help to clinch the diagnosis of underlying disorders.

Table 28.2: Disorders

Findings	Diagnosis	
Firm feel	Normal muscle	
Flabby	Hypotonia	— LMN paralysis, Cerebellar disease Chorea Sleep Drugs (e.g. Diazepam)
Spastic	Hypertonia	Pyramidal lesion Extrapyramidal lesion.
Hard	Myositis ossificans	
Tender and indurated	Polymyositis Trichinosis	

Percussion

a. Percussion of muscle tendon helps to elicit DTR, which
   — is exaggerated in UMN lesion.
   — is depressed in LMN lesion.
   — show delayed relaxation phase (Hung up jerk) in hypothyroidism
   — show pendular jerk in cerebellar disease.
b. Percussion of muscle helps to elicit myotonia.
   e.g. By percussing over thenar eminence, with a knee hammer, one can see dimple lasting for seconds. This is also seen in tongue muscles.

Auscultation

Auscultate for crepitus
- Over the muscle—gas gangrene
- Over the joint—chronic arthritis (e.g. in JRA)
- Along the flexor tendons—tenosynovitis (e.g. in scleroderma).

Power

Evaluation of strength of each muscle group is usually integrated with examination of associated joint for range of motion.

A complete range of motion should be accomplished in each joint, initially without resistance and later as against full resistance.

Muscle strength should be compared bilaterally. Normally, strength is bilaterally symmetric, with full resistance to opposition. Depending on the degree of weakness, strength is graded as follows:

Grade	Description
0	No motion
1 (Trace)	Palpable contraction of muscle but no movement of joint
2 (poor)	Full range-gravity eliminated.

3 (Fair)	Full range against gravity
4 (Good)	Full range against gravity and moderate resistance.
5 (Normal)	Full range against gravity and normal resistance.

A detailed description of method to test the strength of muscles is dealt with in the section on "Examination of nervous system".

Examination of Bones and Joints

In the following section, general principles of examination of bones and joints are discussed. This is followed by detailed discussion on "The examination of individual joints", stressing on the special features to be noted in each joint.

Inspection

The region should be fully exposed and the patient should be positioned to provide the greatest stability to the joints. The region should be inspected from front, back and sides.

Extremeties should be positioned uniformly and observed for overall size, gross deformity, skin folds, alignment, bony enlargement, etc. The two sides should be compared.

Trunk should be observed for kyphoscoliosis or lordosis. Any muscle wasting/prominence, prominence of tendons, obliteration of normal hollows around the joint should be carefully looked for.

Following abnormalities on inspection are of diagnostic significance.

1. Attitude and deformity

Example	a. Effusion into hip joint	—	Flexion, abduction and external rotation (position of maximum capacity)
	b. Effusion into elbow/knee	—	Slight flexion
	c. External rotation of lower limb	—	Paralysis, Perthes disease
	d. Swollen, flexed elbow supported by the other hand	—	Supracardylar fracture of humerus

2. Swelling in relation to bones and joints

Site	Diagnosis
Epiphysis	Osteoclastoma
Metaphysis	Osteosarcoma, acute osteomyelitis
Diaphysis	Ewing's sarcoma
Joints	Effusion, synovial thickening
Tendons	Tenosynovitis

3. Skin over bones and joints should be inspected for

— Redness, edema	— Arthritis (cf ; Arthralgia)
— Sinus which drains pus containing bone chips	— Chronic pyogenic osteomyelitis (Sprouting granulation tissue)
	— TB osteomyelitis (Undermined margin and bluish surrounding)
— Ecchymosis	— Fracture, hemarthrosis

Palpation

Bones, joints, tendons and the surrounding muscles should be palpated systematically and following points are noted.

Local temperature This is best felt with the dorsum of fingers. The sound side should be felt first and then diseased side.

Temperature is elevated in   — Acute arthritis (cf ; arthralgia)
                                         — Acute osteomyelitis
                                         — Osteosarcoma

Local temperature is lowered in   — Compartment syndrome.

Tenderness Joint line, bones in the vicinity of joint and bony attachment of various ligaments are carefully palpated for tenderness and graded as follows.

Grades of tenderness:

Grade   I   — Child says that the joint is tender
Grade   II   — Child winces with pain
Grade III   — Child winces and withdraws the affected part
Grade IV   — Child will not allow the joint to be touched.

Noting the presence of tenderness and grading the tenderness helps in long-term follow-up of chornic arthritis (persistent tenderness over joint line is a good indicator of persistence of inflammation).

In case of fracture, tenderness should be elicited by palpation of bone through healthy soft tissue otherwise damaged soft tissue will mislead the clinician by virtue of its own tenderness.

Site of tenderness	*Inference*
Joint line	Arthritis (cf; Arthralgia)
Metaphysis	Acute osteomyelitis, osteosarcoma
Site of tendinous or ligamentous attachment to bone (*Enthesopathy*)	Ankylosing spondylitis
Tibial tubercle	Osgood-Schlatter disease.

Swelling

Bony swellings   — Fixed to bone
                         — Bony hard (Exception-variable consistency is diagnostic hallmark of osteosarcoma)

Joint effusion   — Swelling confined to joint and takes its shape
                         — Fluctuation positive
                         — Edges not clearly felt

Synovial thickening   — Similar to effusion but the edges can be rolled under the palpating fingers and they feel elastic and spongy/baggy (Gentle palpation is necessary since on firm pressure the synovium collapse).

Enlarged bursa   — Soft and cystic and corresponds to anatomical position of the bursa.

Ulcer or sinus If it is fixed to underlying bone indicates chronic pyogenic osteomyelitis or tubercular osteomyelitis.

The whole length of bone should be palpated to note if there is any irregularity such as sharp elevation and gap. This is a *definite sign of fracture.*

Crepitus Sensation of grating felt (heard)

Causes i. Fracture — Crepitus when the bone ends are moved against each other
   ii. Osteoarthritis
   iii. Tenosynovitis
   iv. Surgical emphysema.
   v.   Gas gangrene
   vi. Charcot's joint
   vii. Hematoma

Movements

Following points are to be noted:
1. All movements around a particular joint should be tested.
2. Both passive and active movements should be tested.
3. Movement against gravity and resistance should be tested.
4. Range of movements in each direction is noted. Though there is a normal range of movement for each joint, the range of movement varies according to the individuals. Hence, the range of movement on the affected side should always be compared with that of normal side.
5. When a joint appears to have an increase/limitation in the range of movement, *goniometer* is used to precisely measure the angle and compare it with the normal side.
6. A few joints exhibit some range of movement though the joint concerned is ankylosed. This is due to movement of neighboring joint (e.g. scapula with shoulder joint, lumbal spine with hip joint). Hence, the neighboring joint has to be fixed in order to know the true range of movement.
7. Any pain/crepitus associated with movements is noted.
8. Any movement in abnormal direction is noted (indicates fracture).

Measurements

Measurement of length and circumference of limbs are taken and compared on either side. For most people, not more than 1 cm discrepancy in the length and circumference should be found.

Circumference Circumference of a limb is taken across the muscle belly from a fixed bony point on either side. Measuring circumference helps to know the presence of wasting (e.g. disuse wasting in arthritis) or hemihypertrophy.

Length Following measurements are useful.
- — Upper segment-lower segment (diagnosis of skeletal dysplasias)
- — Arm span height (diagnosis of skeletal dysplasias)
- — Limb length (diagnosis of skeletal dysplasias, fracture, dislocation)

Method of measuring limb length

Upper limb   :   Angle of acromion (The point where the spine of scapula turns forward to become acromion process) to the distal ulnar prominence.

		Length is decreased in fracture neck of humerus, supracondylar fracture of humerus
Arm	:	Angle of acromion to lateral epicondyle of humerus .
Forearm	:	Lateral epicondyle to lower end of radius.
Lower limb	:	Patient lies in supine position. Affected and normal limbs are kept in identical position (e.g. if there is adduction deformity of affected limb, the normal limb is also adducted till the pelvis becomes horizontal, i.e. a line joining the two anterior superior iliac spines becomes perpendicular to midline).
		Measurement is taken from anterior superior iliac spine to the medial malleolus of ankle, crossing the knee on the medial side.
		Length is decreased in dislocation of hip.
Thigh	:	Anterior superior iliac spine to the joint line of knee on medial side.
Leg	:	Joint line of knee to medial malleolus of ankle.

Examination of Neighboring Joints

It is always mandatory to examine the neighboring joints as pain felt in the joint may be referred pain from the neighboring joint. For example, in diseases of hip, pain may be felt in knee and vice versa.

Percussion and auscultation They do not carry much significance.

Percussion	Helps to elicit tenderness, e.g. spinal tenderness is elicited by percussing with a rubber hammer.
	Percussion along the flexor tendon elicites exquisite tenderness in flexor tenosynovitis.
	Percussion of flexor aspect of wrist elicites tingling sensation along the inner three fingers, in case of carpal tunnel syndrome (*Tinel sign*).
Auscultation	Helps to detect fine crepitus which may be missed by the palpating fingers.

Examination of Individual Joints

Temporomandibular Joint

Inspection The examiner should inspect the region infront of tragus both at rest and during mastication. Arthritis with effusion into temporomandibular joint, produces swelling just infront of tragus.

Palpation The examiner should locate the temporomandibular joint by placing the finger tips just anterior to the tragus and allowing fingertips to slip into the joint space as the patient's mouth opens.

Tenderness (Arthritis), clicking (loose meniscus), crepitus (osteoarthritis), etc. should be noted. Tenderness can also be elicited by putting finger into external auditory canal and pressing forward.

Range of motion
1. *Open and close the mouth.* Normal range is about 3-6 cm between upper and lower incisors.
2. Move the mandible *side to side.* Normal range is *1-2 cm* in each direction.
3. *Protrude and retract* the chin. Both movements should be possible.
   Restriction of movements (especially jaw opening) could be due to:
   • Tetanus
   • Parotitis
   • Dental abscess
   • Painful stomatitis

Percussion Over the joint helps to elicit tenderness

Auscultation Over the joint helps to detect crepitus, click, etc.

Examination of Neck and Spine
The major land marks on the back include:
1. Spinous process of C7-The most prominent bone seen at the root of neck when neck is flexed.
2. Scapulae
3. Iliac crest
4. The paravertebral muscles
5. T7-which corresponds to the angles of scapula
6. L4-which corresponds to the highest point of iliac crest
7. S2-which corresponds to the posterior inferior iliac spine (seen as a dimple).
   In a normal child, expect the head to be positioned directly over the gluteal cleft and the vertebrae to be straight, as indicated by symmetric skin folds, symmetric shoulder, scapulae and the iliac crest levels. The curves of the cervical and lumbar spines should be concave and the curves of thoracic spine should be convex. Children normally have less cervical lordosis and more lumbar lordosis than adults. Flexible increase in thoracic kyphosis is common in adolescents.

Inspection
The child should be inspected from posterior, anterior and lateral aspects. The following points are to be noted. Table 28.3 describes the causes related to corresponding deformities.

Scoliosis may be *fixed/structural* (When the patient bends forward, the curve becomes more prominent with a bulge (Rib hump, in case of thoracic scoliosis; bulging of lumbar muscles, with prominence of the pelvis, in case of lumbar scoliosis) lateral to the convexity of the curve and crowding of ribs on its concave side).

Palpation
This is carried out in standing and prone positions by passing the palm from above downwards palpating the central furrow, paraspinal bulge, sides of cervical spine, iliac crest, sacroiliac joints and buttocks). Following points are noted.

Table 28.3: Causes related to corresponding deformities

Attitude and deformity	Causes
a. Lateral flexion of neck to one side, with the chin pointing towards the opposite side (Torticollis)	1. Sternomastoid tumor 2. Caries cervical spine 3. Fracture dislocation of cervical spine 4. Tender cervical LN 5. Sandifer syndrome 6. URI 7. Cerebellar tumor
b. Short neck with low hair line	Klippel-Feil anomaly
c. Short neck with scoliosis	Hemivertebrae
d. Loss of concavity of cervical curve	JRA, caries spine
e. Prominent upper margin of sacrum and iliac crest	Spondylolisthesis
f. Loss of lumbar lordosis	Ankylosing spondylosis
g. A dimple at the lower end of spine just above the gluteal cleft, which is tan blue in color and has hair around it.	Pilonidal sinus
h. A bunch of hair over the lower end of spine/dermoid sinus/vascular naevus/lipoma.	Spina bifida occulta
i. A swelling in the midline (usually in the thoracolumbar region)	Spina bifida cystica
j. Cold abscess in various places such as paravertebral region, behind the sterno-mastoid muscle, on the lateral chest wall, at the petit's triangle, buttocks, etc.	Pott's spine
k. Prominent convexity of thoracic curvature (Kyphosis)	
Types i. Rounded kyphosis Postural kyphosis	Scheurmann's disease (Idiopathic kyphosis)
ii. Knuckle kyphosis Prominence of single spinous process	Collapse of one vertebra (e.g. caries spine)
iii. Angular kyphosis (Gibbus) Prominence of more than one spinous process	Flattening or collapse of more than one vertebral bodies (e.g. late stage of caries spine Morquio disease.
l. Exaggerated concavity of lumbar spine (Lordosis) Lordosis is mainly compensatory, being secondary to–	– Flexion deformity of hip – DDH – Obesity

m. Lateral curvature of spine, associated with rotational deformity of vertebral bodies (scoliosis)
The primary curve is associated with a compensatory curve above (which keeps the shoulders horizontal) and below (which keeps the pelvis horizontal)
The scoliosis is named according to the level and the side to which the convexity of the primary curve is directed (Fig. 28.2A)
e.g. Right thoracic scoliosis indicates that
	classification of scoliosis (*Cobb's classification*)
	
	i. *Postural* (Functional) e.g. secondary to leg length discrepancy.
	ii. *Structural*
	  • Idiopathic
	  • osteopathic (hemivertebra)
	  • Neuropathic
	    e.g. UMN lesions (CP)
	    LMN lesions (SMA)
	  • Myopathic (DMD)

Contd...

Contd...

Attitude and deformity	Causes
the convexity of the main the curve is towards right side and is at the thoracic level.	*Severity of scoliosis* is estimated by the degree of lateral deviation on X-ray (Figs 28.2B and C)
Scoliosis may be *postural/mobile/transient* (Scoliosis disappears when the patient is asked to bend forward or when made to lie in lateral position on the concave side. If secondary to leg length discrepancy, it disappears when the child is asked to sit down. In case of a small child, the curve disappears when the child is lifted vertically by the arms).	i. < 40° – Mild ii. 40-60° – Moderate iii. 60-80° – Severe iv. > 80° – Extremely severe

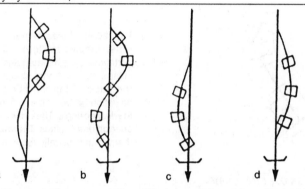

Fig. 28.2A: Diagrammatic representation of the types of idiopathic scoliosis: (a) the dorsal type, (b) the combined dorso lumbar type, (c) the lumbar type, (d) the dorso lumbar type

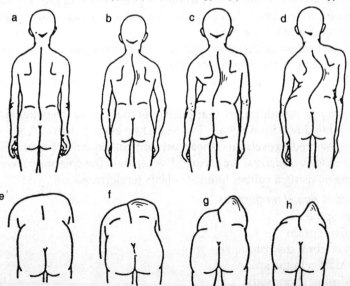

Fig. 28.2B: Diagrammatic representation of the severity of scoliosis (external manifestations): (a)-(b) mild scoliosis; (c)-(d) scoliosis of moderate severity; (e)-(f) severe scoliosis; (g)-(h) extremely severe scoliosis

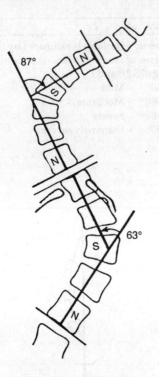

Fig. 28.2C: Measurement of scoliosis (after Lippmann-Cobb). The neutral vertebrae are estimated and a perpendicular is dropped from a straight line across the base of the vertebral body. The deviation between these two lines gives the desired angle. These two methods give quite different values. The latter method is that which is usually recommended

a. *Tenderness over the spine*

The following methods are used to elicit tenderness.

   i. *Direct pressure tenderness* A thumb is pressed along the spinous processes, from above downwards. The patient winces with pain when the tender point is reached.

   ii. *Twist tenderness* Pressure applied upon the spinous process, in an attempt to rotate the vertebra elicits tenderness.

  iii. *Deep thrust tenderness* Gentle blow on either side of the spine with ulnar aspect of the first elicits tenderness.

  iv. *Anvil test* A sudden jerk is applied over the head or the patient is asked to jump down from a chair. This test is however, dangerous, and should be reserved to exclude rather than confirm tenderness over the spine.

   v. *Percussion tenderness* Applying brisk tap over the spinous process with finger/using a rubber hammer elicits tenderness

Causes of spinal tenderness

   i. Caries spine

  ii. Fracture, sprain

 iii. Intervertebral disc prolapse

 iv. Secondaries in the spine

  v. Ankylosing spondylitis

 vi. Hysterical spine—This is always associated with cutaneous hypersensitivity. Thus, the patient winces with pain as soon as the skin is touched.

Tenderness of sacroiliac joint This is elicited by one of the following maneuvers

i. *Compressing* the two iliac crests together.

ii. *Genslen's test* Hip and knee joint of the affected side are completely flexed so as to fix the pelvis. Hip joint of the normal side is hyper extended over the edge of the examining table. This exerts rotational strain on the sacro-iliac joint and results in pain in that region.

iii. *Pretzel test* One lower limb should be crossed across the other lower limb. Opposite upper limb should be crossed across the upper trunk. Now, holding the thigh and shoulder of these limbs, a quick jerk is given so as to move them towards midline. This stretches the sacroiliac joint on the side of the thigh which is being moved and will elicit even minimal tende-rness of the sacroiliac joint. Table 28.4 gives a comparative account of difference between sacroiliac joint lesion and intervertebral disc prolapse.

Table 28.4: Difference between sacroiliac joint lesion and intervertebral disk prolapse

Sacroiliac joint lesion	Disc prolapse (Sciatica)
1. Pain on forward bending in the standing position but not in sitting position (when pelvis becomes fixed)	1. Pain on forward bending in both standing and sitting position
2. Rotatory movement of spine is painful	2. Rotatory movement is painless
3. SLRT (straight leg raising test). The patient lies in supine position, completely relaxed. There should be no lumbar lordosis. The lower limb is flexed at the hip without flex-ing at the knee.Pain starts with the maneu-ver and continues to worsen as the leg is being elevated. There is no aggravation in pain on dorsiflexion	3. Pain starts at a particular angle (Usually < 40°) and pain is aggra-vated by dorsiflexion at the ankle

Swelling This may be

a. Cold abscess at various sites (as described above)

b. Meningomyelocele—usually in the lumbosacral region, in midline. Impulse on crying is positive. Pressure on meningomyelocele by using one hand elicits an impulse which is felt by the other hand placed over anterior fontanelle.

c. Sacrococcygeal teratoma.

Movements

I. *Neck* Neck movements (Fig. 28.3A) should be done with caution, as sudden death may result from dislocation of atlantoaxial joint.

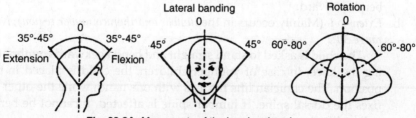

Fig. 28.3A: Movements of the head and neck

Normal range

a. *Flexion*—Bend the head forward, chin towards chest   —   45°
b. *Extension*—Bend the head backward, chin towards ceiling   —   45°
· c. *Lateral bending*—Bend the head to each side, ear to each   —   45°
    (Nodding) shoulder, without raising the shoulder
    (Movements occur at atlanto occipital joint)
d. *Rotation of head*—Turn the head to each side, chin to   —   70°
    (Atlanto-axial joint) shoulder.

II. **Thoraco-lumbar region** (Fig. 28.3b)
  a. Flexion (Mainly occurs in *lumbar region; Normal range-75 to 90°)* The patient
    bends forwards, with the knee extended, and try to touch the toe. Most
    children can touch their toes.

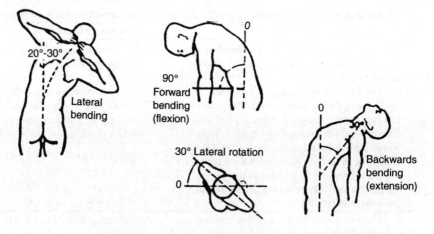

Fig. 28.3B: Movements of the spinal column

    However, this movement can be brought about by excessive hip flexion,
with the spine remaining stiff. Hence, to know the actual movement at
the spine, *modified Schober's test* is done as follows; with the child standing
erect, mark 2 points at a distance of 10 cm above and 5cm below the lumbosacral junction, in the midline. Now ask the child to bend forward and
touch the feet. Measure the distance between the 2 points. Normally, the
back should stretch at least 7 cm between the two points, during this
maneuver. A simpler clinical method is to place 2 fingers on adjacent spinous processes and to estimate the separation of fingers when the patient
bends forward.
  b. *Extension* (Mainly occurs in the *lumbar and thoracolumbar region*); *Normal
    range 30°.*
      The child is asked to stand straight and bend backwards, without flex-
ing the knee. In case of younger children, the child is placed in prone
position. The clinician lifts his legs with one hand, while the other hand
fixes the dorsal spine. If lumbar spine is affected, it cannot be bent but
will be lifted as one piece.

c. *Lateral flexion* (Mainly in the *thoracic region*); *Normal range = 20-30°*

The child stands straight and slides each hand down the thigh and leg whilst the clinician holds firmly his pelvis from the back. In younger children, these movements are demonstrated by lifting the legs as in testing extension and then by carrying the legs first to one side and then to the other, in order to bend the spine sideways. The other hand of the clinician is placed on the thoracic spine so as to detect the movement of the spine.

d. *Rotation* (Mainly in the *thoracic spine*) ; *Normal range = 30°*

Patient sits so as to fix his pelvis. He is then asked to swing the trunk in a circular motion, to the right and left.

Costovertebral joints Range of movement at costovertebral joints is assessed by noting the degree of chest expansion, i.e. measuring the chest circumference in full inspiration and full expiration and noting the difference between the two. *Normally, it is 2½ inches (Adults)*. This measurement is helpful in following up cases of ankylosing spondylitis.

Neurological Examination

Examination of back is incomplete without neurological examination, to assess the presence of any paraperesis, bowel and bladder involvement, sensory disturbances, etc.

Examination of Shoulder Joint and Shoulder Girdle

The child must be stripped upto the waist and should stand in front of the examiner, with both the arms hanging by the side of the trunk. The examiner must palpate contour and symmetry of the shoulders, the shoulder girdle, the clavicles and scapulae.

Inspection

Below mentioned Table 28.5 gives inference corresponding to their findings

Table 28.5: Findings and inference

Findings	*Inference*
1. **Attitude (Position)**	
Arm held by the side of the chest, flexed and medially rotated, being supported by the other hand.	Disease of the shoulder girdle such as # clavicle, dislocation of shoulder
2. **Contour of the shoulder**	
• Undue flattening and loss of rounded-ness of the shoulder just below acromion process	a. Dislocation of shoulder
	b. Wasting of deltoid (Due to arthritis)
• Swelling of the shoulder just below acromion process.	i. # Neck of femur
	ii. Subdeltoid bursitis
• Swelling extending beyond the anterior and posterior margins of deltoid and along the long tendon of biceps indicates	Effusion of shoulder joint

Contd...

Contd...

Findings	Inference
Palpation	
1. Swelling, tenderness, crepitus of the bones forming shoulder girdle.	Fracture of the corresponding bone
2. Tenderness just below the acromion process	Supraspinatus tendinitis
3. Tenderness just below the acromion process with the arm adducted, and which disappears when arm is abducted	Painful arc syndrome (Tender spot disappears under when arm is abducted. acromion process)

Movements (Fig. 28.4)

Abduction and adduction movements are parallel to the frontal plane of the body, flexion and extension are parallel to the sagittal plane while medial and lateral rotation are motions that lie parallel to the transverse plane (Table 28.6).

Table 28.6: Methods and normal range of different types of movements

Movements	Method	Normal range
1. Flexion	Raise both arms forward and straight up over the head	True flexion (Glenohumeral movement -90°; Scapulohumeral movement-next 80°. Total-upto 170°.
2. Extension	Extend and stretch both arms behind the back	35° (End point of extension is that at which further posterior motion of the arm cannot be obtained)
3. Abduction	Lift both arms laterally and straight up over the head	True abduction (glenohumeral movement)-90° Scapulohumeral movement -next 90° Total-upto 180°.
4. Adduction	Swing each arm across the front of the body	20-40°
5. Internal rotation	With the arm hanging by the side of the trunk and elbow flexed to 90°, the forearm is rotated so as to touch the abdomen with the palm	70-90°
6. External rotation	Opposite movement as internal rotation	40-50°

Patient is asked to carry out all movements simultaneously on both sides (for comparison) without and against examiner's resistance in opposite direction. Any difference from the normal side is noted (This applies to movements at all other joints of body).

Examination of Elbow

The patient is asked to stand straight with his arms at the side of the body with the palms looking forwards (anatomical position). Elbow is to be inspected from front, behind and from the sides. Bones around the elbow namely, extensor surface of ulna, olecranon process, medial and lateral epicondyles of humerus are to be systematically palpated (Table 28.7).

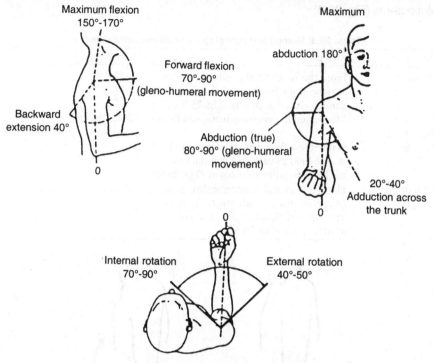

Fig. 28.4: Movements at shoulder joint

Table 28.7: Examination of elbow

	Findings	Inference
Inspection		
1. *Attitude*	Elbow held in position of flexion, being supported by the other hand.	Injury to the elbow
2. *Carrying angle* (outward deviation of the extended and supinated forearm from the axis of the arm).		
	10-15° (20° in females)	Normal
	> 15° (>20° in females)	Cubitus valgus
	< 10°	Cubitus varus.
3. Obliteration of hollows on either side of the olecranon		Effusion into elbow joint
4. Swelling over the olecranon process		Olecranon bursitis (Student's/miner's elbow)
5. Unduely prominent olecranon process		Supracondylar # of humerus. Posterior dislocation of elbow.

Palpation

Swelling, tenderness, crepitus of bones around elbow. — Fracture of the corresponding bones

Localised tenderness at the lateral epicondyle — Tennis elbow

Localized tenderness at the medical epicondyle — Golfer's elbow

Localized tenderness with swelling over olecrenon— Student's elbow

Movements (Fig. 28.8)

Table 28.8: Method and normal range of different movement

Movement	Method	Normal range
Flexion	From the anatomical position anterior surface of the forearm is brought in contact with that of arm (Fig. 28.5A).	160°
Extension (Fig. 28.5A)	Movement in reverse direction as flexion	180° (Forearm in line with arm) hyperextension-0-5°
Pronation	With elbow flexed at right angle and thumb held in vertical position, rotate the hand to palm side down. (Fig. 28.5B)	90°
Supination	Hand movement in reverse direction, (*pronation and supination actually occur at inferior radioulnar joint and not at elbow joint*) (Fig. 28.5B)	90°

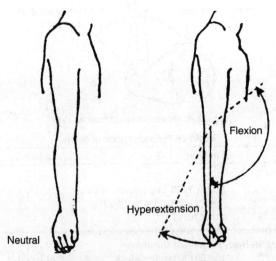

Fig. 28.5A: Movement of the elbow

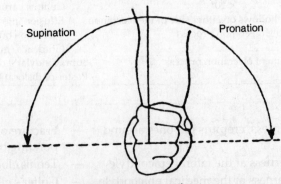

Supination and pronation
Fig. 28.5B: Movements of the forearm

Examination of Wrist (Table 28.9)

Inspection

Table 28.9: Inference of different findings on inspection of wrist

Inspection findings	*Inference*
1. *Attitude* — Wrist flexion	In all affections of wrist joint, the joint will remain in flexed position.
— Dinner fork	Colles fracture
2. *Swelling* limited within the extent of the joint and seen both anteriorly and posteriorly.	Joint effusion.
3. *Swelling* extending beyond the extent of joint, along the tendon sheath, tense, non tender.	Tenosynovitis.
4. A small, circumscribed tense, nontender swelling either on the dorsal (more common) or on the ventral aspect of wrist, along the tendons.	Ganglion.

Palpation

Swelling with tenderness, crepitus, abnormal movement   Fracture
Tenderness with or without swelling along the joint line is   Arthritis.
elicited by squeezing each small joint individually.

Movements (Fig. 28.6A)

a. *Extension* (Fig. 28.6B) Normal range—35-60°.

Patient is asked to bring the hands in midline and place the palms and fingers in contact with each other (Indian method of salute). With the hands in apposition, he is asked to raise both elbow to the maximum extent. The angle between the hand and the forearm indicates the range of extension and has to be compared on either side.

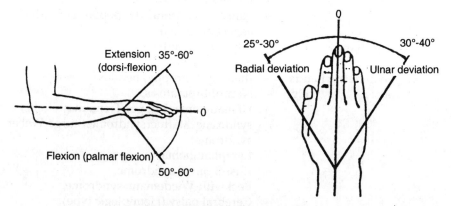

Fig. 28.6A: Movement at the wrist joint

b. *Flexion* Normal range—50-60°.

Dorsum of both hands are placed in contact with each other and the elbows are lowered as far as possible. The angle between the hand and forearm indicates the range of flexion movement.

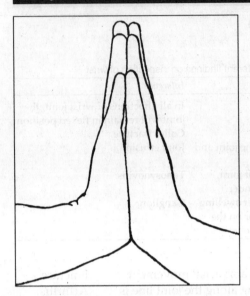

Fig. 28.6B: Minor limitation of the left wrist extension compared with the right. Note the slightly different angulation of the left forearm

c. *Abduction* Normal range—30-40°

Ulnar deviation of wrist in frontal plane.

d. *Adduction* Normal range—25-30°

Radial deviation of wrist in frontal plane

Examination of Hand

Examination of hand is extremely important in diagnosing many underlying diseases. The following section gives a simple guideline to the method of examination of hands.

Inspection

The child is asked to stretch both hands and hold them side by side, infront of the examiner and the hands should be carefully observed both in its dorsal and palmar aspects. The following points are noted;

I. *Size*
  a. **Small hands** e.g. – Down's syndrome
    – Achondroplasia
    – de Lange's syndrome
    – Holt-Oram syndrome
    – Fanconi syndrome (Hypoplasia of radial aspect of hands).
  b. **Large hands** e.g. – Pituitary gigantism
    – Soto syndrome.
  c. **Asymmetric hands** – (hemihypertrophy/hemidystrophy)
    e.g. – Neurofibromatosis,
    – Hemangioma (Klippel-Trenaunay-Weber syndrome, Maffuci syndrome, Sturge-Weber syndrome)
    – Lymphangioma,
    – Russel-Silver syndrome,
    – Beckwith-Wiedemann syndrome,
    – Cerebral palsy (Hemiplegic type).
  d. **Swollen hands** (edema)
    – Thrombophlebitis (due to IV line),
    – Kwashiorkor
    – Sickle cell crisis
    – Cellulitis
    – Tuberculous osteomyelitis (spina ventosa)

II. *Shape (deformity)*

a. *Claw hand* (Griffin hand, Main en griffe) (Fig. 28.7).

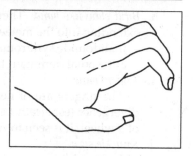

There is hyperextension at the metacarpophalangeal joint and flexion at the interphalangeal joints, due to paralysis of lumbricals and interossei.

Causes

Fig. 28.7: Claw hand

1. Ulnar nerve paralysis (mainly affects little and ring fingers).
2. Median nerve paralysis (mainly affects index and middle fingers).
3. Klumpke's paralysis (produces total claw hand i.e. all fingers are involved).
4. Syringomyelia.

b. *Drop hand* (Wrist drop)

Inability to extend the wrist, due to damage to the radial nerve, producing paralysis of wrist extensors, e.g. plumbism.

c. *Ape hand* (ape thumb/simian hand)

Normally, there is a slight flexion of the thumb so that thumb is not in line with the plane of the other fingers, but when there is damage to median nerve below elbow (resulting in paralysis of opponens pollicis) thumb falls in line with the other fingers. This is called Ape hand.

d. *Pointing index* (Oath hand)

In case of injury to the median nerve (at or proximal to elbow), if the patient is asked to clasp the hands, the index finger of the affected side fails to flex (*Ochsner's clasping test*). This is because, injury to median nerve at this site produces paralysis of lateral ½ of flexor digitorum superficials and profundus (hence flexion of index finger doesn't occur).

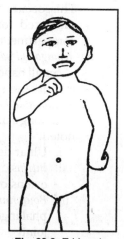

e. *"Policeman receiving the tip" deformity (Erb's paralysis)* (Fig. 28.8)

The arm hangs by the side of the body and internally rotated. Forearm is extended at the elbow and pronated. This is due to lesion at the Erb's point (C5-6) usually as a result of birth injury.

Fig. 28.8: Erb's palsy

f. *Spade-hand*

Hand is coarse and thick with pad-like thenar and hypothenar eminences, and has a squarish contour. It is seen in
– Acromegaly
– Myxedema.

g. *Skeleton-hand*

Hand is bony, due to atrophy of muscles, e.g. syringomyelia.

h. *Bifid claw-like hand* There is a cleft between the 3rd and 4th digits, extending into the metacarpal region. It is seen in
   - thalidomide syndrome
   - autosomal dominant trait.

i. *Trident hand*

   The fingers are of nearly equal length and there is an abnormal divergence (espeically between the 3rd and 4th fingers), like the spokes of a wheel. It is seen in Achondroplasia.

j. *Knuckle sign*

   In pseudohypoparathyroidism, there is hypoplasia of the 4th and 5th metacarpal bones, so that when the hand is fisted, there is dimpling of the corresponding knuckles.

k. *Mitten hand with fused fingers*

   It is seen in Apert's syndrome.

l. *Obstetrical hand (Accoucheur's hand)*

   There is flexion of wrist. Fingers are flexed at metacarpophalangeal joints and extended at interphalangeal joints. Thumb is flexed and adducted into the palm.

   Conditions
   - Hypocalcemic tetany
   - Muscular dystrophy
   - Athetosis.

m. *Volkman's ischemic contracture*

   There is pronation of the hand, flexion of the wrist, extension at metacarpohalangeal joints, and flexion at interphalangeal joints.

   This occurs when the patient has been manipulated and tightly plastered for supra condylar fracture of humerus, resulting in compartment syndrome.

n. *Mongoloid hand*

   Small hand, short stubby fingers, clinodactyly of little fingers. Palm is short and shows a single palmar crease. Seen in Down's syndrome.

o. *Rheumatoid hand:*

   In long standing rheumatoid arthritis, the following deformities are noted:
   i. Ulnar deviation of fingers (*ulnar drift*)
   ii. *Intrinsic plus deformity*—flexion at metacarpophalangeal joints and extension at interphalangeal joints.
   iii. *Boutonniere (button hole)* deformity—flexion at the proximal interphalangeal joints and hyperextension at the distal interphalangeal joint.
   iv. *Swan neck deformity*—Hyperextension at the proximal interphalangeal joint and flexion at the distal interphalangeal joint.
   v. *Finger drop*—failure to extend fingers.
   vi. *Z deformity of thumb.*

p. *Finger anomalies*
   i. *Polydactyly* (Tables 28.10 and 28.11)

Presence of supernumerary fingers, either on the radial side (preaxial) or ulnar side (post axial). It can be an isolated conditions or seen in association with the following disorders.

Table 28.10: Abrnomalities associated with polydactyly

Absence of abductor muscles	Ellis-van Creveld syndrome
Acral-renal syndrome	Epidermolysis bullosa
Albinism	Familial brachydactyly
Anophthalmia microphthalmia	Focal dermal hypoplasia
Apert's syndrome	Goltz syndrome
Aplasia cutis congenita	Hereditary abnormalities
Aplasia of tibia	Hydrometrocolpos
Biemond's syndrome	Ichthyosis simplex
Bifid tongue	Klippel-Trenaunay-Weber syndrome
Blepharoptosis	Lateral facial cleft
Bloom's syndrome	Laurence-Moon-Biedl syndrome
C syndrome	Lissencephaly
Cebocephaly	Maternal radiation
Cheilognathoglossoschisis	Meckel's syndrome
Cleft hand	Medial and oblique facial cleft
Cleft lip	Milroy's disease
Cleft palate	Orodigito facial dysostosis
Congenital ichthyosiform erythroderma	Pili annulati
Conradi's syndrome	Smith-Lemli-Opitz syndrome
Cyclops	Syndactyly
Ectodermal hypohydrotic dysplasia	Ventriculoseptal defect

Table. 28.11: Syndromes featuring polydactyly

Frequent finding	*Occasional finding*
Carpenter syndrome	Bloom syndrome
Ellis-van Creveld syndrome	Conradi-Hunermann syndrome
Meckel-Gruber syndrome	Goltz syndrome
Polysyndactyly syndrome	Klippel-Trenaunay-Weber syndrome
Towne syndrome	Oral-Facial-digital syndrome
Trisomy 13 syndrome	Partial trisomy 10q syndrome
Short rib-polydactyly syndrome	Rubinstein-Taybi syndrome
	Smith-Opitz syndrome
	Trisomy 4p syndrome

ii. *Syndactyly* (Table 28.12)
  Fusion of fingers.
  Causes-it can be an isolated conditions or seen in association with the following disorders.
  Chromosomal disorders associated with syndactyly
  B-D translocation   Trisomy 18
  Extra metacentric chromosome   Trisomy 21 (Down's syndrome)
    triploidy
iii. *Ectrodactyly* Absence of fingers.
iv. *Arachnodactyly*

Table 28.12: Abnormalities associated with syndactyly

Absent ulna	Lip pits
Acrocephalosyndactylism	Maternal radiation
Aglossia-adactylia	Maternal riboflavin deficiency
Alopecia congenita	Meckel's syndrome
Apert's syndrome	Micrognathia-polydactyly
Aplasia cutis congenita	Genital anomalies
Bloom's syndrome	Mobius syndrome
Brachydactyly	Multiple congenital deformities
Cleft hand	Neurofibromatosis
Cleft lip	Oblique facial cleft
Cleft palate	Oculodentodigital dysplasia
Congenital heart disease	Orodigitofacial dysostosis
Conradi's disease	Osteogenesis imperfecta
Crouzon's disease	Papillon-Leage-Psauma syndrome
Cryptophthalmia	Pectoral muscle absence
Deficiency of long bones	Pierre Robin syndrome
Ectodermal dysplasia (hypohydrotic)	Pili annulati
Focal dermal hypoplasia	Poland's syndrome
Glossopalatine ankylosis	Polydactyly
Goltz syndrome	Popliteal pterygium
Hallermann-Streiff syndrome	Prader-Willi syndrome
Hemihypertrophy	Pseudo ainhum
Hereditary abnormalities	Silver's syndrome
Hypertelorism	Synostosis
Incontinentia pigmenti	Thalidomide poisoning
Klippel-Trenaunay syndrome	Thrombocytopenia-absentradius
Lateral facial cleft	Ventriculoseptal defect
Laurence-Moon-Biedl syndrome	Waardenburg's syndrome

Long hands with spidery fingers

Causes – Marfan's syndrome
Homocystinuria,
Hypogonadism,
Congenital contractual arachnodactyly.

v. *Clinodactyly* (Tables 28.13 to 28.15)

Shortened little fingers, with radial deviation, due to hypoplasia of radial aspect of middle phalanx. The little finger either shows a single crease or its distal crease lies proximal to the proximal crease of ring fingers (normally distal crease of little finger lies distal to the proximal crease of ring finger).

Causes — Clinodactyly can be an isolated finding (in 0.3% of normal population) or in association with following disorders.

vi. *Camptodactyly*

Flexion deformity of little finger. It is inherited through a dominant gene and is seen in 1.9 percent of normal population. However, this is also a part of various syndromes such as Down's, Carpenter and Aarskog syndrome.

Table 28.13: Abnormalities associated with clinodactyly of the little finger

Absent pectoral muscle	Myositis ossificans progressiva
Acral-renal syndrome	Oculodentodigital syndrome
Ankyloglossum superins syndrome	Oral-facial-digital syndrome
Bird-headed dwarf (Seckels')	Osteo-onychodysplasia
Bloom's syndrome	Otopalatodigital syndrome
Brachydactyly (type A_3)	Popliteal pterygium syndrome
Cornelia de Lange syndrome	Prader-Willi syndrome
Familial brachydactyly	SC syndrome
Fanconi's syndrome	Silver's syndrome
Focal dermal hypoplasia	Smith-Lemli-Opitz syndrome
Holt-Oram syndrome	Symphalangism
Kirner's deformity	Thrombocytopenia—absent radius (TAR)
Larsen's syndrome	Treacher-Collins syndrome
Laurence-Moon-Biedl syndrome	Turner's syndrome
Meckel's syndrome	Zellweger's syndrome

Table 28.14: Chromosomal disorders associated with clinodactyly

Extrametacentric chromosome	Pseudo 18
4p-	Translocation 17-18
Trisomy 6-12	Trisomy 21
Ring 13	XXXXX
Mosaic trisomy 15	XXXXY-Klinefelter
Partial deletion of chromosome#5	

Table 28.15: Abnormalities associated with clinodactyly and short, little fingers

Cornelia de Lange syndrome	Papillon-Leage-Psaume syndrome
Embryo poisoning with Cytoxan	Proximal symphalangism
Gargoylism	Russel dwarf
Nail patella syndrome	Silver's syndrome
Oral-facial-digital syndrome	Turner's syndrome

vii. *Short fingers of equal length:* It is seen in
 • Achondroplasia (Banana bunch fingers)
 • Hypothyroidism.

viii. *Mallet fingers*
  Persistent flexion at the terminal phalanx. It is due to rupture or extensor tendon at the insertion or avulsion fracture of the base of terminal phalanx.

ix. *Hypoplasia of metacarpal bones of all fingers*: It is seen in
 • Coffin-Siris syndrome
 • Cri du chat syndrome

x. *Thumb anomalies*
 Table 28.16 gives syndromes associated with thumb anomalies.

xi. *Steinberg sign*
  When the thumb is adducted across the palm and the fist is closed, the tip of the thumb is seen to protrude past the ulnar border of the palm. This is seen in Marfan's syndrome but absent in homocystinuria.

xii. *Wrist sign*
  Thumb and the little finger appreciably overlap when encircling the wrist.

Table 28.16: Syndromes associated with thumb anomalies

Abnormality	Syndrome
Triphalangeal thumb	Holt-Oram syndrome
Thumb aplasia	13q syndrome
Broad thumb	Rubinstein-Taybi syndrome
Proximal placement of thumb	18 q syndrome
Flexed thumb	Arthogryposis
Bifid thumb	Translocation 3/13.

xiii. *Brachydactyly*
Broad fingers—It is seen in Down's syndrome
q. *Anomalies of nail* (Discussed elsewhere).

III. *Surface*
- a. *Color – Pallor*
  - Anemia—pallor of palm indicates severe anemia, pallor is first seen in the skin creases.
  - – Hypothyroidism,
  - – Edema, shock.
  - – *Dusky* – Polycythemia
  - – *Blue* – Cyanosis
  - – *Pigmentation* – Addison's disease (mainly pigmentation involves skin creases)
    - – folate deficiency (knuckle pigmentation)
  - – *Yellow* – Jaundice-It is associated with yellow sclera
    - – carotinemia-not associated with yellow sclera
- b. *Erythemia of thenar and hypothenar eminence (palmar erythema)*
  - – Cirrhosis of liver.
  - – Autonomic instability
  - – Beriberi, hyperthyroidism and other high out put failure states.
- c. *Rash*—measles, SLE, Rubella, sec. syphilis.
- d. *Purpuric lesions* – Henoch-Schonlein purpura,
  - – meningococcemia.
- e. *Raynaud's phenomenon*—On exposure to cold, there is an attack of local syncope (characterized by pallor, tingling and numbness) followed by local asphyxia (characterised by cyanosis with burning sensation) involving the fingers. The two attacks are repeated until there occurs local gangrene of the finger tips.
- f. *Gottron papules* Seen over the extensor surface of the joints, particularly knuckles. They are atrophic and scaly lesions. They are initially erythematous and later on develop hyperpigmentation or vitiligo. It is seen in dermatomyositis.
- g. *Papulovesicular lesions in the intertriginous area* Seen in scabies.
- h. *Vesicular lesions* Herpes simplex
  Epidermolysis bullosa
  Congenital syphilis.

i. *Pustules* Seen in infected scabies, impetigo contagiosa.
j. *Nodular lesions along the flexor tendons*—JRA.
k. *Janeway lesions*—Painless, hemorrhagic lesions and over the palms (and soles), seen in infective endocarditis.
l. *Vasculasitic ulcers at the tip of fingers*—Scleroderma.
m. *Dermatoglyphics* (Table 28.17)

It is the study of configuration of characteristic ridge pattern on the volar surface of the hand.

Table 28.17: Abnormalities in dermatoglyphics give a clue to the underlying diagnosis

Flexion Creases	1. Simian crease (Figs 28.11A and B)	
	Single transverse palmar crease running across the entire palm. (For abnormalities, see Table 28.18)	Bilateral simial crease is seen in 45% patients with Down's syndrome (For other conditions see the table)
	2. Sydney crease	
	Here, there are 2 transverse creases The proximal crease runs across the entire palm	Congenital rubella syndrome
	3. 2 creases across the palmar aspect of distal interphalangeal joint	Sickle cell anemia
atd angle	Increased *atd* angle	– Down's syndrome (70-80°) – Trisomy 13 (90°)
Fingerprint	All or most fingers have	
	– Ulnar loop	Down's syndrome
	– Whorl	Rubella, Turner's syndrome
	– Arches	Trisomy 18
Ridge count (Fig. 28.12)	Increased	Rubella and Turner's syndrome (169) (because they have more whorls).
	Decreased	Klinefelter's syndrome (27)

The 3 components of dermatoglyphics are

1. *Flexion creases* Usually there are 3 flexion waves-2 horizontal and one oblique over the palm. There are 2—3 flexion creases over the proximal interphalangeal joints and one over the distal inter-phalangeal joint of fingers.
2. *Ridge arrangements of palm* The ridges of palm run in different directions. The region where 3 ridge systems meet is called triradius (Fig. 28.9). There is one triradius located near the base of the 4th metacarpal bone at some point on its axis. This is called axial triradius and designated as "t"

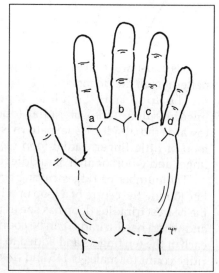

Fig. 28.9: Axial triradius

There are 4 other triradii located one each under the index, middle, ring and little finger. These are called digital triradii and are designated as *a, b, c and d* respectively. The angle between the lines at and adt is called *atd* angle and is normally 40-50°.

3. *Fingerprint pattern* (Fig. 28.10) There are 4 characteristic patterns over the pulp of fingers. They are loop, whorl, arch and mixed.

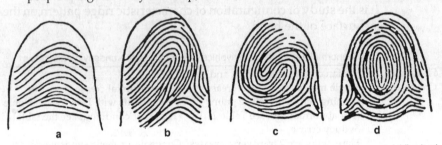

Fig. 28.10: Dermatoglyphic patterns of fingers: (a) arch, (b) loop, (c) double loop and (d) whorl

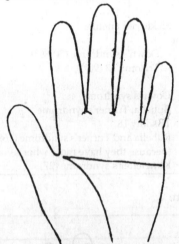

Fig. 28.11A: Simiancrease

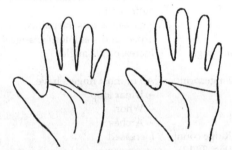

Fig. 28.11B: (a) example of normal flexion crease on palm, and (b) transpalmar crease on palm

It is unusual to find the same finger print pattern in all the fingers.

The loop may be ulnar (opening towards ulnar side) or radial (opening towards radial side). Usual pattern is ulnar loop of little finger, radial loop of index finger and whorl or arch of middle finger.

The number of ridges cutting across a line joining the centre of a loop or whorl to the nearest triradius (loop has one tri radius and whorl has 2 triradii) can be counted in each of the ten fingers and added to get the ridge count. The average value of ridge count for males is 145 and that for females is 127.

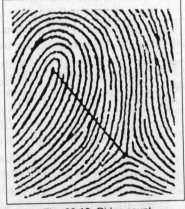

Fig. 28.12: Ridge count

Table 28.18: Abnormalities associated with a single palmar crease

Acrocephalosyndactyly	Mental retardation (10%)
Anencephaly	Nonmongol mental defectives (13%)
BBB syndrome	Noonan's syndrome
C syndrome	PKU (25%), institutionalized
Cleft lip/palate (4%)	Pseudohypoparathyroidism
Coffin-Siris syndrome	Psoriasis
Cornelia de Lange syndrome	Rubella syndrome
Epilepsy	Rubinstein's syndrome
First arch syndrome	Schwartz's syndrome
Hirschsprung's disease	Seckel's dwarf
ISC syndrome	Smith-Lemli-Opitz syndrome
Kidney-liver-hand syndrome	Thalidomide poisoning
Lenz's syndrome	Thrombocytopenia, absent radius
Lissencephaly	Treacher-Collins syndrome
Manic-depressive psychosis	Zellweger syndrome
Maple syrup urine disease	

Palpation

Holding the child's hand gives a lot of information besides boosting emotional bond between the examiner and the child. The following informations are obtained.

a. *Hand shake*   The following abnormalities can be noted;
   i. *Subduced hand shake*
      - Weakness of grasp (neuropathy or myopathy)
      - Painful grasp (arthritis, osteomyelitis, tenosynovitis)
      - Mental depression
      - Sick child (warm hand shake is a sign of recovery from illness).
   ii. *Milk maid sign*   On sustained grasp, there is an alternate squeezing and relaxation (inability to sustain grasp) seen in chorea.
   iii. *Inability to relax grasp*   It is seen in myotonia.
   iv. *Warm hands*
      - Fever
      - Thyrotoxicosis
      - Beriberi
      - Inflammatory state (e.g. JRA)
   v. *Cold hands*
      - Shock (cold and moist)
      - Anxiety (cold and moist)
      - Raynaud's syndrome.
   vi. *Excessive dryness*
      - Fever
      - Cretinism
      - Dehydration
      - Ichthyosis.
b. Testing the *sensation over the hand* helps to know the integrity of ulnar, radial and median nerves.
   Index finger   – median nerve
   Little finger   – ulnar nerve

Web space betweent the 1st and — radial nerve
2nd metacarpal bones on the
dorsal surface of the hand.

c. *Tenderness along the joint line* It is elicited by squeezing each small joint individually.
d. *Swelling*
    i. *Compound palmar ganglion* A swelling on the palm that shows cross fluctuation (across the flexor retinaculum) with another swelling on the palmar aspect of wrist.
        Seen in *ulnar bursitis* secondary to tuberculosis or rheumatoid arthritis.
    ii. *Osler's nodes* Tender, pink or bluish, pea-sized nodules over the pads of the fingers as well as thenar and hypothenar eminence. They are usually recognised by blanching the area with pressure from a glass slide. Seen in *bacterial endocarditis*

Movements

Normal range of movements (Fig. 28.13)
Normal range of movements at different joints of fingers (except thumb)

	MP Joint	Proximal IP	Distal IP
Flexion	90°	0°-100°	0°-80°
Extension	10°	0-100° in reverse direction as flexion	0°-80° in reverse direction as flexion

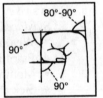

Fig. 28.13: Movements of the finger joints

Screening method to detect movements
• Ability to grip a ball and release it,.
• Ability to touch finger tips to the palm.

Movements of thumb (Fig. 28.14)
Hand is laid flat on the table, with the palm facing upwards.

Flexion — The thumb moves parallel to the palm, towards little finger.
Extension — Movement in the direction opposite to that of flexion.
Abduction — The thumb moves upwards at right angle to the palm of the hand.
Adduction — Movement in opposite direction as abduction.
Opposition — The thumb swings across the palm to touch the tips of the other fingers. Opposition is detected in a young child by its ability to a perform pincer grasp.

Movement of fingers
Flexion at metacarpophalangeal (MCP) joint	– 80-90°
Extension at MCP	– 0-20°
Flexion at proximal interphalangeal joint (PIP)	– 90-100°
Extension at PIP joint	– 0-90°
Flexion at distal interphalangeal joint (DIP)	– 0-90°
Extension at DIP joint	– 0-90°

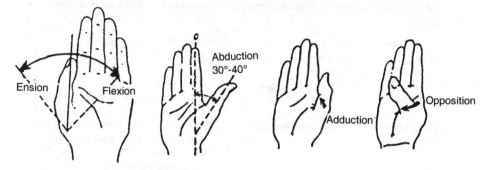

Fig. 28.14: Movements of the thumb

Hand movements are brought about by *ulnar, median and radial nerves*. A simple way to detect the integrity of motor components of these nerves is to test the mobility of thumb.

Paralysis	Lesion
i. Abduction and extension	– Radial nerve
ii. Adduction	– Ulnar nerve
iii. Opposition	– Median nerve

Abnormal movements They can be noticed; tremors, chorea, athetosis, dystonia, and asterexis, etc.

Triggering/locking of fingers They indicate tonosynovitis of flexor tendons (as occurs in rheumatoid arthritis).

Handedness Since definite handedness may not be established till 2½ to 3 years of age, a consistent approach with one hand at a very early age should arose suspicion of hemiplegia.

Examination of Hip Joint
Diseases of hip are fairly common in children (for example DDH, Perthes disease, toxic synovitis) and diagnosis of a limping child often comes as a challenge to a pediatrician. Hence, it is extremely important to have a thorough knowledge regarding the method of examination of hip.

Inspection
The child should be stripped completely so as to expose the entire spine, pelvis and both lower limbs.

Attitude Inspection in standing posture, Table 28.19 given a clue to the diagnosis.

Trendelenburg's test It is done to determine the stability of hip joint.

Normally, in standing position, each leg bears ½ the body weight. When a person stands on one leg, the pelvis has to be titled, raising the side of the pelvis which is not bearing body weight, so that the centre of gravity passes through the weight bearing limb and the body is maintained in balanced position.

Table 28.19: Diagnosis of attitude on the basis of abnormalities and their inference

Findings	Inference
a. The child stands, lurching on one side, bearing the entire body weight on one limb.	Pathology in the opposite hip (Pain/instability)
b. Posture of the non-weight bearing limb.	
i. Slight flexion, abduction and lateral rotation	Synovitis of hip joint e.g. Toxic synovitis, stage I tubercular arthritis
ii. Slight flexion, adduction and medial rotation	a. Destruction of articular cartilage, with resultant spasm of adductors and flexors of hip. e.g. Stage II TB arthritis b. Dislocation of pathological femoral head e.g: Stage III TB arthritis septic arthritis traumatic posterior dislocation of hip.
iii. Marked external rotation, with slight adduction	Slipped capital femoral epiphysis (SCFE)
c. An asymmetric number of thigh skinfolds	DDH on the side with increased skin folds.
d. An attitude of lordosis (with undue protrusion (developmental dysplasia of hip) of abdomen anteriorly and buttocks posteriorly with an increase in the width of the space just below the perineum.	Bilateral DDH

This mechanism, i.e. the stability of the hip joint is maintained by

Fulcrum   —   Head of femur within actabular cavity
Lever   —   Neck of femur
Power   —   Abductors of hip joint (G. medius)

If any one of these is abnormal, the hip of the weight bearing limb fails to tilt the pelvis, which sags down and balance cannot be maintained.

Test The child stands on unaffected limb. The buttock on the opposite (affected) side automatically rises. This is taken as *Trendelenburg's test negative*.

Next, the child stands on the affected side. The pelvis on the opposite (normal) side sinks (as shown by gluteal folds and iliac crest). This is *Trendelenburg's test positive*.

Conditions producing positive Trendelenburg's test:
1. Femoral head not contained within acetabular cavity. (Unstable fulcrum), e.g. Developmental and pathological dislocation of hip.
2. When lever system is not intact, e.g. fracture neck of femur, Perthes' disease.
3. Paralysis of Gluteus medius (Power failure)
   e.g.   Poliomyelitis
          Muscular dystrophies

The child is next inspected in supine position
A. *Determination of fixed deformity.* Any pathology in hip joint results in fixity of hip joint in various positions (flexion, abduction, adduction, etc.) due

to muscle spasm or fibrosis. These deformities (called *fixed deformities*) are masked by compensatory tilting of the lumbar spine and pelvis.

Presence of fixed deformities are usually demonstrated with the patient lying on the bed.

- *Fixed adduction and abduction deformity* The deformity is normally masked by compensatory scoliosis of the lumbar spine.

  The deformity is detected as follows A line is drawn joining the two anterior superior iliac spines. Normally this line is perpendicular to the midline of the body. In adduction deformity, the anterior superior iliac spine on the affected side will be at a lower level, whereas in abduction deformity it will be at a higher level.

  The angle of deformity is detected as follows The affected limb is held just above the ankle and is gradually adducted/abducted according to the existing deformity till the interspinous line becomes perpendicular to the midline of the body. The angle of deformity is the angle through which the limb has to be moved so as to bring the interspinous line to this position.

- *Fixed flexion deformity* This is masked by lumbar lordosis. In recumbent position, patient is asked to completely extend the affected limb. This results in lumbar lordosis, which is detected by passing a hand behind the lumbar spine.

  The angle of deformity is determined by *Thomas test*. In this test, the normal hip is flexed until the lumbar lordosis is completely obliterated. This automatically results in flexion of the affected thigh. The angle through which the thigh moves is the angle of fixed flexion deformity.

- *Fixed medial and lateral rotation* This deformity cannot be concealed by compensatory movement of the lumbar spine. It is determined by noting the direction of patella/of the toes when the foot is held at right angle to the leg. Normally there is slight lateral rotation of the lower limb (Patella and toes point slightly laterally). If the patella and the toes point towards ceiling, it indicates slight medial rotation.

B. *Galeazzi sign/Allis sign* (Fig. 28.15) When the supine infant's feet are placed together on the examining table with the hips and knees flexed, both the knees are in the same horizontal level. Uneven knee levels indicates real shortening of thigh (e.g. Seen in developmental dysplasia of hip) due to dislocation of femoral head from the acetabulum.

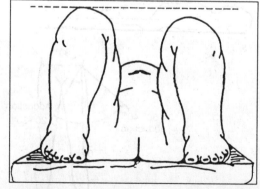

Fig. 28.15: Positive Galeazzi sign of unequal knee height, demonstrating shortening of the left lower extremity due to posterior dislocation of the left hip

Palpation

Tenderness
a. Tenderness of the hip joint is elicited by applying steady pressure inwards over the 2 greater trochanters. This indicates arthritis of hip.
b. Tenderness over the greater trochanter—trochanteric fracture.
c. In transcervical and sub capital fractures, tenderness can only be elicited when the shaft of the femur is rotated.

Swelling
a. Abnormal swelling and bruising indicates hematoma (# neck of femur) or abnormal position of femoral head (dislocation).
b. Tender, fluctuating swelling associated with signs of inflammation, felt just below mid inguinal point indicates suppurative arthritis.
c. Cold abscess can be felt as fluctuant, nontender swelling, medial to the greater trochanter, medial to femoral vessels, in the gluteal region, ischiorectal fossa.

Vascular sign of Narath Normally femoral artery is felt against the head of femur. In case of congenital dislocation, the head of the femur is dislocated and the bony support is missing. Hence, there is a great difficulty in feeling the artery. This is known as vascular sign of Narath.

Movements (Figs 28.16A and B)
Before testing the movements, pelvis has to be steadied during movements by holding the iliac crest. True range of movement is the one which is brought about without causing any movement of pelvis.
Flexion While supine, the child is asked to raise the leg
  • with the knee flexed—Normal range upto 120°
  • with the knee extended—Normal range upto 90°

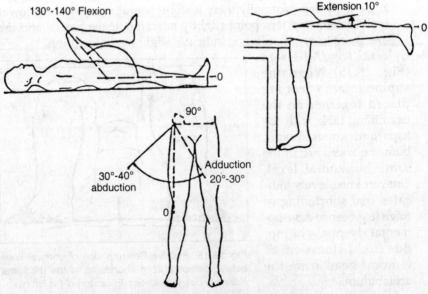

Fig. 28.16A: Movements of the hip

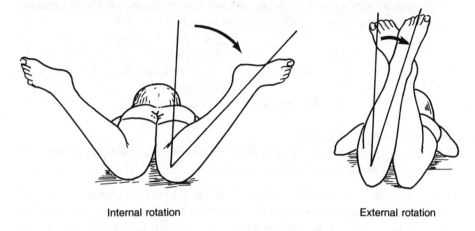

Internal rotation   External rotation

Fig. 28.16B: Internal and external rotation

Extension While prone, the child is asked to lift the leg, with knee extended – Normal range upto 15°

Abduction With the child in supine position, both the hip and knee are flexed and the feet are brought together. The knees are now bent outwards simultaneously on both sides. The range of abduction noted and compared on either side. Normal range 40°.

Adduction The patient is asked to lift the affected limb and then cross it over its fellow. Normal range—30° (i.e. the limb can be made to cross the middle 1/3rd of the opposite thigh).

Rotation (Rotation in extension): With the patient in supine position, the palm of the hand is placed over the thigh and the thigh is rolled to and fro observing the foot as an index of the degree of rotation. Normal Range-internal rotation-40°, external rotation-30°.

    Alternate method (Rotation in flexion): With the patient in prone position, knee is flexed to 90°. Fixing the hip with one hand and grasping the ankle with the other hand, the ankle is moved medially (To test for the external rotation at hip) and then laterally (To test for the internal rotation at hip) (Fig. 28.16B).

    Normal range   — Internal rotation in flexion   30°
                       External rotation in flexion   45°

In neonates, lateral rotation normally exceeds medial rotation. The reverse is true during early childhood. By the time skeletal maturity is reached, symmetric arcs of medial and lateral rotation are seen.

Though all movements are generally restricted in diseases of the hip, certain movements are predominantly restricted in certain diseases.

e.g.	Disease	Restricted movements
	SCFE	Abduction and internal rotation
	Perthes' disease	Abduction and internal rotation
	DDH	Abduction
	Early TB arthritis	Abduction

Examination of Hip Stability

Stability of hip joint is jeopardised in DDH. So the following 3 tests are performed when the condition is suspected.

Telescopic test The pelvis is fixed with one hand touching the greater trochanter. The hip is now flexed to 90° and the knee is grasped with the other hand of the clinician who pushes the thigh downwards along the axis of the thigh with this hand, while the other hand notes whether the greater trochanter is moving downwards. This positive telescopic test is seen in DDH as well as pathological dislocation of the hip and also in Charcot's joint.

Ortolani's test This test must be carried out in a relaxed child, preferably after feeding. Flex the knees and encircle them with the hands so that the thumbs lie along the medial sides of the thighs and the fingers over the trochanters. Now flex the hips to right angle and starting from a position where the thumbs are touching, smoothly and gently abduct the hips. If a hip is dislocated, as full abduction is approached the femoral head will be felt slipping into the acetabulum and an audible click may accompany the displacement (Figs 28.18A to C).

Barlow's test Fix the pelvis between symphysis and sacrum with one hand. With the thumb of the other hand make an attempt to dislocate the hip by gentle but firm backward pressure. Check on both sides. If the head of the femur is felt to subluxate backwards, its reduction should be achieved by forward finger pressure or wider abduction. The movement of reduction should also be appreciated with the fingers (Fig. 28.17 and Figs 18A to C).

Examination of Knee

Examination of knee should be done in standing, sitting, supine and prone positions. It should be noted that examination of knee is not complete without examining hip and vice-versa (Because, with pathology in one joint, pain is refered to the other joint. Important points on inspection are depicted in Table 28.20.

Palpation

1. One should palpate the bony points, patella and ligamentous attachments for tenderness, crepitus, bony gaps, etc. which indicate fracture of bones, sprain of ligaments, etc.

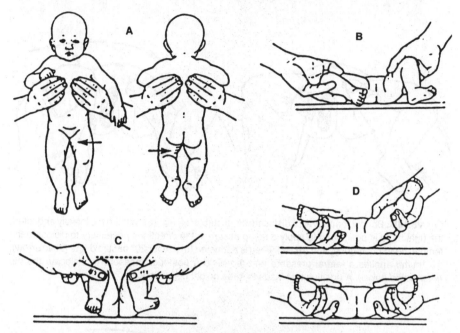

Fig. 28.17: Signs of developmental dysplasia of the hip: (A) Asymmetry of gluteal and thigh folds, (B) Limited hip abduction, as seen in flexion, (C) Apparent shortening of the femur, as indicated by the level of the knees in flexion, (D) Ortolani click, heard when affected leg is abcucted in infant under 4 weeks of age

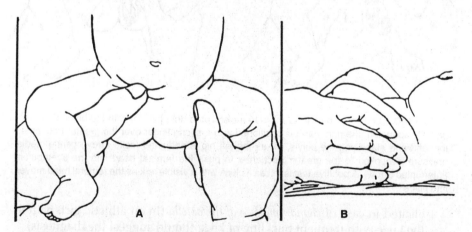

Fig. 28.18A: Hand position for examining the left hip: (a) the right thumb is positioned proximally on the medial femur with the hand encircling the knee (important for the Barlow maneuver). The left hand stabilizes the pelvis, and (b) position of the long fingers on the greater trochanter (important for the Ortolani maneuver)

If the knee is kept extended and the patella is pressed down against the femoral condyle while moving it laterally, exquisite tenderness is

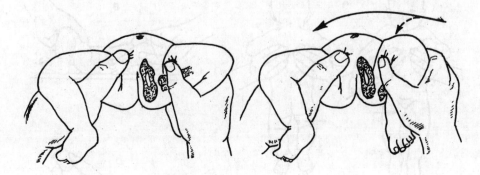

Fig. 28.18B: Barlow maneuver to dislocate an unstable left hip: (a) with the hip initially abducted, the right hand is positioned to apply a soft pressure in the directions necessary to dislocate the femoral head posteriorly, and (b) as the leg is adducted to at least 20° past mid-line *(solid arrow)*, the thumb applies a lateral pressure and the hand a posterior pressure to dislocate the hip *(interrupted arrow)*. A positive test leads to knee height discrepancy

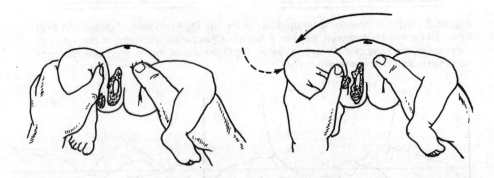

Fig. 28.18C: Ortolani maneuver to relocate a dislocated right hip: (a) with the hip in neutral or partially adducted, the right hand is positioned with the long finger over the greater trochanter, the left hand stabilizing the pelvis, (b) as the left hip is abducted (solid arrow) gentle medial pressure is applied to the greater trochanter to push the femoral head into the acetabulum (interrupted arrow). A positive test is felt as a clunk with a visible jerk as the femoral head moves into place

elicited in case of *chondromalasia of the patella* (In an athletic girl, pain in the knee with frequent buckling of knee should suggest the diagnosis).

Swelling
a. *Knee effusion*
  i. *Minimal effusion* The patient is asked to stand and gentle pressure is applied over one of the obliterated hollows on either side of ligamentum patellae (so as to displace the fluid) and now the pressure is released, the hollow will be filled slowly.

  A 2nd method is to elicit *patellar tap* with the patient standing.

Table 28.20: Examination of knee on the basis of inspection, attitude and swelling

Inspection

1. *Attitude*

   a. *Position of moderate flexion* (This is the position in which the joint can accommodate maximum fluid within its cavity)
   - Acute septic arthritis
   - Early stage of TB arthritis

   b. *Triple dislocation* (Flexion, posterior subluxation and lateral rotation of tibia, due to spasm of hamstrings)
   Late stage of TB arthritis (Due to destruction of cruciate and collateral ligaments)

   c. *Genu recurvatum* (i.e. knee hyperexension with weight bearing (i.e. standing)
   - Weakness of quadriceps
   - In girls there can be normally 5-10° of hyperextension Physiological (< 2years)

   d. *Genu varus* (Bow leg)-Normally there is an outward angulation of 15° between the long axis of femur and tibia when the child stands (i.e. in weight bearing position). In genu varus, there is inward angulation between the two. This is tested as follows:
   Due to *in utero* positioning. Pathological: rickets,

   The child is asked to stand, with the medial malleoli touching each other. The distance between the medial condyles of tibia on either side, is measured
   Achondroplasia, Metaphysial dysplasia, Blount's disease.

   Distance > 5 cm indicates genu varus. (Figs 28.23A and B)
   Trauma to medial condyle of femur or tibia or tumor from lateral condyle of femur.

   e. *Genu valgum* (Knock knee)
   The child is asked to stand, with the medial condyles touching each other. If the distance between the 2 medial malleoli is > 5 cm, it indicates genu valgum (Figs 28.24A and B)
   Physiological-2-5 yrs
   Pathological: rickets
   Trauma to lateral femoral/tibial condyle,
   Tumor arising from medial condyle
   Congenital dislocation of patella, cerebral palsy.

2. *Swelling*

   a. Horse-shoe shaped swelling extending above the patella, on both sides of patella and the ligamentum patellae, obliterating the normal depressions.
   Knee joint effusion

   b. Similar swelling as above, but also extending over the patella and its ligament.
   Superficial cellulitis

   c. Swelling on the posterior aspect of knee, which becomes more prominent and tense on extension of the knee but disappears on flexion.
   Morrant Baker's cyst (associated with TB or osteoarthritis)

   d. Swelling infront of lower part of patella and ligamentum patellae.
   Prepatellar/infrapatellar bursitis.

3rd method — *Bulge sign*—With the knee extended examiner should milk the medial aspect of the knee upwards 2-3 times. This pushes the fluid into the lateral aspect of suprapatellar pouch. Now the examiner should tap the lateral edge of the patella and observe for the bulge of returning fluid into the hollow area medial to the medial border of the patella. (Make sure it is not the patella that is moving).

ii. *Moderate effusion* — *Patellar tap* is positive. Patient lies in supine/ standing position. With one hand, suprapatellar pouch is pressed so as to drive the whole of its fluid into the joint space. With the index finger of the other hand, patella is pushed backwards towards the femoral condyles with a sharp and jerky movement. The floating patella can be felt to touch the femoral condyle.

iii. *Massive effusion* — *Patellar tap*
— *Fluctuation*—Demonstrated by pressing the suprapatellar pouch with one hand and feeling the impulse with the thumb and the index finger of the other hand placed on either side of ligamentum patellae.

b. *Thickened synovial membrane*

This is also present as a fluctuating swelling similar to knee effusion and is differentiated from effusion as follows:
   i. Spongy or Kashmir Velvette feel
   ii. Absence of patellar tap.
   iii. Edge of the swelling can be rolled under the finger (cf: Effusion-No edge is felt). Gentle palpation is necessary to appreciate synovial thickening since the synovium collapses on firm pressure .

c. *Popliteal aneurysm* —An expansile swelling in the popliteal fossa.

d. *Popliteal cyst* (Morrant Baker's cyst) It is a herniation of the synovial membrane posteriorly through the fibres of the oblique popliteal ligament to form a swelling in the middle of the posterior aspect of the knee. The swelling becomes prominent on extension and disappears on flexion. The condition is often associated with tuberculosis/ osteoarthritis of the joint.

Movements (Fig. 28.19)

	Normal range
Flexion	— Until calf touches the back of thigh (130°)
Extension	— Until thigh and calf are in straight line. Hyperextension of 5-10° may be possible.
Adduction, abduction and rotation	— Usually absent with the knee in full extension. But with the knees flexed to 90°, minimal movements (upto 15°) are possible.

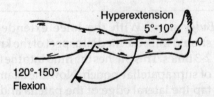

Fig. 28.19: Movements of the knee joint

Tests for Stability

Stability is maintained mainly by collateral ligament and cruciate ligaments. Tear of these ligaments alters the stability. Following tests are done to know the integrity of different ligaments of knee joint.

Adduction and abduction test The patient lies in supine position, the lower limb is elevated by holding the ankle with one hand. Knee is held with the other hand. With the hand on the knee as fulcrum, the leg is adducted and abducted using the hand over the ankle.

Results   Normal—No adduction/abduction is possible.

Tear of medial collateral ligament—abnormal abduction.

Tear of lateral collateral ligament—abnormal adduction.

If the ligament is sprained, the joint will remain stable but the patient complaints of excruciating pain during the exercise.

Drawer's test The patient lies in supine position. Knee is flexed to 90°, keeping the foot on the table. The upper part of tibia is held with one hand and alternately pulled forwards and pushed backwards.

Results   Normal—No movement is possible.

Rupture of anterior cruciate ligament—increased anterior mobility.

Rupture of posterior cruciate ligament—increased posterior mobility.

Apley's grinding test The patient lies in prone position. Knee joint is flexed to 90° (Table 28.21). Patients femur is fixed by keeping the clinician's knee over the patients thigh. Now, the following movements are made and any pain during the different movements is noted.

Table 28.21: Different movements with respect to various torn cartilages

Movements	Torn cartilage
1. Compression and external rotation of leg (by holding the foot with one hand)	Medial semilunar cartilage
2. Compression and internal rotation of leg	Lateral semilunar cartilage
3. Pulling the leg upwards and rotating externally	Medial collateral ligament
4. Pulling the leg upwards and rotating internally	Lateral collateral ligament

Examination of Ankle and Foot

Examination of ankle should be done in both weight bearing (sitting and standing) and non-weight bearing (supine) postures. Child is also made to walk and foot print is taken (Tables 28.22 and 28.23).

Inspection

Attitude and deformity

Table 28.22: Examination of ankle and foot on the basis of inspection of attitude and deformity

Description	Inference
1. Mild plantar flexion with the foot slightly off the ground	Arthritis of ankle
2. The foot shows plantar flexion (Equinus), inversion, varus i.e., the sole faces inwards and forefoot adduction. Foot is smaller, heel is poorly developed, lateral malleolus is unduely prominent while medial malleolus is burried. There is a transverse crease across the sole of medial side while the lateral surface shows callosities.	Talipes equinovarus. It may be an isolated finding or associated with syndromes (Table 28.23).

Table 28.23: Syndromes associated with club feet

Frequent
> Amyoplasia congenita disruptive sequence
> Diastrophic dysplasia syndrome
> Distal arthrogryposis syndrome
> Escobar syndrome
> Femoral hypoplasia—unusual facies syndrome
> Fetal aminopterin effects
> Freeman-Sheldon syndrome (varus with contracted toes)
> Hecht syndrome
> Larsen syndrome
> Meckel-Gruber syndrome
> Moebius sequence
> Partial trisomy 10q syndrome
> Pena-Shokoe syndrome
> Triploidy syndrome
> Trisomy 9 mosaic syndrome
> Trisomy 9p syndrome
> Trisomy 20p syndrome
> Zellweger syndrome
> 4p-syndrome
> 9p-syndrome
> 13q-syndrome
> 18q-syndrome

Occasional
> Aarskog syndrome
> Bloom syndrome
> Conradi-Hunermann syndrome
> Dubowitz syndrome
> Ehlers-Danlos syndrome
> Ellis-van Creveld syndrome (valgus)
> Generalized gangliosidosis syndrome
> Homocystinuria syndrome (pes cavus, everted feet)
> Hunter syndrome
> Mietens syndrome
> Nail-patella syndrome
> Noonan syndrome
> Popliteal web syndrome
> Radial aplasia-thrombocytopenia syndrome
> Rilley-Day syndrome

Contd...

Contd...

Schwartz syndrome
Seckel syndrome
Steinert myotonic dystrophy syndrome
Trisomy 4p syndrome
Trisomy 13 syndrome
Trisomy 18 syndrome
Weaver syndrome
XXXXX syndrome
Zellweger syndrome
18 p syndrome

1. The foot shows dorsiflexion at the ankle (calcaneus) and eversion, i.e. the sole faces outwards (valgus)	**Talipes calcaneovalgus** This is uncommon and it is important to exclude congenital dislocation of hip in this condition.
2. The great toe is abducted at the metatarso-phalangeal joint. The medial surface of the head of 1st metatarsal bone forms a prominence	**Hallux valgus** 1. Congenital 2. Wearing of short, pointed shoes.
3. The lesser toes (4th and 5th) show flexion at the proximal interphalangeal joint with lateral rotation and varus alignment.	**Curly toes** Usually familial and bilateral May be associated with callosities.
4. Toes shows extension at metatarso-phalangeal joint and flexion at proximal interphalangeal joint.	**Hammer toe** Usually familial, bilateral and involve 2nd toe. May be associated with painful calluses.
5. Toes showing extension at metatarso-phalangeal joint and flexion at both proximal and distal interphalangeal joints.	**Claw toe** Usually associated with *pes cavus* and is secondary to an underlying neurological disease such as Charcot-Marie-Tooth disease.
6. Distal interphalangeal joint shows flexion	**Mallet toe** Idiopathic, may be associated with dorsal callosity and nailbed irritation.
9. Overlapping of toes.	• Overlap of 2nd toe over the 1st, is associated with hallux valgus. • Overlapping of 5th over 4th toe is idiopathic. • Trisomy 13 and 18.
10. Fusion of toes	Syndactyly
11. Presence of supernumerary toes	Polydactyly.

Pes planus Normally where a child stands on a flat surface, the lateral border touches the floor, while the medial border touches the floor only in the region of forefoot and hind foot. This is because of the concavity produced by medial longitudinal arch. In children with *pes plannus*, the surface of the foot is flat and hence, touches the floor throughout (Figs 28.20A to C).

Etiology

1. *Mobile flat foot* This is common in neonates and toddlers. It can persist till 6 years. This is due to laxity of bone-ligament complex that forms the arch and the presence of fat in the medial longitudinal arch.

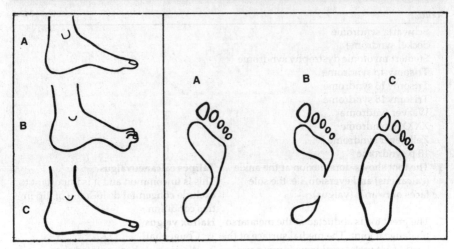

Figs 28.20A to C: Deformities of the arch of the foots (A) normal foot,
(B) Claw-foot, and (C) flat foot

In older children this is due to generalized ligamentous laxity (autosomal dominant trait).

Children with flexible flat foot are usually asymptomatic

2. Fixed flat foot   Etiology — Tendo-Achilles contracture
                                         — Congenital vertical talus
                                         — Cerebral palsy

Pes cavus It is an uncommon condition in which there is an increased concavity of the arch of the foot, so that the instep is unduly high. When the child stands on a flat surface, the medial border is unduly high. The lateral border is also high so that the plantar surface of foot doesn't touch the floor in its central part. It is typically associated with clawing of toes (Figs 28.20A to C).
Etiology

1. Idiopathic   : Most common-usually noticed by 8-10 years in an otherwise fit child.

2. Neuromuscular diseases   : In this, there is weakness of intrinsic muscles of foot which are overpowered by the extrinsic muscles which cause the toes to assume the claw position and the foot to bunch, e.g. Friedreich's ataxia.

3. Contracture of plantar fascia   : Myopathy.

Swelling

a. Swelling extending on either side of the   — Effusion into ankle joint,
tendo-achilles, as well as across the front   Pedal edema
of the joint.

b. Swelling extending along the long axis   — Tenosynovitis
of the leg on either side of tendo-achilles
and the foot, far beyond the joint level.

Palpation

1. Ankle should be palpated for tenderness, irregularity, unnatural mobility, crepitus to diagnose fracture, sprain, corns, callosities, bursitis, etc.
2. Subtalar tenderness is elicited by gripping the ankle firmly and moving the foot into inversion and eversion.
3. Small joints of foot should be tested individually by squeezing the individual joints.
4. Swelling associated with tenderness, redness and heat, at the metatarsophalangeal joint of the great toe indicates Gouty arthritis. A draining trophus may occasionally be present.
5. Fluctuation between the swelling on either side of the tendo-Achilles may be obtained in effusion of the joint. With the other hand, an impulse can be felt in front of the joint, simultaneously.
6. Dependent edema manifests as swelling that pits on pressure and extends below and above the ankle joint. Fluctuation is absent.
7. A thickened tendo-Achilles indicates hyperlipidemia.

Movements (Fig. 28.21)

The range of motion is assessed by asking the patient to perform the following movements while sitting. With the foot in neutral position (i.e. the long axis of foot makes a right angle with the long axis of leg in mid sagittal plane). The following movements are assessed.

a. *Dorsiflexion (Ankle joint)* Point the foot towards the ceiling. *Normal range* is 20-30°.

b. *Plantar flexion (Ankle joint)* Point the foot towards the floor. *Normal range* is 40-50°.

c. *Inversion (Supination) (Subtalar joint)* With the ankle fixed by holding the calcaneum, tilt the foot towards the midline so that the plantar surface of foot faces towards the other foot. *Normal range is* 30°.

d. *Eversion (Pronation) (Subtalar joint)* After the fixing the ankle by holding the calcaneum, tilt the foot away from the midline. *Normal range* is 30-35°.

e. *Abduction and adduction* Rotating the ankle, turn the foot towards (adduction) and then away from (abduction) the other foot, while the examiner stabilises the leg, *normal range* of abduction and adduction are 10° and 20° respectively.

f. *Bend and straighten the toes* Bend and straighten the toes to note flexion and extension respectively (Especially at great toe). *Normal range* of flexion and extension at great toe is 65° and 60° respectively. Restriction in movement is often seen in JRA, gout and ischemic conditions.

Functional Assessment

This is best tested by means of ADL **(Activities of daily living).**

Evaluation of ADL is helpful in assessing children with chronic conditions such as severe rheumatoid arthritis or neuromuscular disease. ADL evaluation

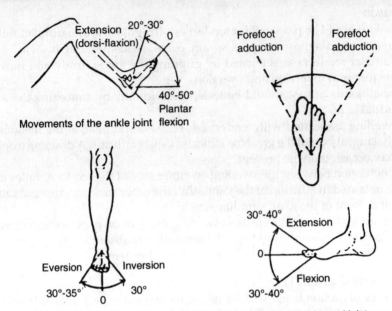

Fig. 28.21: Movement of the ankle joint, movement at the subtarsal joint, and movement of the metatarsophalangeal joints

is also used for functional classification of severely handicapped children. The functional categories are:
a. Fully dependent.
b. Mostly dependent-minimal help required.
c. Wheel chair-bound-but can take care of certain items.
d. Totally dependent on others.

Functional Tests Used in Following Children with Dermatomyositis
1. Elevation of neck from lying in supine position.
2. Elevation of extended lower limb (in seconds).
3. Ability to get up from lying, without help.
4. Ability to get up from sitting, with arms folded in front.

Functional Tests Used in Following Children with Rheumatoid Arthritis
1. Duration of morning stiffness.
2. Time to walk 50 feet.
3. Grip strength.
4. Gait.

Grip Strength
A blood pressure cuff is rolled and given to the child to hold in the hands. Ten fingers should go around the cuff. The bulb is squeezed by the examiner to reach a measurement of 20 mm Hg on the manometer. Now the child is asked to squeeze the bag as strongly as possible with the right hand. After the child lets go and rests, this is repeated two more times, and the best of the three

measurements is taken as the value. This is now repeated on the left side. *Normally, children six to ten years old can squeeze up to 120 mmHg, and adolescents can squeeze the mercury out of the unit.* The grip strength measures a composite of pain, tenderness, limitation of range of movements, and weakness of muscles of the hand. However, in long-term follow-up of children with arthritis, it is a good indicator of improvement or worsening.

Systemic Examination

Systemic examination is done keeping in mind, the signs/complications of underlying disease under consideration.

CNS : Seizures, psychosis, neurodeficits—in SLE,
         proximal weakness—Dermatomyositis.

CVS : Hypertension—HSP
         CCF–Rheumatic fever, SLE
         Shock–Fracture with hemorrhage into internal organs.

RS : Pleuritis—RA, SLE,

PA : Hepatosplenomegaly, tenderness—SLE.

APPENDIX

QUICK ORTHOPEDIC EXAMINATION

Orthopedic examination in children should be carried out in the following way which has been recommended by *American Academy of Pediatrics, Sports Medicine Branch* (Table 28.24).

Table 28.24: The 2-minute orthopedic examination

Instructions	Observation
• Stand facing examiner	• Acromioclavicular joints
	• General habitus
• Look at ceiling, floor, over both shoulders	• Cervical spine motion
• Shrug shoulders (examiner resists)	• Trapezius strength
• Abduct shoulders to 90 degrees (examiner resists at 90 degrees)	• Deltoid strength
• Full external rotation of arms	• Shoulder motion
• Flex and extend elbows	• Elbow motion
• Arms at sides, elbows 90 degrees flexed; pronate and supinate wrists	• Elbow and wrist motion
• Spread fingers; make fist	• Hand or finger motion and deformities
• Tighten (contract) quadriceps; relax quadriceps	• Symmetry and knee effusion
	• Ankle effusion
• "Duck walk" four steps (away from examiner with buttocks on heels)	• Hip, knee, and ankle motion
• Turn back to examiner	• Shoulder symmetry, scoliosis
• Keep knees straight, touch toes	• Scoliosis, hip motion, hamstring tightness
• Raise up on toes, raise heels	• Calf symmetry, leg strength

Quick Modified Orthopedic Examination

A detailed examination of the musculoskeletal system is often difficult as well as time consuming in a busy clinic. Hence, pediatrician should adopt a shortcut to quickly, but precisely assess the musculoskeletal system. Any abnormality detected by this method should necessitate detailed formal examination (Tables 28.25 and 28.26).

The following is a simple guideline to quick orthopedic examination (Modified from guidelines AAP, sports medicine branch).

Neonatal Examination

Genetic and fetal insults can produce musculoskeletal anomalies. The fetus is exposed to various postural pressures that can be manifested in the infant as musculoskeletal anomalies. Hence, a careful evaluation of the musculoskeletal system should be part of every newborn examination. Early diagnosis and prompt referal are essential elements of care in many of the orthopedic problems of infancy and early childhood. Review of the history of pregnancy and identification of possible familial musculoskeletal disorders should precede examination. Systematic evaluation of the head, neck, trunk, and extremities will disclose most of the common disorders of the musculoskeletal system. The following outline is offered only as a guide for neonatal neuromusculoskeletal examination; format is less important than thoroughness.

History

1. Family history of musculoskeletal disease.
2. Exposure to teratogenic substances, irradiation, or infections during pregnancy.

Table 28.25: Modified orthopedic examination

Instructions	Observation
1. Stand facing the examiner	a. General habitus
	b. Shoulder symmetry
	c. Neck symmetry
	d. Carrying angle.
2. Look at ceiling, floor, side to side and nod the head	Cervical spine motion
3. Swing shoulders (Examiner resists)	Trapezius strength
4. Abduct shoulders to 90° (Examiner resists at 90°)	Deltoid strength
5. Raise the arms above shoulder and touch the palms with each other	Abduction and internal rotation.
6. Bring the arms behind the back and clasp the hands with each other.	Adduction and external rotation.
7. Fold the hands in Indian greeting position and press hard	Elbow flexion and wrist extension
8. Flex and extend elbow	Elbow motion
9. Arms at sides, elbows 90° flexed; pronate and wrists	Elbow motion supinate
10. Spread the fingers	Deformities
11. Bend the fingers "as if you are going to scratch some one"	Interphalangeal joint motion
12. Close the first	Metacarpophalangeal joint motion.
13. Pick up small objects using thumb and index finger (pincer grasp)	Opposition
14. Tighten quadriceps. Relax quadriceps	Symmetry of knee effusion; Ankle effusion.
15. Squat down without support	Hip and knee flexion
16. Get up without support	Hip and knee extension
17. Walk normally with wet foot	Foot print (pes planus/cavus)
18. "Duck walk" four steps (away from the examiner, with the buttocks on heels)	Hip, knee and ankle motion
19. Walk on forefoot and toes	Plantar flexion
20. Walk on heels	Dorsiflexion
21. Raise up on toes, raising the heels	Calf symmetry, leg strength
22. Walk on lateral border of foot	Inversion
23. Walk on medial border of foot	Eversion.
24. Turn, facing the back to the examiner. Stand straight with the lower limb placed side by side.	Scoliosis
	Shoulder symmetry
	Genu varus
	Genu valgum
25. Pick up an object from the floor, without bending the knees	Scoliosis
	Flexion of spine (separation of fingers placed on adjacent spinous process)
Hip flexion	Hamstring tightness
26. Bend laterally sliding the hand along the ipsilateral lower limb.	Lateral flexion

3. Bleeding during pregnancy
4. Lack of normal fetal movement
5. Breech position
6. Traumatic delivery, birth asphyxia, neonatal sepsis

Fig. 28.26: Quick functional assessment and musculoskeletal assessment

Activity to observe	Indicator of weakened muscle groups
Rising from lying to sitting position	• Rolling to one side and pushing with arms to raise to elbows; grabbing a siderail or table to pull to sitting
Rising from chair to stand	• Pushing with arms to supplement standing weak leg muscles; upper torso thrusts forward before body rises
Walking	• Lifting leg farther off floor with each step; shortened swing phase; foot may fall or slide forward; arms held out for balance or move in rowing motion
Climbing steps	• Holding handrail for balance; pulling body up and forward with arms; uses stronger leg
Descending steps	• Lowering weakened leg first; often descends sideways holding rail with both hands; may watch feet
Picking up item from floor	• Leaning on furniture for support; bending over at waist to avoid bending knees;uses one hand on thigh to assist with lowering and raising torso
Tying shoes and putting on and pulling up trousers or stockings	• Using foot stool to decrease spinal flexion. Difficulty may indicate decreased shoulder and upper arm strength; these activities often performed in sitting position until clothing is pulled up
Putting on sweater	• Putting sleeve on weaker arm or shoulder first; uses internal or external shoulder rotation to get remaining arm in sleeve
Zipping dress in back	• Difficulty with this indicates weakened shoulder rotation
Combing hair	• Difficulty indicates problems with grasp, wrist flexion, pronation and supination of forearm, and elbow rotation
Pushing chair away from table while seated	• Standing and easing chair back with torso; difficulty indicates problems with upper arm, shoulder, lower arm strength, and wrist motion
Buttoning collapses button or writing name	• Difficulty indicates problem with manual dexterity and finger-thumb opposition

Physical examination

Head and neck
1. Skull symmetry and shape
2. Neck configuration any torticollis, equality of skin folds.
3. Normal range of passive motion

Trunk
1. Anterior and posterior surfaces closed; no signs of neural tube defects
2. Observe for any cutaneous dimpling, nevi, or hairy patches (spina bifida occulta) or a transilluminant midline swelling over the spine (spina bifida cystica).
3. Observe for trunk symmetry (underlying spinal deformity)
4. Palpate along the spine, with the trunk flexed. Observe for any midline defect (spina bifida occulta).
5. Palpate both clavicles noting irregularity, crepitus, tenderness.

Extremities
1. Observe for the symmetry of posture (normally there is a symmetric flexion of upper limb and lower limb on either side) and symmetry of gluteal, genital and axillary folds. If asymmetric, place the newborn in fetal position to observe how that might have contributed to any asymmetry of posture and shape of extremities.
2. Observe for the equality of limb length and circumference.
3. Observe all parts of both extremities and note if any deformity is present.
4. Observe the spontaneous movements at different joints of both upper and lower limbs, noting especially the symmetry and movements.
5. Do Moro's reflex and findout if it is symmetric. Asymmetry indicates fracture clavicle or Erb's palsy on one side.
6. Do full range of passive movements at different joints of upper and lower limbs, noting any pain, restriction, increased range or abnormal direction of movement.
7. Observe the hands. Normally hands should open periodically. When the hand is fisted, the thumb should be positioned inside the fingers. Open the fist, observe the dermatoglyphics, count the number of fingers, noting polydactyly, syndactyly, clinodactyly, etc.
8. Note features of DDH such as hip instability, (Ortoloni's and Barlow's test), restricted abduction and Allis test.
9. Observe the foot. Note if there is any deformity (e.g. CTEV), polydactyly, syndactyly, etc. All babies are flat-footed and many newborns have a slight varus curvature of the tibias (tibial torsion) or forefoot adduction (metatarsus adductus) from fetal positioning. Hence, the midline of the foot may bisect the 3rd and 4th toes, rather than the 2nd and 3rd toes. Forefoot should be flexible, straightening with abduction. It is necessary to follow apparent problems carefully, but seldom is it necessary to intervene. As growth and development take place, the expected body habitus is usually achieved.

Adolescent Sports Medicine

Risk Factors for Sports Injury
- Poor physical conditioning
- Failure to warm up muscles adequately
- Intensity of competition
- Collision and contact sports participation
- Rapid growth
- Overuse of joints

Screening Musculoskeletal Examination for Child and Adolescent Sports Participation
- Observe posture and general muscle contour bilaterally
- Observe gait
- Ask patient to walk on tiptoes and heels
- Observe patient hop on each foot
- Ask patient to duck walk four steps with knees completely bent
- Inspect spine for curvature and lumbar extension, fingers touching toes with knees straight
- Palpate shoulder and clavicle for dislocation
- Check the following joints for range of motion neck, shoulder, elbow, forearm, hands, fingers and hips
- Test knee ligaments for drawer sign

Technique of Examination of the Extremities

Observe for spontaneous activity or in response to stimulation inspect the limbs for
- Symmetry in lengths of arms and of legs
- Symmetry in circumferences of arms and of legs
  - Symmetry of muscle mass
  - Evidence of muscular or vascular anomalies
- Proportion of limb-to-trunk lengths
- Presence of contractures or abnormal webbing
- Symmetry and size of hands and feet
- Proportion of each hand and foot to the rest of the extremity
- Number, size, and symmetry of fingers and toes
- Presence and appearance of fingernails and toenails
- Distribution of the palmar and plantar creases
  a. Measure any regions that appear disproportionate or asymmetric, using a specific anatomic landmark to define the site of measurement.
  b. Determine range of motion across the joints in any areas that appear abnormal.
  c. Feel and compare the pulses.
  d. Palpate for tenderness, fluctuation, and temperature changes in areas of discoloration or swelling.
  e. Palpate for hip stability.
  f. Palpate for symmetry, tenderness, crepitation, or swelling along the clavicles.
  g. If not already completed as part of the regional trunk examination, examine the spine for integrity, mobility, and the presence of any overlying cutaneous lesions or subcutaneous masses.
  h. Examine the joints.

DISORDERS OF THE DEVELOPING MOTOR SYSTEM ON ALL LEVELS, LEADING TO IMMOBILIZATION AND ARTHROGRYPOSIS MULTIPLEXA CONGENITA (AMC)

The term AMC refers to multiple joint contractures present at birth. AMC is not a specific disorder but is the consequence of neurologic, muscular, connective tissue and skeletal abnormalities or intrauterine crowding, which may lead to limitation of fetal joint mobility and the development of contractures. The following is the list of conditions associated with AMC.
1. Disorders of the developing neuromuscular system
   - Loss of anterior horn cells

- Radicular disease with collagen proliferation
- Peripheral neuropathy with neurofibromatosis
- Congenital myasthenia
- Neonatal myasthenia (maternal myasthenia gravis)
- Amyoplasia congenita
- Congenital muscular dystrophy
- Central core disease
- Congenital myotonic dystrophy
- Glycogen accumulation myopathy
2. Disorders of developing connective tissue or connective tissue disease
3. Muscular and articular connective tissue dystrophy
4. Articular defects by mesenchymal dysplasia
5. Increased collagen synthesis
6. Disorders of developing medulla or medullar disease
   - Congenital spinal epidural hemorrhage
   - Congenital duplication of the spinal canal
7. Disorders of brain development (e.g. porencephaly) or brain disease (e.g. congenital encephalopathy)

DIFFERENTIAL DIAGNOSIS OF A LIMP IN CHILDHOOD (Fig. 28.22)

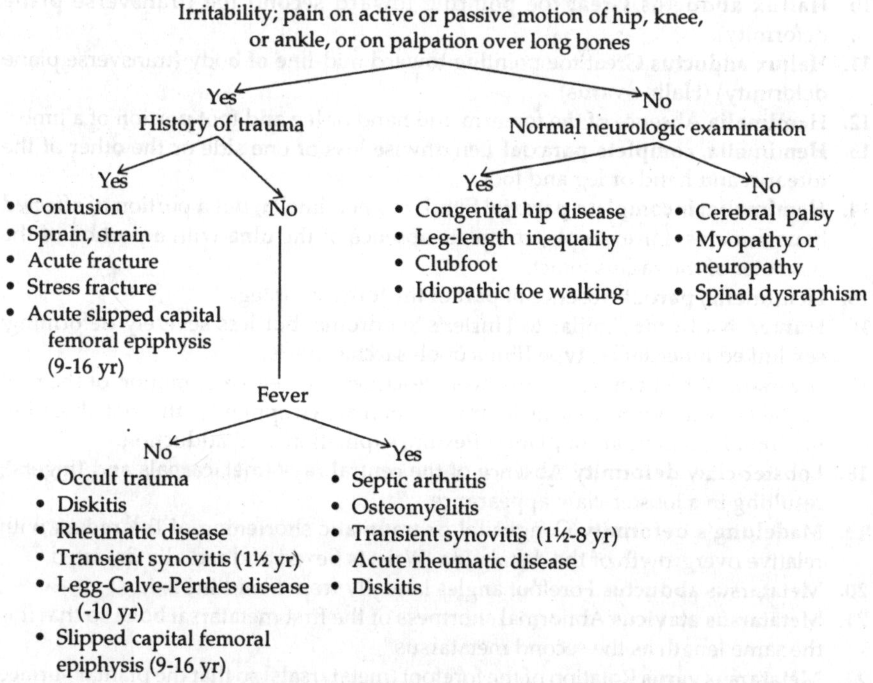

Irritability; pain on active or passive motion of hip, knee,
or ankle, or on palpation over long bones

Yes ← → No

History of trauma   Normal neurologic examination

Yes → No   Yes → No

- Contusion
- Sprain, strain
- Acute fracture
- Stress fracture
- Acute slipped capital femoral epiphysis (9-16 yr)

- Congenital hip disease
- Leg-length inequality
- Clubfoot
- Idiopathic toe walking

- Cerebral palsy
- Myopathy or neuropathy
- Spinal dysraphism

Fever

No ← → Yes

- Occult trauma
- Diskitis
- Rheumatic disease
- Transient synovitis (1½ yr)
- Legg-Calve-Perthes disease (-10 yr)
- Slipped capital femoral epiphysis (9-16 yr)

- Septic arthritis
- Osteomyelitis
- Transient synovitis (1½-8 yr)
- Acute rheumatic disease
- Diskitis

Fig. 28.22: Differential diagnosis of a limp in childhood

TERMINOLOGY

The following are the few terms used in evaluation of musculoskeletal disorders.
1. **Apodia** Absence of the foot
2. **Arthrogryposis** Persistent flexure or contracture of a joint; usually related to a congenital neuromuscular disorder.

3. **Camptodactyly** Bent finger; commonly referred to as a congenital flexion deformity of the proximal interphalnageal joint, usually of the little finger. It is associated with some syndromes involving multiple pterygia or trismus but is most often a minor variant that is inherited as an autosomal-dominant disorder.

4. **Clubfoot** Foot deformity resulting in the appearance of a golf club. The components include forefoot adduction with medial displacement of the talus, ankle equinus, and heel varus. The result is that the foot turns in with the heel pulled medially.

5. **Coxa valga** Hip deformity in which the angle of the axis of the head and neck of the femur and the axis of its shaft (neck shaft angle) is increased.

6. **Coxa vara** Reduced neck and shaft angle, usually caused by failure of normal bone growth; coxa adducta.

7. **Genu valgum** Synonym knock-knee. Deformity in which knees are close together, with ankle space increased. Even though valgum would indicate bending away from the midline, the valgum refers to the distal portion, which, when the knees are bowed in, forces the ankles away from the mid-line.

8. **Genu varum** Deformity in which knees are bowed out and ankles are close in; may be associated with internal tibial torsion (ITT).

9. **Genu recurvtum** Ability of the knee to bend backward; caused by trauma, prolonged intrauterine pressure, or general joint laxity.

10. **Hallux abductus** Great toe pointing toward second toe (transverse plane deformity).

11. **Hallux adductus** Great toe pointing toward mid-line of body (transverse plane deformity) (Hallux varus).

12. **Hemimelia** Absence of the forearm and hand or leg and foot portion of a limb.

13. **Hemimelia, complete paraxial** Lengthwise loss of one side or the other of the forearm and hand or leg and foot.

14. **Hemimelia, incomplete paraxial** Similar to hemimelia, but a portion of affected bone remains, for example, complete absence of the ulna with a portion of the diameter of the radius intact.

15. **Hemimelia, partial** Absence of part of the forearm or leg.

16. **Hunter syndrome** Similar to Hurler's syndrome, but less severely deforming; sex-linked inheritance; type II mucopolysaccharidosis.

17. **Inversion** When applied to the heel, describes the degree of motion of the heel pushed inward with ankle in neutral position; when applied to the foot, describes the combined motions of plantar flexion, supination, and adduction.

18. **Lobster-claw deformity** Absence of the central rays (metacarpals and fingers), resulting in a lobster-claw appearance.

19. **Madelung's deformity** Congenital or traumatic shortening of the radius with relative overgrowth of the distal ulna. Wrist is flexed and radially deviated.

20. **Metatarsus abductus** Forefoot angles laterally from a midline axis.

21. **Metatarsus atavicus** Abnormal shortness of the first metatarsal bone so that it is the same length as the second metatarsus.

22. **Metatarsus varus** Rotation of the forefoot (metatarsals) so that the plantar surface faces medially.

23. **Phocomelia complete** Presence of only a hand or foot.

24. **Phocomelia, distal** Hand directly attached to upper arm; or foot directly attached to thigh.

25. **Phocomelia, proximal** Presence of hand and forearm with absence of upper arm, or leg and foot with absence of thigh.

26. **Poland syndrome** Absence of the pectoral head of the pectoralis major muscles associated with the deformities in the thumb ray or fingers. Simple absence of a portion of the pectoralis muscle is more common and functionally unimportant. The absence causes loss of an anterior axillary fold and cephalad positioning of the nipple.

27. **Polydactyly** Congenital deformity, excess number of digits. It is most commonly postaxial, occurring on the ulnar side of the fifth digit (postminimus polydactyly). Tends to be hereditary.

28. **Postaxial** A position relating to embryologic development of the caudad portion of an extremity, thus including the third through fifth fingers; the ulnar side. On the lower extremity because of opposite rotation in human, the postaxial structures include the third through fifth toes; the fibular side.

29. **Preaxial** A position relating to embryologic development of the cephalad portion of an extremity, thus including the thumb and index finger; the radial side. On the lower extremity because of opposite rotation in human, the preaxial structures include the great and first toes; the tibial side.

30. **Rocker-bottom flatfoot, congenital** *Synonyms* Congenital vertical talus, congenital convex pes valgus. Condition present at birth; abnormal equinus position of talus with valgus position of the heel, resulting in a foot that looks like a rocker and has a prominence below the medial ankle.

31. **Rocker-bottom foot** Deformity of the foot such that the arch is disrupted and looks like a rocker bottom. This may be a complication of clubfoot treatment or myelomeningocele.

32. **Syndactyly** Fusion of two or more fingers in which there may be involvement of soft tissue only (simple) or the may include a fusion of bone or cartilage (complex). It is found most often between the second and third toes and the third and fourth fingers. It occurs as an isolated defect or as part of syndromes (deLange, Smith-Lemli-Optiz or Poland anomaly). Complete syndactyly occurs in Apert's syndrome.

33. **Talipes calcaneovalgus** Abnormally dorsiflexed hindfoot with turning out of the heel.

34. **Talipes equinovarus** Turning of the heel inward with increased plantar flexion. More precisely, a clubfoot, often having the components of talipes equinovarus with metatarsus adductus. This condition can result from paralysis or from unknown causes.

35. **Valgus** The distal part is away from the mid-line, e.g. genu valgus (knock-knee) (Fig. 28.23A).

36. **Varus** The distal part is toward the mid-line, e.g. genu varus (bowlegged) (Fig. 28.23B).

OUTLINE OF MUSCULOSKELETAL SYSTEM EXAMINATION

In a patient presenting with musculoskeletal abnormality, the following points on history and examination must be noted.

History

Age

Remember certain diseases common in different age groups.

Sex

Remember certain diseases common in males and females.

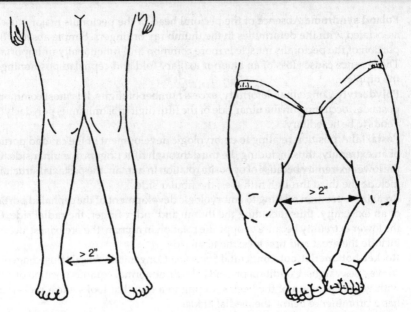

Figs 28.23A and B: (A) Genu valgum (knock-knee), and (B) genu varum (bowleg)

Chief Complaints

a. *Pain*
   i. *Onset*—Acute, insidious, following trauma.
   ii. *Character*—Dull aching, throbbing
   iii. *Site*—Bones, joints, muscle, tendinous attachments of (remember referred pain).
   iv. *Relieving and aggravating factors*—Sleep, (night cry), rest, movement, drugs (aspirin, steroids).

b. *Joints involved*
   i. *Number of joints*-Mono/pauci/polyarticular
   ii. *Types of joint*-Major/small/unusual joints.

c. *Any abnormal movements*
   i. Restricted/absent/increased range.
   ii. Movement in abnormal direction
   iii. Abnormal gait
   iv. Involuntary movement/features of myotonia

d. *Change in skeletal contour*
   i. Short stature/long stature
   ii. Deformity
   iii. Swelling

e. *Miscellaneous* Joint locking, weakness, wasting, fatigue, fracture following trivial trauma, etc.

Past History

History of trauma, TB, osteomyelitis, surgery on bones/joints, chronic illness (example CRF).

Family History
i. Bleeding tendency (Hemophilia).
ii. Bony deformities (Resistant rickets, osteogenesis imperfecta, DDH, CTEV, scoliosis)
iii. Arthritis (Gout, anklosing spondylitis)

Birth and Developmental History
i. History of reduced fetal movements, prematurity, perinatal asphyxia, weak cry, poor suck (myopathy)
ii. Abnormal presentation, large baby, birth injury (fracture, nerve damage)
iii. Delayed motor milestones.

Examination
- Gait
- General physical Examination
- Local examination (Muscles, bones and joints).
- Functional assessment
- Systemic examination

Gait
Note any abnormal gait as the patient walks into the examination room.

General Physical Examination

a. *Vital signs*   Signs of inadequate peripheral perfusion (pulse, BP, capillary refill time, temperature)

b. *Anthropometry*   Length/height
Upper segment /lower segment
Arm span/height
Length of proximal (rhizo), middle (meso) and distal (Acro) segments of limit.

c. *Head to toe examination*
i. *Eyes* Blue sclera, conjunctivitis, iridocyclitis, phlycten, cataract, retinopathy.
ii. *Skin* Rash, cutaneous bleeds, draining sinuses, tight skin, subcutaneous, nodules
iii. *Nails* Clubbing, splinter hemorrhages, pitting, nail bed telangiectasia.
iv. *Mucosal lesions* Mucosal bleeding, enlarged, bleeding gums.
v. *Lymphadenopathy*

Local Examination

a. *Examination of Muscles*
i. Inspection   : Absence, wasting, hypertrophy of muscles
Any involuntary movements.
ii. Palpation   : Firm, flabby, spastic, hand, tender and indurated
iii. Percussion   : Myotonia, DTR.
iv. Auscultation   : Crepitus
v. Power   : Note the strength of each muscle and each muscle group that carries out a particular movement.

b. *Examination of bones and joints*
i. Inspection   – *Attitude and deformity*—Inspect the skeleton and extremities for symmetry, alignment, skinfolds, any gross deformity.

	– *Swelling* in relation to bones and joints
	– *Skin*-redness, early miosis, edema, sinus.
ii. Palpation	– Bones, joints, tendon and surrounding muscles should be systematically palpated for, tendernesss, swelling, ulcer, sinus, crepitus.
iii. Movements	– Movements should be compared on either side
	– Active and passive movements
	– Movements against gravity and resistance
	– Range of movement in each direction
	– Any pain or crepitus during movements
	– Any movement in abnormal direction
iv. Measurements	– Circumference of the limbs
	– Length (US:LS, arm span height, limb length)
v. Percussion	– Note any tenderness
vi. Auscultation	– Note any crepitus

Examination of Individual Joints

Temperomandibular Joint

Inspection	: Swelling infront of tragus
Palpation	: Tenderness, crepitus, clicking
Movement	: Jaw opening, closure, side to side movement, protrusion and retraction

Percussion and Auscultation

Neck and Back

Inspection	: Attitude and deformity, alignment, symmetry of skin folds.
Palpation	: Tenderness (Spine, sacroiliac joint),
	Swelling (cold abscess, meningomyelocele), etc.
Movement	: *Neck*-Flexion, extension, lateral bending, rotation
	: *Thoracolumbar region* Flexion, extension, lateral flexion, rotation
	: *Costo-vertebral joints* Degree of chest expansion.

Percussion and auscultation

Neurological examination— Paraplegia, sensory deficit, bowel and bladder involvement.

Shoulder Joint

Inspection	: Attitude, deformity, contour of shoulder
Palpation	: Swelling, tenderness
Movements	: Flexion, extension, abduction, adduction, rotation
Measurements	: Circumference of the arm, length of arm.

Percussion and auscultation

Elbow Joint

Inspection	: Attitude, deformity, carrying angle, swelling.
Palpation	: Swelling, tenderness, crepitus.
Movements	: Flexion, extension, pronation, supination.
Measurements	: Circumference of arm and forearm Length of arm and forearm

Percussion and auscultation

Wrist Joint

Inspection	: Attitude, swelling
Palpation	: Tenderness, crepitus
Movements	: Flexion, extension, adduction, abduction
Measurements	: Circumference of forearm, length of forearm.

Percussion and auscultation

Hand

Inspection : *Size*—Small, large, asymmetric, swollen hands.
Shape—Any shape abnormality.
Finger anomalies—Polydactyly, syndactyly, etc.
Nails—Any nail anomalies.
Surface—Color (pallor, dusky, blue, yellow)
Rashes, skin bleeds, papules, nodules, pustules, etc.
Raynauds phenomena
Dermatoglyphics

Palpation : Hand shake, sensation over the hand, tenderness, swelling

Movements : Flexion, extension, adduction, abduction, any involuntary movements, handedness.

Percussion and auscultation

Hip Joint

Inspection : Attitude in weight bearing and non-weight bearing postures
Trendelenburg's test (Fig. 28.24)
Any fixed deformity
Galeazzi's sign (in DDH)

Palpation : Tenderness, swelling, vascular sign of Narath (hip dislocation)

Movements : Flexion, extension, adduction, abduction, rotation.

Tests for hip stability (in DDH) : Telescopic test, Ortolani's test, Barlow's test.

Measurements : Thigh circumference, length of lower limb and thigh.

Percussion and Auscultation

Knee Joint

Inspection	: Attitude, deformity, swelling
Palpation	: Swelling, tenderness
Movements	: Flexion, extension, adduction, abduction, rotation.
Test for knee stability	: Adduction and abduction test, Drawer's test, Apley's grinding test.
Measurements	: Circumference of thigh and leg. Length of lower limb.

Percussion and Auscultation

Ankle and Foot

Inspection	: Attitude and deformity, swelling
Palpation	: Tenderness, irregularity, unusual mobility, crepitus, swelling
Movements	: Dorsiflexion, Plantar flexion, inversion, eversion, forefoot adduction, forefoot abduction, flexion and extension of toes.
Measurements	:

Percussion and auscultation

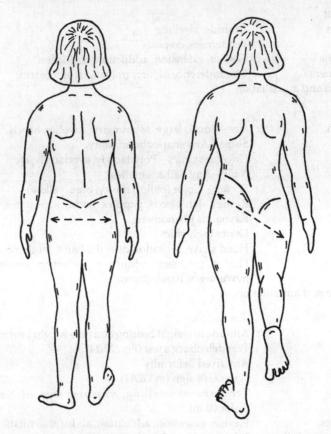

Fig. 28.24: Trendelenburg sign. When standing on affected side normal side drops

FUNCTIONAL ASSESSMENT (Activities of daily living)
Useful in following up of patients with chronic musculoskeletal problems.

Systemic Examination
- CNS
- CVS
- RS
- PA

CHAPTER 29 Development—Its Assessment and Different Aspects

INTRODUCTION

Growth and Development comprise the basic science in the field of Pediatrics. Pediatricians owe responsibility for care of the child and should thus be familiar with the methods of study and assessment of growth, their normal patterns and milestones of normal development, thus enabling them to recognize any deviations from norm at the earliest. Thus, a careful developmental history should enable us to detect deficiencies or disorders and to give appropriate and timely attention and care.

Growth and development are sometimes used interchangeably. But growth implies increase in size of organs and body and development implies differentiation and maturation of function. The former indicates quantitative growth and the latter indicates qualitative growth. Development is influenced by the physical, emotional and social environment. In early childhood, congnitive growth and development are difficult to differentiate from neurologic and behavioral maturation. In later childhood, it can be measured by communicative skills and cognitive abilities.

The development of each child is unique and the pattern of development may be profoundly different for each child within the broad limits of 'normality'.

Factors Affecting Child Development

Growth and development constitute a continuous process from fertilization till maturity. Besides genetic factors, growth is influenced by nutrition, illness, social, economic and psychological environment.

Various factors determining the development of the child are detailed below.

Genetic Factors

Even though genetic factors are thought to be biologic and of utmost importance, they are intimately inter-woven with the environment.

Physical Factors

Prenatal as well as postnatal physical insults affect growth and development.

Nutritional Factors

Nutritional factors influence growth and development. Chronic malnutrition causes stunting of physical growth. Prental and early postnatal malnutrition affects development and reduces the ability of the individual to adapt to the environment.

Emotional Factors
Emotional factors like position of the child in the family, the child rearing practices in the family and community, etc. affect growth and development.

Socio-cultural Factors
Socio-cultural factors either limit or expand the range of behavior of children. The schedule for acquisition of skills, such as sitting, walking, etc. which were earlier thought to be the result of maturation alone are now found to be influenced by the conventional expectations. Socio-economic factors are also reflected in the nutritional status of the child.

Interaction between Various Factors and Child Development
There is an interplay between genetic, nutritional and environmental factors that influence growth, development and intelligence. However, the contribution of each of them is difficult to separate and evaluate. The effect of malnutrition in reducing the intellectual achievement is so difficult to separate from other associated retarding social and environmental factors. Genetic endowment, nutrition and environment are the important determinants of the overall development. Some claim that genetic factors accounted for 80 percent of development and only 20 per cent is accounted by the other factors. But some others are of the opinion that this is an underestimate of the other factors. The child's ultimate intelligence is the result of the interaction between host, nutrition and environment.

Tests for Developmental Assessment
Maturity, behaviour and mental functions can be evaluated by the assessment of development and intelligence. The neurodevelopmental status of children should be assessed in order to understand the deviation, impairment or retardation and to plan appropriate recommendations and interventions. Observation based on casual examination should be interpreted with caution because a child who is irritable, hungry, sleepy or ill, does not perform at his or her expected level. A future examination may be needed in such children. For infants born prematurely, the developmental level may be compared to 'corrected chronological age' during the first two years of life.

The role of developmental assessment is to understand, whether the child is progressing as per norms set by large majority of children of the same age group. However, it is not a predictor of future IQ and any deviation from normal should be brought to the notice of the parents in reassuring way. The developmental tests mainly measure maturity and behaviour in four functional areas namely gross motor, fine motor, adaptive, language and personal-social. The four functional areas are closely related and overlapping. But in defective development, they show some dissociation. A child may be advanced in one area and retarded in the other. Thus, each function must be evaluated separately. A battery of developmental tests are available.

The Denver Developmental Screening Test (DDST)

The DDST was originally designed as a screening test (Frankenburg, 1967). It is now being increasingly used as a tool for routine developmental assessment (Glascoe, 1992). The Denver developmental reference chart is suitable for quick assessment of all the four areas of development in children from birth to 6 years of age (Frankenburg, 1981). This will take 10-30 minutes only.

The DDST meets most of the required criteria for an ideal screening test and is widely used\for population screening. The test is mainly concerned with the measurement of attainment of various milestones. The scale has 15 items including all 4 parameters-personal-social, finemotor-adaptive, language, gross motor. The milestones are shown in graphic from. It has a line interesting 4 areas of development and the chronogical age is mentioned in each line. The items through which the chronological age line passes are tested. The scale provides 25th, 50th, 75th and 90th centiles for all the items. Failure to perform a test passed by 90th percentile of child is considered significant.

The original DDST was criticized for under identification of developmental disability especially in the area of language. The revised DDST-II has greater sensitivity particularly for language delays.

Gesell's Developmental Schedule

This measures the four functional areas of development (i.e. motor, adaptive, language, and personal-social) in children beween 0-5 years of age. It will take 30-40 minutes. It is more concerned with the diagnosis and evaluation of abnormalities than the attainment of various milestones (Gesell *et al*, 1962). For quick assessment, Gessel has provided the concept of key areas, which are the basic stages of maturity like 4, 16, 28, 40 weeks, 12, 18, 30 months respectively. It is necessary to test the child in two adjacent age levels, while assessing at their key ages. On the basis of the performance, a child may be said to be normal, retarded or accelerated in development with respect to chronological age. The scale provides an estimation of developmental quotient (DQ) for each area separately and also for the overall DQ. The formula is as follows:

$$DQ = \frac{\text{Maturity Age}}{\text{Chronological Age}} \times 100$$

A child having DQ between 65-75 is considered at risk of developmental delay. This test has clinical diagnostic orientation and is a more satisfactorily clinical screening test.

Bayley Scale of Infant Development (BSID)

This scale provides the motor scale, the mental scale and the infant behavior record in children 2 to 30 months of age. An overall development index is based upon the combined scores on the motor and mental scales. It takes approximately 30-60 minutes (Bayley, 1969). This scale provides 3 complementary scales for assessing the developmental status of children (in motor, mental and infant behavior). This test has been standardised by Phatak (Baroda scale) which further has been simplified by MKC Nair *et al* at Trivandrum (Trivandrum Development Scale TDSC).

Availability of the Kit The kits and manuals are available from Psychological Corporation, New York, USA or through their Indian agents—Anand Agencies, 1433. A Shukrasarpeth, Pune-411002.

Advantages
a. Bayley scale is the only developmental assessment tool for babies less than 30 months of age which is standardised for Indian population.
b. Bayley scale gives an objective score for mental and motor performances and hence most appropriate for research purposes.
c. Raw score can be converted to percentile performance position and hence appropriate for comparing wide range of performance.

Disadvantages
a. The Bayley sample is drawn from a population of normal children and hence there are problems for using the scale among abnormal babies.
b. Babies with problem may perform at lower levels because many of the mental items are closely interlinked with motor capability.

Baroda Developmental Screening Test
This is a screening test based on BSID, Baroda norms (Phatak *et al*, 1984). The Baroda norms were standardized on Indian children. An abbreviated BSID is also available for follow up of high risk neonates (Phatak, 1990).

Trivandrum Developmental Screening Chart (TDSC) (Fig. 29.1)
Based on 17 selected items from BSID Baroda norms, the test was designed in the Child Development Centre, SAT Hospital, Trivandrum for children upto 24 months of age. This simple tool can be administered and interpreted by any person with minimal training. It takes 5 to 7 minutes only (Nair *et al* 1991).

This is a simple developmental screening chart designed and validated at the child development centre, and is being used in large scale community developmental screening programs using anganwadi workers. There are 17 test items in the chart, carefully chosen after repeated trial and error method. The range of each test item is taken from the norms given in the Bayley Scales of Infant Development. The left hand side of each horizontal dark line represents the age at which 3 percent of children passed the item and the right end represents the age at which 97 percent of the children passed the item in the Baroda sample. A ventrical line is drawn or a pencil is kept vertically at the level of the chronological age of the child being tested. If the child fails to achieve any item that falls short on the left side of the vertical line, the child is considered to have a developmental delay. Any obvious abnormality or asymmetry is also considered abnormal.

TDSC is a simple tool that can be administered by anganwadi workers or any person with minimal training. It was validated both at the hospital and community level against the standard DDST. Among the 17 tests, items for testing hearing and vision are also included. This is a developmental assessment in a community setting.

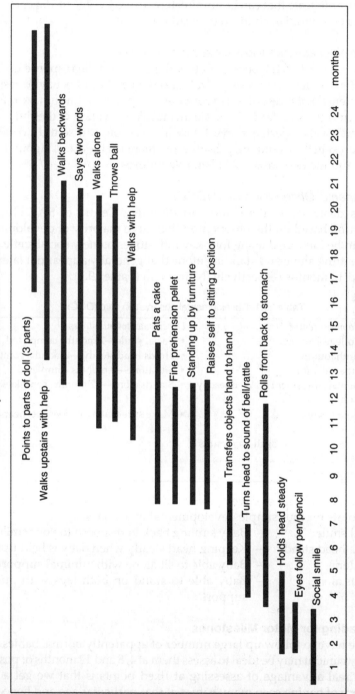

DEVELOPMENT CARD

Make sure your child sees, hears and listens

Note: To use this chart, keep a pencil vertically on the age of the child. All milestones falling to the left of the pencil should have been achieved by the child.

Based on BSID Baroda norms and Trivandrum Developmental Screening Chart (TDSC).

Fig. 29.1: Development card

Developmental Screening Test
This is a simple scale that can be administered upto the age of 15 years. It was standardized on Indian children (Bharathraj, 1983).

Brazelton Neonatal Behavioural Assessment Scale
This scale is based on the observation of the baby and the response to 20 primitive reflexes (Brazelton, 1981). Evaluates the newborn's behavior response on these items. Each response is scored on a 9 point continuum. A rating of 5 mid point is the standard. The scale includes observation of the child, when asleep and awake, alertness, eye following, response to sound, irritability, social interest in the examiner, passive movements of the arms, vigour, tremulousness and the response to 20 primitive reflexes.

Developmental Observation Card (DOC)
This was designed in the Child Development Centre of SAT Hospital, Trivandrum, based on the observation that large majority of developmental delays can be identified using four key milestones namely social smile, head holding, sitting alone and standing alone that generally appear not later than 2, 4, 8 and 12 months respectively (Nair, 1992) (Table 29.1).

Table 29.1: Developmental observation card (DOC)

Child development centre	*Developmental milestones*
Medical College Campus	• Social smile—2 months completed
Thiruvananthapuram	• Holds head steady—4 months completed
Bring the baby for	• Sits alone—8 months completed
Developmental assessment on Wednesday	• Stands alone—12 months completed
at 9 AM	
Appointment (Date)..................	• Make sure that baby does see, hear and listen.

	At birth	4 months
Weight	....	....
Head circumference	....	....

The large majority of developmental delays could be identified by using cut off points for four simple developmental milestones.
1. Social smile   — Baby smiling back in response to your smile.
2. Holds head steady — Keeping head steady when baby is held upright.
3. Sits alone   — Baby able to sit alone with minimal support.
4. Stands alone   — Baby able to stand on both legs with minimal support.

CDC Grading for Motor Milestones
When we have to follow up large number of apparently normal babies in the well baby clinic, it may be ideal to assess them at 4, 8 and 12 months of postnatal life. The real advantage of assessing at fixed points is that we get a lot of experience of having seen many babies at that particular age and hence get a mental impression of normal, and delay. It is even more advantageous to have

grading of three important motor mile stones so that we can objectively record the developmental status as well as communicate with each other better. The grading for head holding, sitting and standing developed at the Child Development Centre (CDC), Medical College, Trivandrum, is given below:

Head Holding

Grade 0 : No head holding at all
Grade 1 : Head erect and steady momentarily
Grade 2 : Supine-lifts head when pulled up by arms
Grade 3 : Prone-elevates self by arms
Grade 4 : Holds head steady when moved around
Grade 5 : Head balanced always.

Setting

Grade 0 : Not sitting at all
Grade 1 : Sits momentarily
Grade 2 : Sits 30 seconds or more leaning forward
Grade 3 : Sits with the child's back straight
Grade 4 : While sitting can manipulate a toy
Grade 5 : Self raises to sitting position.

Standing

Grade 0 : Not standing at all
Grade 1 : Stand holding a furniture momentarily
Grade 2 : Take few steps both hands held
Grade 3 : Without support, stand alone (legs apart)
Grade 4 : Stands himself, up by throwing weight on arms
Grade 5 : Without support takes few steps.

Although it would be ideal to have a follow up at completed 2 months (social smile), 4 months (head holding), 8 months (sitting) and 12 months (standing), every baby should have atleast one developmental assessment at completed four months which may be coupled with 2nd or 3rd dose of DPT and polio vaccine.

Grades 0, 1 and 2 are to be considered definitely abnormal and need a detailed neurodevelopmental evaluation. Grades 3, 4 and 5 are considered normal and do not require any further followup routinely. If a baby has apparently Grade 3 head holding (only lifting head without raising on arms) without Grade 2, this is to be considered abnormal, because this may be due to neck extensor hypertonia. Occasionally, it may be possible that Grade 4 standing is achieved before the child is able to stand alone and this need not be considered abnormal.

However, these developmental tests have very low predictive value regarding future IQ and have several limitations. The cross cultural use of these scales is also not often ideal. Indian children have motor skills ahead of others. But the language and personal-social skills are often behind. Developmental assessment furnishes information on the stage of development and gives the parents a chance to perceive in what stage the child is and the degree of retardation if there is any. But the selection of the test is very important.

Assessment of Intelligence

This is generally done in children above three years of age. Intelligence tests measure several brain functions including auditory, memory, visual-spatial capability and receptive and expressive language. The Intelligence Quotient (IQ) is computed usign the following formula:

$$\frac{\text{Mental age}}{\text{Chronological age}} \times 100$$

The calculated IQ is an average of various mental functions measured. Stanford Binet, who designed the first IQ test did not intend it as a measure of congnitive ability, but as a simple tool to predict school performance. IQ may not reflect the optimal cerebral function or potential of the individual. It is insensitive to the adverse effects of socio-cultural and environmental factors that affect the potential. Adaptations to the environment, social skills, etc. also adaptation in the community, both vocationally and socially. In spite of all the limitations, IQ remains the major diagnostic criterion used to deal with the retraded children. The levels of intellectual retardation according to IQ are given in the Table 29.2.

Table 29.2: Showing various levels of retardation—according to IQ

Level of retardation	IQ	Remarks
Borderline/average	70-85	Vulnerable to educational problems
Mild/educable	50-69	Often need special classes
Moderate/trainable	35-49	Trainable in workshop setting
Severe	20-34	Trainable for self care skills
Profound	< 20	Need custodian care.

These IQ ranges are based on the American Association on Mental Deficiency (AAMD) terminology and classification and the American Psychiatric Society Diagnostic and Statistical Manual III (DSM III). According to the WHO International Classification of Disease (ICD), Borderline retardation is not included.

Even the retarded children should be given stimulation and educational services either in regular classes with extra resources or in special classes. Education does not mean studying academic subjects alone, but also means learning self care activities and social skills. The various available intelligence tests are detailed below.

Stanford Binet Intelligence Scale

This takes into account verbal ability, perceptual skills, short-term memory, and hand and eye co-ordination. It takes 45-60 minutes (Terman *et al*, 1937). This test provides an estimate of basal age, mental age and intelligence quotient (IQ). This test has also certain limitations as it is crosscultural and the items are mainly dependent on formal schooling. An Indian adaptation by Kulshreshta and Kamat is available. Age range is 2 years to adult.

Binet Kamat Test

This is an Indian adaptation of the Stanford Binet scale (Kamat, 1967). This is also available in Hindi (Kulshrestha, 1971).

Wechsler Intelligence Scale for Children (WISC)

This is an Indian adaptation of WISC. Since the items are mostly influenced by formal schooling system, it may not give the real capabilities in non-school going children (Wechsler, 1949).

Wechsler Intelligence Scale for Children—revised

This has an age range of 5-15 years. Time taken is approximately 45-60 mintues. The IQ obtained from the Wechsler scale is viewed as a measure of the child's general ability compared with other children of similar age. This scale has two large subsections—verbal and performance, each consisting of several subjects. An Indian adaptation of this test in the verbal part as well as a few performance scales (e.g. Codign), is available but is highly loaded with items influenced by formal schooling systems. Hence, its use is not proper in non-schoolgoing urban low socio-economic and rural children, as it will not give a real picture of their capabilities (Table 29.3).

Table 29.3: Different WISC subscales with respect to different type of abilities

Scales	Ability
Verbal	
Information	Ability to retain and utilise general knowledge
Comprehension	Ability to reason about social situations
Arithmetic	Numerical ability
	Simple mental arithmetic problems
Similarities	A test of classification and abstract reasoning
Vocabulary	Definition of word meanings
Performance	
Picture completion	Visual scanning of pictures in order to discover the piece that is missing
Picture arrangement	Re-arrangement of a series of picture cards into a logical sequence to tell a story
Block design	Analysis of visually presented patterns and their reproduction by use of colored blocks
Object assembly	Perceptual reasoning
	Requires construction of a carboard forms (e.g. manikin, horse, etc) from its constitutent parts
Cording	Speed of thought and perceptuo-motor functioning.

Malin Intelligence Scale for Indian Children

This is an Indian adaptation of WISC. Since the items are mostly influenced by formal schooling system, it may not give the real capabilities in non-school going children (Malin, 1969).

Goodenough's Draw-A-Man Test for Indian Children

This is a paper pencil test for children between 3-15 years of age. The child is asked to draw a man. There is no time limit. The child is asked to draw a man and he/she receives 1 point for each of the items present in the drawing. For each 4 points, 1 year is added to the basal age of 3 (Fig. 29.2) (Phatak, 1987). Thus, if a child drawing shows that 9 items are present, he scores 9 point and his mental age score is 5.5 years. This provides an estimate of IQ which can be calcualted as: IQ = Mental Age/Chronological Age × 100. In India, Phatak has made a modification of this test. It provides age norms for ages 4-15 years in the form of average standard scores, education, IQ's and their percentiles (Fig. 29.2).

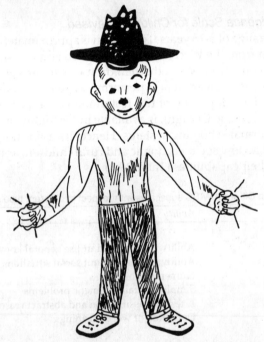

Fig. 29.2: Goodenough draw-a-man test (e.g. A 7-year 5 months old child can be able to draw the above given figure)

Tests of Cognitive Functions

Based on Piaget's theory of intellectual development, cognitive functions can be measured in four major stages of development namely, sensori-motor stage (0-2 years), preoperational stage (2-7 years), concrete operational stage (7-11 years) and formal operational stage (above 11 years). The cognitive development of Indian children has been shown to follow a similar pattern. However, this is not an estimate of IQ.

Intelligence tests when culturally appropriate, measure major cognitive and mental abilities. The Indian modification of WISC, Stanford Binet test, Draw-a-man test, etc. are suitable for Indian children. Nutritional status, socioeconomic factors, and maternal IQ, etc. have been found to influence growth, development and intelligence. Malnutrition and other retarding environmental variables also adversely influence the cognitive development and school performance.

Developmental Milestones

During eliciting the developmental history one should ask for the following points and should be recorded.

- Gestational age — For preterm babies use corrected age. A baby born at 32 weeks of gestation brought in one month after birth should be considered as at 36 weeks of gestation.
- Birth weight
- Weight chart
- Dentition
- Milestones-Compare with siblings
- Toilet training
- School performance
- Interaction with peers and adults
- Participation in organised activity.

Principles of Development

1. Development is due to maturation of brain.
2. Craniocaudal progression of achievements of milestones.
3. Gross motor functions are replaced by fine motor function.
4. Reflex activities are replaced by voluntary activities.
5. Normal variations are common.
6. Critical age for development of a particular milestone. Any amount of stimulation cannot make it appear earlier.
7. Girls are faster in language development.
8. Children in developing countries are rather faster in attainment of milestones.
9. For proper development, normal sensory inputs, normal brain and a stimulating and encouraging atmosphere are important.

Some Peculiarities

1. Some children do not roll over but directly sit.
2. Some children do not crawl but hop.
3. Crawling and creeping should be differentiated. Crawling is bear walking on all four limbs that comes around 9-10 months, whereas creeping is swimming along the floor that comes around 4 months of age.

Developmental milestones: Features of neurodegenerative disorders are regression of attained milestones and failure to attain new milestones.

1. Predominant gray matter disorders are characterised by
   — Dementia, fits, blindness and later motor.
2. Predominant white matter disorders are characterised by
   — Motor delay, gait disturbances and later mental retardation and fits.

Differential Development

a. *Predominant speech delay*
   - Familial
   - Emotional deprivation
   - Twins
   - Mental retardation
   - Cerebral palsy
   - Left handedness
   - Aphasia
   - Hearing loss (monoaural or binaural)
   - Infantile autism
   - Fragile X syndrome.

b. *Predominant motor delay*
   - Individual variation
   - Familial variation
   - Rickets
   - Protein energy malnutrition
   - Werdnig-Hoffmann's syndrome
   - Prader-Willi syndrome
   - Chronic illness
   - Congenital dislocation of hip
   - Cerebral palsy
   - Hypotonic child
   - Ataxia
   - Hemiplegia
   - Paraplegia.

c. *Definitive handedness before 3 years of age*
   - Weakness on the other side

d. *Early advanced social development*
   - It is seen in Down's syndrome but does not persist beyond infancy.

e. *Delayed visual maturation or lack of eye to eye contact*
   - Mental retardation
   - Autism
   - Infantile spasms

f. *Global delay*
   - Cerebral malformations
   - Chromosomal anomalies
   - Intrauterine infection
   - Perinatal disorders.
   - Progressive encephalopathy.

g. *Advanced head control, rolling over and bearing weight*
   - Spastic cerebral palsy.

h. *Delayed sphincter control*
   - Familial factors
   - Mental subnormality
   - Psychological factors
   - Bad toilet training
   - Organic diseases of spine, CNS and urinary system

i. *Delayed reading*
- Emotional and environmental factors
- Delayed maturation
- Poor teaching
- Visual, auditory, spatial difficulties
- Genetic factors

j. *Early signs of cerebral palsy (development peculiarities)*
- Advanced head control due to spasticity
- Advanced rolling over due to spasticity
- Advanced bearing weight on legs-Dealange's sign
- No progression of disease
- Others-excessive crying, feeding difficulty and handling difficulty.

k. The most sensitive early maker of mental retardation is language development.

l. *Developmental milestones*—features of neurodegenerative disorders.
   The important features of neurodegenerative disorder is regression of attained milestones and failure to attain milestones.
- Predominant grey matter disorder are characterised by dementia, convulsions, blindness and later motor, delay.
- Predominant white matter disorders are characterised by motor delay, gait disturbances and later mental retardation and convulsion.

Behavioral Pattern in the Fields of Development

1. Down syndrome	—	Lovable, friendly, happy love music and dance.
2. Fragile X syndrome	—	Shyness, autism
3. Prader-Willi syndrome	—	Stubborn, excessive appetite
4. Angelman syndrome	—	Bouts of laughing
5. Lesch-Nyhan syndrome	—	Self-mutilation

Developmental Handicap

- Hearing handicap leads to speech delay
- Visual handicap causes adaptive delay
- Motor handicap causes delay in motor milestone
- Emotional deprivation causes speech and communication delay
- Global developmental delay means — all the four areas of development are affected (motor, adaptive, speech, social).

Warning Signs of Developmental Delay for Further Evaluation

4-6 weeks:
- Not responding to nearby voices by 8 weeks
- Absent "startle"
- No social smile by 3 months

At 3 months:
- Not showing interest in people and playthings by 3-4 months.
- No head control by 5 months.
- No vocalisation

At 6 months:
- — Persistent Moro's and asymmetric tonicneck reflexes.
- — Not visually alert.
- — Not reaching for objects.

At 9 monhts:
- — No hand transfer
- — Not sitting
- — No repetitive babble even by 10 months.

At 1 year:
- — Not starting a variety of speech sounds
- — Not pulling to standing position

At 1½ year:
- — Not moving about to explore
- — Not speaking single word by 21 months.

At 2 years:
- — Avoiding eye contact.
- — Handedness before 2 years-looks for weakness of opposite hand.
- — No sentence by 27 months.

At 3 years:
- — Not following simple directions
- — Monotonous play by self.

At 4 years:
- — No intelligible speech
- — Not drawing a human figure.

At 5 years:
- — No grammatical speech.

DEVELOPMENTAL ASSESSMENT

Prerequisites: Summary (Tables 29.4 to 29.7).

Prior to assessment of development, the following prerequisite are essential for the tests.

1. Child should be in a familiar surrounding
2. Child should get adjusted with stranger
3. Child should be made to get familiarised with test objects
4. There should not be any prompting by parents
5. Gestational age should be taken into account in preterm baby.
6. Margin should be given for physical handicaps—spasticity, hearing defect and vision defect.

A concise list of the milestones of development from birth to late adolescence are given in Table 29.4.

Sexual Maturity Rating (SMR)

Introduction The Tanner staging is widely used for assessing SMR (Fig. 29.3A). Five stages are described separately for boys and girls in different secondary sexual characters. Pubic hair (Fig. 29.3B) and breast development for girls and pubic hair, penis and testis development for boys. These stages are shown in (Tables 29.8 and 28.9).

Table 29.4: Milestones of development (From birth to adolescence)

Neonatal Period (1st 4 weeks)

Prone	Lies in flexed attitude, turns head from side to side; head sags on ventral suspension
Supine	Generally fixed and a little stiff
Visual	May fixate face or light in line of vision; "doll's-eye" movement of eyes on turning of the body
Reflex	Moro response active; stepping and placing reflexes, grasp reflex active
Social	Visual preference for human face

At 4 weeks

Prone	Legs more extended; holds chin up; turns head: head lifted momentarily to plane of body on ventral suspension
Supine	Tonic neck posture predominates; supple and relaxed; head lags on pull to sitting position
Visual	Watches person; follows moving object
Social	Body movements in cadence with voice of other in social contact; beginning to smile

At 8 weeks

Prone	Raises head slightly farther; head sustained in plane of body on ventral suspension
Supine	Tonic neck posture predominates; head lags on pull to sitting position
Visual	Follows moving object 180 degrees
Social	Smiles on social contact; listens to voice and coos

At 12 weeks

Prone	Lifts head and chest, arms extended; head above plane of body on ventral suspension
Supine	Tonic neck posture predominates; reaches toward and misses objects; waves at toy
Sitting	Head lag partially compensated on pull to sitting position; early head control with bobbing motion; back round
Reflex	Typical Moro response has not persisted; makes defensive movements or selective withdrawal reactions
Social	Sustained social contact; listens to music, says "aah, ngah"

At 16 weeks

Prone	Lifts head and chest, head in approximately vertical axis; legs extended
Supine	Symmetric posture predominates, hands in midline; reaches and grasps objects and brings them to mouth
Sitting	No head lag on pull to sitting position; head steady, tipped forward; enjoys sitting with full truncal support
Standing	When held erect, pushes with feet
Adaptive	Sees pellet, but makes no move to it
Social	Laughs out loud; may show displeasure if social contact is broken; excited at sight of food

At 28 weeks

Prone	Rools over, pivots; crawls or creep-crawls (Knobloch)
Supine	Lifts head; rools over; squirming movements
Sitting	Sits briefly, with support of pelvis; leans forward on hands; back rounded
Standing	May support most of weight; bounces actively
Adaptive	Reaches out for and grasps large object; transfers objects from hand to hand; grasp uses radial palm; rakes at
Language	Polysyllabic vowel sounds formed
Social	Prefers mother; babbles; enjoys mirror; responds to changes in emotional content of social content

Contd...

	At 40 week
Sitting	Sits up alone adn indefinitely without support, back straight
Standing	Pulls to standing position, "cruises" or walks holding on to furniture
Motor	Creeps or crawls
Adaptive	Grasps objects with thumb and forefinger; pokes at things with forefinger; picks up pellet with assisted pincer hidden toy; attempts to retrieve dropped object; releases object grasped by other person
Language	Repetitive consonant sounds (mama, dada)
Social	Responds to sound of name; plays peek-a-boo or pat-acake; wave bye-bye

	At 52 weeks (1 year)
Motor	Walks with one hand held (48 weeks); rises independently, takes several steps (Knobloch)
Adaptive	Picks up pellet with unassisted pincer movement of forefinger and tumb; releases object to other person
Language	A few words besides "mama, "dada"
Social	Plays simple ball game; makes postural adjustment to dressing.

	15 months
Motor	Walks alone; crawls up stairs
Adaptive	Makes tower of 3 cubes; makes a line with crayon; inserts pellet in bottle
Language	Jargon; follows simple commends; may name a familiar object (ball)
Social	

	18 months
Motor	Runs stiffy; sits on small chair; walks up stairs with one hand held; explores drawers and waste baskets
Adaptive	Makes a tower of 4 cubes imitates scribbling; imitates vertical stroke; dumps pellet from bottle
Language	10 words (average); names pictures; identifies one or more parts of body
Social	Feeds self; seeks help when in trouble; may complain when wet or soiled; kisses parent with pucker

	24 months
Motor	Runs well; walks up and down stairs, one step at a time; opens doors; climbs on furniture; jumps
Adaptive	Tower of 7 cubes (6 at 21 months) circular scribbling imitates horizontal stroke; folds paper once imitatively
Language	Puts 3 words together (subject, verb, object)
Social	Handles spoon well; often tells immediate experiences; helps to undress; listens to stories with pictures

	30 months
Motor	Goes up stairs alternating feet
Adaptive	Tower of 9 cubes; makes vertical and horizontal strokes, but generally will not join them to make a cross; imitates circular stroke, forming closed figure
Language	Refers to self by pronoun "I", knows full name
Social	Helps put things away; pretends in play

	36 months
Motor	Rides tricycle; stands momentarily on one foot
Adaptive	Tower of 10 cubes; imitates construction of bridge of 3 cubes copies a circle; imitates a cross
Language	Knows age and sex; counts 3 objects correctly; repeats 3 numbers or a sentence of 6 syllables
Social	Plays simple games (in parallel with other children); helps in dressing (unbuttons clothing and puts on shoes) was hands

Contd...

48 months	
Motor	Hops on one foot; throws ball overhand; uses scissors to cut out pictures; climbs well
Adaptive	Copies bridge from model; imitates construction of gate of 5 cubes; copies cross and square; draws a man with 2 parts besides head; names longer of 2 line
Language	Counts 4 pennies accurately; tells a story
Social	Plays with several children with beginning of social interaction and role playing goes to toilet alone

60 months	
Motor	Skips
Adaptive	Draws triangle from copy; name names heavier of 2 weights
Language	Names 4 colors; repeats sentence of 10 syllables; counts to pennies correctly
Social	Dresses and undresses; asks questions about meaning of words domestic role playing.

Comparisons in Adolescence—Early, Middle and Late

Adolescence may be subdivided as early, middle and late.

Early adolescence This starts with onset of puberty (SMR2) and has age onset of 10.5-14 year in boys and 10-13 years in girls. Middle adolescence corresponds to SMR 3 and 4 and coincides with the most dramatic growth change. Age of onset in boys is 12.5-15 years, girls-12-14 years. Late adolescence (SMR5) starts at 14-16 years in boys and 14-17 years in girls. A brief categorization of adolescence into early, middle and late is given in Table 29.10.

Dental Development

Dentition is assessed by counting the number of erupted teeth. A tooth which has at least partly emerged through the gum is considered erupted. The eruption of deciduous teeth is to be assessed by direct inspection without the aid of a mirror.

Dental Maturity (Figs 29.4A and B)

Like skeletal maturity, dental maturity can also be related to a set of standard values by counting the number of teeth erupted. Deciduous teeth are present from ages 6 months to 2 years and permanent teeth from 6 years to 13 years. It is to be remembered that dental development is less affected by the environment than is skeletal development and thus there is less need for maintaining indigenous standards. The counting of the teeth is a crude way of assessing maturity, but the stages of calcification of teeth seen in jaw radiographs are a very reliable guide. Boys and girls show similar maturity with respect to primary dentition but girls are in advance of boys in permanent dentition.

For a rough estimate, these are shown in the Table 29.11.

Total number of deciduous teeth is 20. They start erupting from 6 months of age and the process is completed by 2 to 2 1/2 years of age. A simple formula to calculate the number of deciduous teeth is

Age in months – 6 = No. of deciduous teeth (not more than 20 !)

Table 29.5: Growth and development during preschool years

Age	Physical	Gross motor	Fine motor	Language
3 yrs.	• Usual weight gain of 1.8 to 2.7 kg (4 to 6 pounds) • Average weight of 14.6 kg (32 pounds) • Unsual gain in height of 7.5 cm (3″) • Average height of 95 cm (37.25″) • May have achieved night-time control of bowel and bladder	Rides tricycle. Jumps off bottom step. Stands on one foot for a few seconds Goes up stairs using alternate feet, may still come down using both feet on step Broad jumps May try to dance, but balance may not be adequate.	Builds tower of nine or ten cubes Builds bridge with three cubes Adeptly places small pellets in narrow-necked bottle In drawing, copies a circle, imitates a cross, names what has been draw sticks figure but may make circle with facial features.	Has vocabulary of about 900 words. Uses primarily "telegraphic" speech Uses complete sentences of three to four words Talks incessantly regardless of whether any one is paying attention. Repeats sentences of six syllables. Asks many questions.
4 yrs.	• Pulse and respiration rates decrease slightly • Growth rate is similar to that of previous year • Average weight of 16.7 kg (36.75 pounds) • Average height of 103 cm (40.5″) • Length at birth is doubled • Maximum potential for development of amblyopia	Skips and hops on one foot. Catches ball reliably Throws ball overhand Walks downstairs using alternate footing.	Uses scissors successfully to cut out picture following outline. Can lace shoes but may not be able to tie bow. In drawing, copies a square, traces a cross and diamond, adds three parts to stick figure.	Has vocabulary of 1500 words or more Uses sentences of four to five words. Questioning is at peak. Tells exaggerated stories. Knows simple songs. May be mildly profane if associates with older children. Obeys four prepositional phrases, such as under, on top of, beside in, back of, or in front of. Names one or more colors. Comprehends analogies, such as, "If ice is cold, fire is..."
5 yrs.	Pulse and respiration rates decrease slightly. Average weight of 18.7 kg (41.25 pounds). Average height of 110 cm (43.25″). Eruption of permanent dentition may begin. Handedness is established (about 90% are right-handed)	Skips and hops on alternate feet. Throws and catches ball well. Jumps repeatedly. Skates with good balance. Walks backward with heel to toe. Jumps from height of 12″ and lands on toes. Balances on alternate feet with eyes closed.	Ties shoelaces. Uses scissors, simple tools, or pencil very well. In drawing, copies a diamond and triangle; adds seven to nine parts to stick figure; prints a few letters, numbers, or words, such as first name.	Has vocabulary of about 2100 words. Uses sentences of six to eight words, with all parts of speech. Names coins (e.g. nickle, dime). Name four or more colors. Describes drawing or pictures with much comment and numeration. Knows names of days of week, months, and other time-associated words. Knows composition of articles, such as, "A shoe is made of...." Can follow three commands in succession

Contd...

Contd...

Age	Socialization	Cognition	Family relationships
3 (yrs)	Dresses self almost completely if helped with back buttons and told which shoe is right or left. Has increased attention span. Feeds self completely. Can prepare simple meals, such as cold cereal and milk. Can help to set table, can dry dishes without breaking any. May have fears, especially of dark and going to bed. Knows own sex and sex of others. Play is parallel and associative, begins, to learn simple games but often follows own rules; begins to share.	Is in preconceptual phase. Is egocentric in thought and behaviour. Has beginning understanding of time; uses many time oriented expressions; talks about past and future as much as about present; pretends to tell time. Has improved concept of space as demonstrated in understanding of prepositions and ability to follow directional command. Has beginning ability to view concepts from another perspective.	Attempts to please parents and conform to their expectations. Is less jealous of younger sibling; may be opportune time for birth of additional sibling. Is aware of family relationships and sex role functions. Boys tend to identify more with father or other male figure. Has increased ability to separate easily and comfortably from parents for short periods.
4 (yrs)	Very independent. Tends to be selfish and impatient. Aggressive physically as well as verbally. Takes pride in accomplishments. Has mood swings. Shows off dramatically, enjoys entertaining others. Tells family tales to other with no restraint. Still has many fears play is associative. Imaginary playmeter are common. Uses dramatic, imaginative, and imitative devices. Sexual exploration and curiosity demonstrated through plays, such as being "doctor" or "nurse".	Is in phase of intuitive thought. Casuality is still related to proximity of events. Understands time better, especially in terms of sequence of daily events. Unable to conserve matter. Judges everything according to one dimension, such as height, width, or order. Immediate perceptual clues dominate judgement. Is beginning to develop less egocentrism and more social awareness. May count correctly but has poor mathematic concept of numbers. Obeys because understanding of right and wrong.	Rebels if parents expect too much, such as impeccable table manners. Takes aggression and frustration out on parents or siblings. "Do's" and "don'ts" become important. May have rivalry with older or younger siblings; may resent older sibling's privileges and younger sibling's invasion of privacy and possessions. May run away from home. Identifies strongly with parent of opposite sex. Is able to run simple errands outside the home.
5 (yrs)	Less rebellious and quarrelsome than at age 4 years. More settled and eager to get down to business. Not as open and accessible in thoughts and behavior as in earlier years. Independent but trustworthy; not foolhardy more responsible. Has fewer ears; relies on fouter authority to control world. Eager to do things right and to please; tires to "live by the rules". Has better manners. Cares for self totally except for teeth, occasionally needing supervision in dress or hygiene. Not ready for concentrated close work or small print because of slight farsightedness and still unrefined eye hand coordination. Play is associative; tries to follow rules but may cheat to avoid losing.	Begins to question what parents think by comparing them with age mates and other adults. May notice prejudice and bias in outside world. Is more able to view other's perspective, but tolerates differeneces rather than understanding them. May begin to show understanding of conservative of numbers through counting objects regardless of arrangement. Uses time-oriented words with increased understanding. Very curious about factual information regarding world.	Gets along well with parents. May seek out parent more often than at age 4 years for reassurance and security, especially when entering school. Begins to question parent's thinking and principles. Strongly identifies with parent of same sex, especially boys with their fathers. Enjoys activities such as sports, cooking, shopping with parent of same sex.

Table 29.6: Growth and development from 6 to 12 years

Age	Physical and motor	Mental	Adaptive	Personal-social
6 yrs	Growth and weight gain continues slowly. Weight: 16 to 23.6 kg (35.4 to 58 pounds); height > 106.6 to 123.5 cm (42 to 48"). Central mandibular incisors erupts. Loses first tooth. Gradual increases in dexterity. Activity age; constant activity. Often returns to finger feeding. More aware of hand as a tool. Likes to draw, print, and color vision reaches maturity.	Develops concept of numbers. Counts 13 pennies. Knows whether it is morning or afternoon. Defines common objects such as fork and chair in terms of their use. Obeys triple commands in succession. Knows right and left hands. Says which is pretty and which is ugly of a series of drawings of faces. Describes the objects in a picture rather then simply enumerating them. Attends first grade.	At table, uses knife to spread butter or jam on bread. At play, cut, folds, pastes paper toys. sews crudely if needle is threaded. Takes bath without supervision; performs bed time activities alone. Reads from memory; enjoys oral spelling game. Like table games, checkers, simple card games. Giggles a lot. Sometimes steals money or attractive items. Has difficulty owning up to misdeeds. Tries out own abilities.	Can share and cooperate better. Has great need for children of own age. Will cheat to win. Often jealous of younger brother or sister. Does what adults are seen doing. May have - occasional temper tantrums. Is a boaster. Is more independent, probably influence of school. Has own way of doing things. Increases socialization.
7 yrs	Begins to grow at least 2 inches a yr. Weight: 17.7 to 30 kg (39 to 66.5 pound); height: 111.8 to 129.7 cm (44 to 51"). Maxillary central incisors and lateral mandibular incisors erupt. More cautious in approaches to new performances. Repairs performances to master them. Jaw begins to expand to accommodate permanent teeth.	Notices that certain parts are missing from pictures. Can copy a diamond. Repeats three numbers backward. Develops concept of time; reads ordinary clock or watch correctly to nearest quarter hour; uses clock for practical purposes. Attends the second grade. More mechanical in reading; often does not stop at the end of a sentence, skips words such as it the, and be.	Use table knife for curting meat; may need help with tough or difficult pieces. Brushes and combs hair acceptably without help. May steal. Likes to help and have a choice. Is less resistant and stubborn.	Is becoming a real member of the family group. Takes part in group play. Boys prefer playing with boys; girls prefer playing with girls. Spends a lot of time alone; does not require a lot of companionship.
8-9 yrs	Continues to grow at 5 cm (2") a year Weight: 19.6 to 39.6 kg (43 to 87 pounds); height: 117 to 141.8 cm (46 to 56"). Lateral incisors (maxillary) and mandibular cuspids erupt. Move-	Gives similarities and differences between two things from memory. Counts backward from 20 to 1; understands concept of reversibility. Repeats days of the week and	Makes use of common tools such as hammer, saw, or screw driver. Uses household and sewing utensils. Helps with routine household tasks such as dusting, sweeping. Assumes	Is easy to get along with at home. Likes the reward system. Dramatizes Is more sociable. Is better behaved. Is interested in boy-girl relationship but will not admit. Goes about

Contd...

Contd...

Age	Physical and motor	Mental	Adaptive	Personal-social
	ment fluid; often graceful and poised. Always on the go; jumps, chases, skips. Increased smoothness and speed in fine motor control; uses cursive writing. Dresses self completely. Likely to overdo; hard to quiet down after recess. More limber; bones grow faster than ligaments.	months in order; knows the date. Describes common objects in detail, not merely their use. Makes change out of a quarter. Attends third and fourth grades. Reads more; may plan to wake up early just to read. Reads classic books, but also enjoys comics. More aware of time; can be relied on to get to school on time. Can grasp concepts of parts and whole (fractions). Understands concepts of spaces, cause and effects, nesting (puzzles) conservation (Permance of mass and volume). Classifies objects by more than one quality; has collections. Produces simple paintings or drawings.	responsibility for share of household chores. Looks after all of own needs at table. Buys useful articles; exercises some choice in making purchases. Runs useful errands likes pictorial magazines. Likes school; wants to answer all the questions. Is afraid to failing a grade; is ashamed of bad grades. Is more critical of self. Takes music and sport lessions.	home and community freely, alone, or with friends and groups. Plays mostly with groups of own sex but is beginning to mix. Develops modestly compares self with others. Enjoys Scouts, group sports.
10-12 yrs	**Boys: Slow growth in height and rapid weight gain; may become obese in this period. Weight: 24.3 to 58 kg (54 to 128 pounds); height 127.5 to 162.3 cm (50 to 64''). Posture is more similar to an adult's; will overcome lordosis. Girls: pubescent changes may begin to appear; body lines soften and round out. Remainder of teeth will erupt and tend toward full development (except wisdom teeth).**	**Writes brief stories. Attends fifth to seventh grades.** Writes occasional short letters to friends or relatives on own initiatives. Uses telephone for practical purposes responds to magazine, radio, or other advertising. Reads for practical information or own enjoyment stories or library books of advanture or romance, or animal stories.	**Makes useful articles or does easy repair work. Cooks or sews in small way. Raises pets. Washes and dries** own hair. Is responsible for a thorough job of cleaning hair, but may need reminding to do so. May sometimes be left alone at home for an hour or so. Is successful in looking after own needs or those of other children left in his or her care.	**Is fond of friends. Chooses friends more selectively; may have a best friend.** Loves conservation. Develops beginning interest in opposite sex. Is more diplomatic. Likes mother and wants to please her in many ways. Demonstrates affection. Like dad, too; he is adored and idolized. Respects parents. Loves friends; talks about them constantly.

Table 29.7: Growth and development during early, middle and late adolescence

	Early adolescence (11-14 yrs)	Middle adolescence (14-17 yrs)	Late adolescence (17-20 yrs)
Growth	Rapidly accelerating growth Reaches peak velocity Secondary sex characteristics appear	Growth decelerating in girls Stature reaches 95% of adult height Secondary sex characteristics well advanced	Physical mature Structure and reproductive growth almost complete
Cognition	Explores newfound ability for limited abstract thought Clumsy groping for new values and energies Comparision of "normality" with peers of same sex	Development capacity for abstract thinking Enjoys intellectual powers, often in idealistic terms Concern with philosophic, political and social problems	Established abstract thought Can perceive and act on long range operations Able to view problems comprehensively Intellectual and functional identity established
Identity	Preoccupied with rapid body changes Trying out of various roles Measurement of attractiveness by acceptance or rejection of peer Conformity to group norms	Modifies body image Very self centered; increased narcissim Tendency toward inner experience and self discovery Has a rich fantasy life Idealistic Able to perceive future implications of current behavior and decisions; variable application.	Body image and gender role definition nearly secured Mature sexual identity Phase of consolidation of identity Stability of self-esteem Comfortable with physical growth Social roles defined and articulated
Relationship with parents	Defining independence dependence boundaries Strong desire to remain dependent on parents while tying to detach No major conflicts over parental control	Major conflicts over independence and control Low point in parent child relationship Greatest push for emancipation; disengagement Final and irreversible emotional detachement from parents; mourning	Emotional and physical separation from parents completed Independence from family with less conflict Emancipation nearly secured

Contd...

Contd...

	Early adolescence (11-14 yrs)	Middle adolescence (14-17 yrs)	Late adolescence (17-20 yrs)
Relationship with peers	Seeks peer affiliations to counter instability generated by rapid change Upsurge of close idealized friendships with members of the same sex. Struggle for mastery takes palace within peer group	Strong need for identity to affirm self-image Behavior standards set by peer group Acceptance by peers extremely important-fear of rejection Exploration of ability to attract the opposite sex	Peer group recedes in importance in favor of individual friendship Testing of male female relationships against possibility of permanent alliance. Relationships characterized by giving and sharing
Sexuality	Self-exploration and evaluation Limited dating, usually group Limited intimacy	Multiple plural relationships Decisive turn towards heterosexuality (If is homosexual, knows by this time) Exploration of self appeal Feeling of being in love Tentative establishment of relationships	Forms stable relationships and attachment to another Growing capacity for mutuality and reciprocity Dating as a male female pair Intimacy involves commitment rather than exploration and romanticism
Psychologic health	Wide mood swings Intense daydreaming Anger outwardly expressed with moodiness, temper outbursts, and verbal insults and name calling	Tendency toward inner experiences; more introspective Tendency to withdraw when upset or feelings are hurt Vascillation of emotions in time and range Feelings of inadequacy common; difficulty in asking for help	More constancy of emotion Anger more apt to be concealed

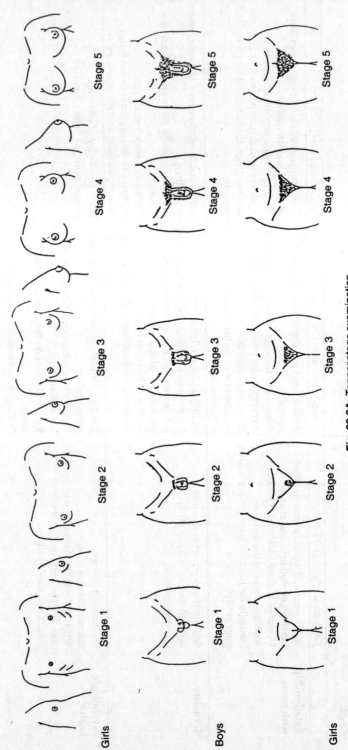

Fig. 29.3A: Tanner stage examination

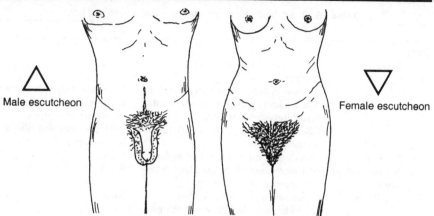

Fig. 29.3B: Normal sexual hair distribution in adult men and women. Changes may signal hormonal abnormalities

Male escutcheon

Female escutcheon

Table 29.8: Sexual maturity rating in girls

SMR	Pubic hair	SMR	Breast
1.	Preadolescent	1.	Preadolescent
2.	Sparse, lightly pigmented, straight, medial border of labia.	2.	Breast and papilla elevated as small mound, areolar diametere increased.
3.	Darker, beginning to curl, increased amount.	3.	Breast and areola enlarged, no counter separation.
4.	Coarse, curly, abundant but less amount than adult.	4.	Areola and papilla form secondary mound.
5.	Adult feminine triangle, spread to medial surface of thighs.	5.	Mature; nipple projects, areola part of general breast contour.

Table 29.9: Sexual maturity rating in boys

SMR	Pubic hair	Penis	Testes
1.	None	(Preadolescent)	(Preadolescent)
2.	Scanty, long slightly pigmented	Slight enlargement	Enlarged scrotum, pink, texture altered.
3.	Darker, starts to curl, small amount.	Longer	Larger
4.	Resemble adult, the amount less; coarse, curly	Larger, glans and breadth increase in size.	Larger, scrotum dark
5.	Adult distribution spreads to medial surface of thighs	Adult size	Adult size

In primary dentition, the 1st teeth to appear are the lower central incisors. If there is no eruption of teeth by approximately 13 months (mean + 3SD) dentition is said to be delayed. The common causes are familial, idiopathic, hypothyroid, malnutrition and hypoparathyroidism.

Skeletal Maturity

Skeletal maturity implies how far the bones of a particular area have progressed towards maturity not in size but in shape and in their relative positions to one

Table 29.10: Adolescence subdivided as early, middle and late

	Girls	Boys
Early		
i. Physical	Weight gain 2 kg/year height gain 6-8 cm/year	Same
	Increase in body fat, subscapular skin fold thickness increases by one-third.	Increase of muscle bulk more than fat
	Breast development (SMR 2)	Enlargement of testes
	Changes of uterus, vagina, Pubic hair on medial aspect	Pubic hair-fine and silky at base of penis.
ii. Dentition	Shedding of canines and first molar	Same
iii. Neurodevelopement	Mature response to all standard neuro-developmental assessment.	Same
iv. Cognitive	Generates hypothesis to be tested, thinks logically (concrete operations).	Same
v. Psychosocial development	Independence from family, attachment to peer groups, especially same sex, friendships thriving on joint activity but lacking depth and mutually.	Same
Middle		
i. Physical development	Growth spurt occurs, increase in heigth 8 cm/yr. (at 12 years).	Increase in height 10 cm/yr (at 14 years).
	Orderly progression of skeletal growth from distal to proximal parts of body starting with feet.	Same
	Sex differences in skeletal growth, increased bi-trochanteric diameter is estrogen determined.	Increased bi-acromial diameter-androgen deter-mined
	Breast development, increase in breast and areola with secondary mound.	Increase in size of penis and scrotum. Scrotum darkness. Gynecomastia may occur.
	Public hairs curl, darken coarse. Menarche.	Same
ii. Neurodevelopement	Maturity already reached	Same
	Decrease in sleep latency time and increased day time sleepiness.	Same
iii. Cognitive development	Emergence of abstract thought, more questioning.	Same
iv. Psychosocial development	School and peer groups gain importance. Sex difference in peer relationship. Boys—achievement and independence, Girls—loyalty, commitment and intimacy of shaped information. Eriksonian search for identiy, sexual adequacy.	Same
Late		
(Boys and Girls common)		
a. Physical development	Body approximates young adult proportion and size. Development of secondary sexual characteristics completed. Consolidation of sexual identity.	
b. Neuro-development	Completed already. Congnitive, moral, social development may continue to evolve through rest of life.	
c. Psychosocial	Rebellious attitude replaced by gradual return to family. Absolute and moralistic attitudes of thinking tempered to empathy, intimacy. Practical independence. Family base remains secure. Career decisions made.	

Fig. 29.11: Age of appearance of individual teeth

Name of primary tooth	Age of appea-rance (months)	Name of secondary tooth	Age of appea-rance (years)
Central incisors	6-7	1st molar	6
Lateral incisors	7-10	Central incisor	7
1st molar	12	Lateral incisor	8
Canine	18	1st premolar	9
2nd molar	24	2nd molar	10
		Canine	11
		2nd molar	12
		3rd molar	18

Table 29.12: Time of appearance in roentgenograms of centres of ossification in infancy and childhood

Boys-age at appearance	Bones and Epiphyseal centres	Girls-age at appearance
3 weeks	Humerus, head	3 weeks
	Carpal bones	
2 months ± 2 months	Capitate	2 months ± 2 months
3 months ± 2 months	Hamate	2 months ± 2 months
30 months ± 16 months	Triangular	21 months ± 14 months
42 months ± 19 months	Lunate	34 months ± 13 months
67 months ± 19 months	Trapezium	47 months ± 14 months
69 months ± 15 months	Trapezoid	49 months ± 12 months
66 months ± 15 months	Scaphoid	51 months ± 12 months
No standards available	Pisiform	No standards available
	Metacarpal bones	
18 months ± 5 months	II	12 months ± 3 months
20 months ± 5 months	III	13 months ± 3 months
23 months ± 6 months	IV	15 months ± 4 months
26 months ± 7 months	V	16 months ± 5 months
32 months ± 9 months	I	18 months ± 5 months
	Fingers (epiphyses)	
16 months ± 4 months	Proximal phalanx, 3rd finger	10 months ± 3 months
16 months ± 4 months	Proximal phalanx, 2nd finger	11 months ± 3 months
17 months ± 5 months	Proximal phalanx, 4th finger	11 months ± 3 months
19 months ± 7 months	Distal phalanx, 1st finger	12 months ± 4 months
21 months ± 5 months	Proximal phalanx, 5th finger	14 months ± 4 months
24 months ± 6 months	Middle phalanx, 3rd finger	15 months ± 5 months
26 months ± 6 months	Distal phalanx, 4th finger	15 months ± 5 months
28 months ± 16 months	Distal phalanx, 3rd finger	18 months ± 4 months
28 months ± 6 months	Proximal phalanx, 4th finger	18 months ± 5 months
32 months ± 7 months	Distal phalanx, 1st finger	20 months ± 5 months
37 months ± 9 months	Distal phalanx, 5th finger	23 months ± 6 months
37 months ± 8 months	Distal phalanx, 2nd finger	23 months ± 6 months
39 months ± 10 months	Middle phalanx, 5th finger	22 months ± 7 months
152 months ± 18 months	Sesamoid (adductor pollicis)	121 months ± 13 months

Contd...

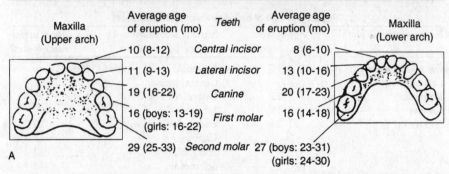

Maxilla (Upper arch)	Average age of eruption (mo)	*Teeth*	Average age of eruption (mo)	Maxilla (Lower arch)
	10 (8-12)	Central incisor	8 (6-10)	
	11 (9-13)	Lateral incisor	13 (10-16)	
	19 (16-22)	Canine	20 (17-23)	
	16 (boys: 13-19) (girls: 16-22)	First molar	16 (14-18)	
A	29 (25-33)	Second molar	27 (boys: 23-31) (girls: 24-30)	

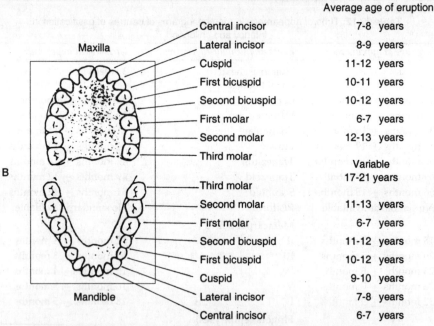

Maxilla		Average age of eruption
	Central incisor	7-8 years
	Lateral incisor	8-9 years
	Cuspid	11-12 years
	First bicuspid	10-11 years
	Second bicuspid	10-12 years
	First molar	6-7 years
	Second molar	12-13 years
	Third molar	Variable 17-21 years
	Third molar	
	Second molar	11-13 years
	First molar	6-7 years
	Second bicuspid	11-12 years
	First bicuspid	10-12 years
	Cuspid	9-10 years
Mandible	Lateral incisor	7-8 years
	Central incisor	6-7 years

Figs 29.4a and b: (a) Sequence of eruption of primary teeth. Range represents ± standard deviation or 67% of subjects studied, (b) sequence of eruption of secondary teeth

Contd...

Boys-age at appearance	Bones and Epiphyseal centres	Girls-age at appearance
	Hip and Knee	
Usually present at birth	Femur, distal	Usually present at birth
Usually present at birth	Tibia, proximal	Usually present at birth
4 months ± 2 months	Femur, head	4 months ± 2 months
46 months ± 11 months	Patella	29 months ± 7 months

another, as seen in a radiograph. The number of centres of ossification present and the stage of development of each gives an estimation of the skeletal maturity (Figs 29.5A and B) (Table 29.12).

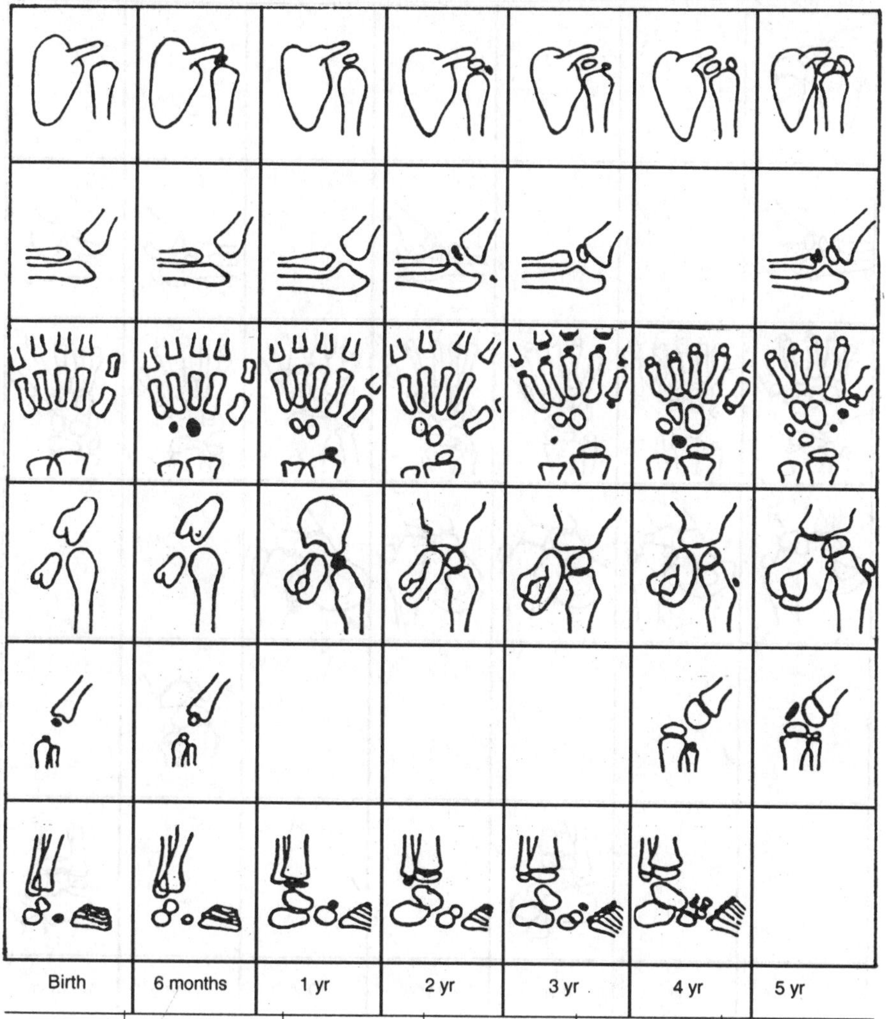

| | Birth | 6 months | 1 yr | 2 yr | 3 yr | 4 yr | 5 yr |

	Birth	1 yr	2 yr	3 yr	4 yr	5 yr
Sholder 0		Head of humerus (3 months)	Great tuberosity			
Elbow 0			Capitellum			Head of radius
Hand 0		Hamale (1 mos.) Capitale (6 mos.) E.p. radius		Triquetrum E.p. metacarpals E.p. phalanges	Lunatum	Trapesium Scaphoid
Hip 0		Head of femur (9 months)			Great trochanter	
Knee Ep femur and tibia					Head of fibula	Patella
Foot Cuboid		Ext. cuneiform E.p. tibia	E.p. fibula	Int. euneiform E.p. metalarsals	Mid cuneiform Navicular	

Fig. 29.5A: The new centers of ossification (age birth to 5 yr.) which appear at each year are shown in black

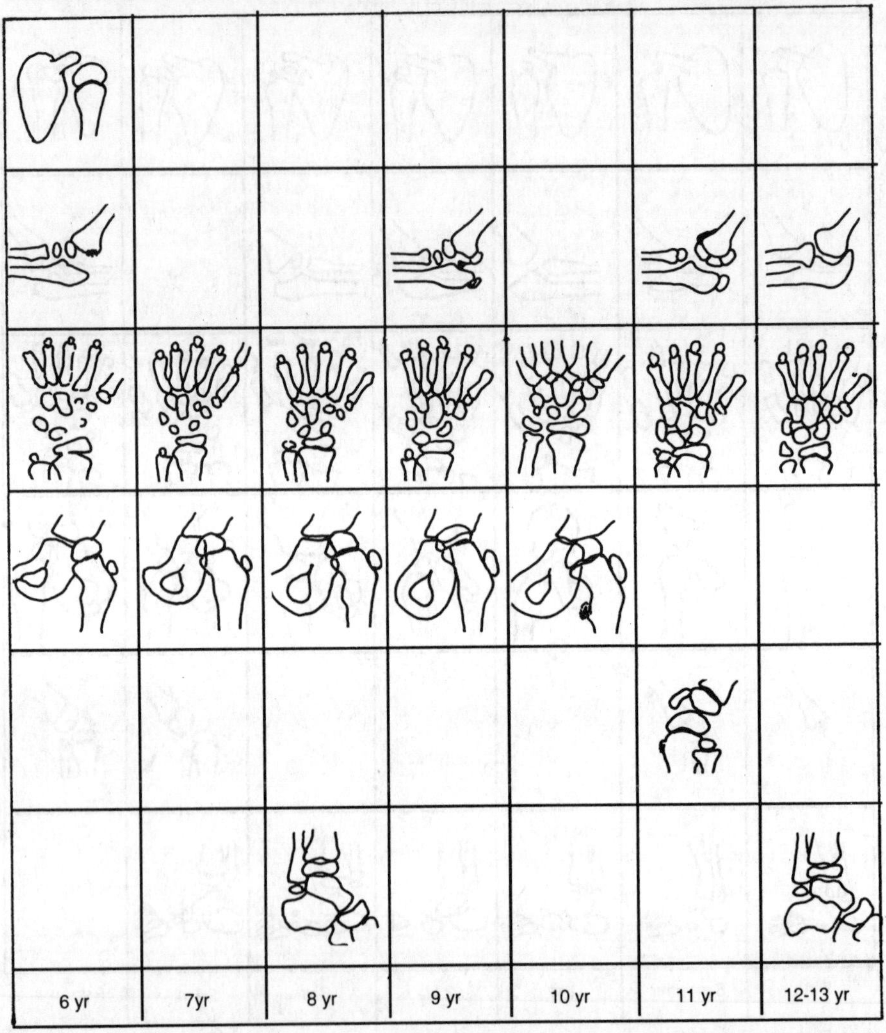

| 6 yr | 7yr | 8 yr | 9 yr | 10 yr | 11 yr | 12-13 yr |

6 yr	7 yr	8 yr	9 yr	10 yr	11 yr
Union head and tuberosity					
Int. epiondyle			Trochlea Olecranon		Ext. epicondyle
Trapesoid E.p. ulna				Pisiform	Styloid ulna
	Union ischium and pubis			E.p. lesser trochanter	
					Tibial tuberele
		E.p. os calcis			

Fig. 29.5B: The new centers of ossification (age 6 to 13) which appear at each year are shown in black

For a rough estimate of bone age from the left hand X-ray: Centres of ossification appears as: Capitate, hamate (1-year), lower end of radius (2-year). triquetral (3-year), lunate (4-year), scaphoid (5-year), lower end of ulna, trapezium, trapezoid (6-years), pisiform (12-years) for the elbow joint, the appearance of centres of ossification of the lower end of the humerus are: Medial epicondyle (5-year), trochlea (1-year), capitulum (1-year), lateral epicondyle (12-year). The epicondyle for the upper end of radius and ulna appear at 4 year and 8 year respectively.

Thumb rule

1. The number of carpal bones at wrist = age in years plus one.
2. There are five ossification centres at birth in term babies. Two at knee joint (upper end of tibia and lower end of femur) and 3 in the foot (talus, cuboid, calcaneus).

APPENDIX I

Summary of Growth and Development

This summary of growth and development offers a broad overview of the significant physical, psychosocial and mental achievements during childhood. It begins with a comparison of cognitive and personality development throughout the life span according to different theorists. Following are summaries of the specific developmental milestones associated with each major age group of children (Tables 29.13 and 29.14).

Table 29.13: Developmental milestones in summary

Motor	Adaptive behavior
Head control-3 months	Follows object 90°-1 month
Rolling over-5 months	Follows objects 180°-3 months
Sitting with support-6 months	Reaching objects with both hands-4 months
Sitting without support-7 months	— 6 months (Ulnar grasp-5-7 months, radial grasp 6-8 months).
Pivoting-9 months	Transfer objects-7 months
Standing with support-9 months	Pincer grasp-9 months
Crawls-10 months	Release objects-11 months
Stands without support-10 months	Scribbles circle-15 months
Walks with support-11 months	Balances one cube over other-15 months
Walks without support-13 months	Vertical strokes-18 months
Climbs stairs, furnitures-15 months	Draws a square-3 years
Runs-20 months	Draws a circle-4 years
Climbs downstair 20 months	Identifies long, short, heavy light coins-5 years
Jumps-2 years	Draws rhomboid-6 years.
Stands on one leg-3 years	Simple arithmetics 6 years.
Rides tricycle-3 years	
Hops-5 years	

Language	Social behavior
Cooing-2 months	Social smile-2 months
Babbing-5 months	Recognises mother-3 months
Monosyllables without meaning-7months	Laughs aloud-4 months
Monosyllables with meaning-9 months	Limitation-6 months
Ten words-1 year	Recognises stranger-6 mts
Combining words-15 months	Regard image in mirror-7 months
Jargon-15 months	Peak-a boo-9 months
3 word sentence-2 years	Drinks from a cup-9 months
(50% intelligible)	Eats and drinks himself-11 months
Recites rhymes-3 years	Obeys commands-15 months
Can tell name-3 years	Part of body-18 months
Speaks well-4 years	Helps to dress-2 years
(Nouns, pronouns, adjectives, verbs)	Listening to story-2years
rules of Grammar	Knows his sex-3 years
Narrates stories-4 years	Bladder control-3 years
Read, write, recites 5-6 years	Plays with friends-4 years
Poems remember, accidents	Knows good and bad-5 years
(ready for school)-6 years	Put shoes, ties and laces-6 years.

Table 29.14: Personality, moral, and cognitive development

	Radius of significant relationships (Sullivan)	Psychosexual stages (Freud)	Psychosocial stages (Erikson)	Cognitive stages (Piaget)	Moral judgment stages (Kohlberg)
I Infancy (birth to 1 year)	Maternal person (unipolar-bipolar)	Oral sensory	Trust vs mistrust	Sensorimotor (birth to 18 months)	Preconventional (premoral) level Punishment and obedience orientation
II Toddlerhood (1-3 years)	Parental persons (tripolar)	Anal-urethral	Autonomy vs shame and doubt	Preoperational thought, preconceptual phase (transductive reasoning, for example, specific to specific) (2 to 4 years)	Preconventional (premoral) level Naive instrumental orientation
III Early childhood (3-6 years)	Basic family	Phallic-locomotion	Initiative vs guilt	Preoperational thought, intuitive phase (transductive reasoning) (4 to 7 years)	
IV Middle childhood (6-12 years)	Neighborhood, school	Latency	Industry vs inferiority	Concrete operations (inductive reasoning and beginning logic)	Conventional level Good-boy, nice-girl orientation Law-and-order orientation
V Adolescence (13-18 years)	Peer groups and out-groups Models of leadership Partners in friendship, sex, competition, cooperation	Genitality	Identity and repudiation vs identity confusion	Formal operations (deductive and abstract reasoning)	Postconventional or principled level Social-contract orientation Universal ethical principle orientation (no longer included in revised theory)
VI Early adulthood	Divided labor and shared household		Intimacy and solidarity vs isolation		
VII Young and middle adulthood	Mankind "My kind"		Generativity vs darity vs isolation		
VIII Later adulthood			Ego integrity vs despair		

APPENDIX II

Assessment of Language and Speech

Major developmental characteristics of language and speech (Table 29.15).

Table 29.15: Assessment of language and speech
(Major developmental characteristics of language and speech for given years)

Age	Normal language development	Normal speech development	Intelligibility
1 year	Says two to three words with meaning Imitates sounds of animals	Omits most final and some initial consonants Substitutes consonants "m", "w", "p", "b", "k", "g", "n", "t", "d", and "h", for more difficult sounds	Usually no more than 25% intelligible to unfamiliar listener Height of unintelligible jargon at age 18 months
2 years	Uses two to three-words phrases. Has vocabulary of about 300 words Uses "I", "me", "you"	Uses above consonants with vowels, but inconsistently and with much substitution Omission of final consonants	At age 2 years, 50% intelligible in context
3 years	Says four to five-words sentences. Has vocabulary of about 900 words Uses "who", "what", and "where" in asking questions Uses plurals, pronouns, and prepositions	Masters "b", "t", "d", "k", and "g", sounds "r", and "l", may still be unclear, omits or substitutes "w" Repetitions and hesitations common	At age 3 years, 75% intelligible
4-5 years	Has vocabulary of 1500 to 2100 words Able to use most grammatic forms correctly such as past tense of verb with "yesterday" Uses complete sentences with nouns, verbs, prepositions, adjectives, adverbs, and conjunctions	Masters "f" and "v", may still distort "r", "l", "s", "z", "sh", "ch", "y", and "th" Little or no omission of initial or last consonant	Speech is 100% intelligible, although some sounds are still imperfect
5-6 years	Has vocabulary of 3000 words, comprehends "if", "because", and "why"	Master "r", "l", and "th", may still distort "s", "z", "sh", "ch", and "j" (usually mastered by age 7½ to 8 years)	

APPENDIX III

Assessment of Vision

Major developmental characteristics of vision at different months (Table 29.16).

Table 29.16: Major developmental characteristics of vision at different months

Age (months)	Development
Birth	Visual acuity 20/100 Pupillary and corneal (blink) reflexes present Able to fixate on moving object in range of 45° when held 8 to 10 inches away Cannot integrate head and eye movements well (doll's eye reflex-eyes lag behind if head is rotated to one side)
1	Can follow in range of 90° Can watch parent intently as he or she speaks to infant Tear glands begin to function Visual acuity is hyperopic because infant has less spheric eyeball than adult
2-3	Has peripheral vision to 180° Binocular vision begins at age 6 weeks and is well established by age 4 months Convergence on near objects begins by age 6 weeks and is well developed by age 3 months Doll's eye reflex disappears
4-5	Able to fixate on a ½ inch block Recognizes feeding bottle Looks at hand while sitting or lying on side Looks at mirror image Able to accommodate to near objects
5-7	Adjusts posture to see an object Able to rescue a dropped toy Develops color preferences for yellow and red Able to discriminate between simple geometric forms Prefers more complex visual stimuli Develops hand-eye coordination Pats image of self in mirror
7-11	Can fixate on very small objects Depth perception begins to develop Lack of binocular vision indicates strabismus
11-12	Visual acuity approaches 20/20 Visual loss may develop if strabismus is present Can follow rapidly moving objects
12-14	Able to identify geometric forms, for example, places round object into hole Displays intense and prolonged interest in pictures
18-24	Accommodation well-developed Able to fixate on small objects for up to 60 seconds
36-48	Able to copy geometric figures, for example, circle, cross Reading readiness may be present, but usually at 48 to 72 months
48-60	Maximal potential for amblyopia Able to copy a square
60-72	Less potential for amblyopia Recognizes most colors Depth perception fully developed

APPENDIX IV

Assessment of Hearing

Major developmental characteristics of hearing (Table 29.17).

Table 29.17: Major developmental characteristics of hearing after specific number of months

Age (months)	Development
Birth	Responds to loud noise by startle reflex Responds to sound of human voice more readily than to any other sound Becomes quite with low-pitched sounds, such as lullaby, metronome, or hearbeat
2-3	Turns head to side when sound is made at level of ear
3-4	Locates sound by turning head to side and looking in same direction
4-6	Can localize sounds made below ear, which is followed by localization of sound made above ears will turn head to the side and then look up or down Begins to imitate sounds
6-8	Locates sounds by turning head in a curving arc Responds to own name
8-10	Localizes sounds by turning head diagonally and directly toward sound
10-12	Knows several words and their meaning, such as *no*, and names of members of the family Learns to control and adjust own response to sound, such as listening for sound to occur again
18	Begins to discriminate between harshly dissimilar sounds, such as sound of doorbell and train
24	Refines gross discriminative skills
36	Begins to distinguish more subtle differences in speech sounds, such as between *e* and *er*
48	Begins to distinguish such similar sounds as *f* and *th* or between *f* and *s* Listening becomes considerably refined Able to be tested with an audiometer

APPENDIX V

Development of Localisation of Sounds (Fig. 29.6 and Table 29.18)

Table 29.18: Development in localisation of sound

Age	Response
3 months	Baby stills; eyes deviate towards the side of sounds; early head turning may occur.
4-5 months	Eyes and head turning towards the side of sound well established.
6 months	Eyes and head turn laterally and then drop to locate sound source in low position.
7-8 months	Eyes and head move in towards sound source.
9 months	Eyes and head turn directly towards sound source. This occurs later to sounds in superior than in inferior positions. Visual searching for sound source may be seen.

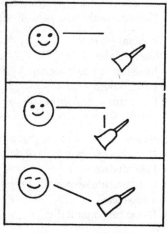

Fig. 29.6: Auditary localisation

APPENDIX VI

Assessment of Child for Hearing Impairment

Family History
- Genetic disorders associated with hearing impairment
- Family members, especially siblings, with hearing disorders

Prenantal History
- Miscarriages
- Illnesses during pregnancy (rubella, syphilis, diabetes)
- Drugs taken
- Exposure to childhood diseases
- Eclampsia

Delivery
- Duration of labor, type of delivery
- Fetal distress
- Presentation (especially breech)
- Drugs used
- Blood incompatibility

Birth History
- Birth weight < 1500 g
- Hyperbilirubinemia at level exceeding indications for exchange transfusion
- Severe asphyxia
- Prematurity
- Congenital perinatal viral infection (Cytomegalovirus, rubella, herpes, Syphilis, toxoplasmosis)
- Congenital anomalies involving head and neck

Past Health History
- Immunizations
- Serious illness (e.g.bacterial meningitis)
- Seizures
- High unexplained fevers
- Ototoxic drugs
- Hyperbilirubinemia (if preterm)
- No history (adopted child)
- Colds, ear infections, allergies
- Treatment of ear problems
- Visual difficulties
- Exposure to excessive noise (such as monitor alarms, gunshot)

Hearing
- Parental concerns regarding hearing loss (what cues, at what age)
- Response to name calling, loud noises, sounds of different frequencies (crinkling paper, whisper, bell, rattle)
- Results of previous audiometric testing

Speech Development
- Age of babbling, first meaningful words, phrases

- Intelligibility of speech
- Present vocabulary

Motor Development
- Age of sitting, standing, walking
- Level of independence in self-care, feeding, toileting, grooming

Adaptive Behavior
- Play activities
- Socialization with other children
- Behaviors: temper tantrums, stubbornness, self-vexation, vibratory stimulus
- Educational achievement
- Recent behavioral and/or personality changes

Clues for Detecting Hearing Impairment

Orientation Response
- Lack of startle or blink reflex to a loud sound
- Persistence of Moro reflex beyond 4 months of age (associated with mental retardation)
- Failure to be awakened by loud environmental noises during early infancy
- Failure to localize a source of sound by 6 months of age
- General indifference to sound
- Lack of response to the spoken word; failure to follow verbal directions
- Response to loud noises as opposed to the voice

Vocalizations and Sound Production
- Monotone quality, unintelligible speech, lessened laughter
- Normal quality in central auditory loss
- Lessened experimental sound play and squealing
- Normal use of jargon during early infancy in central auditory loss, with persistent use later on
- Absence of babble or inflections in voice by age 7 months
- Failure to develop intelligible speech by age 24 months
- Vocal play, head banging, or foot stamping for vibratory sensation
- Yelling or screeching to express pleasure, annoyance, or need

Visual Attention
- Augmented visual alertness and attentiveness
- Responding more to facial expression than verbal explanation
- Being alert to gestures and movement
- Use of gestures rather than verbalization to express desires, especially after age 15 months
- Marked imitativeness in play

Social Rapport and Adaptations
- Less interest and involvement in vocal nursery games
- Intense preoccupation with things rather than persons
- Avoidance of social interactions; often puzzled and unhappy in such situations
- Inquiring, sometimes confused facial expression
- Suspicious alertness, sometimes interpreted as paranoia, alternating with cooperation

- Marked reactivity to praise, attention, and physical affection
- Shows less interest than peers in casual conversation
- Is often inattentive unless the environment is quiet and the speaker is close to the child
- Is more responsive to movement than to sound
- Intently observes the speaker's face, responding more to facial expression than verbalization
- Often asks to have statements repeated
- May not follow directions exactly

Emotional Behavior
- Use of tantrums to call attention to self or needs. Frequently stubborn because of lack of comprehension. Irritable at not making self-understood. Shy, timid and withdrawn. Often appears "dreamy", in a word of his/her own or markedly inattentive.

APPENDIX VII

Developmental Milestones Associated with Feeding (Table 29.19)

Table 29.19: Different developmental milestones associated with feeding

Age (months)	Development
Birth	Has sucking, rooting, and swallowing reflexes Feels hunger and indicates desire for food by crying; expresses satiety by falling asleep
1	Has strong extrusion reflex
3-4	Extrusion reflex is fading Begins to develop hand-eye coordination
4-5	Can approximate lips to the rim of a cup
5-6	Can use fingers to feed self a craker
6-7	Chews and bites May hold own bottle, but may not drink from it (prefers for it to be held)
7-9	Refuses food by keeping lips closed; has taste preferences Holds a spoon and plays with it during feeding May drink from a straw Drinks from a cup with assistance
9-12	Picks up small morsels of food (finger foods) and feeds self Holds own bottle and drinks from it Drinks from a household cup without assistance but spills some Uses a spoon with much spilling
12-18	Drools less Drinks well from a household cup, but may drop it when finished Holds cup with both hands Begins to use a spoon but turns it before reaching mouth
24	Can use a straw Chews food with mouth closed and shifts food in mouth Distinguishes between finger and spoon foods Holds small glass in one hand; replaces glass without dropping Uses spoon correctly but with some spilling
36	Spills small amount from spoon Begins to use fork; holds it in fist Uses adult pattern of chewing, which involves rotary action of jaw
48	Rarely spills when using spoon Serves self finger foods Eats with fork held with fingers
54	Uses fork in preference to spoon
72	Spreads with knife
84	Cuts tender food with knife

APPENDIX VIII

Injury Prevention during Infancy
In Relation to Developmental Accomplishments

Injury Prevention

Aspiration
- Keep buttons, beads, syringe caps, and other small objects out of infant's reach
- Keep floor free of any small objects
- Do not feed infant hard candy, nuts, food with pits or seeds, or whole or circular pieces of hot dog
- Exercise caution when giving teething biscuits, because large chunks may be broken off and aspirated
- Do not feed infant while infant is lying down
- Inspect toys for removable parts
- Keep baby powder, if used, out of reach
- Avoid storing large quantities of cleaning fluid, paints, pesticides, and other toxic substances
- Discard used containers of poisonous substances
- Do not store toxic substances in food containers

Suffocation
- Keep uninflated balloons out of reach
- Remove all crib toys that are strung across crib or playpen when child begins to push up on hands or knees or is 5 months old

Falls
- Restrain in a high chair
- Keep crib rails raised to full height

Poisoning
- Make sure that paint for furniture or toys does not contain lead
- Place toxic substances on a high shelf or in locked cabinet
- Hang plants or place on high surface rather than on floor
- Discard used button-sized batteries; store new batteries in safe area
- Know telephone number of local poison control center (usually listed in front of telephone directory)

Burns
- Keep faucets out of reach
- Place hot objects (cigarettes, candles, incense) on high surface
- Limit exposure to sun; apply sunscreen

Motor vehicles
- See under birth-4 months

Bodily damage
- Give toys that are smooth and rounded, preferably made of wood or plastic
- Avoid long, pointed objects as toys
- Avoid toys that are excessively loud
- Keep sharp objects out of infant's reach

Major Developmental Accomplishments (Age 8-12 months)
- Crawls/creeps
- Stands, holding onto furniture

- Stands alone
- Cruises around furniture
- Walks
- Climbs
- Pulls on objects

Injury Prevention

Aspiration
- Keep lint and small objects off floor and furniture and out of reach of children
- Take care in feeding solid table food to ensure that very small pieces are given
- Do not use beanbag toys or allow child to play with dried beans
- See also under 4-7 months

Suffocation/drowning
- Keep doors of ovens, diswashers, refrigerators, coolers, and front-loading clothes washers and dryers closed at all times
- If storing an unused appliance, such as a refrigerator, remove the door
- Supervise contact with inflated balloons; immediately discard popped balloons and keep uninflated balloons out of reach
- Fence swimming pools
- Always supervise when near any source of water, such as cleaning buckets, drainage areas, toilets
- Keep bathroom doors closed
- Eliminate unnecessary pools of water
- Keep one hand on child at all times when in tub

Motor vehicles
- See under birth-4 months
- Throws objects
- Is able to pick up small objects; has pincer grasp
- Explores by putting objects in mouth
- Dislikes being restrained
- Explores away from parent
- Increasing understanding of simple commands and phrases

Falls
- Fence stairways at top and bottom if child has access to either end
- Dress infant in safe shoes and clothing (soles that do not "catch" on floor, tied shoelaces, pant legs that do not touch floor)
- Avoid walkers, especially near stairs
- Ensure that furniture is sturdy enough for child to pull self to standing position and cruise

Poisoning
- Administer medications as a drug, not as a candy
- Do not administer medications unless so prescribed by a practitioner
- Replace medications and poisons immediately after use; replace caps properly if a child-protector cap is used
- Have syrup of ipecac in home; use only if advised

Burns
- Place guards in front of or around any heating appliance, fireplace, or furnace
- Keep electrical wires hidden or out of reach

- Place plastic guards over electrical outlets; place furniture in front of outlets
- Keep handing tablecloths out of reach (child may pull down hot liquids or heavy or sharp objects)

Injury Prevention during Infancy in Relation to Development

(Age: Birth-4 months)

Major Developmental Accomplishments
- Involuntary reflexes, such as the crawling reflex, may propel infant forward or backward and the startle reflex may cause the body to jerk

Injury Prevention

Aspiration
- Not as great a danger to this age group, but should begin practicing safeguarding early (see under 4-7 months)
- Never shake baby powder directly on infant; place powder in hand and then on infant's skin; store container closed and out of infant's reach
- Hold infant for feeding; do not prop bottle
- Know emergency procedures for choking
- Use pacifier with one-piece construction and loop handle

Suffocation/drowning
- Keep all plastic bags stored out of infant's reach; discard large plastic garment bags after tying in a knot
- Do not cover mattress and loose blankets; no pillows
- Make sure crib design follows federal regulations and mattress fits snugly
- Position crib away from other furniture and away from radiators
- Avoid sleeping in bed with infant
- Do not tie pacifier on a string around infant's neck
- Remove bibs at bedtime
- Never leave infanat alone in bath
- Do not leave infant under 12 months alone on adult or youth mattress

Falls
- Always raise crib rails
- Never leave infant on a raised, unguarded surface
- When in doubt as to where to place child, use the floor
- Restrain child in infant seat and never leave child unattended while the seat is resting on a raised surface
- Avoid using a high chair until child can sit well with support
- May roll over
- Increasing eye-hand coordination and voluntary grasp reflex

Major Developmental Accomplishments (Age: 4-7 months)
- Rolls over
- Sits momentarily
- Grasps and manipulates small objects
- Resecures a dropped object
- Has well-developed eye-hand coordination
- Can focus on and locate very small objects
- Mouthing is very prominent
- Can push up on hands and knees

- Crawls backward

Poisoning
- Not as great a danger to this age group, but should begin practicing safeguards early

Burns
- Install smoke detectors in home
- Use caution when warming formula in microwave ove; always check temperature of liquid before feeding
- Check bathwater
- Do not pour hot liquids when infant is close by, such as sitting on lap
- Beware of cigarette ashes that may fall on infant
- Do not leave infant in the sun for more than a few minutes; keep exposed areas covered
- Wash flame-retardant clothes according to label directions
- Use cool-mist vaporizers
- Do not leave child in parked car
- Check surface heat of car restraint before placing child in seat

Motor vehicles
- Transport infant in federally approved, rear-facing car seat
- Do not place infant on the seat or in lap
- Do not place child in a carriage or stroller behind a parked car

Body damage
Avoid sharp, jugged objects
Keep diaper pins closed and away from infant

Injury Prevention during Early Childhood (Table 29.20)

Table 29.20: Injury prevention of different development abilities related to risk injuries

Developmental abilities related to risk of injury	Injury prevention

Walks, runs, and climbs
Able to open doors and gates
Can ride tricycle
Can throw ball and other object
	Motor vehicles
	Use federally approved car restraint; if restraint is not available, use lap belt
	Supervise child while playing outside
	    Do not allow child to play on curb or behind a parked car
	    Do not permit child to play in pile of leaves, snow, or large carboard container in trafficked area
	Supervise tricycle riding
	Lock fences and doors if not directly supervising children
	Teach child to obey pedestrian safety rules:
	    Obey traffic regulations; walk only at crosswalks and when traffic signal indicates it is safe to cross
	    Sand back a step from curb until it is time to cross
	    Look left, right, and left again and check for turning cars before crossing street

Contd...

Contd...

Developmental abilities related to risk of injury	Injury prevention
	Use sidewalks; when there is no sidewalk, walk on left, facing traffic
	Wear light colors at night, and attach fluorescent material to clothing
Able to explore if left unsupervised Has great curiosity Helpless in water; unaware of its danger; depth of water has no significance	*Drowing* Supervise closely when near any source of water, including buckets Keep all bathroom doors and lids on toilets closed Have fence around swimming and water safety (not a substitute for protection)
Able to reach heights by climbing, stretching, standing on toes, and using objects as a ladder Pulls objects Explores any holes or opening Can open drawers and closets Unaware of potential sources of heat or fire Plays with mechanical objects	*Burns* Turn pot handles toward back of stove Place electric appliances, such as coffee maker, frying pan, and popcorn machine, toward back of counter Place guardrails in front of radiators, fireplaces, or other heating elements Store matches and cigarette lighters in locked or inaccessiblearea; discard carefully Place burning candles, incense, hot foods, ashes, embers, and cigarettes out of reach Do not let tablecloth hang within child's reach Do not let electric cord from iron or other appliance hang within child's reach Cover electrical outlets with protective devices Keep electrical wires hidden or out of reach Do not allow child to play with electrical appliance, wires, or lighters Stress danger of open flames; teach what "hot" means Always check bathwater temperature; adjust hot-water heater temperature to 120°F or lower; do not allow children to play with faucets Apply a sunscreen with SPF 15 or higher when child is exposed to sunlight
Explores by putting objects in mouth Can open drawers, closets, and most containers Climbs Cannot read warning labels Does not knowsafe dose or amount	*Poisoning* Place all potentially toxic agents in a locked cabinet or out of reach (including plants) Replace medications and poisons immediately; replace childresistant caps properly Refer to medications as drugs, not as candy Do not store large surplus of toxic agents Promptly discard empty poison containers; never reuse to store a food item or other poison Teach child not to play in trash containers Never remove labels from containers of toxic substances Have syrup of ipecac in home; use only if advised Know number and location of nearest poison control center (usually listed in front of telephone directory)
Able to open doors and some windows Goes up and down stairs Depth perception unrefined	*Falls* Keep screens in windows, nail securely, and use guardrail

Contd...

Contd...

Developmental abilities related to risk of injury	Injury prevention
	Place gates at top and bottom of stairs
	Keep doors locked or use child resistant doorknob covers at entry to stairs, high porch, or other elevated area, such as laundry chute
	Remove unsecured or scatter rugs
	Apply nonskid mat in bathtub or shower
	Keep crib rails fully raised and mattress at lowest level
	Place carpeting under crib and in bathroom
	Keep large toys and bumpr pads out of crib or playpen (child can use these as "stairs" to climb out), then move to youth bed when child is able to crawl out of crib
	Avoid using walkers, especially near stairs
	Dress in safe clothing (soles that do not "catch" on floor, tied shoelaces, pant legs that do not hang on floor)
	Keep child restrained in vehicles; never leave unattended in shopping cart or stroller
	Supervise at playgrounds; select play areas with soft ground cover and safe equipment
Puts things in mouth	***Choking and suffocation***
May swallow hard or nonedible pieces of food	Avoid large, round chunks of meat, such as whole hot dogs (slice lengthwise into short pieces)
	Avoid fruit with pits, fish with bones, dried beans, hard candy, chewing gum, nuts, popcorn, grapes, marshmallows
	Choose large sturdy toys without sharp edges or small removable parts
	Discard old refrigerators, ovens, and so on; if storing old applience, remove doors
	Keep automatic garage door transmitter in inaccessible place
	Select safe toy boxes or chests without heavy, hinged lids
Still clumsy in many skills	***Bodily damage***
Easily distracted from tasks	Avoid giving sharp or pointed objects-such as knives, scissors, or toothpicks-especially when walking or running
Unaware of potential danger from strangers or other people	Don not allow lillipops or similar objects in mouth when walking or running
	Teach safety precautions (e.g. to carry fork or scissors with pointed end away from face)
	Store all dangerous tools, garden equipment, and firearms in locked cabinet
	Be alert to danger of animals, including household pets
	Use safety glass and decals on large glassed areas, such as sliding glass doors

Contd...

Contd...

Developmental abilities related to risk of injury	Injury prevention
	Teach personal safety:
	Teach name, address, and phone number and to ask for help from appropriate people (cashier, security guard, policeman) if lost; have identification on child (sewn in clothes inside shoe)
	Avoid personalized clothing in public places
	Teach child to never go with a stranger
	Teach child to tell parents if anyone makes child feel uncomfortable in any way
	Always listen to child's concerns regarding others' behavior
	Teach child to say "no" when confronted with uncomfortable situations

APPENDIX IX

Injury Prevention during School-age Years (Table 29.21)

Table 29.21: Injury prevention during school-age years

Developmental abilities related to risk of injury	Injury prevention
Is increasingly involved in activities away from home Is excited by speed and motion Is easily distracted by environment Can be reasoned with	**Motor vehicles** Educate child regarding proper use of seat belts while a passenger in a vehicle Maintain discipline while a passenger in a vehicle (e.g. keep arms inside, do not lean against doors or interfere with driver) Emphasize safe pedestrian behavior Insist on wearing safety apparel (e.g. helmet) where applicable, such as riding bicycle, motorcycle, moped, and all-terrain vehicles
Is apt to overdo May work hard to perfect a skill Has cautious, but not fearful, gross motor actions Likes swimming	**Drowing** Teach child to swim Teach basic rules of water safety Select safe and supervised places to swim Check sufficient water depth for diving Swim with a companion Use an approved flotation device in water or boat Advocate for legislation requiring fencing around pools Learn CPR
Has increasing independence Is adventuresome Enjoys trying new things	**Burns** Instruct child in behavior in areas involving contact with potential burn hazards (e.g. gasoline, matches, bonfires or barbecues, lighter fluid, firecrackers, cigarette lighters, cooking utensils, chemistry sets); avoid climbing or flying kites around high-tension wires Instruct child in proper behavior in the event of fire (e.g. fire drills at home, school, & so on) Teach child safe cooking (use low heat, avoid any frying, be careful to steam burns, scalds, or exploding foods, especially from microwaving)
Adheres to group rules May be easily influenced by peers Strong allegiance to friends	**Poisoning** Educate child regarding hazards of taking nonprescription drugs and chemicals, including aspirin and alcohol

Contd...

Contd...

Developmental abilities related to risk of injury	Injury prevention
	Teach child to say "no" if offered illegal or dangerous drugs or alcohol
	Keep potentially dangerous products in properly labeled receptacles-preferably out of reach
Has increased physical skills	***Bodily damage***
Needs strenuous physical activity	Help provide facilities for supervised activities
Is interested in acquiring new skills and perfecting attained skills	Encourage playing in safe places
Is daring and adventurous, especially with peers	Keep firearms safely locked up except during adult supervision
Frequently plays in hazardous places	Teach proper cre of, use of, and respect for devices with potential danger (power tools, fire-crackers, and so on)
Confidence often exceeds physical capacity	Teach children not to tease or surprise dogs, invade their territory, take dogs' toys, or interfere with dogs' feeding
Desires group loyalty and has strong need for friends' approval	Stress eye, ear, or mouth protection when using potentially hazardous objects or devices or when engaged in potentially hazardous sports
Attempts hazardous feats	Teach safety regarding use of corrective devices (glasses); if child wears contact lenses, monitor duration of wear to prevent corneal damage
Accompanies friends to potentially hazardous facilities	Stress careful selection, use, and maintenance of sports and recreation equipment, such as skateboards and in-line skates
Delights in physical activity	Emphasize proper conditioning, safe practices, and use of safety equipment for sports or recreational activities
Is likely to overdo	Caution against engaging in hazardous sports, such as those involving trampolines
Growth in height exceeds muscular growth and coordination	Use safety glass and decals on large glassed areas, such as sliding glass doors
	Teach name, address, and phone number and to ask for help from appropriate people (cashier, security guard, police) if lost; have identification on child (sewn in clothes, inside shoe)
	Teach personal safety:
	Avoid personalized clothing in public places
	Never go with a stranger
	Tell parents if anyone makes child feel uncomfortable in any way
	Always listen to child's concerns regarding others' behavior
	Say "no" when confronted with uncomfortable situations

APPENDIX X

Injury Prevention during Adolescence (Table 29.22)

Table 29.22: Injury prevention during adolescence

Developmental abilities related to risk of injury	Injury prevention

Need for independence and freedom
Testing independence
Age permitted to drive a motor vehicle (varies)
Inclination for risk taking
Feeling of indestructibility
Need for discharging energy, often at expense of logical thinking and other control mechanisms
Strong need for peer approval
May attempt hazardous feats
Peak incidence for practice and participation in sports
Access to more complex tools, objects, and locations
Can assume responsibility for own actions
	Motor/nonmotor vehicles
	Pedestrian—Emphasize and encourage safe pedestrian behavior
	Passenger—Promote appropriate behavior while riding in a motor vehicle
	Driver—provide competent driver education; encourage judicious use of vehicle, discourage drag racing, "playing chicken"; maintain vehicle in proper condition (brakes, tires, etc.)
	Teach and promote safety and maintenance of two-wheeled vehicles
	Promote and encourage wearing of safety apparel such as helmet, long trousers
	Reinforce the dangers of drugs, including alcohol, when operating a motor vehicle
	Drowning
	Teach nonswimmer to swim
	Teach basic rules of water safety:
	  Judicious selection of place to swim
	  Sufficient water depth for driving
	  Swimming with companion
	Burns
	Reingorce proper behavior in areas involving contact with burn hazzards (gasoline, electric wires, fires)
	Advise regarding excessive exposure to natural or or artificial sunlight (ultraviolet burn)
	Discourage smoking
	Encourage use of sunscreen
	Poisoning
	Educate in hazards of drug use, including alcohol
	Falls
	Teach and encourage general safety measures in all activities
	Bodily damage
	Promote acquisition of proper instruction in sports and use of sports equipment
	Instruct in safe use of and respect for firearms and other devices with potential danger (e.g. power tools, firecrackers)
	Provide and encourage use of protective equipment when using potentially hazardous devices
	Promote access to and/or provision of safe sports and recreational facilities
	Be alert for signs of depression (potential suicide)
	Descourage use of and/or availability of hazardous sports equipment (trampoline, surfboards)
	Instruct regarding proper use of corrective devices such as glasses, contact lenses, hearing aids
	Encourage and foster judicious application of safety principles and prevention

APPENDIX XI

PARENTAL GUIDANCE

Guidance during Infancy

First 6 Months
- Understand each parent's adjustment to newborn, especially mother's postpartal emotional needs
- Teach care of infant and assist parents to understand his or her individual needs and temperament and that the infant expresses wants through crying
- Reassure parents that infant cannot be spoiled by too much attention during the first 4 to 6 months
- Encourage parents to establish a schedule that meets needs of child and themselves
- Help parents understand infant's need for stimulation in environment
- Support parents' pleasure in seeing child's growing friendliness and social response, especially smiling
- Plan anticipatory guidance for safety
- Stress need for immunization
- Prepare for introduction of solid foods

Second 6 Months
- Prepare parents for child's "stranger anxiety".
- Encourage parents to allow child to cling to them and avoid long separation from either
- Guide parents concerning discipline because of infant's increasing mobility
- Encourage use of negative voice and eye contact rather than physical punishment as a means of discipline
- Teach injury prevention because of child's advancing motor skills and curiosity
- Encourage parents to leave child with suitable caregiver to allow some free time
- Discuss readiness for weaning
- Explore parents feelings regarding infant's sleep patterns

Guidance during Toddler years

Ages 12 to 18 Months
- Prepare parents for expected behavioral changes of toddler, especially negativism and ritualism
- Assess present feeding habits and encourage gradual weaning from bottle and increased intake of solid foods
- Stress expected feeding changes of physiologic anorexia, presence of food fads and strong taste preferences, need for scheduled routine at mealtimes, inability to sit through an entire meal, and lack of table manners
- Assess sleep patterns at night, particularly habit of a bedtime bottle, which is a major cause of dental caries, and procrastination behaviors that delay hour of sleep
- Prepare parents for potential dangers of the home, particularly motor vehicle, poisoning, and falling injuries; give appropriate suggestions for safeproofing the home
- Discuss need for firm but gentle discipline and ways in which to deal with negativism and temper tantrums; stress positive benefits of appropriate discipline
- Emphasize importance for both child and parents of brief, periodic separations
- Discuss new toys that use developing gross and fine motor, language, cognitive, and social skills

- Emphasize need for dental supervision, types of basic dental hygiene at home, and food habits that predispose to caries; stress importance of supplemental fluoride

Ages 18 to 24 Months
- Stress importance of peer companionship in play
- Explore need for preparation for additional sibling; stress importance of preparing child for new experiences
- Discuss present discipline methods, their effectiveness, and parents' feelings about child's negativism; stress that negativism is important aspect of developing self-assertion and independence and is not a sign of spoiling.
- Discuss signs of readiness for toilet training; emphasize importance of waiting for physical and psychologic readiness.
- Discuss development of fears, such as darkness or loud noises, and of habits, such as security blanket or thumb-sucking; stress normalcy of these transient behaviors
- Prepare parents for signs of regression in time of stress
- Assess child's ability to separate easily from parents for brief periods of separation under familiar circumstance
- Allow parents opportunity to express their feelings of weariness, frustration, and exasperation; be aware that it is often difficult to love toddlers at times when they are not asleep
- Point out some of the next year, such as longer attention span, somewhat less negativism, and increased concern for pleasing others

Ages 24 to 36 Months
- Discuss importance of imitation and domestic mimicry and need to include child in activities
- Discuss approaches toward toilet training, particularly realistic expectations and attitude toward accidents.
- Stress uniqueness of toddlers' thought processes, especially through their use of language, poor understanding of time, causal relationships in terms of proximity of events, and inability to see events from another's perspective
- Stress that discipline still must be quite structured and concrete and that relying solely on verbal reasoning and explanation leads to confusion, misunderstanding, and even injuries
- Discuss investigation of preschool or daycare center toward completion of second year

Guidance during Preschool Years

Age 3 Years
- Prepare parents for child's increasing interest in widening relationships
- Encourage enrollment in preschool
- Emphasize importance of setting limits
- Prepare parents to expect exaggerated tension-reduction behaviors, such as need for "security blanket".
- Encourage parents to offer child choice when child vacillates
- Expect marked changes at 3½ years, when child becomes less coordinated (motor and emotional), becomes insecure, and exhibits emotional extremes
- Prepare parents for normal dysfluency in speech and advise them to avoid focusing on the pattern
- Prepare parents to experctextra demands on their attention as a reflection of child's emotional insecurity and fear of loss of love

- Warm parents that equilibrium of 3-years-old will change to aggressive, out-of-boundsbehavior of 4-year-old
- Anticipate more stable appetite with more food selections
- Stress need for protection and education of child to prevent injury (see Injury prevention)

Age 4 Years
- Prepare for more aggressive behavior, including motor activity and offensive language
- Prepare parents to expect resistance to parental authority
- Explore parental feelings regarding child's behavior
- Suggest some kind of respite for primary caregivers, such as placing child in preschool for part of the day
- Prepare for increasing sexual curiosity
- Emphasize importance of realistic limit-setting on behavior and appropriate discipline techniques
- Prepare parents for highly imaginary 4-year-old who indulges in "tall tales" (to be differentiated from lies) and for child's imaginary playmates
- Expect nightmares or an increase in them and suggest they make sure child is fully awakened from a frightening dream
- Provide ressurance that a period of calm begins at 5 years of age

Age 5 Years
- Expect tranquil period at 5 years
- Prepare child for entrance into school environment
- Make sure immunizations are up-to-date before entering school
- Suggest that nonemployed mothers or fathers consider own activities when child begins school
- Suggest swimming lessons

Guidance during School-age Years

Age 6 Years
- Prepare parents to expect strong food preferences and frequent refusal of specific food items
- Prepare parents to expect increasingly ravenous appetite
- Prepare parents for emotionality as child experiences erratic mood changes
- Help parents anticipate continued susceptibility to illness
- Teach injury prevention and safety, especially bicycle safety
- Encourage parents to respect child's need for privacy and to provide a separate bedroom for child, if possible
- Prepare parents to expect increased involvement with peers and interest in activities outside the home
- Help parents understand the need to encourage child's interactions with peers

Ages 7 to 10 Years
- Prepare parents to expect improvement in health with fewer illnesses, but warm them that allergies may increase or become apparent
- Prepare parents to expect an increase in minor injuries
- Emphasize caution in selecting and maintaining sports equipment and reemphasize safety
- Prepare parents to expect increased involvement withpeers and interest in activities outside the home

- Emphasize the need to encourage independence while maintaining limit-setting and discipline
- Prepare mothers to expect more demands at 8 years
- Prepare fathers to expect increasing admiration at 10 years; encourage father-child activities.
- Prepare parents for prepubescent changes in girls

Ages 11 to 12 years
- Help parents prepare child for body changes if pubescence
- Prepare parents to expect a growth spurt in girls
- Make certain child's sex education is adequate with accurate information
- Prepare parents to expect energetic but stormy behavior at 11, to become more even tempered at 12
- Encourage parents to support child's desire to "grow up" but to allow regressive behavior when needed
- Prepare parents to expect an increase in masturbation
- Instruct parents that the amount of rest child needs may increase
- Help parents educate child regarding experimentation with potentially harmful activities

Health Guidance
- Help parents understand the importance of regular health and dental care for child
- Encourage parents to teach and model sound health practices-including diet, rest, activity, and exercise
- Stress the need to encourage children to engage in appropriate physical activities
- Emphasize providing a safe physical and emotional environment
- Encourage parents to teach and model safety practices

Guidance during Adolescence
- Accept adolescent as a human being
- Respect adolescent's ideas, likes and dislikes, wishes
- Provide opportunity for choosing options and accept natural consequences of these choices
- Allow teenager to learn by doing, even when choices and methods differ from those of adults
- Provide adolescent with clear, reasonable limits
- Clarify house rules and consequences for breaking them
- Use family conferences to negotiate house rules
- Allow increasing independence within limitations of safety and well-being
- Be available but avoid pressing young person too far
- Respect adolescent's privacy
- Try to share adolescent's feelings of joy or sorrow
- Respond to feelings, as well as words
- Give space to a teenager who is in a bad mood
- Be available to answer questions, give information, and provide companionship
- Listen and try to be open to adolescent's views, even when they disagree with parental views
- Try to make communication clear
- Assist adolescent in selecting appropriate career goals and preparing for adult role
- Provide undemanding love
- Be aware that:
- Adolescent is struggling for independence

- Adolescent is sensitive to feelings and behavior that affect him or her
- Message given to adolescent may not be message received
- Friends are extremely important to adolescent
- Adolescent has a strong need "to belong"
- Adolescent sees things in black or white, good or bad

APPENDIX XII

PLAY AND IT'S RELATION TO DEVELOPMENT

Functions of Play

Sensorimotor Development
- Improves fine and gross motor skill and coordination
- Enhances development of all the senses
- Encourages exploration of the physical nature of the world
- Provides for release of surplus energy

Intellectual Development
- Provides multiple sources of learning
- Exploration and manipulation of shapes, sizes, textures, colors
- Experience with numbers, spatial relationships, abstract concepts
- Opportunity to practice and expand language skills
- Provides opportunity to rehearse past experiences to assimilate them into new perceptions and relationships
- Helps children to comprehend the world in which they live and to distinguish between fantasy and reality

Socialization and Moral Development
- Teach adult roles, including sex role behavior
- Provides opportunity for testing relationships
- Develops social skills
- Encourages interaction and development of positive attitudes toward others
- Inforces approved patterns of behavior and moral standards

Creativity
- Provides an expressive outlet for creative ideas and interests
- Allows for fantasy and imagination
- Enhances development of special talents and interests

Self-awareness
- Facilitates the development of self-identity
- Encourages regulation of own behavior
- Allows for testing of own abilities (self-mastery)
- Provides for comparison of own abilities with those of others
- Allows for opportunity to learn how own behavior affects others

Therapeutic Value
- Provides for release from tension and stress
- Allows for expression of emotions and release of unacceptable impulses in a socially acceptable fashion
- Encourages experimentation and testing of fearful situations in a safe manner
- Facilitates nonverbal and indirect verbal communication of needs, fears, and desires

APPENDIX XIII

DEVELOPMENTAL CHARACTERISTICS OF CHILDREN'S RESPONSES TO PAIN

Developmental Characteristics of Children's Responses to Pain

Young Infants
- Generalized body response of rigidity or thrashing, possibly with local reflex withdrawal of stimulated area
- Loud crying
- Facial expression of pain (brows lowered and drawn together, eyes tightly closed, mouth open and squarish)
- Demonstrates no association between approaching stimulus and subsequent pain

Older Infant
- Localized body response with deliberate withdrawal of stimulated area
- Loud crying
- Facial expression of pain and/or anger (same facial characteristics as pain but eyes may be open)
- Physical resistance, especially pushing the stimulus away *after* it is applied

Young Children
- Loud crying, screaming
- Verbal expressions of "Ow", "Ouch", or "It hurts"
- Thrashing of arms and legs
- Attempts to push stimulus away before it is applied
- Uncooperative; needs physical restraint
- Requests termination of procedure
- Clings to parent, nurse, or other significant person
- Requests emotional support, such as hugs or other forms of physical comfort
- May become restless and irritable with continuing pain
- All these behaviors may be seen in anticipation of actual painful procedure

School-age Children
- May see all behaviors of young child, especially during painful procredure but less in anticipatory period
- Stalling behavior, such as "Wait a minute" or "I'm not ready"
- Muscular rigidity, such as clenched fists, white knuckles, gritted teeth, contracted limbs, body stiffness, closed eyes, wrinkled forehead

Adolescents
- Less vocal protest
- Less motor activity
- More verbal expressions, such as "It hurts" or "You're hurting me"
- Increased muscle tension and body control.

APPENDIX XIV

AGE SPECIFIC APPROACHES TO PHYSICAL EXAMINATION OF CHILDREN BASED ON DEVELOPMENTAL CHARACTERISTICS

Infant

Position
- *Before sitting* prone or supine in mother's lap, mother in view or in couch
- *Afte sitting* sitting in mother's lap, mother in full view

Preparation
- Undress completely if room is warm
- Distract by using light, rattle and talking, allow them to hold something in hand, smile and talk with gentle voice, breastfeed
- Examine, ears, eyes, mouth last
- Take help of mothers in restraining children for examination of throat and ears.

Procedure
- If quiet ascultate heart, lungs and abdomen
- Record heart rate and respiratory rate
- Palpate and percuss heart, lung and abdomen
- Head to foot examination including reflexes
- Examine ears, mouth, eyes and Moro's reflex last

Toddler

Position
Sitting or standing facing examiner preferably mother or parent holding one hand and in parent's lap
   Toddlers are afraid of being examined in lying down position or from behind, as, often injections are administered in these positions

Preparation
- Allow them to handle equipment and do a quick examination
- Praise the child
- Remove clothes gently and piecemeal
- Take parents help in restraining

Procedure
- Inspect body through play.
- Minimum handling.
- Introduce equipment slowly.
- Ascultate, percuss, palpate when quiet.
- Traumatic procedures done last.
  e.g. throat, eye and ear examination

Preschool Child

Position
- Standing or sitting.
- May be quiet in prone or supine.
- Parents presence is important.

Preparation
- Request self undressing.
- Underpants may be left if shy.
- Offer equipments.

Procedure
- If cooperative, head to foot.
- If uncooperative, like toddler.

Schoold Child

Position
- Prefer sitting.
- Cooperative in any position.
- Younger children like parent's presence and older may like privacy.

Preparations
- Request self undressing
- Allow underpants
- Explain use of equipments

Procedure
- Head to foot
- Genitalia last
- Respect their privacy and modesty.

Adolescents

Position
- Same as school children
- Parents presence--leave the option to child

Preparation
- Undress in private
- Give gown or covering sheet
- Expose only areas to be examined
- Respect privacy and their modesty
- Explain findings and reassure each time
- Genitalia are examined last, (only if required).

APPENDIX XV

MEASUREMENT OF INTELLIGENCE

Intelligence as a concept has been understood in different ways by different psychologists, they had emphasized that:
- Intelligence is the ability to learn.
- Intelligence is an ability to deal with abstract.
- Intelligence is an ability to make adjustments or adapt to new situation.

Wechsler gave a comprehensive definition of intelligence, that is, "Intelligence is the aggregate or global capacity of an individual to act purposefully, to think rationally and to deal effectively with the environment."

Intelligence is measured with the help of psychological tests. Psychologists have devised many such tests for the measurement of intelligence. Measurement of intelligence is expressed in terms of Intelligence Quotient (IQ). The use of this index was first suggested by William Stern. The ratio of an individuals Mental Age (MA) to his Chronological Age (CA) is found by the formula

$$IQ = \frac{MA}{CA} \times 100$$

IQ indicates rate of mental development or degree of brightness.

Mental age This concept was introduced by Binet, means level of development in mental ability expressed as equivalent to chronological age.

SCALES FOR INFANTS AND PRESCHOOL CHILDREN

Several scales are devised to evaluate mental development of children ranging in age from one month to six years. These scales are not tests as the term is commonly understood, they are norms and inventories of development of behavior. The scales commonly used in clinical practice are:

Gesell's Developmental Schedule

The test consists of selected items for assessing maturity in infants are preschool children in the four developmental areas:

1. Motor behavior	:	Includes both gross bodily control and finer motor coordination like head balance, postural reaction and locomotion.
2. Adaptive behavior	:	Includes perceptual, orientational, manual and verbal adjustments.
3. Language development	:	Includes all means of communication such as facial expression, gestures, postural movements and vocalization.
4. Personal-Social behavior	:	Includes the child's personal reactions to others play behavior, social smile, feeding and toilet training.

Gesell's Developmental schedule provides an estimate of Developmental Age (DA) and Developmental Quotient (DQ). It is used for the age group of 4-72 months.

Data on GDS items should be obtained through direct observation of the child's response and supplemented by information gathered from the mother. If the item is adequately performed by the child it should be marked right (✓), if the child fails it should marked wrong (×).

With the help of the items marked right find out DA for each of the four developmental areas and overall DA by adding all the DAs and divide by 4. Compute

DQ by dividing DA by CA and multiplying by 100 for each developmental areas and overall DQ.

Example DAs-DQs of a 2 year old child are as follows

Developmental area	DA	DQ
1. Motor months	6 Months	25
2. Adaptive behavior	9 Months	33
3. Language development	6 Months	25
4. Personal-social months	12 Months	50

Overall DA = 6 months + 9 months + 6 months + 12 months/4 = 8.2 months
Overall DQ = 34.

DEVELOPMENTAL SCREENING TEST

Devised by Bharathraj, is a non-verbal test designed to measure the mental development of children from birth to 15 years. The information is obtained by the use of semi-structured interview with the parents/caretaker. This test is particularly useful for assessing children who are non-cooperative, those with multiple impairment or those with severe behavior problems.

VINELAND SOCIAL MATURITY SCALE

The Vineland Social Maturity Scale (VSMS) was developed by EA Doss. Adapted to Indian conditions by Dr AJ Malin. VSMS measures the differential social capacities of an individual. It provides an estimate of Social Age (SA) and Social Quotient (SQ). SA shows high correlation with Binet mental age.

It is designed to measure social areas;
1. Self help general (SHG)
2. Self help eating (SHE)
3. Self help dressing (SHD)
4. Self direction (SD)
5. Occupation (OCC)
6. Communication (COM)
7. Locomation (LOC)
8. Socialization (SOC)

The scale consists of 89 test items grouped in to year levels. VSMS can be used for the age group of 0-1 year to 15 years.

Data on VSMS items should be obtained through direct observation of the child's responses and supplemented by information gathered from the mother. If the item is adequately performed by the child it should be marked right ($\checkmark$), if the child fails it should be marked wrong (×). Scoring is total number of the items marked right and to find out social Age from the norms give in VSMS manual.

Example: If the total score on VSMS is 28

SA = 19.7 months

CA = 3.6 years

$$SQ = \frac{SA}{CA} \times 100 = 47$$

SCALES FOR CHILDREN

Sequine form Board Test

This test was developed by Sequine, a French physician. Sequine Form Board Test (SFB) is the most commonly used performance test for measuring psychomotor and

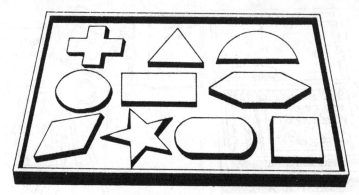

Fig. 29.7: Sequine form board

visuo-perceptual abilities for children between 4 to 20 years. It is also used as a quick measure of intelligence in children between 3-11 years and for mentally retarded adults.

The test consists of a form board. The board has 10 wooden blocks of different shapes (Fig. 29.7). The blocks are stacked in three piles like:

	Examiner's left	Middle	Examiner's right
Top of the board	Hexagon	Triangle	Diamond
	Oval	Cross	Circle
	Rectangle	Square	Star
Bottom of the board		Half circle	

Ask the child to place those blocks in a corresponding wholes as fast as possible. Three trials are given and note down the time taken in each trial. Convert the time taken in to mental age with the help of the norms given in the SFB manual.

Example	:	1st trial	35 sec
		2nd trial	30 sec
		3rd trial	27 sec

Scoring : Shortest of 3 trials or total of 3 trials whichever is less. In this simple way the MA on total of 3 trials is 7 years.

Binet Scale (Fig. 29.8)

The first intelligence test devised by Binet-Simon in 1905 to identify mentally deficient children. In 1908 the test was standardized and the concept of mental age employed for the first time. Many revisions were done. In 1916 the revision was called as Stanford-Binet because the revision was done in Stanford University. This test had been revised and adapted to Indian conditions and is available as Binet-Kamat Test. It has been translated in Hindi, Marathi, Gujarati and Kannada.

Binet-Kamat test is an extensively used verbal test for mentally retarded persons. It gives a pattern analysis for seven primary abilities; language, memory, conceptual thinking, reasoning, numerical reasoning, visuo-motor co-ordination and social intelligence.

The test consists of 90 items, covering age group of 3 years to 22 years. At each age level it has six items with some alternate items (which may replace one of six). The scoring in each item gets 2 months credit if answered correctly. For example, if the

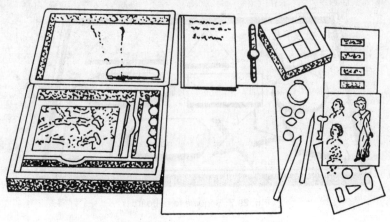

Fig. 29.8: Binet-Kamat test materials

child answers all the six items at the 3 years level, this means the child's mental age is 3 years. This is called as basal year, then we have to proceed further till the child fails in all six items of a particular age level. This is called as terminal year, here we have to stop the test. The credits are added to the basal year so the total score is the mental age (Table 29.23).

Table 29.23: Binet-Kamat record sheet

	Mental age				
Test items	3	4	5	6	7
1	+	+	+	+	−
2	+	+	+	−	−
3	+	+	−	−	−
4	+	−	−	−	−
5	+	−	−	−	−
6	+	−	−	−	−
Alt					
1			−	−	
2		−			
3		−			

MA= 3 years + 6 months + 4 months + 2 months = 4 years
CA = 12 years
IQ = 33

APPENDIX XVI

ASSESSMENT OF DEVELOPMENT DENVER II* (Figs 29.9 and 29.10)

The Denver II is a major revision and a restandardization of the Denver Developmental Screening Test (DDST) and the Revised Denver Developmental Screening Test (DDST-R). It differs from the earlier screening tests in items included, the form, the interpretation, and the referral. Like the other tests, it assesses gross motor, language, fine motor, adaptive, and personal-social development in children from 1 month to 6 years.

Item Differences

The previous total of 105 items has been increased to 125, including an increase from 21 DDST to 39 Denver II language items.

Previous items that were difficult to administer and/or interpret have either been modified or eliminated. Many items that were previously tested by parental report now require observation by the examiner.

Each item was evaluated to determine if significant differences exist among sex, ethnic group, maternal education, and place of residence. Items for which clinically significant differences exit were replaced or, it retained, are discussed in the Technical Manual. When evaluating children delayed on one of these items, the diagnostician can look up norms for the subpopulations to determine if the delay may be due to sociocultural differences.

Test Form Differences

The age scale is similar to the American Academy of Pediatrics suggested periodicity schedule for health maintenance visits to facilitate use of the Denver II at these times.

In children born prematurely, the age is adjusted only until the child is 2 years old.

The items on the test form are arranged in the same format as the DDST-R.

The norms for the distribution bars were updated with the new standardization data but retain the 25th, 50th, 75th, and 90th percentile divisions (see practice Alert, p 29).

The test form contains a place to rate the child's behavioral characteristics (compliance, interest in surroundings, fearfulness, and attention span).

Interpretation and Referral

Explain to the parents that the Denver II is not an intelligence test but a systematic appraisal of the child's present development. Stress that the child is not expected to perform each item.

To determine relative areas of advancement and areas of delay, sufficient items should be administered to establish the basal and celling levels in each sector.

By scoring appropriate items as "pass", "refusal", or "no opportunity", and relating such scores to the age of the child, each item can be interpreted as described in Table 29.24.

To identify cautions, all items intersected by the age line are administered.

---

* To ensure that the Denver II is administered and interpreted in the prescribed manner, it is recommended that those intending to administer the Denver II receive the appropriate training, which can be otained with the forms and instructional manual from Denver Developmental Materials, PO Box 6919, Denver, CO 80206-0919, USA: (303) 355-4729.

Denver II

Examiner:
Date:

Name:
Birth date:
ID No.

Months

2   4   6   9   12   15   18   24

Years

3   4   5   6

Personal-Social

Fine motor-adaptive

Language

Gross motor

Test Behavior
(Check boxes for 1st, 2nd or 3rd test)

Typical	1	2	3
Yes			
No			

Compliance (see Note 31)	1	2	3
Always complies			
Usually complies			
Rarely complies			

Interest in Surroundings	1	2	3
Alert			
Somewhat disinterested			
Seriously disinterested			

Feartulness	1	2	3
None			
Mild			
Extreme			

Attention Span	1	2	3
Appropriate			
Somewhat distractable			
Very distractable			

Months

2   4   6   9   12   15   18   24

Years

3   4   5   6

Fig. 29.9

DIRECTIONS FOR ADMINISTRATION

1. Try to get child to smile by smiling, talking or waveing. Do not touch him/her.
2. Child must stare at hand several seconds.
3. Parent may help guide toothbrush and put toothpaste on brush.
4. Child does not have to be able to tie shoes or button/zip in the back.
5. Move yarn slowly in an arc from one side to the other, about 8° above child's face.
6. Pass if child grasps rattle when it is touched to the backs or tips of fingers.
7. Pass if child tries to see where yarn went. Yarn should be dropped quickly from sight from tester's hand without arm movement.
8. Child must transfer cube from hand to hand without help of body, mouth, or table.
9. Pass if child picks up raisin or with any part of thumb and finger.
10. Line can very only 30° or less from lester's line.
11. Make a fist with thumb pointing upward and wiggle only the thumb. Pass if child imitates and does not move any fingers other than the thumb.

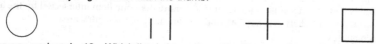

12. Pass any enclosed form. Fail continuous round motions (pass 3 of 3 or 5 of 6).
13. Which line is longer? (Not bigger). Turn paper upside down and repeat.
14. Pass any lines crossing near midpoint.
16. Have child copy first. If failed, demonstrate.

When giving items 12, 14, and 15, do not name the forms. Do not demonstrate 12 and 14.
16. When scoring, each pair (2 arms, 2 legs, etc.) counts as one part.
17. Place one cube in cup and shakegently near child's ear, but out of sight. Repeat for other ear.
18. Point to picture and have child name it (No credit is given for sounds only).
   If less than 4 pictures are named correctly, have child point to picture as each is name by tester.

19. Using doll, tell child: Show me the nose, eyes, ears, mouth, hands, feet, tummy, hair. Pass 6 of 8
20. Using picture, ask child: which one flies?...says meow?...talks?...barks?...gallops? Pass 2 of 5, 4 of 5.
21. Ask child: What do you do when you are cold?...tired?...hungry? Pass 2 of 3, 3 of 3.
22. Ask child:What do you do with a cup? What is a chair used for? What is a pencil used for? Action words must be included in answers.
23. Pass if child correctly places and says how many blocks are on paper (1,5).
24. Tell child: Put block on table; under table; In front of me, behind me. Pass 4 of 4. (Do not help child by pointing, moving head or eyes).
25. Ask child: What is a ball?...lake?...desk?...house?...banana?...curtain?...fence?...celling? Pass if defined in terms of use, shape, what it is made of, or general category (such as banana is fruit, not just yellow). Pass 5 of 8, 7 of 8.
26. Ask child: If a horse is big. A mouse is ___? If fire is hot, ice is ___? If the sun shine during the day, the moon shines during the ___? Pass 2 of 3.
27. Child may use wall or rail only, not person. May not crawl.
28. Child must throw ball overhand 3 feet to within arm's reach of tester.
29. Child must perform standing broad jump over width of test sheet (8½ inches).
30. Tell child to walk forward, ⊂⊃⊂⊃ → heel within 1 inch of toe. tester may demonstrate. Child must walk 4 consecutive steps.
31. In the second year, half of normal children are non-compliant.

OBSERVATIONS:

Fig. 29.10: Directions for administration

To screen solely for developmental delays, only the items located totally to the left of the child's age line are administered.

Criteria for referral are based on the availability of resources in the community.

Table 29.24

Denver II Scoring

Interpretation of Denver II scores	Interpretation of test
Advanced: Passed an item completely to the *right* of the age line (passed by less than 25% of children at an age older than the child)	**Normal:** No delays and a maximum of one caution
OK: Passed, failed, or refused an item intersected by the age line between the 25th and 75th percentiles	**Suspect:** One or more delays and/or two or more cautions
Caution: Failed or refused item intersected by the age line on or between the 75th and 90th percentiles	**Untestable:** Refusals on one or more items completely to the left of the age line or on more than one item intersected by the age line in the 75% to 90% area
Delay: Failed an item completely to the *left* of the age line may also be considered delays, since the reason for the refusal may be inability to perform the task	**Recommendations for referral for suspect and untestable tests** Rescreen in 1 to 2 weeks to rule out temporary factors. If rescreen is suspect or untestable, use clinical judgment based on the following: number of cautions and delays; which items are cautions and delays; rate of past development; clinical examination and history; availability of referral resources.

APPENDIX XVII

Revised Denver Prescreening Developmental Questionnaire[*] (Figs 29.11A and B)
The Revised Prescreening Developmental Questionnaire (R-PDQ) is a revision of the original PDQ. Advantages of the R-PDDQ include the addition and arrangement of items to be more age-appropriate, simplified parent scoring, and easier comparison with Denver Developmental Screening Test (DDST) norms for professionals. The R-PQD is a parent answered prescreen consisting of 105 questions from the DDST, although only a subset of questions are asked for each age group. With less educated parents, the form may need to be read to the caregiver.

Preparation and scoring of the R-PDQ include the following:

1. Calculate the child's age as detailed in the Denver II manual and choose the appropriate form[**] for the child: orange (0 to 9 months), purple (9 to 24 months), gold (2 to 4 years), white (4 to 6 years), (See sample of 0 to 9 months from Fig. 0.00).
2. Give the appropriate form to the child's caregiver and have person note relationship to the child. Have the caregiver answer questions until: (1) 3 NOs are circled (they do not have to be consecutive); or (2) all of the questions on both sides of the form have been answered.
3. Check form to see that all appropriate questions have been answered.
4. Review "YES" and "NO" responses. Ensure that the child's caregiver understood each question and scored the items correctly. Give particular attention to the scoring of questions that require verbal responses by the child and that require the child to draw.
5. Identify "delays" (item passed by 90% of children at a younger age than the child being screened). Ages at which 90% of children in the DDST sample passed the items are indicated in parentheses in the "For Office Use" column. These ages are shown in months and weeks up to 24 months, and in years and months after 24 months. Highlight "delays" by circling the 90% age in parentheses to the right of the item that the child was not able to perform.
6. Children who have no "delays" are considered to be developing normally.
7. If a child has one "delay", give the caregiver age-appropriate developmental activities to pursue with the child,[†] and schedule the child for rescreening with the R-PDQ 1 month later. If on rescreening a month later the child has one or more "delays", schedule second-stage screening with the Denver II as soon as possible.
8. If a child has two or more "delays" on the first-stage screening with the R-PDQ, schedule a second-stage screening with the Denver II as soon as possible. If, on second-stage screening with the Denver II, a child receives other than normal results, schedule the child for a diagnostic evaluation.

---

[*] Forms and complete instructions are available from Denver Developmental Materials, Inc., PO Box 6919, Denver, CO 80206-0919, USA; (303) 355-4729.
[**] Suggested Denver Developmental Activities are available from Denver Developmental Materials, Inc.

APPENDIX XVIII

The Goodenough Draw-A-Man Test (See Fig. 29.2)

The Goodenough draw-a-mantest is on of the simplest developmental tests that may be done in the office. The rules and scoring criteria are given below.

Basal age = 3 years. For each four criteria, add 1 year to arrive at mental age, between ages 3 and 10 years. Instruct child to draw *a complete person;* no further instructions.

$$\frac{\text{Maturation age}}{\text{Chronological age}} \times \frac{100}{1} = \text{IQ}$$

Twenty-eight criteria for scoring:

1. Head present
2. Legs present
3. Arms present
4. Trunk present
5. Length of trunk greater than breadth
6. Shoulder indicated
7. Both arms and legs attached to trunk
8. Legs attached to trunk and arms to trunk at correct point
9. Neck present
10. Outline of neck continuous with that of head or trunk, or both
11. Eyes present
12. Nose present
13. Mouth present
14. Both nose and mouth in two dimensions, two lips shown
15. Nostrils indicated
16. Hair shown
17. Hair on more than circumference of head, nontransparent, better than scribble.
18. Clothing present
19. Two articles of clothing, nontransprent
20. Entire drawing, with sleeves and trousers shown, free from transparency.
21. Four or more articles of clothing definitely indicated
22. Costume complete without incongruities
23. Fingers shown
24. Correct number of fingers shown
25. Fingers in two dimensions, length greater than breadth, angle subtended not greater than 180 degrees
26. Opposition of thumbs shown
27. Hand shown as distinct from fingers or arms
28. Arm joint shown; either elbow, shoulder, or both.

0-9 Months (R-PDQ)

REVISED DENVER PRESCREENING

Child's Name _____

Person Completing R-PDQ: _____

Relation to Child _____

_____

	For Office Use

CONTINUE ANSWERING UNTIL 3 "NOs" ARE CIRCLED

1. Equal movements

   When your baby is lying on his/her back, can (s)he move each of his/her arms as easily as the other and each of the legs as easily as the other? Answer No if your child makes jerky or uncoordinated movements with one or both of his/her arms or legs.

   Yes   No   (0)   FMA

2. Stomach lifts head

   When your baby is on his/her stomach on a flat surface, can (s)he left his/her head off the surface?

   Yes   No   (0-3)   GM

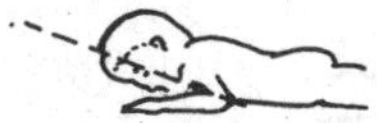

3. Regards face

   When your baby is lying on his/her back, can (s)he look at you and watch your face?

   Yes   No   (1)   PS

4. Follows to midline

   When your child is on his/her back, can (s)he follow your movement by turning his/her head from one side to facing directly forward?

   Yes   No   (1-1)   FMA

5. Responds to bell

   Does your child respond with eye movements, change in breathing or other change in activity to a bell or rattle sounded outside his/her line of vision?

   Yes   No   (1-2)   L

6. Vocalizes not crying

   Does your child make sounds other than crying, such as gurgling, cooing or babbling?

   Yes   No   (1-3)   L

7. Smiles responsively

   When you smile and talk to your baby, does (s)he smile back at you?

   Yes   No   (1-3)   PS

   Contd...

Fig. 29.11A: Revised prescreening developmental questionnaire

DEVELOPMENTAL QUESTIONNAIRE

For Office Use

Today's Date: _____ yr _____ mo _____ day

Child's Birthdate: _____ yr _____ mo _____ day

Subtract to get Child's Exact Age: _____ yr _____ mo _____ day

R-PDQ Age: (_____ yr _____ mo _____ completed wks)

		For Office Use

8. **Follows past midline**
When your child is on his/her back, does (s)he follows your movement by turning his/her head from one side almost all the way to the other side?

Yes   No   (2-2)   FM

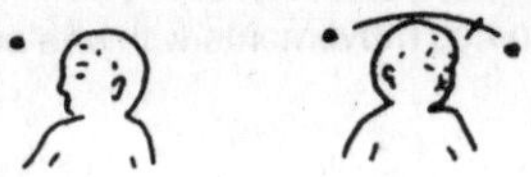

9. **Stomach head up 45°**
When your baby is on his/her stomach on a flat surface, can (s)he left his/her head 45°?

Yes   No   (2-2)   GM

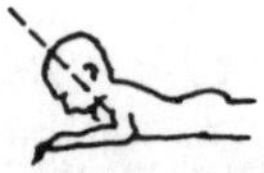

10. **Stomach, head up 90°**
When your baby is on his/her stomach on a flat surface, can (s)he lift his/her head 90°?

Yes   No   (3)   GM

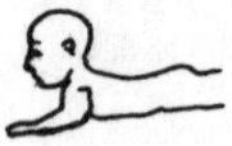

11. **Laughs**
Does your baby laugh out loud without being tickled or touched?

Yes   No   (3-1)   L

12. **Hands together**
Does your baby play with his/her hands by touching them together?

Yes   No   (3-3)   FMA

13. **Follows 180°**
When your child is on his/her back, does (s)he follow your movement from one side *all the way* to the other side?

Yes   No   (4)   FMA

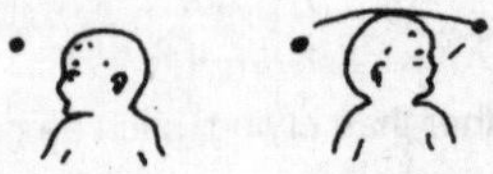

14. **Grasps rattle**
It is important that you follow instructions carefully. Do not place the pencile in the palm of your child's hand. When you touch the pencil to the back or tips of your baby's fingers, does your baby grasp the pencil for a few seconds?

Yes   No   (4)   FMA

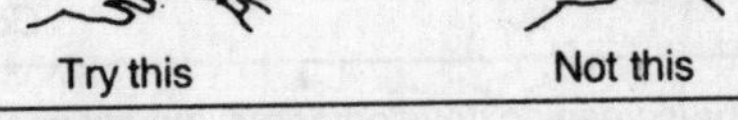

Try this   Not this

Fig. 29.11B: Revised prescreening developmental questionnaire

APPENDIX XIX

Neonatal Reflexes (Table 29.25)

Table 29.25: Some important reflexes in newborn

Reflex	Method of eliciting	Time of Appearance	Time of Disappearance	Remarks
Grasp	Palmar: By introducing finger or suitable object into the palm from the ulnar side	Birth	6 months	• Persistence beyond stipulated period is a sign of cerebral palsy (CP)
	Plantar: By gently stroking the sole of the foot behind the toes.	Birth	10 months	• Absent in generalised neurological depression, hemisyndrome, Erb's palsy clavicle fracture.
Moro	Head dropped by 300	28 week	2-3 months	• Incomplete before 35 weeks of gest.
				• Exaggerated (even in presence of hypotonia)/absent in CP
	Components			• Absent in hypotonia.
	— Abduction-Extension			• In hypertonia, arm may fail to open and arm movements are incomplete. movements are incomplete.
	— Opening of fingers			• Asymmetrical Moro may be seen in: Erb's palsy, fracture of humerus, clavicle, spastic hemiplegia
	— Abduction of arm, flexion of arms embracing phenomenon.			• In kernicterus sudden extension of arm is not followed by flexion but downward rolling of eye balls, lid lag and peculiar grim
				• Adduction phase is poor in term growth retarded babies.
Startle	Sudden voice or tapping	1month	3-5 months	• It is similar to Moro reflex but elbow is flexed istead of extension and hands remain closed.

Contd...

Contd...

Reflex	Method of eliciting	Time of Appearance	Time of Disappearance	Remarks
Asymmetric tonic neck	Prerequisites: lying awake and at rest, supine position. Method:-head turned to one side: arm and leg same side get extended and knee of contralateral side is flexed.		2-3 months	• Persists beyond 3 months in spastic children and in cerebral palsy even after 5 months. • Absent in medullary or spinal cord damage. • May be weak or absent in small for date babies.
Walking reflex	Infant held vertically and his sole is pressed against the surface of the table: infant makes walking movements.	After birth in FT-AGA babies. Present from 28 weeks but weak and PT baby walks on toes	2 months without neck extended and for several months with neck extended	• Reflex not full developed till 40 weeks of fetal life. • Absent in breech deliveries and in depressed babies • Not of much importance • Poor or absent in small for dates.
Rooting reflex	On touching (with finger or breast) cheek or angle of mouth: Opening of mouth and turning towards the point of stimulus	Birth	9 months	• It enables him to find the breast with being directed to it. • Absent in-bulbar palsy and hypotonia
Crossed extensor reflex	Passively extend one lower limb Pressing the knee down and stimulate the sole of the foot of this fixed limb: Flexion and slight abduction of the unstimulated lower limb occurs.	Few days after birth	1 month	• Absent in spinal cord damage and weak in peripheral nerve damage.
Galant (trunk incurvation)	Stroke a pin or thumb nail along the para vertebral line (about 3 cm from the midline) from the shoulder to the buttock: The back should curve with concavity to the stimulated side.	5-6 days	7-9 months	• Unilateral in hemisyndrome. • Absent in spinal cord damage.
Perez	Elicited as for galant but by stroking over central vertebral spine: Infant arches backward, the buttocks rise and anus dilates.	5-6 days	7-8 months	• Same as in Galant reflex.

Contd...

Contd...

Reflex	Method of eliciting	Time of Appearance	Time of Disappearance	Remarks
Placing reflex	With the baby held upright between the hand of examiner, dorsal part of foot is brought lightly in contact with edge of table: Normally the baby flexes knee and places foot on the table.	4 days	6 weeks	• Absent in general neurological depression hypotonia and paresis of the lower limb.
Crawling reflex	Infant in prone position: Crawling movements may occur spontaneously, but can be reinforced by pressing with thumb gently on the sole. The crawling reflex is more easily elicited in the immature infant than the walking reflex.	4 days	4 months	
Bicep jerk		2 days		• Absent in general neurologic depression, hypotonia. Exaggerated in hyperexcitability.
Knee jerk		2 days		
Ankle jerk		Birth		
Ankle clonus		Birth		
Parachute reflex	Child held in ventral suspension and suddenly lowered to the cough: arms are distended as a defensive reaction	6-9 months	Remains life long	• Absent/Abnormal in cerebral palsy
Landau's reflex	Seen in ventral suspensin, when head, spine and legs are extended. If the head is flexed, the hip, knees and elbow also show flexion	3 months	Difficult to elicit after 1year may persist upto 2 year.	• Absent in-hypotonia, hypertonia and severe subnormality.
Labyinthine reflex	Baby held upright with examiners hand under infants arm. Spin around so that baby turns with the examiner first in one direction and then in other direction: eyes should turn towards the direction in which the baby is being turned.	Birth		• Absent in disturbed vestibular function and in ophthalmoplegia

Contd...

Contd....

Reflex	Method of eliciting	Time of Appearance	Time of Disappearance	Remarks
Doll's eye	Turn head slowly to right or left Watching position of the eye (normally eyes do not move with head).	Birth	2 months	• Absent in ophthalmic muscle
Acoustic blink	Clap the hands about 30 cm from the infant's head avoid producing an air stream across the face, rapid habituation is observed: Eyes blink.	After a few days		• Absent in impaired hearing
Optic blink	Shine a bright light at the eyes: eyes blink.	At birth		• Absent in generalised neurologic depression and in impaired vision.
Glabellar tap	A sharp blow on the glabella produces momentary tight closure of the eyes.	Birth	Variable persistance	• Absent in apathy, facial palsy and hyper rexcitability.
Sucking child	By stroking the lips	Birth	4 months (awake) 7 months (asleep)	• Absent in depressed child or sick
Neck righting reflex	Rotation of the trunk occurs in the direction in which the head of the supine infant is turned	4-6 months	24 months	• Absent or decreased in infants with spasticity.

30 Psychiatric Assessment

Psychiatric assessment is more time-consuming in child psychiatry than in other branches of psychiatry or medicine. It has three components:
- The diagnostic assessment interview
- Psychological assessment
- Information about the child and parents from other professionals.

Diagnostic Assessment Interview

This has many similarities with traditional methods, though with important modifications. Interview skills are essential in understanding and treating the emotional and behavioral problems in children. Training in interview skills should be an important part of medical undergraduate and postgraduate training. It is of general importance that the interviewing doctor manages to:
- Clarify the nature of the problem and the reason for referral.
- Obtain adequate factual information.
- Elicit emotional responses and attitudes to past and current events
- Observe behavior during the interview
- Establish the trust and confidence of the child and family
- Provide the parents with a summary of problems and a provisional plan of treatment at the end of the initial assessment interview.

Diagnostic Interview Schedule

A flexible approach is essential in order to ensure that the interview fulfils its two main objectives: firstly, to obtain an accurate account of the problems and their associated features; and secondly, to establish a good relationship with the child and the family. Finally, it is good practice to encourage as much eye to eye contact and interaction with the family as possible rather than spend the interview writing copious notes-keep note-taking to a minimum.

Arrangement/layout of their Interview Room

General Points

The interview room should be large enough to seat the family comfortably and also allow the children to use the play material in a relaxed manner.

Arrange the seating so that everyone can see each other easily without barriers, for instance, a desk between the clinician and the family.

Have a variety of play materials available suitable for a wide age range of children. Common items are crayons and paper, dolls house, play telephones, miniature domestic and zoo animals, jigsaws, simple games and books (for a rough estimate of reading ability).

The Initial Phase of the Interview
- Meet the family in waiting room in a friendly, welcoming manner.
- Introduce yourself and get the family to introduce themselves.
- Take the family to the interview room (don't go too fast or you will lose them!)
- Show the children the available toys and suggest seating arrangements
- Make introduction again to ensure everyone knows everyone else.
- Outline the purpose of the interview and the proposed duration (never normally longer than 1 hour)

It is often helpful to begin by checking factual details (e.g., ages, names and schools), as this allows the introduction of topics such as schooling, neighborhood, etc.

Ask someone to tell you about the problem.

Before beginning detailed questioning, it is crucial to put the family at ease and begin to develop their trust and confidence, and to show them that you understand them and their problem. The clinician must develop a repertoire of verbal and communication skills based on his own style, personality and experience to facilitate this process.

The hardest therapeutic task is to win the support and co-operation of both the parents and the child, a difficult balancing act. It is likely that one group, the parents or the child, will feel understood and the other misunderstood.

Detailed History Taking and Examination
Once the child and family are sufficiently at ease, it is possible to begin to obtain information on the topics mentioned below.

Basic data   Name, address, date of birth, date seen.
1. Presenting problems: frequency; severity; onset; course; exacerbating/ameliorating factors; effect on family; help given so far.
2. Other problems or complaints
   i. General health-eating, sleeping, elimination, physical complaints, fits or faints.
   ii. Interests, activities and hobbies.
   iii. Relationship with parents, siblings and relationship with other children: special friends.
   iv. Mood: happy, sad, anxious
   v. Level of activity, attention span, concentration.
   vi. Antisocial behavior.
   vii. Schooling: attainments, attendance, friendships, relationship with teachers.
   viii. Sexual knowledge, interest and behavior (when relevant).

3. Any other problems not previously mentioned.
4. Family structure: Parents occupations/current physical and psychiatric state/previous physical and psychiatric history.
5. Family function: Quality of parenting / parent child relationship/siblings relationships/pattern of family relationships.
6. Personal history: Temperamental characteristics/developmental milestones/past illnesses and injuries/separations greater than one week/ previous schooling.
7. Observation of child's behavior and emotional state.
    i. Appearance: Nutritional state; signs of neglect or injury.
    ii. Activity level: Involuntary movements; concentration
    iii. Mood: Expressions or signs of sadness, misery, anxiety.
    iv. Reaction to and relationship with the doctor: Eye contact; spontaneous talk; inhibition and disinhibition.
    v. Relationship with parents; affection/resentment; ease of separation.
    vi. Habits and mannerisms.
    vii. Presence of delusions, hallucinations, thought disorder.
8. Observation of family relationships:
9. Physical examinations.
    a. Screening neurological examiantion.
        i. Note any facial asymmetry
        ii. Eye movements; ask child to follow a moving finger and observe eye movement for jerkiness, lack of co-ordination.
        iii. Finger thumb apposition: ask child to press the tip of each finger against the thumb in rapid succession; observe clumsiness, weakness.
        iv. Copying pattern; drawing a man.
        v. Observe grip and dexterity in drawing.
        vi. Jumping up and down on the spot.
        vii. Hopping.
        viii. Hearing: Capacity of child to repeat numbers whispered 2 meters behind him.
    b. Further medical examiation (if relevant).

Conclusion of Interview

At the end of the interview, the clinican has the following tasks to perform with the family:
    i. To summarise his own assessment of the problems based on their opinions and his observations.
    ii. To indicate whether further assessment interview and/or special investigations are requried.
    iii. To outline provisional treatment plan where indicated.
    vi. To indicate that he will be writing to the referrer to inform him of his findings.
    v. To ensure that the family has understood what has been said.

Formulations

At the completion of the assesement, the clinician should be able to make a formulation. This is a summary of the important features of the individual case and is set out in the following.

Principles of Formulation

- Summary of main problems
- Diagnosis and differential diagnosis
- Aetiology, with relative contribution of constitutional and environment factors
- Further information required (including special investigations)
- Probables short-term and long-term outcome
- Initial treatment plan

Summary of Psychological History

1. Affective development
   - Mood
   - Behavior
   - Relation with siblings, peers and others
   - Temperament, discipline, adaptation
   - Attachment with parents
   - Activity of the child
2. Cognitive
   - Language
   - Speech
   - School function.
3. Habits and day to day function.
   - Sleep
   - Toilet
   - Habits
   - Sexuality
4. Household and family relation
5. Child's self image.

General Scheme of Examination

CHAPTER

31 General Scheme of Examination

GENERAL SCHEME OF PHYSICAL EXAMINATION

General Remark

a. Age
b. Sex
c. Built (Height) and nourishment (Weight)
d. General Appearance
- Sickness — Facial expression
- Toxicity — Febrile
  - Pallor
  - Coated tongue
  - Sunken eyes
  - Beads of sweat over the philtrum
- Shock — Altered consciousness
  - Tachycardia
  - Hypotension
  - Cold and clammy peripheries
- Respiratory distress — Nasal flare
  - Tachypnea
  - Retraction of chest
  - Sounds (Stridor, wheezing, hoarseness, muffled sounds)
  - Type of cough-Croupy, wheeze.
- Dehydration — Depressed anterior fontanelle
  - Sunken eyes
  - Loss of skin turgor
  - Signs of shock
- Altered level of consciousness
  - Confused
  - Disoriented
  - Drowsy
  - Stupor
  - Semicoma, coma
- Increased intracranial pressure
  - Bulging anterior fontanelle
  - Altered consciousness

- High pitched cry
- Unconsolable
- Altered vitals

- Pain
  - Irritable, anxious
  - Splinting
  - Rigid posture
  - Facial expression

- Posture/Abnormal movements
  - Decerebrate
  - Decorticate
  - Opisthotonus
  - Emprosthotonus
  - Inability to move the limbs
  - Tremor
  - Chorea
  - Athetosis, hemiballismus
  - Spasms
  - Fits
  - Tics

- Pallor/cyanosis

Vital Signs

a. Pulse — Normal rate at different ages
b. Respiratory rate/type — Normal rate and type at different ages.
c. Blood pressure — Method, normal cuffsize, normal values at different ages.
d. Temperature — Method, type of temperature.

Anthropometry

Weight
Proper Recording: Scales (Beam, Salter, Spring and Electronic)
- IAP grading chart
- Weight age chart
- Plot on NCHS
- Plot on Agarwal chart
- Plot on road to health chart
- Welcome grading, Gomez grading

Height
Proper Recording: (Infantometer, Standing Height)
- Height for age
- Plot on NCHS chart
- Plot on Agarwal chart

Head Circumference
Proper Recording:
- Plot on NCHS chart
- Plot on Agarwal chart
- Plot on SD chart

Chest Circumference
Proper Recording and compare with head circumference.

Midarm Circumference (1-5 years)
Proper Recording: Interpretation

Normal	>13.5 cms
Borderline PEM	12.5-13.5 cms
Severe PEM	< 12.5 cms

   *Anthropometric Indices:
   Kanawati, Mclarain, Rao's and Dugdale's Index.

Genetic Anthropometry (In Special Situations)

Size of anterior fontanelle	Ear length and breadth
Head length and width	Ear routine
Pupillary distance	Upper segment/lower segment II
Innercanthal distance	Segment
Outercanthal distance	Arms span
Slant of eye fissure	Hand length
Corneal size,	Finger length
Nasal width and length	Foot length
Philtrum length,	Testis volume
Mouth width	Penile length
Chest circumference	Anal placement
Thoracic index	Skin fold thickness
Internipple distance	Angle and thumb attachment
Sternal length	Carrying angle
Torso length	Limb length and girth
	Ponderal index

Head to Foot Examination (Regional)

Head
- Inspection   : Shape, size, position of bony landmarks swellings, discoloration, scalp.
- Palpation   : Continuity of bones, tenderness, sutures, fontanelles (location, size, tension). Craniotabes, texture and consistency of hair, soft tissue masses. Measurement of head circumference.
  Tachycerebrae.

- Percussion : Macewan's sign
- Auscultation : Bruit
- Transillumination : (Subdural effusions, hydrocephalus, arachnoid cyst, porencephaly, hydrancephaly, Alobarholoprusencephaly, enlarged cisterna magna, Dandy Walker cyst, cerebral destruction).
  Conventional method/using chun gun.

Face

Table 31.1

General	Infections	Nutrition
Sickness	Tetanus	Kwashiorkor
Shock	Mumps	Marasmus
Dehydration	Measles	Angular stomatitis
Toxicity	Roseola	Xerophthalmia
Mental retardation	Infantaum	
Distress	Adenoid face	
Pallor/cyanosis		

Table 31.2

Renal	Endocrinal	CNS
• Acute glomerulonephritis	• Cretinism	• Myasthenia gravis
• Nephrotic syndrome	• Cushing's syndrome	• 7th nerve palsy
	• Steroid face	Myopathy
		Hydrocephalus
		Microcephaly

Table 31.3

Genetic	Hematology
Down's syndrome	Thalassemia
Turner's syndrome	Chloroma
Sturge-Weber syndrome	
Pierre-Robin sequence	
Whistling face syndrome	
Hallerman-Streiff syndrome	
Goldenhar syndrome	
Tuberous sclerosis	
Apert's syndrome	

Eyes

Structure

- Periorbital anatomy
- Spacing and size
  Position – Hypotelorism, hypertelorism, shallow orbit
  Size – Anophthalmia, microphthalmos, microcornea, megalocornea, buphthalmos, prominent supraobital ridges.

Number	-	Anophthalmos, cyclopia, synophthalmia, cryptophthalmia.

- Eyelids, lashes, eye brows.

Position	-	Telecanthus
Direction	-	Upslanting and downslanting palpebral fissure.
Size	-	Blepharoptosis, ptosis, blepharophimosis.
Shape	-	Ectropion, ankyloblepharon, coloboma.
Consistency	-	Edema.

- Abnormalities

Absence	-	Madarosis
		Localized loss of lashes
		Absent brow hair
Size or number	-	Numerous or long distichiasis
Shape of eyebrows		
	-	Synophrys
		Medial flaring
		High arch
	-	Nasolacrimal puncta and duct pathway.
	-	Palpebral fissure
	-	Conjunctiva
	-	Sclera
	-	Anterior segment
		Cornea
		Irides
		Lens
Shape	–	Keratoconus, cornea plana
Color of irides	-	Heterochromia of iris
		Nonpigmented iris
		Brushfield's spots
Pigmented deposition		
Color of pupil	-	Leucocoria
Clarity	-	Corneal opacity (diffuse, localized)
		Sclerocornea
		Presence of vessels in iris (gestation related)
Absence or malposition		
	-	Aniridia, absence of lens lens opacity, dislocation, coloboma iris, lens.

- Fundoscopic examination.
- Functions   (assessed through examination of structure)

        Visual acuity
        Pupil reactivity
        Extraocular muscle activity.

Ears

External

Inspect both ears
- Preauricular area: Skin appendages, fistula, pits and skin markings.
- Postauricular area: Ecchymoses, swelling, fistulae and skin markings.
- Auricle: Size, shape and symmetry (anterior and posterior surface).
  For example: Aural atresia, sinus, appendage, microtia, lop ear, cup ear.
- Tragus: Size in proportion to the size of the ear
  Attachment of ear lobe.
- External auditory meatus: Patency and size.
  Determine position and rotation
  Palpate the auricle
      Texture
      Firmness of cartilage and recoil
      Masses.
- Otoscopy: clear debris.
    - Examine canal surface for integrity, color, size and direction.
    - Inspect ear drum for visual characteristics
      Color, lustre, translucence, light reflex, vascularity, contour (bulge, retraction), landmark, mobility on positive and negative pressure.
    - Determine the mobility of eardrum by insufflation.
    - Other conditions: Otorrhea
      Hemotympanum
      Amber serous effusion.

Nose Examination

Assess the nose and nasal cavity for
- Size and shape
- Masses or clefts
- Secretions
- Patency, airflow and flaring.
- Assess size and shape by evaluating the components individually and as the nose relates to the rest of the facial structures.
- Nasofrontal angle   : Normal, flat, deep.
- Nasal root protrusion   : Average, high, low.
- Nasal bridge   : High, low, broad, beaked or bulbous
- Nasal tip   : Normal, flat, bifid.
- Shape of each nasal ala   : Normal, slightly flat, markedly flat, angles slighly or markedly.
- Nasal ala configuration   : Cleft, hypoplastic, hypotrophic, coloboma.
- Size of nostril   : Symmetric or asymmetric.

Throat and Mouth
- Inspect mouth, perioral region and oral pharynx for:
  Size, shape, color, continuity of philtrum, lips, gums, palate, buccal mucosa tongue, tonsils and floor and mouth.

- Dentition—Number, type (deciduous/permanent), abnormal occlusion, dental age.
- Examine pharynx and tonsils
- Presence of anomalous structures of masses
- Tongue—Aglossia, microglossia, hemiatrophy macroglossia, hemi-hypertrophy, large tongue, increased mobility, ankyloglossia, glossoptosis, clefts.

    Note palatal movements, gag reflex, voice.

Neck

- Position of head and neck
- Appearance of skin
- Symmetry of cervical musculature
- Range of movements of cervical spine:
    - Flexion-anterior and lateral
    - Extension
    - Rotaion
- Presence of: – Masses
    - Lymph nodes
    - Webbing
    - Thyroid gland (assess the size)
- Position of trachea
- Neck rigidity (True/false)

Chest

- Respiratory rate
- Contour and shape of chest and abdomen
- Bilateral symmetry
- Depth and ease of respiration
- Coordination of chest and abdominal movements during breathing
- Retraction or bulge
- Precordial activity
- Skin over chest-dermal lesions
- Nipple-discharge
- Rickety rosary, Harrison's sulcus
- Breast-mass, areola, Tanner's staging in older children
- Assess cry and other sounds made by children
- Palpate   - Subcutaneous skin,
                    Apex,
                    Vibration, pulsation, etc.
- Percuss chest (lungs, heart, liver, spleen)
- Transillumination of chest in newborn
- Auscultation of heart and lungs

Abdomen

- Contour, size
- Symmetry

- Skin
- Umbilicus
- Bowel sounds
- Masses
- Percussion
- Auscultation

Genitalia and Perineum
- Determine sex
- Locate anus relative to genital landmarks
- Patency and tone of anus
- Inspect vaginal opening and discharge
- Size of clitoris, labia minora and majora
- Palpate labia majora for masses
- Palpate size and shape of penis and scrotum
- Visualize urethral opening and urine stream
- Testis size
- Transilluminate-scrotal enlargement
- Palpate inguinal region
- Femoral pulsation
- Assess for hernia

Back
- Symmetry between two sides
- Position and symmetry of scapula
- Length, shape and integrity of spine
- Dermal sinus, swelling, etc. over vertebral column
- Palpate spine—tenderness, swelling
- Auscultate chest and flanks
- Check for scoliosis

Extremities
- Symmetry in length of arms and legs
- Symmetry in girth of arms and legs
- Symmetry of muscle mass
- Muscular or vascular anomalies
- Limb to trunk relation
- Hands and feet—symmetry and size
- Proportion of hand and foot to rest of the limb
- Number, size, symmetry of fingers and toes
- Nails
- Palmar and plantar creases
- Range of movement at joints
- Arterial pulses
- Examine swellings, discoloration
- Examine—Hips and clavicles

Skin

Inspect and palpate skin:

- Colour
- Moisture
- Temperature
- Texture and creasing
- Mobility and turgor
- Lesions-masurements
    - Configuration
    - Elevation and depression
    - Palpate characteristics
      Color
      Localization on body
      Pattern of distribution
- Inspect and palpate finger nails and toe nails:
    - Color
    - Shape
    - Size
    - Lesions
- Inspect and palpate hair:
    - Color
    - Distribution
    - Pattern of growth
    - Texture
    - Unusual concentration
- Take scraping of skin and culture when indicated
- Photograph findings when indicated.

Systemic Examination

- Central nervous system examination
    - Higher mental function,
    - Cranial nerves,
    - Motor system
    - Sensory system
    - Cerebellar signs,
    - Meningeal signs
    - Autonomic nervous system
    - Superficial and deep reflexes
    - Primitive and somatic reflexes
    - Skull and spine
- Cardiovascular system examination, per abdomen examination, respiratory system
    - Inspection, palpation, percussion, auscultation

Developmental Assessement

Case Oriented Examination

Summary

SUMMARY OF PHYSICAL EXAMINATION
   i. General remarks
   ii. Vital signs
   iii. Anthropometry
   iv. Regional examination (Head to foot)
   v. Systemic examination
   vi. Case oriented examination
   vii. Developmental examination
   viii. Summary of examination findings

Skill Development
A student of pediatrics should develop the following skills by constant practice.
1. Do physical examination on newborns, infants and children by inspection, palpation, percussion, auscultation (Standard clinical methods).
2. Weigh children—Interpretation—Plot on growth charts and road to health card.
3. Other anthropometric measurement—Use infantometer, tape, Shakir strip, Bangle test, Quack stick.
4. Use and interpret growth chart
5. Restrain child for throat, ear, eye examination
6. Use of auroscope, ophthalmoscope, nasal speculum
7. Recording vital signs and interpreting according to age
8. Vision assessment/hearing assessment
9. Use of calipers, peak flow meter, Snellen's chart, magnifying lens, orchidometer, skinfold caliper.
10. SMR staging
11. Assessment of dentition, skin fold thickening
12. Assessment of gestational age in newborn
13. Universal precaution for prevention of infection/HIV
14. Assessment of dehydration
15. Digital rectal examination/proctoscopy
16. Use sense of smell for recognition of certain conditions.
17. Recognize the importance of sounds made by children e.g. types of cry, stridor, wheeze, grunt, croup, etc.

Equipments Required for Examination of Children
1. Thermometers
2. Measuring tape
3. Sphygmomanometer
4. Peak flow meter
5. Infantometer
6. Weight scale
7. Nasal speculum
8. Tongue depressor
9. Auroscope

10. Ophthalmoscope
11. Growth charts/Road to health chart
12. Percussion hammer
13. Torch
14. Transillumination—Torch/Chun gun
15. Snellen's chart
16. Tuning Fork (500-1000 Hz for auditory examination 100-400 for vibratory sense)
17. Skin fold calipers (Harpender)
18. Magnifying lens
19. Stethoscope
20. Others
    - Goniometer
    - Orchiodometer
    - Wood's lamp
    - Vaginal speculum
    - Proctoscope
    - Monitoring equipments - Vital signs, Pulse oxymetry

Normal Values (Table 31.4)

Table 31.4: Shows normal values of pulse, respiration and blood pressure in children of different age groups

	Pulse rate (BPM)	Respiratory rate (per min)	Blood pressure (mmHg)
Newborn	80-180	40-60	80/60
Infants	80-160	30	90/70
1 to 4 years	80-120	24-26	95/70
4 to 8 years	80-110	20-22	100/70
8 to 12 years	70-110	18-20	110/70
> 12 years	60-90	18-20	120/80

Anthropometry (Table 31.5)

Table 31.5: Depicts weight, height ang HC in children of different age groups

	Weight (kg)	Height (cm)	HC (cm)
Birth	3	50	35
6 months	6	—	1/1st 6 months 0.5/for next 6 months
1 year	9	75	45
2 years	12	87.5	
Above 2 years	2/Every year till 12	0.4/100 cm then 6 cm every 13 years	3-47 years 7-49 years -51 years

Chart 31.1: Illustrates a graphical representation of physical and sexual growth pattern of affluent Indian boys in age group of 1 to 18 years

Boys: 1-18 years

Name: _____ Record No: _____ Date of Birth: _____

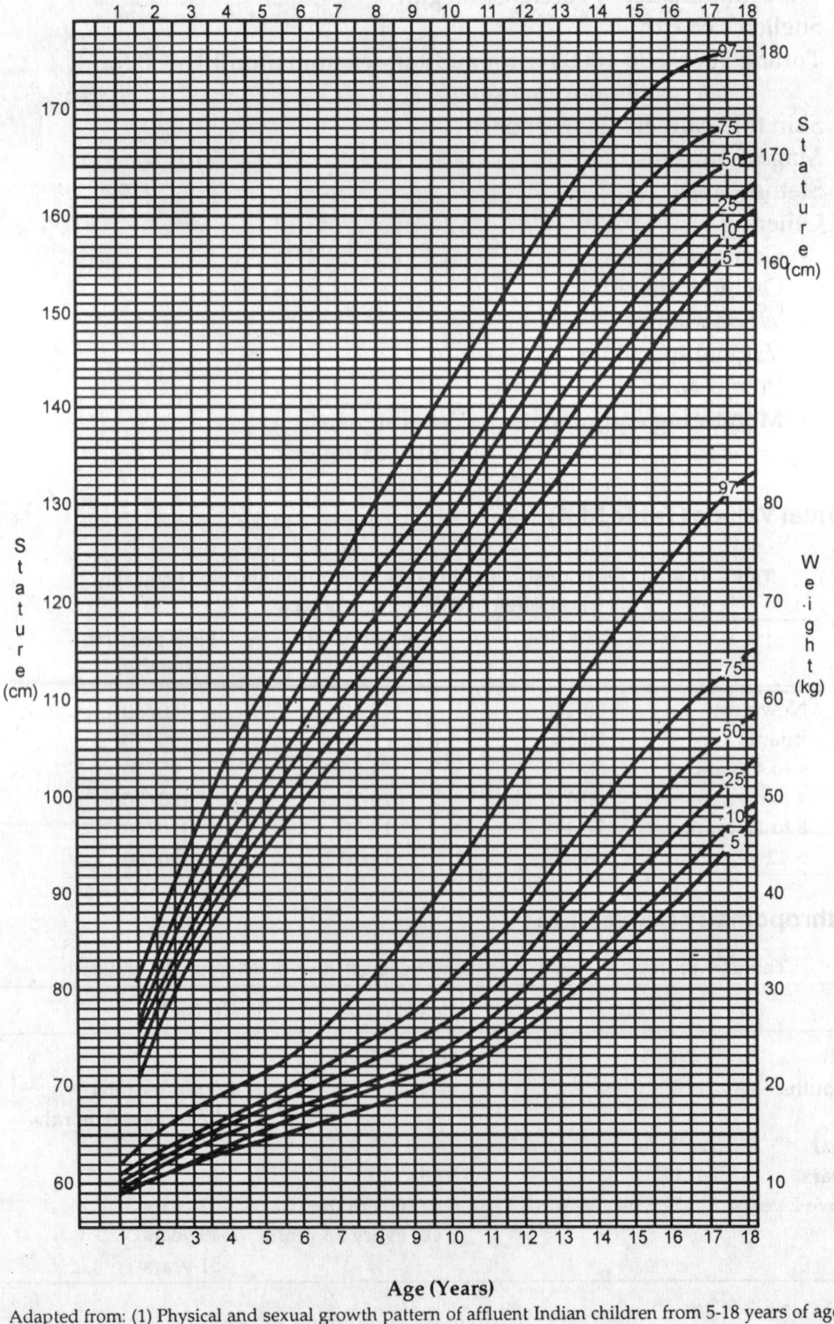

Age (Years)

Adapted from: (1) Physical and sexual growth pattern of affluent Indian children from 5-18 years of age. *Ind Pediatr.* 1992; 29: 1203. (2) Physical growth in affluent Indian children (Birth to 6 years). *Ind. Pediatr.* 1994; 31: 377. Dept. of Endocrinology, SGPGMS, Lucknow

Chart 31.2: Illustrates a graphical representation of physical and sexual growth pattern of affluent Indian girls in age group of 1 to 17 years

Girls: 1-17 years

Name: _____ Record No: _____ Date of Birth: _____

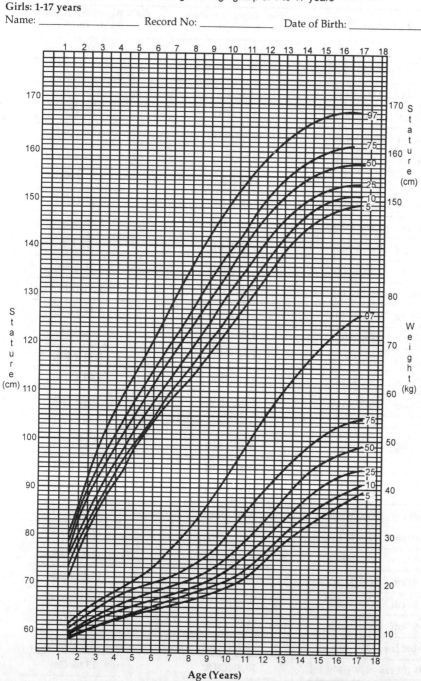

Adapted from: (1) Physical and sexual growth pattern of affluent. Indian children from 5-18 years of age. *Ind Pediatr.* 1992; 29: 1203. (2) Physical growth in affluent Indian children (Birth to 6 years). *Ind. Pediatr.* 1994; 31: 377. Dept. of Endocrinology, SGPGMS, Lucknow

Table 31.6: Illustrates weight percentiles of boys and girls less than four years and prepubescent ones according to their recumbent length, respectively

Recumbent Length	Boys: Weight Precentiles kg and (Ib)	Girls: Weight Precentiles kg and (Ib)
	50th	50th
Boys and girls younger than four years		
48—50 cm (19-19¼ in)	3.15 (7)	3.29 (7¼)
50-52 cm (19¼-20½ in)	3.48 (7¼)	3.55 (7¼)
52-54 cm 20½-21¼ in)	3.88 (8½)	3.89 (8½)
54-56 cm (21¼-22 in)	4.34 (9½)	4.29 (9½)
56-58 cm (22-22¼ in)	4.84 (10¼)	4.76 (10½)
58-60 cm (22¼-23½ in)	5.38 (11¼)	5.27 (11½)
60-62 cm (23½-24½ in)	5.94 (13)	5.82 (12¼)
60-64 cm (24½-25¼ in)	6.52 (14¼)	6.39 (14)
64-66 cm (25¼-26 in)	7.11 (15¼)	6.97 (15¼)
66-68 cm (26-26¼ in)	7.70 (17)	7.55 (16¼)
68-70 cm (26¼-27½ in)	8.27 (18¼)	8.11 (17¼)
70-72 cm (27½-28¼ in)	8.82 (19½)	8.64 (19)
72-74 cm (28¼-29¼ in)	9.33 (20½)	9.14 (20¼)
74-76 cm (29¼-30 in)	9.81 (21¼)	9.59 (21¼)
76-78 cm (30-30¼ in)	10.27 (22¼)	10.02 (22)
78-80 cm (30¼-31½ in)	10.70 (23½)	10.41 (23)
80-82 cm (31½-32¼ in)	11.12 (24½)	10.80 (23¼)
82-84 cm (32¼-33 in)	11.53 (25½)	11.18 (24¼)
84-86 cm (33-33¼ in)	11.93 (26¼)	11.56 (25½)
86-88 cm (33¼-34¼ in)	12.34 (27¼)	11.95 (26¼)
88-90 cm (34¼-35½ in)	12.76 (28¼)	12.36 (27¼)
90-92 cm (35½-36¼ in)	13.20 (29)	12.80 (28¼)
92-94 cm (36¼-37 in)	13.65 (30)	13.27 (29¼)
94-96 cm (37-37¼ in)	14.14 (31¼)	13.77 (30¼)
96-98 cm (37¼-38½ in)	14.66 (32¼)	14.31 (31½)
98-100 cm (38½-39¼ in)	15.21 (33½)	14.87 (32¼)
100-102 cm (39¼-40¼ in)	15.81 (34¼)	15.46 (34)
102-104 cm (40¼-41 in)	16.45 (36¼)	

Contd...

Contd...

Recumbent Length	Boys: Weight Precentiles kg and (lb)	Girls: Weight Precentiles kg and (lb)
	50th	50th
Boys and girls prepubescent		
90-92 cm (35½-36¼ in)	13.41 (29½)	13.14 (29)
92-94 cm (36¼-37 in)	13.89 (30½)	13.63 (30)
94-96 cm (37-37¼ in)	14.38 (31¼)	14.12 (31¼)
96-98 cm (37¼-38½ in)	14.89 (32¼)	14.62 (32¼)
98-100 cm (38½-39¼ in)	15.43 (34)	15.13 (33¼)
100-102 cm (39¼-40¼ in)	15.98 (35¼)	15.65 (34½)
102-104 cm (40¼-41 in)	16.65 (36½)	16.20 (35¼)
104-106 cm (41-41¼ in)	17.13 (37¼)	16.75 (37)
106-108 cm (41¼-42½ in)	17.74 (39)	17.33 (38¼)
108-110 cm (42½-43¼ in)	18.37 (40½)	17.94 (39½)
110-112 cm (43¼-44 in)	19.02 (42)	18.56 (41)
112-114 cm (44-45 in)	19.70 (43½)	19.22 (42¼)
114-116 cm (45-45¼ in)	20.39 (45)	19.91 (44)
116-118 cm (45¼-46½ in)	21.11 (46½)	20.64 (45½)
118-120 cm (46½-47¼ in)	21.85 (48¼)	21.42 (47¼)
120-122 cm (47¼-48 in)	22.63 (50)	22.25 (49)
122-124 cm (48-48¼ in)	23.45 (51¼)	23.13 (51)
124-126 cm (48¼-49½ in)	24.32 (53½)	24.09 (53)
126-128 cm (49½-50½ in)	25.24 (55¼)	25.11 (55¼)
128-130 cm (50½-51¼ in)	26.22 (57¼)	26.22 (57¼)
130-132 cm (51¼-52 in)	27.26 (60)	27.40 (60½)
132-134 cm (52-52¼ in)	28.38 (62½)	28.68 (63¼)
134-136 cm (52¼-53½ in)	29.58 (65¼)	30.06 (66¼)
136-138 cm (53½-54¼ in)	30.86 (68)	31.54 (69½)
138-140 cm (54¼-55 in)	32.23 (71)	
140-142 cm (55-56 in)	33.70 (74¼)	
142-144 cm (56-56¼ in)	35.27 (77¼)	
144-146 cm (56¼-57½ in)	36.95 (81½)	

Chart 31.3A: Gives a graphical representation of length (stature) and weight by age in boys, while each curve corresponds to the indicated percentile level

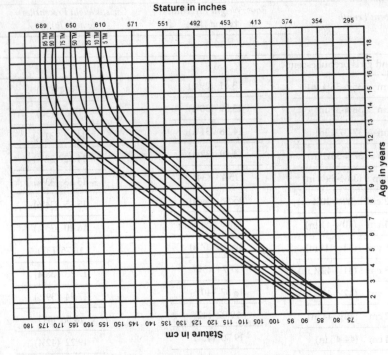

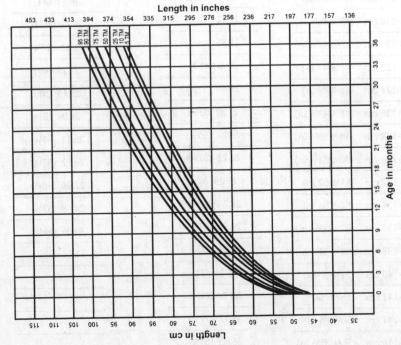

Chart 31.3A (Contd...)

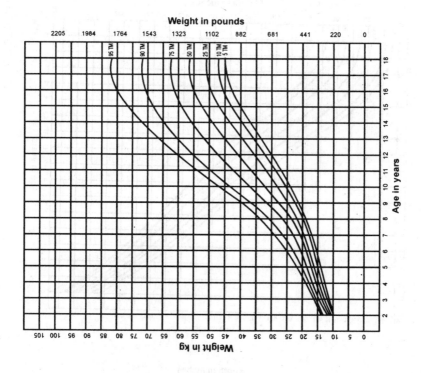

Weight in pounds

Weight in kg

Age in years

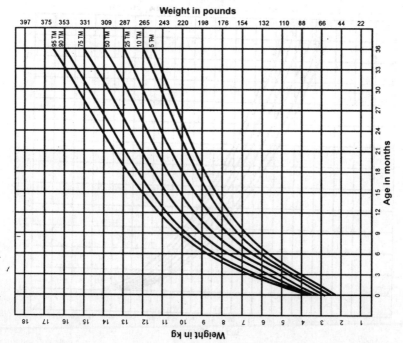

Weight in pounds

Weight in kg

Age in months

Chart 31.3A (Contd...)

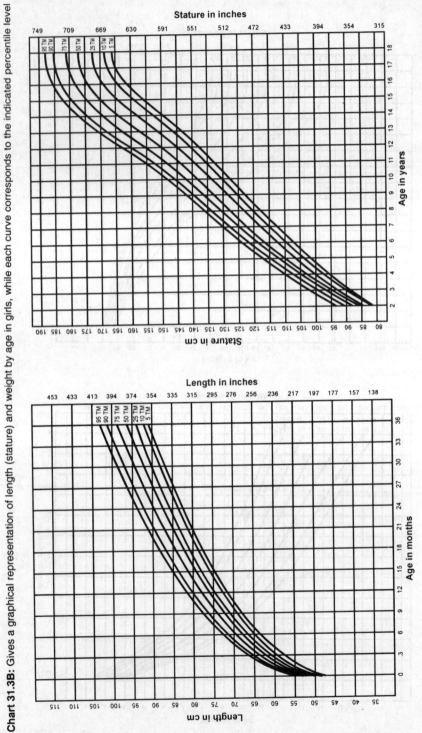

Chart 31.3B: Gives a graphical representation of length (stature) and weight by age in girls, while each curve corresponds to the indicated percentile level

Chart 31.3B (Contd...)

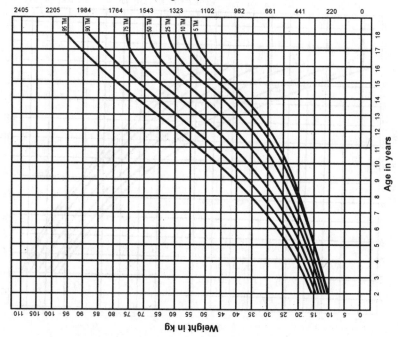

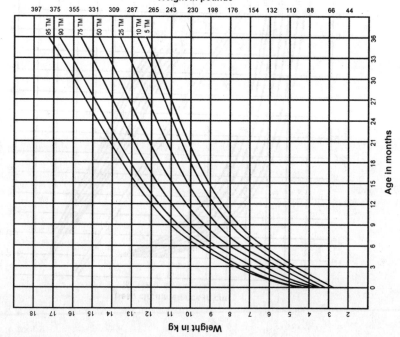

Chart 31.3B (Contd...)

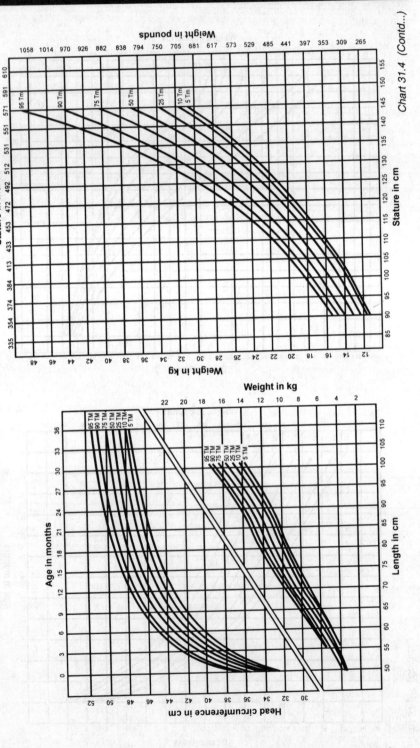

Chart 31.4: A graphical representation of weight by length and head circumference by age in infants and young boys and girls

Chart 31.4 (Contd...)

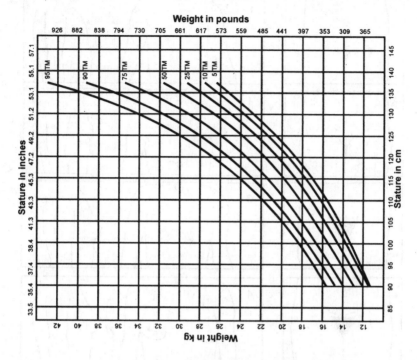

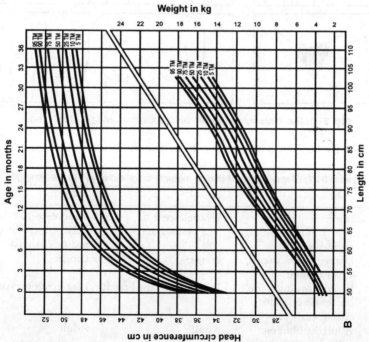

Chart 31.4 (Contd...)

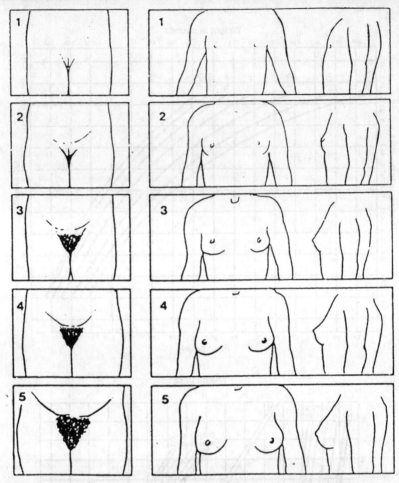

Fig. 31.1: Sex maturity stages (A) Girls' pubic hair, and (B) Girls' breasts

Table 31.7 depicts genital maturity in boys in different stages.

Table 31.7: Classification of genital maturity stages in boys (Tanner ratings)

Stage	Pubic hair	Penis	Testes
1	None	Preadolescent	Preadolescent
2	Scanty, long, slightly pigmented	Slight enlargement	Enlarged scrotum, pink texture changed
3	Darker, begins to curl, small amount	Longer	Longer
4	Resembles adult type, but less in quantity; coarse, curly	Larger, glans and breadth	Larger, scrotum darker
5	Adult distribution, spread to medial thighs	Adult	Adult

Adapted from Daniel WA Jr. *Adolescents in health and disease*. St. Louis: Mosby, 1977.

Table 31.8 depicts genital maturity in girls in different stages.

Table 31.9 gives a stepwise assessment of a dehydration in patients brought in different conditions.

Chart 31.5 represents black letters graduating in size to test visual acuity.

Table 31.10 in a complete dental formula gives age at eruption, shedding and calcification of primary and secondary teeth.

Table 31.11 illustrates development milestones in locomotion and language corresponding to adaptive and social behavior.

Chart 31.6 is a WHO prototype growth chart which can be used as a tool to assess infant and child health.

Table 31.12 represents height percentile for boys and girls of affluent Indian and NCHS in different age group familes.

Table 31.8: Classification of genital maturity stages in girls (Tanner ratings)

Stage	Pubic hair	Pubic hair	Testes
1	Preadolescent	Preadolescent	
2	Sparse, slightly pigmented, straight, at medial border of labia	Breast and papilla elevated as small mound, areolar diameter increased	
3	Darker, beginning to curl, increased amount	Breast and areola enlarged, without contour separation	
4	Coarse, curly, abundant, but amount less than in adult	Areola and papilla form secondary mound	
5	Adult feminine triangle, spread to medial surface of thighs (Fig. 31.1)	Mature, nipple projects, areola part of general breast contour	

Adapted from Daniel WA Jr. *Adolescents in Health and Disease* St. Louis: Mosby, 1977.

Table 31.9: How to assess patients for dehydration

	First, Assess Your Patient for Dehydration		
	A	**B**	**C**
1. Look at: Condition	Well, alert	*Restless, irritable*	*Letharglc or uncon-sclous; floopy*
• Eyes	Normal	Sunken	Very sunken and dry
• Tears	Present	Absent	Absent
• Mouth and tongue	Moist	Dry	Very dry
• Thirst	Drinks normally, not thirst	*Thirsty, drinks eagerly*	*Drinks poorly or not able to dirnk*
2. Feel: Skin pinch	Goes back quickly	*Goes back slowly*	*Goes back very slowly*
3. Decide:	The patient has **No signs of dehy-dration**	If the patient has 2 or more signs inclu-ding at least one * sign*, there is **Some dehydration**	If the patient has 2 or more signs inclu-ding at least one * sign*, there is **Severe dehydration**
4. Treat:	Use treatment Plan A	Weight the patient, if possible, and use Treatment Plan B	Weight the patient and use Treatment Plan C **Urgently**

* Key Signs

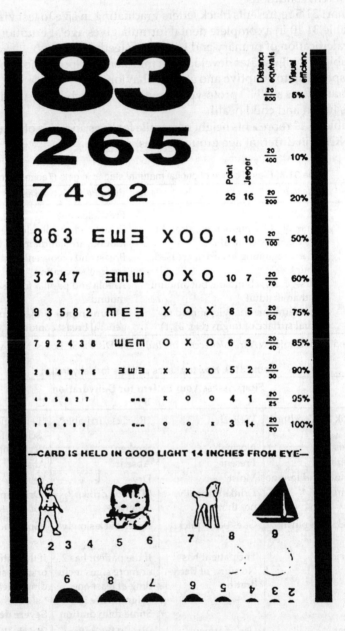

Chart 31.5: Snellen's chart

Table 31.10: Dental formula for primary and secondary teeth

| | Calcification | | Age at Eruption | | Age at Shedding | |
	Begins at	Complete at	Maxillary	Mandibular	Maxillary	Mandibular
Primary teeth						
Central incisors	5th fetal month	18-24 months	6-8 months	5-7 months	7-8 months	6-7 months
Lateral incisors	5th fetal month	18-24 months	8-11 months	7-10 months	8-9 months	7-8 months
Cuspids (canines)	6th fetal month	30-36 months	16-20 months	16-20 months	11-12 months	9-11 months
First molars	5th fetal month	24-30 months	10-16 months	10-16 months	10-11 months	10-12 months
Sedond molars	6th fetal month	36 months	20-30 months	20-30 months	10-12 months	11-13 months
Secondary Teeth						
Central incisors	3-4 months	9-10 years	7-8 years	6-7 years		
Lateral incisors	Max, 10-12 months Mand, 3-4 months	10-11 years	8-9 years	7-8 years		
Cuspids (canines)	4-5 months	12-15 years	11-12 years	9-11 years		
First premolas (bicuspids)	18-21 months	12-13 years	10-11 years	10-12 years		
Second premolas (bicuspids)	24-30 months	12-14 years	10-12 years	11-13 years		
First molars	Birth	9-10 years	6-7 years	6-7 years		
Second molars	30-36 months	14-16 years	12-13 years	12-13 years		
Third molars	Max, 7-9 years Mand, 8-10 years	18-25 years	17-22 years	17-22 years		

Dental Formula: Age in months – 6 = No. decidious teeth

Table 31.11: Developmental milestones

Motor			Adaptive bevavior		
Head control	-	3 months	Follows object 90°	-	1 months
Rolling over	-	5 months	Follows object 180°	-	3 months
Sitting with support	-	6 months	Reaching objects with both hands	-	4 months
Sitting without support	-	7 months	Reaches objects with one hand		
			Ulnar grasp	-	5-7 months
			Radial grasp	-	6-8 months
Pivoting	-	9 months	Transfers objects	-	7 months
Standing with support	-	9 months	Pincer grasp	-	9 months
Crawls	-	10 months	Releases objects	-	11 months
Standing without support	-	11 months	Scribbles circle	-	15 months
Walks with support	-	15 months	Balances one/cube over	-	15 months
Walks without support	-	20 months	other months		
Climbs stairs, furniture	-	20 months	Vertical strokes	-	18 months
Jumps	-	2 years	Draws a triangle	-	3 years
Stands on one leg	-	3 years	Draws a square	-	4 years
Walks backward	-	3 years	Identifies long, short heavy, light coins	-	5 years
Rides tricycle	-	3 years	Draws rhomboid	-	6 years
Hops	-	5 years	Simple arithmetics	-	6 years

Language			Personal social behavior		
Cooing	-	2 months	Social smile	-	2 months
Babbling	-	5 months	Recognizes mother	-	3 months
Monosyllables without meaning	-	7 months	Laughs aloud	-	4 months
Monosyllables with meaning	-	9 months	Imitation	-	6 months
Ten words	-	1 year	Recognizes stanger	-	6 months
Combining words Jargon speech	-	15 months	Regards image in mirror	-	7 months
3 words sentence (50% intelligilible)	-	2 years	Peek-a-boo	-	9 months
Recites rhymes	-	3 years	Drinks from a cup	-	9 months
Can tell name	-	3 years	Eats and drinks himself	-	11 months
Speaks well (Nouns, Pronouns, Adjectives, Verbs) Rules of grammar	-	4 years	Obeys commands	-	15 months
Narrates stories	-	4 years	Part of body	-	18 months
Reads, Writes, Recites Poems remembers (Ready for school)	-	5-6 years	Helps to dress	-	2 years
			Listening to story	-	2 years
			Knows his sex	-	3 years
			Bladder control	-	3 years
			Plays with friends	-	4 years
			Knows good and bad	-	5 years
			Puts shoes, ties and laces	-	6 years

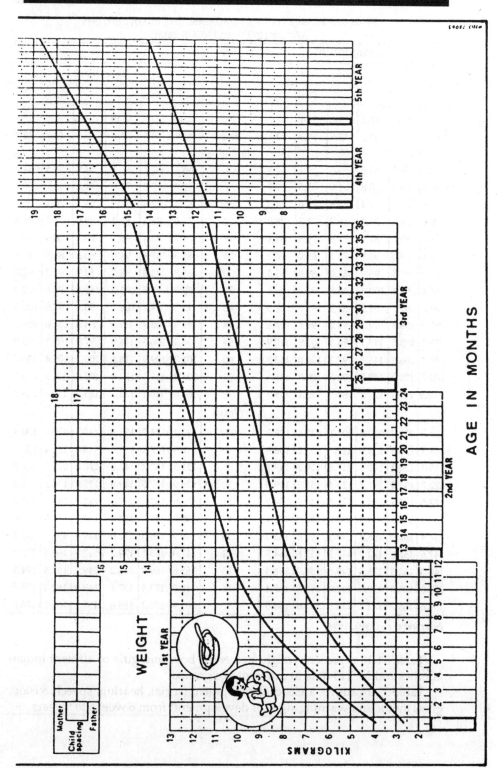

Table 31.12: Length or height percentiles (cm) for boys and girls
(Affluent Indian and NCHS data)

Affluent Indian						Age	NCHS					
Percentiles							Percentiles					
Boys			Girls				Boys			Girls		
3rd	50th	97th	3rd	50th	97th		3rd	50th	97th	3rd	50th	97th
47.6	50.4	53.2	47.5	50.3	53.1	Birth	46.2	50.5	54.8	45.8	49.9	53.9
						(Months)						
56.3	59.4	63.8	55.8	59.1	62.9	3	56.1	61.1	66.1	54.9	59.5	64.2
62.5	65.9	70.8	61.6	65.5	69.7	6	62.8	67.8	72.9	61.0	65.9	70.9
66.8	70.6	75.4	65.6	70.0	74.5	9	67.4	72.3	77.3	65.3	70.4	75.6
70.1	74.3	78.8	68.6	73.5	78.0	12	71.0	76.1	81.2	69.0	74.3	79.6
75.6	80.7	84.9	73.8	79.8	84.4	18	76.7	82.4	88.1	75.1	80.9	86.7
80.1	86.0	90.5	78.2	85.0	90.2	24	81.3	87.6	94.0	80.3	86.5	92.6
84.0	90.5	95.9	82.0	89.9	95.3	30	85.8	92.3	98.7	84.9	91.3	97.7
87.3	94.4	100.8	85.3	93.3	99.9	36	89.9	96.5	103.2	88.8	95.6	102.3
90.2	97.7	105.2	88.3	96.7	104.0	42	91.5	99.1	106.7	90.6	97.9	105.3
92.8	108.8	109.3	91.2	99.8	107.6	48	94.9	102.9	111.0	94.0	101.6	109.2
95.3	103.7	113.1	94.1	102.9	110.9	54	98.2	106.6	114.9	97.2	105.1	113.0
97.9	106.2	116.4	97.2	106.0	113.8	60	101.3	109.9	118.6	100.1	108.4	116.7
100.7	110.0	119.5	100.6	109.3	116.4	66	104.2	113.1	122.0	102.8	111.6	120.3
10.3.9	113.6	122.2	104.5	113.1	118.7	72	107.0	116.1	125.2	105.4	114.6	123.9
						(Years)						
108.5	119.7	130.8	107.1	117.4	129.3	7	112.1	121.7	131.3	110.3	120.6	130.9
113.3	123.6	135.5	112.3	123.2	136.4	8	116.9	127.0	137.0	115.0	126.4	137.7
118.0	128.2	141.4	117.8	129.2	143.1	9	121.5	132.2	142.8	120.0	132.2	144.5
122.7	133.6	147.7	123.4	135.2	149.0	10	126.0	137.5	149.0	125.4	138.3	151.2
127.5	139.6	154.3	128.8	140.9	154.2	11	130.6	143.3	155.9	131.7	144.8	157.8
132.4	145.8	160.8	133.9	146.0	158.1	12	135.5	149.7	163.8	138.7	151.5	164.4
137.4	152.0	166.9	148.3	150.4	162.0	13	140.9	156.5	172.0	144.6	157.1	169.7
142.6	157.6	172.3	147.5	153.8	164.7	14	147.0	163.1	179.2	147.8	160.4	172.9
148.0	162.5	176.8	145.5	156.0	166.5	15	153.8	169.0	184.2	149.1	161.8	174.5
153.6	166.3	179.8	142.4	156.8	167.4	16	160.0	173.5	187.1	149.9	162.4	175.0
159.6	168.7	181.2	138.5	157.0	168.0	17	163.9	176.2	188.6	151.1	163.1	175.0

Agarwal *et al.* (1992, 1994)

Table 31.13 represent weight percentile boys and girls of affluent Indian families and NCHS data in different age groups.

Table 31.14 shows areas of development (social, hearing, speech, vision, gross motor and warning signs of development) from 6 weeks to 5 years.

Table 31.13: Weight (kg) for boys and girls
(Affluent Indian and NCHS data)

Affluent Indian						Age	NCHS					
Percentiles							Percentiles					
Boys			Girls				Boys			Girls		
3rd	50th	97th	3rd	50th	97th		3rd	50th	97th	3rd	50th	97th
2.5	3.1	4.0	2.5	3.2	3.9	Birth	2.5	3.3	4.2	2.3	3.2	3.9
						(Months)						
4.8	5.7	6.7	4.5	5.4	6.6	3	4.2	6.0	7.6	4.0	5.4	6.9
6.2	7.4	8.6	5.9	7.0	8.4	6	6.0	7.8	9.7	5.6	7.2	8.9
7.2	8.5	10.1	6.8	8.1	9.6	9	7.4	9.2	11.1	6.7	8.6	10.4
7.8	9.3	11.2	7.5	9.0	10.5	12	8.2	10.2	12.2	7.6	9.5	11.5
8.9	10.7	13.1	8.6	10.4	12.2	18	9.3	11.5	13.8	8.6	10.8	13.0
9.8	11.9	14.7	9.4	11.6	13.7	24	10.1	12.6	15.0	9.6	11.9	14.3
10.6	12.9	16.0	10.1	12.6	15.2	30	10.9	13.7	16.2	10.5	12.9	15.7
11.3	13.8	17.2	10.8	13.5	16.7	36	11.8	14.7	17.5	11.3	13.9	17.0
11.9	14.6	18.3	11.3	14.3	18.0	42	12.4	15.7	19.3	12.1	15.1	19.1
12.5	15.4	19.3	11.9	15.1	19.4	48	13.1	16.7	20.5	12.8	16.0	20.4
13.1	16.2	20.3	12.6	15.9	20.6	54	13.9	17.7	21.8	13.4	16.8	21.6
13.8	17.1	21.5	13.4	16.8	21.9	60	14.7	18.7	23.2	14.0	17.7	22.9
14.5	18.1	22.7	14.4	17.8	23.1	66	15.5	19.7	24.7	14.6	18.6	24.3
15.3	19.2	24.2	15.7	18.9	24.3	72	16.3	20.7	26.2	15.3	19.5	25.8
						(Years)						
16.2	21.0	29.7	14.8	19.0	27.5	7	17.9	22.9	29.8	16.7	21.8	29.7
17.5	22.6	33.5	15.9	20.8	32.3	8	19.5	25.3	34.1	18.3	24.8	35.0
19.2	24.4	37.7	17.1	23.5	37.7	9	21.0	28.1	39.2	20.2	28.5	41.3
20.9	27.0	42.7	19.5	26.9	43.4	10	22.7	31.4	45.2	22.5	32.5	48.2
22.9	30.6	48.2	22.3	30.9	49.3	11	24.8	35.3	51.7	25.2	37.0	55.3
25.3	34.8	54.1	25.1	35.0	55.1	12	27.6	39.8	58.7	28.3	41.5	62.0
28.1	39.4	60.0	27.9	39.1	60.7	13	31.2	45.0	65.9	31.7	46.1	68.0
31.2	44.1	65.9	30.7	42.7	65.7	14	35.9	50.8	73.2	35.2	50.3	73.0
34.6	48.5	71.4	33.4	45.7	70.0	15	40.9	56.7	80.1	38.3	53.7	76.8
38.5	52.4	76.3	35.7	47.7	73.3	16	45.7	62.1	86.4	40.8	55.9	79.1
42.8	55.5	80.5	37.6	48.4	75.6	17	49.6	66.3	91.6	42.3	56.7	80.0

Age of Appearance of Ossification Centers

The following (Table 31.15) gives the appearance of ossification centers. The figures under the main head are in years and indicate maximum age at which centres are expected to appears. Figures in parenthesis indicate mean age in months of appearance of these centers.

Table 31.14: Shows areas of development from 6 weeks to 5 years

		Areas		
Social	Hearing and Speech	Vision	Gross motor	Warning signs
		6 weeks old		
Smiles, coos responsively.	Stills to mother's voice, startle to sudden noise.	Follows face 90° and states intently.	Primitive reflexes + Head in line with trunk when lifted.	• None is clicited. • Abnormal Moro's • Presistent squint
		6 to 9 months old		
6 months Enjoys bath, playing boo, chews on items. **9 months** Show objects to mother, pats mirror image.	**6 months** Responds to own name. speaks ma, da. **9 months** Mama, dada, (Double syllabi) understands "No".	**6-7 months** Change in grasp palmar to index transfers objects hand to mouth. **9 months** Pincer grasp, foot regard, fixes on pellet of paper, follows fallen object.	**6 months** Bears some weight on legs, rolling over, in prone head up, weight of hands. **7 months** Sits on supported. **9 months** Crawls and pulls to stand.	• Slow social responses. • Abscnce of babble. • Presistence of hand regard. • Abnormal voluntary hand grasp. • Persistent primitive reflexes.
		12 months old		
Comes when called, finds hidden objects, waves bye–bye, gives toys on request.	Understands some words uses "mama", "dada" (with meaning shakes head "no").	Throws object, watches them fall, picks up crumbs from floor pincer grasp, bans two bricks together.	Shuffing gait like a bear, cruises round, holding on to furniture, walks one hand held, pivots when sitting.	• No tuneful babble. • Hold objects close to eyes. • Immature gait. • No sitting.
		18 months old		
Cup: lifts-drinks puts down, self spoon feeding, pulls at obrty nappy Does-dusting, sweeping.	Points to 3 body parts obeys single commands Says-6 words, jargons, cechoes speech.	Neat pincer picking of threads pins. Scribbles using fisted grasp Turns 2 or more pages at a time, Builds tower of 3-4. (2.5 cm cubes).	Walks well, carries toys, climb stairs, climbs into chair.	• Drools no words • Absent pincer grasp • Not walking
		2 to 2½ years		
Plays alone, tantrums, demanding, day by day, puts on shoes, socks and pant. Turns door handles, uses spoon and fork.	Phrases of 2-3 words, gives name 50 words + naming games, has inner language.	Turns one page at a time imitates a straight line in both vertical and horizontal and a circle. Unscrews lids, tower of 6-8 cubes.	Pushes tricycle with feet, walks down stairs 2 feet per tread, runs, kicks ball, jumps on the spot.	• No speech • Unsteady on feet

Contd...

Contd...

Areas				
Social	Hearing and Speech	Vision	Gross motor	Warning signs

3 to 3½ years

| Goes toilet unassisted dresses or undresses with minimum assistance, knows some nursery rhymes, handles knife and fork, plays with paper. | Gives full name, sex, counts to 10, uses phirals, 3-5 word sentences. | Mature pen grasp copies + and 0. Correctly matches 2 or more colors. Threads large beads. Tower of 9. | Stands on one leg for a few seconds, peddles tricycle, stairs adult style for ascent, jumps off bottom step. | • No phrases.
• Persistent day time wetting/ soiling.
• Clumsy. |

4 to 5 years

| Wips own bottom eats using knife and fork, dresses-except for tie and laces, imaginative play, play in-groups, stares toys and obey rules. | Gives address/ age/telephone no. counts upto 10 by 4 years. 20 by 5 years knows 3 coins, grammatical speech, asks meaning of abstract words. | Matches 4 colors copies cross, square and by 5a triangle, draws a recognisable man | *4 years*
Climbs trees and ladder, enjoys ball games.
5 years
Hops, skip, jump off 3 steps, catches a ball. | • Unable to perform. |

Table 31.15: Age at appearance (years)

Bones	Males Max. (Mean)	Females Max. (Mean)	Fusion	
Carpal bones	0.5 (2 m)	1.0 (2 m)		
Hamate	1.0 (3 m)	1.0 (2 m)		
Triquetral	4.0 (30 m)	3.0 (21 m)		
Lunate	6.0 (42 m)	5.0 (34 m)		
Scaphoid	8.0 (66 m)	5.0 (51 m)		
Trapezium	7.0 (67 m)	6.6 (49 m)		
Trapezoid	13.0 (69 m)	6.6 (49 m)		
Pisiform	13.0 (y)	10.0 (y)		
Metacarpals			Male	Female
2nd	1.7 (18 m)	1.6 (12 m)	17.0	14.9
3rd	1.7 (20 m)	1.6 (13 m)	17.0	14.8
4th	1.7 (23 m)	1.6 (15 m)	16.4	14.9
5th	1.7 (26 m)	1.6 (16 m)	16.4	14.9
1st	4.1 (32 m)	2.0 (18 m)	17.0	14.9
Wrist				
Radius	1.7	3.5	17.4	16.4
Ulna	7.4	3.5	17.4	15.8
Shoulders				
Coracoid	5.6	13.0	18.0	17.0
Acromion	14.0	12.0	18.0	17.6
Phalanges	between "2 and 3 years"			

Contd...

Contd...

Bones	Males Max. (Mean)	Females Max. (Mean)	Fusion	
Elbow				
Radius	6.2	3.5	16.2	14.2
Med. epicondyl	7.4	5.6	16.5	14.3
Lat. epicondyle	6.2	7.5	16.0	13.0
Trochlea	7.9	7.6	16.0	13.0
Capitulum	0.5	0.5	16.0	13.0
Ulna	10.4	8.6	16.4	14.0
Hip and Knee				
Distal end of femur	at birth	at birth	16.0	15.0
Proximal tibia	at birth	at birth	17.0	16.0
Femur head	1.0 (4 m)	1.0 (4 m)	20.0	20.0
Greater trochanter	2.0	—	19.0	—
Lesser trochanter	12.0	—	18.0	—
Patella	5.0 (46 m)	3.0 (29 m)		
Diac crest	16.0	16.0	20.0	19.0
Shoulder				
Clavicles (medial end)	17.0	17.0	25.0	25.0
Upper end—humerus	0.5	0.5	6.0	5.0
Greater tuberosity	3.5	2.9	17.5	16.5

Note: m = months

y = years

Examination
in Special Situations

32 Clinical Approach to Different Ages

Approach to children depends on several factors like age, developmental stage, the situation, the illness of the child, the background of the child and above all the nature of the child. However, it is a common experience that age plays an important role. In the following pages are described some of the guidelines that are age specific (Tables 32.1 to 32.5).

Table 32.1: Clinical approach for infants

Position	Sequence	Preparation
< 4-6 months supine/prone > 6 months sitting in and mother's lap	If quiet-auscultate heart, lung and abdomen. Record HR, RR, palpate abdomen. Exam of ear, eye, mouth last (mouth can be examined while crying). Elicit reflex-Moro's.	Undress if warm environment. Show light, rattle, keys, talk smile (be gentle). Breast feeding puts many infants at ease. Avoid abrupt jerky movements.

Table 32.2: Clinical approach for toddler

Position	Sequence	Preparation
Sitting or standing with parent. Prone or supine in parent's lap.	Inspect body through play, e.g. count finger, minimal physical contact, allow handling equipment. Auscultate abdomen and palpate when quite. Traumatic procedures at the last.	Parent removes child's clothes, Allow handling of instruments, quick examination, Tell about examination, Praise for cooperation.

Table 32.3: Clinical approach for preschool child

Position	Sequence	Preparation
Standing or sitting Prefers parents usually co-operative in prone/supine position. May be examined in standing position if apprehensive in lying down position	If cooperative, proceed in head to foot sequence.	Request self undressing. Respect modesty. Allow him to use equipments and give choices, explain about procedures, e.g. while testing muscle strength you may say, "I am going to see how strong you are".

Table 32.4: Clinical approach for school aged children

Position	Sequence	Preparation
Sitting position, some like parent's presence. Older ones may like privacy.	Head to toe examination and genital examination at the last.	Request self undressing, explain procedures.

Table 32.5: Clinical approach for adolescents

Position	Sequence	Preparation
Sitting position, Older children like privacy.	Head to toe examination and genital examination at the last.	Examine only the parts that are to be examined. Explain findings during examination and emphasise the normality of systems. Reserve genital examination to the last.

33 Evaluation of Emergency Situations

An emergency situation, whether irresponsiveness, an acute medical or surgical condition, intoxication or trauma, demands alteration of the usual sequence of history taking and examination. Life threatening conditions must be rapidly identified and managed within a few seconds, not minutes. Patients are assessed and treatment priorities established based on physiological conditions and stability of vital signs and not any specific diagnosis. In emergency situations in children, it is necessary to remember a few differences between children and adults.

Children are Different from Adults
Children have not only a smaller anatomy, but also differing physiological response when compared to an adult. The differences are listed below.

Skin
The surface area relative to body mass is greater and the skin is thinner, with less subcutaneous fat and is less protective against burns, more likely to develop hypothermia.

Head
- Larger and heavier compared to rest of the body, prone for head injury.
- Fontanelles and sutures are open and palpable; hence it is easier to assess dehydration, bone growth and increased ICT.
- The developing brain is more vulnerable to injury, infections and poisons.
- The dura is attached very firmly to the skull and is more apt to tear and bleed with injury.

Neck
Is shorter and JVP is difficult to observe.

Airway
- Nasal passages are relatively smaller and easily obstructed by discharges or foreign bodies.
- Tongue is relatively larger and is more easily able to obstruct the upper airway.
- Trachea is relatively much narrower and its cartilage more easily collapsable and hence vulnerable to edema, pressure and inflammation. Both flexion and hyper extension can obstruct the trachea.
- Larynx is higher, more anterior and available easily for aspiration.

Chest and Lungs
- Rib cage, more elastic and flexible, less vulnerable for injury, more apt to allow retraction during respiratory distress.
- Lung tissue is fragile and more easily contused.
- Mediastinum is more vulnerable and prone to tension pneumothorax.
- Chest muscles and diaphragm tire easily with prolonged effort.

Heart and Circulation
- Healthy heart -- faster heart rate
- Strong vagal tone is responsible for sinus arrhythmia
- Infants and children have a smaller blood volume, but will lose blood similar to an adult after an injury.
- Even when a significant blood or fluid is lost, children maintain BP longer than adults.
- Bradycardia, initial response to hypoxemia may herald a cardiac arrest.

Abdomen
- Liver and spleen are relatively larger, more vascular and less protected by ribs and more prone to injury.

Extremities
- Bones of children are softer and more prone to fractures compared to those of adults.

Nervous Systems
An infant is able to feel pain anywhere in the body, but cannot localize or isolate it.

In an emergency situation:
- Quickly assess the vital functions efficiently through a rapid primary survey.
- Resuscitation of vital functions may interrupt the primary survey.
- A detailed secondary survey is undertaken next.
- Finally-definitive care is given.

The primary survey: the ABC;
a. Airway maintenance and cervical spine control.
b. Breathing (ventilatory ability is assessed).
c. Circulation is assessed and hemorrhage controlled.
d. Disability (neurologic status) is assessed in terms of patient's degree of responsiveness.
e. Exposure-undress the patient as much as possible, when trauma is suspected to identify all injuries.

The immediate goal of primary survey is to identify life threatening conditions as an airway obstruction, impaired ventilation and hypoxemia, hypovolemic shock, and hemorrhage. It may be interrupted to manage the life threatening condition as soon as it is identified. Once the condition is stabilized, primary survey is continued. The survey should be repeated every 5 minutes in an emergency, since condition may change rapidly.

Findings in Primary Survey that Indicate a Sense of Urgency

Airway and Breathing
- Respiratory rate > 60, sustained especially with O_2.
- Respiratory distress (nasal flaring and retractions)
- Respiratory rate < 20, especially in acute illness or surgery.
- Cyanosis.
- Stridor—indicates upper airway obstruction.
- Head bobbing—indicates imminent respiratory failure.
- Prolonged expiration—indicates airway disease.
- Grunting indicates alveolar collapse or loss of lung volume.

Circulation
- Heart rate > 180 or < 80 (<5 years old)
- Heart rate > 160 (over 5 years)
- Sustained sinus tachycardia
- Bradycardia—indicates impending cardiac arrest.
- Hypotension—indicates hypovolemia-(decompensated)
- Absence of peripheral pulses—poor tissue perfusion.
- Absence of central pulse—ominous sign.
- Capillary refill time > 2 sec.
- Mottling, pallor and peripheral cyanosis.
- Diminished urine output indicate poor renal perfusion.

Neurological Disability
- Diminished level of consciousness
- Agitation, anxiety
- Lethargy
- Irritability to passivity
- Unresponsiveness
- Failure to recognize parents/caretakers
- Hypotonia and/or lost deep tendon reflexes, may indicate hypoperfusion of the brain.
- Generalised convulsions may indicate a seizure disorder, hypoglycemia, hypertensive encephalopathy, drug ingestion, severe renal dysfunction.
- Pupillary dilatation may indicate raised intracranial pressure.

Infant or Child: Really Sick or Reasonably Well

The Yale observation scale is a guide to recognize whether a well appearing child is really well or not. Can be used for a febrile or non-febrile child. The only drawback is the great variability due to subjectivity of observations (Table 33.1).

Secondary Survey

An in depth, head to toe examination to identify anatomical problems, additional conditions that are potentially life threatening condition and patients previously diagnosed condition. This begins only after all life threatening

Table 33.1: Yale observation scales

Observation Item	Score of observation		
	Reasurring(1)	*Worrisome (3)*	*Ominous (5)*
1. Quality of cry	Strong with expected tone, or content and not crying	Whimpening, or sobbing	Weak or moaning or high pitched
2. Reaction to parents	Cries briefly and stops or content, not crying	Cries off and on	Continuous cry, or hardly responds
3. Awake or asleep	If Awake, stays awake, or if asleep and stimulated awakens quickly	Eyes close briefly and then awakens, or Awakens with pro-longed stimulation.	Falls asleep or will not arouse
4. Color	Pink	Pale extremities, or acrocyanosis	Pale or cyanosed, or ashen or mottled.
5. Hydration	Appropriate skin turgor and eyes and mucous membrane moist.	Appropriate skin turgor eyes mosit and mucus membrane dry.	Skin doughy or ten-ted and dry mucuous membrane and/or sunken eyes.
6. Response to social overtures	Smiles or consistently alert (< 2 months)	Brief smile or briefly alert (< 2 months)	No smile, face anxi-ous, dull or expres-sionless or not alert (< 2 months)

The higher the score, more likely the child is ill particularly when score approaches or is greater than 10

conditions have been stabilised. It can be interrupted for repeated primary surveys if any life threatening condition develops.

Special investigations like peritoneal lavage, radiological evaluation and laboratory studies are conducted during this phase. Assessment of eyes, ears, nose, mouth, rectum and pelvis should not be neglected.

Primary Survey: The Procedure

ABC evaluation should be rapidly completed and needs only 30 seconds in a stable patient. But may take several minutes when patient is critically ill, and should be done as quickly and efficiently (Table 33.2).

Airway (Cervical Spine)

Hypoxemia and respiratory arrest in children causes acute deterioration and cardiopulmonary arrest. Thus, establishment and maintenance of a patent airway and support of adequate ventilation are most important components of life support.

Relaxation of the muscles and posterior displacement of the tongue leads to airway obstruction in the unconscious victim. The airway may be opened by:
1. Head tilt-chin lift maneuver (Fig. 33.1).
2. If cervical spine injury is suspected then the same is accomplished by jaw thrust maneuver (Fig. 33.2).

Table 33.2: Algorithm of initial assessment of patient

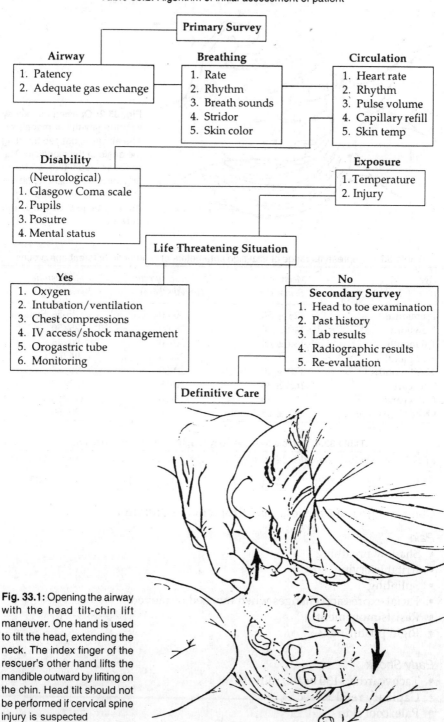

Primary Survey

Airway
1. Patency
2. Adequate gas exchange

Breathing
1. Rate
2. Rhythm
3. Breath sounds
4. Stridor
5. Skin color

Circulation
1. Heart rate
2. Rhythm
3. Pulse volume
4. Capillary refill
5. Skin temp

Disability
(Neurological)
1. Glasgow Coma scale
2. Pupils
3. Posutre
4. Mental status

Exposure
1. Temperature
2. Injury

Life Threatening Situation

Yes
1. Oxygen
2. Intubation/ventilation
3. Chest compressions
4. IV access/shock management
5. Orogastric tube
6. Monitoring

No
Secondary Survey
1. Head to toe examination
2. Past history
3. Lab results
4. Radiographic results
5. Re-evaluation

Definitive Care

Fig. 33.1: Opening the airway with the head tilt-chin lift maneuver. One hand is used to tilt the head, extending the neck. The index finger of the rescuer's other hand lifts the mandible outward by lifiting on the chin. Head tilt should not be performed if cervical spine injury is suspected

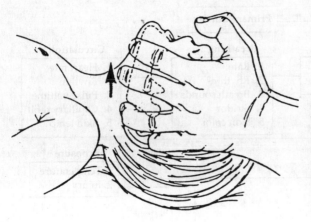

Fig. 33.2: Opening the airway with the jaw-thrust maneuver. The airway is opened by lifting the angle of the mandible. The rescuer uses two or three fingers of each hand to lift the jaw while the remaining fingers guide the jaw upward and outward

Table 33.3: Represents range of vital sign parameters of children in different age groups

Age	Mean pulse Beats/Min	Respiratory rate (Breaths/Min)	Syst/Diastolic BP (mm Hg)
Premature	125 ± 50	30-60	35-56 Systolic
Newborn	140 ± 50	30-60	75/50
1-6 months	130 ± 45	30-40	80/46
6-12 months	115 ± 40	24-30	96/65
12-24 months	110 ± 40	20-30	99/65
2-6 years	105 ± 35	20-25	100/60
6-12 years	95 ± 30	16-20	110/60
Over 12 years of age	82 ± 25	12-16	120/60

Table 33.4: Depicts average body weights corresponding to age

Birth	6 months	12months	24 months	36 months	5 years	10 years	12 years	14 years
3.5 kg	7 kg	10 kg	12 kg	15 kg	20 kg	30 kg	40 kg	50 kg

Classic Signs of Physiological Problems in Children

Pain
- Shallow breathing
- Irritable crying
- Splinting
- Facial expression changes when touched or moved
- Resists movement
- Rigid posturing

Early Shock
- Tachycardia >130 beats/min
- Capillary refill >2 sec
- Pale, cool skin

- Altered level of consciousness
- Normal systolic BP.

Late Shock
- Tachycardia > 130 beats/minute
- Capillary refill > 3-4 second
- Pallor, cold extremities
- Altered consciousness
- Systolic BP < 80 mmHg (except in infants)

Respiratory Distress
- Nasal flaring
- Mottled, dusky skin color
- Tachypnea, shallow breathing
- Altered level of consciousness
- Sounds—stridor, hoarseness, muffled voice, wheezing
- Retractions and asymmetrical chest movements
- Tripod positioning

Increased Intracranial Pressure
- Bulging fontanelle (infants)
- Altered level of consciousness
- High-pitched cry
- Change in vital signs
- Irritable cry, unconsolable.

Altered Level of Consciousness
- Combative
- Decreased responsiveness
- Lethargy
- Weak cry, moaning
- Personality change

Severe Dehydration
- Sunken fontanelle
- Signs of shock
- Parched mucous membranes
- No tears
- Sunken eyeballs.

Airway Management
The goals of airway management are:
- Recognition and relief of obstruction
- Prevention of aspiration of gastric contents
- Promotion of adequate gas exchange
- Substitute artificial respiration if necessary.

Table 33.5: Modified Glasgow coma scale

	Child		Infant	
Eye Opening	Spontaneous	4	Spontaneous	4
	To verbal stimuli	3	To Verbal stimuli	3
	To pain only	2	To pain only	2
	No response	1	No response	1
Verbal Response	Oriented, appropriate	5	Coos and babbles	5
	Confused	4	Irritable cries	4
	Inappropriate words	3	Cries to pain	3
	Nonspecific sounds	2	Moans to pain	2
	No response	1	No response	1
Motor Response	Obeys commands	6	Moves spontaneously and purposefully	6
	Localizes pain	5	Withdraws to touch	5
	Withdrawal to pain	4	Withdraws to pain	4
	Flexion in response to pain	3	Decorticate	3
	Extension in response to pain	2	Decerebrate	2
	No response	1	No response	1

Table 33.6: Represents Adelaide pediatric coma scale:child's reaction to various sensory responses

Eye opening		Best verbal response		Best motor response		Normal score	
Spontaneous	4	Oriented	5	Obeys commands	5	0-6 months	- 9
To speech	3	Words	4	Localises pain	4	6-12 months	- 11
To pain	2	Vocal sounds	3	Flexion to pain	3	1-2 years	- 12
None	1	Cries	2	Extension to pain	2	2-5 years	- 13
		None	1	None	1	> 5 years	- 14

Is the Airway Patent?
Sources of Obstruction
- Posteriorly displaced tongue
- Foreign body
- *Trauma*   Blunt or penetrating
- *Infection*   Epiglottitis, croup, peritonsillary abscess, retropharyngeal abscess, diphtheria
- *Inflammation*   Burn, smoke inhalation
- *Tumor*   Thyroid, hemangioma, hematoma, edema
- *Neurological lesion*   Vocal cord paralysis
- *Congenital anomalies*   Laryngeal web, tracheomalacia.

Symptoms of Obstruction
- Respiratory distress: dyspnea, tachypnea
- Anxiety: tense, worried facies (may signal epiglotitis)
- Difficulty in swallowing
- Pain, may be diffuse or related to area of difficulty
- Cough and associated change in voice
- Restless behavior: Inability to find a comfortable position

Signs of Obstruction
- Hoarse voice and/or cough ("barking quality")
- Stridor: Severity related to extent of obstruction
    - Inspiratory: obstruction at the glottis, epiglottis
    - Expiratory: obstruction below the glottis
- Retraction:
    - Suprasternal: obstruction above trachea
    - Intercostal and subscostal: obstruction in bronchial tree or below
- Drooling (difficulty in swallowing)
- Bleeding: Hemoptysis, hematoma
- Subcutaneous emphysema
- Fracture.

Breathing
- Assess the ventilatory effort of the patient. Note approximate rate and depth of respiration
- Bilateral chest movement should be synchronized with breathing and breath sounds and all entry assessed with a stethoscope
- Signs of respiratory distress should be looked for and oxygen given before continuing the survey
- In cases of trauma, look for bruising, open chest wounds and paradoxical chest movements and airleak syndromes— should be immediately attended to.

Air Exchange
May be deficient from central causes such as apnea or from abnormal chest wall dynamics such as tension pneumothorax.

Methods to Augment Ventilation
Mouth to mouth; mouth to nose rescue breathing (Fig. 33.3)   After inhaling deeply, form a tight mouth to mouth seal and give 2 rescue breaths 1 to 2.5 sec per breath pausing to take a breath. Volume and pressure of the breaths should be sufficient to cause the chest to rise.

Bag and mask ventilation (Fig. 33.4)
- Remember to keep the head and neck in "sniffing" position
- Give ventilation at a rate and pressure for that age and watch for chest wall rise
- Remember to empty or deflate the stomach if IPPV by this method is given beyond 2 minutes as the gastric dilation will cause respiratory embarrasment (limits the downword movement of diaphragm) and also predisposes to regurgitation and aspiration of the stomach contents.

Endotracheal airway (Fig. 33.5)
- Most effective and reliable method of ventilation
- Airway is isolated ensuring adequate ventilation and oxygen delivery

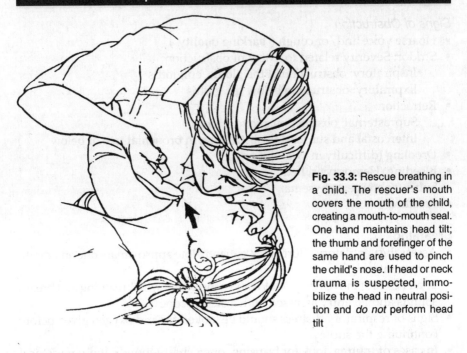

Fig. 33.3: Rescue breathing in a child. The rescuer's mouth covers the mouth of the child, creating a mouth-to-mouth seal. One hand maintains head tilt; the thumb and forefinger of the same hand are used to pinch the child's nose. If head or neck trauma is suspected, immobilize the head in neutral position and *do not* perform head tilt

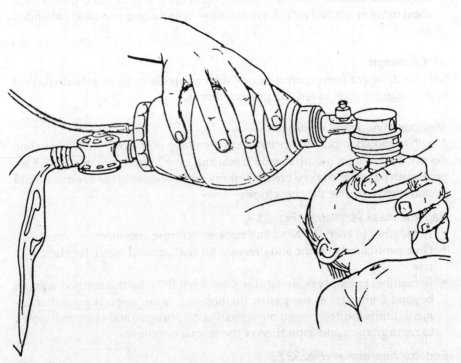

Fig. 33.4: One-handed facemask application technique. Note that the fingers avoid pressure on the soft tissues of the neck, which could cause laryngeal/tracheal compression

- Potential pulmonary aspiration of the gastric contents is reduced.
- Interposition of ventilations with chest compressions can be accomplished effectively.
- Inspiratory time, peak inspiratory pressures can be controlled (on a ventilator).
- Positive end expiratory pressure (PEEP) can be delivered if needed (on ventilator).

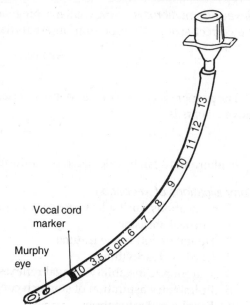

Fig. 33.5: Endotracheal tube with distance markers

Indications for Endotracheal Intubation
- Inadequate CNS control of ventilation.
- Functional or anatomic airway obstruction.
- Loss of protective airway reflexes.
- Excessive work of breathing which may fatigue and cause respiratory insufficiency.
- Need for high peak inspiratory pressure or PEEP to maintain effective alveolar gas exchange.
- Need for mechanical ventilatory support.
- Potential occurence of any of the above and patient transport is needed.

Syndromes Associated with Difficult Intubation

Micrognathia   Cri-du-chat (also narrow larynyx), Di-George syndrome (hypocalcemic tetary); Pierre-Robin syndrome, Treacher-Collins syndrome, Noonan's syndrome, Turner's syndrome. Trisomy 13 and 18.

Macroglossia   Beckwith-Wiedmann syndrome, Trisomy 21, Hurler and Hunter syndrome, hypothyroidism, glycogen storage disease (Pompe disease); Schie syndrome (prognathism, short-neck)

Mid-face hypoplasia   Craniofacial dysostosis (Maxilla and/or mandible) apert, Crouzon, Goldenhar syndrome, cherubism, median cleft face syndrome.

Short Neck Rigid Neck   Ankylosing spondylitis, rheumatoid arthritis, Hurler, Hunter syndrome, Morquio syndrome, Klippel-Feil syndrome.

Temporomandibular joint disease   Rheumatoid arthritis, *polyarteritis nodosa*, systemic lupus erethymatosus, arthrogryposis multiplex, trismus, infection like Lundwig angina.

Airway edema/fibrosis Angio edema, pregnancy, Stevens-Johnson syndrome. The correct size of ET tube (mm internal diameter) may be selected by the formula:

$$ET\ tube\ =\ \frac{Age\ (yr)}{4}\ +\ 4$$

The proper distance (cm) i.e., depth of insertion in centimeters for children above 2 years is

$$\frac{Age\ (yr)}{2}\ +\ 12$$

or alternately can be calculated by multiplied by 3 (the internal diameter).

Compalications of Intubation

a. Complications during laryngoscopy or intubation
   1. Corneal abrasion
   2. Dental or soft tissue trauma
   3. Cardiac dysrhythmia
   4. Autonomic instability—vagal reflexes
   5. Pulmonary aspiration of stomach contents
   6. Esophageal intubation
   7. Arytenoid cartilage dislocation.
b. Complications with tube in place
   1. Increased resistance to breathing
   2. ET tube obstruction (plugging or kinking)
   3. Accidental extubation
   4. Autonomic instability
c. Complications after intubation
   1. Laryngeal damage or edema
   2. Tracheal damage or edema
d. *Other methods of ventilation* Occasionally ventilation can be achieved by an airway by cricothyrotomy or tracheostomy.

Circulation

Once the airway is opened and 2 rescue breaths are given, the circulation is assessed by pulse check. If cardiac contractions are ineffective or absent, there will not be a palpable pulse in the arteries. Apical impulse is not used in pulse check. In children less than 1 year, due to a chubby neck it is very difficult to locate the cartoid pulse, hence brachial pulse is recommended. In children more than 1 year the cartoid artery is well palpated. However, since the blood supply to brain is already impaired carotid pulse check might further aggravate hypoxic injury to brain.

a. If pulse is well felt and spontaneous breathing is absent, continue to take care of ventilation after opening the airway.
b. If the pulse is not palpable or heart rate is less than 60 and signs of poor systemic perfusion present, chest compressions along with ventilation are started; at least 20 cycles are done before deciding on further course of actions.

The details of compressions are as follows (Table 33.7).

Table 33.7: Details of compressions in infants and children

Compressions	Infant (< 1 year)	Child (1-10 years)
1. Pulse check	Brachial/femoral	Cartoid
2. Compression area	Lower ½ of the sternum	Lower ½ of the sternum
3. Compression width	2-3 fingers	Heel of one hand
4. Rate	100-120/min	80-100/mm.
5. Depth	3/4 " to 1"	1-1.5"

Perfusion is also assessed by peripheral pulse volume. Capillary refill and blood pressure are determined. Blood pressure is the least sensitive as compromised circulation may exist despite a well maintained BP.

Circulatory Support

During primary survey may be given by:
1. Control of active hemorrhage
2. Intravenous fluid (Crystalloid or colloid)
   (details under management of shock).

Disability

Rapid and brief neurological evaluation is performed to determine the level of consciousness. The patient is said to be in one of these levels.

A : Alert
V : Verbal stimuli (responds to)
P : Painful stimuli (responds to)
U : Unresponsive

Detailed neurological examination is done in secondary survey.

Exposure

1. Undress the patient fully to assess the injuries in case of trauma or in cases of hyperthermia or heat stroke.

Secondary Survey

Remember to take AMPLE history

A : Allergies
M : Medications of any kind being taken by the patient
P : Past illness such as diabetes, epilepsy, hypertension
L : Last meal
E : Events preceding the precipitating event.

Head and Face

- Examine for maxillofacial trauma by palpation of bony prominences, presence of bloody or cerebrospinal fluid from ears, nose, mouth.
- Dehydration—sunken eyes/fontanelle, dry mucosa
- Poisoining and metabolic problems—odor from mouth, discoloration of mucosa

- Eyes—pupillary size and reaction, fundoscopic appearance and vision if possible.
  Racoon eyes.
- Scalp—lacerations or hematoma, specific signs of basilar skull fractures-Battle sign.

Neck
Palpated gently for obvious signs of fracture, no movement of the neck is done untill neck injury has been excluded.

Chest
Inspected for adequate respiration and palpated for evidence of fracture.

Abdomen
Flanks are observed for hematoma, Cullen's signs and Grey-Turner's sign.

Pelvis
The bony prominences of the pelvis are palpated for tenderness or instability
- Perineum is examined for laceration, hematoma, active bleed or discharge.
- Rectal examination when indicated.
  Detailed neurovascular and orthopedic examination should always follow.

Increased Intracranial Pressure
The skull, a closed space, limits the expansion of brain tissue or fluid volume (blood or CSF); resulting in rising pressure, trauma or disease process.

Causes Infectious: Meningitis, encephalitis.
- Tumor and tumor like conditions:
  - Intracranial space occupying lesion
  - Pseudotumor cerebri.
  - Hypervitaminosis A
  - Head trauma
  - Anatomical defects
  - Subdural or extradural hematoma
- Metabolic and other conditions:
  - Hypoxia
  - Hypercapnia
  - Vasodilatation.

Clinical Signs and Symptoms of Raised ICT

A. Infants	B. Children
Tense bulging fontanelle	Headache
Lack of normal pulsations	Nausea
Separated cranial sutures	Projectile vomiting
Macewan's sign	Diplopia/blurred vision
Irritability	Seizures

Contd...

Contd...

A. Infants	B. Children
High-pitched cry	VI cranial nerve palsy
Increased head size	Bounding, slow pulse
distended scalp veins	Increased systolic BP
Changes in feeding	Personality and behavioral changes
Crying when held or rocked	Irritability, restlessness
Setting sun sign	Indifferent, drowsy
Vasomotor instability.	Declining school performance
	Excessive sleep and fatigue
	Weight loss/memory loss
	Poor response to commands
	Lethargy and drowsiness
	Late signs are decreased conciousness, decreased motor and sensory com- commands
	Pupillary change
	Decerebrate/decorticate posturing.

SHOCK

Definition A state of hypoperfusion where the cardiac output is unable to meet the oxygen demands of the tissues.

Circulation and perfusion are assessed by:
1. Heart rate (pulse)
2. Blood pressure
3. Peripheral circulation
4. Skin perfusion
5. Level of consciousness
6. Urine output.

Heart Rate and Blood Pressure
See Chapter on Vital Signs.

Peripheral Circulation and Skin Perfusion
– Evaluate temperature of the extremities
– Capillary refill
– Skin color.

Cold toes and extremities are suggestive of low-cardiac output. Capillary refill of more than 2 seconds in pediatric age group, also indicates tissue hypoperfusion. Both these can give false values in hypothermia. Other sites for capillary refill assessment are, gums, mouth, forehead and sternum.

Indicators of Poor Skin Perfusion
• Pallor
• Mottling
• Poor capillary refill

Table 33.8: Represents signs and symptoms of certain life threatening conditions

	Definition	Causes	Signs and symptoms
1. Upper airway obstruction	Compromise of airway space, resulting in impaired respiratory exchange	– Foreign body – Infections – Tumor (goiter) – Trauma – Smoke inhalation – Aspiration of chemicals	– Patients grasps neck – Fatigue – Severe dyspnea – Tachypnea – Stridor – Hoarseness – Dysphagia – Drooling – Anxiety – Tripod positioning.
2. Hypovolemic shock	Loss of fluid from intravascular space resulting in inadequate perfusion.	– GI Bleed – Trauma – Dehydration – GI fluid loss – Renal fluid loss – Cutaneous fluid loss (burns, sweat) – Ascites	– Anxiety – Pallor – Diaphoresis – Oliguria – Coma (altered sensorium) – Circulatory collapse – Tachycardia – Hypotension – Delayed capillary refill.
3. Hypoxemia	Severely reduced blood levels in major organs resulting from respiratory distress, poor perfusion, lung injury with increased permeability of alveoli	– Aspiration – Trauma – Increased ICT – Drug overdose – DIC – Infection – Shock – Upper Airway obstruction – Lower-Asthma	– Severe dyspnea oxygen – Cyanosis – Altered mental status – Tachypnea – Tachycardia

Contd...

Contd...

Definition	Causes	Signs and symptoms
4. Status epilepticus	Seizures of any type that are protracted and recurrent without recovery of consciousness	– Generalized or focal – Grand mal or petit mal epilepsy – Metabolic encephalopathy – Encephalitis	– Obvious convulsive movements with unresponsiveness. – Hypotension – Arrhythmias – Fever
5. Status asthmaticus	A severe and prolonged attack of asthma resisting usual therapeutic approaches	A wide variety of physical chemical and pharmacological stimuli	– Dyspnea – Able to speak only few words in between breath – Tachycardia (>130 b/min.) – Tachypnea – Hypertension – Wheeze – Pulsus paradoxus.
6. Ventilatory failure	Compromised exhalation of CO_2 because of alveolar hypoventilation	Upper airway obstruction CNS causes Neurologic disorders Drug overdose Increased ICT C3-5 involvement Phrenic nerve palsy GB syndrome Poliomyelitis Severe kyphoscoliosis Trauma with flail chest Pulmonary contusion.	**Cardinal signs** Restlessness, tachypnea tachycardia, diaphoresis **Early less obvious signs** Mood changes Headache Altered depth and pattern of respiration. Flaring of nose Chest retractions Expiratory grunt Wheeze, prolonged expiration Exertional dyspnea Confusion and irritability Increased BP

Contd...

Contd...

Definition	Causes	Signs and symptoms
		Severe hypoxia Hypotension Dimness of vision Decreased respiration Cyanosis Somnolence Stupor Coma Dyspnea Bradycardia
7. Congestive cardiac failure	Disparity between cardiac output and tissue perfusion.	

Table 33.9: Depicts cardiac failures due to different types of congestions

A. Due to reduced myocardial function	B. Due to pulmonary congestion	C. Due to systemic venous congestion
Tachycardia Sweating Reduced urine output Fatigue Weakness Restlessness Anorexia Pale, cool limbs Weak peripheral pulses Decreased BP Gallop rhythm Cardiomegaly	Tachypnea Dyspnea Retractions Flaring nares Exercise intolerance Cough Hoarseness Cyanosis Wheezing Grunting	Weight gain Hepatomegaly Edema Ascites Neck vein distention

- Peripheral Cyanosis
- Skin temperature reduced.

Level of Perfusion of CNS

As the perfusion becomes impaired, the level of consciousness decreases.
a. Alert
b. Sleepy/combative
c. Failure to recognize parents
d. Failure to respond to pain
e. Fluctuating level of consciousness
   also
   - Absent DTRs
   - Small pupils
   - Cheyne-Stokes breathing

Urine Output

Normal kidney perfusion 1 to 2 ml/kg
- Urine output less than 1 ml/kg/hr in absence of renal disease is a signs of poor perfusion
- Placing an indwelling catheter assists in determining accurate urine output.
- Used to evaluate the success of volume expansion.

The following Table 33.10 shows 3 main types of shock viz. hypovolemic, distributive and cardiogenic and their features.

Table 33.10: Clinical features of three main types of shocks

Hypovolemic	Distributive	Cardiogenic
Most common cause in	Due to sepsis or anaphylaxis	Myocarditis
infants and children	Evidence of infection	Severe congenital heart diseases
10-15% loss of blood	Tachycardia	Cardiomyopathy
Volume is compensated	Tachypnea	Drug toxicity
	Fever or hypothermia	Severe electrolyte imbalance
Signs of Early	Peripheral vasodilatation	After cardiac surgery
Compensated Shock		
Persistent tachycardia	**Septic Syndrome**	**Signs and Symptoms**
Cutaneous vasocons-	Signs of sepsis	Results of low cardiac output
triction	Pulmonary failure	Delayed capillary refill
Reduced pulse pressure	GI or hepatic dysfunction	Cool extremities
BP maintained	Oliguria and renal failure	Mottling of the skin
Neurologically normal		Diminished peripheral pulses.
	Septic Shock	
25% or More Loss	Sepsis syndrome with hypo-	
Decompensated	tension	
Hypotension significant		
tachycardia	**Anaphylaxis**	
Delayed capillary refill	Severe allergic response	
Altered mental status	Stridor, wheeze	
Oliguria	Tachycardia, hypotension,	
Moderate tachypnea	Arrhythmia	
Cool extremities	Vomiting diarrhea	
Mottling and pallor	Angio edema	
	Urticaria	

Management of Shock

Hypovolemia is the most common cause of shock in children worldwide. It results from intravascular volume depletion, hemorrhage, trauma, diarrhea, vomiting, renal loss, deprivation leads to cellular hypoperfusion, metabolic acidosis and cell death.

Blood pressure is an insensitive index of hypovolemia as it is caused only after profound failure of homeostasis in shock syndrome.

Table 33.11 shows different clinical observation corresponding to different level percent (age) of dehydration.

Table 33.11: Assessment estimation of dehydration

Dehydration (% of Body weight)	Clinical observation
5%	Increased Heart rate (10-15%) above baseline
	Dry mucous membrane
	Concentrated urine
	Poor tear formation
10%	Decreased skin turgor
	Oliguria
	Soft sunken eyes
	Sunken anterior fontanelle
15%	Decreased BP, tachypnea, tachycardia
	Poor tissue perfusion and acidosis
	Delayed capillary refill (>2 sec)

Fluid Management

A. Effective circulating volume-Fluid boluses
B. Replacement of old and ongoing losses
C. Provision of normal maintenance fluid and electroclyte requirements

Table 33.12 represents treatment algorithin for fluid resuscitation of shock.

Fluid deficit is calculated by multiplying the assessed percentage of dehydration by the child's weight. Three types of dehydration are described.

a. Isotonic (130-150 mEq/l Na$^+$)
b. Hypotonic (< 130 mEq/l Na$^+$)
c. Hypertonic (> 150 mEq/l Na$^+$)

Specific Therapy for Hemorrhagic Shock

Table 33.13 shows various classes of hemerrhagic shock.

Class I   1. Replace the volume loss with RL or NS. One or 2 boluses of 10 to 20 ml/kg over 20 minutes till peripheral pulses are well felt.

2. Replace ongoing losses, control hemorrhage.

Class II: Treated the same way as class I hemorrhage except that blood is frequently required as well as ongoing losses are replaced ml for ml with blood.

Class III or IV: Hemorrhage requires 10 to 15 ml/kg whole blood as well as Ringer's lactate. It will also need other measures to improve perfusion—like drugs.

Table 33.12: Treatment algorithm for fluid resuscitation of shock

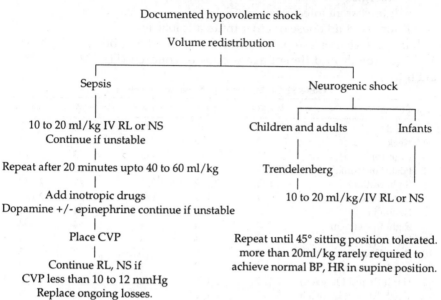

Table 33.13: Classification of hemorrhagic shock

	I	II	III	IV
Est. Blood vol deficit	10-15%	20-25%	30-35%	>40%
Pulse (b/min)	>100	>150	>150	>150
Respiration	Normal	Increased	Tachypnea	Tachypnea or apnea
Capillary refill	<5 sec	5-10 Sec	10-15 Sec	>20 sec
BP	Normal	Decreased Pulse pressure	Decreased	Severely decreased
Mental status	Normal	Anxious	Confused	Unconscious
Orthostatic hypotension	+	++	+++	+++
Urine output	1-3 ml/kg	0.5 ml-1 ml/kg	< 0.5 ml/kg	None

Remember Fluid boluses are contraindicated in cardiogenic and septic shock. In cardiogenic shock, rapid fluid bolus worsens the existing shock. In septic shock, the sepsis correction is the priority with adequate antibiotics and inotropes.

Management of Burns Patient

Assessment of Burn Injury

History:

1. When, where and how the injury occured?
   How long patient was exposed to smoke or fire ?
2. Past medical history:
   - Pre-existing medical problems
   - Tetanus immunization history

- Allergies
- Intercurrent infections

3. History of child abuse or other traumatic injuries

Burn surface area estimation of modified Lund and Bowder Table 33.14 showing growth in different age groups of children (Figs 33.6 and 33.7A and B).

Table 33.14: Modified Lund and Bowder chart

Area	0-1 year	1-4 years	5-9 years	10-14 years	15 years
1. Head	19	17	13	11	9
2. Neck	2	2	2	2	2
3. Anterior trunk	13	13	13	13	13
4. Posterior trunk	13	13	13	13	13
5. Right buttock	2 1/2	2 1/2	2 1/2	2 1/2	2 1/2
6. Left buttock	2 1/2	2 1/2	2 1/2	2 1/2	2 1/2
7. Genitalia	1	1	1	1	1
8. Right upper arm	4	4	4	4	4
9. Left upper arm	4	4	4	4	4
10. Right lower arm	3	3	3	3	3
11. Left lower arm	3	3	3	3	3
12. Hand Rt and Lt. (each)	2 1/2	2 1/2	2 1/2	2 1/2	2 1/2
13. Thigh Rt. and Lt. (each)	5 1/2	6 1/2	8	8 1/2	9
14. Leg Rt. and Lt. (each)	5	5	5 1/2	6	6
15. Rt. foot	3 1/2	3 1/2	3 1/2	3 1/2	3 1/2
16. Lt. foot	3 1/2	3 1/2	3 1/2	3 1/2	3 1/2

DEHYDRATION:

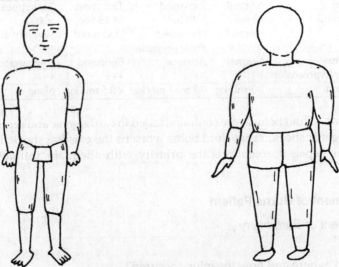

Fig. 33.6: Burn surface area estimation

Table 33.15 shows management of life threatening burns by various methods.

Table 33.16 shows secondary survey in various forms of burns.

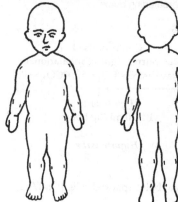

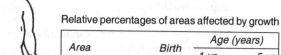

Relative percentages of areas affected by growth

Area	Birth	Age (years)	
		1 yr	5 yr
A = ½ of head	9½	8½	6½
B = ½ of one thigh	2¼	3¼	4
C = ½ of one leg	2½	2½	2¼

Fig 33.7A: Estimation of distribution of burns in children from birth to age 5 years

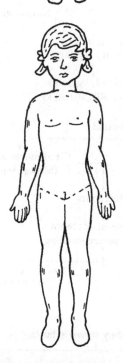

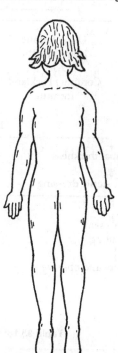

Relative percentages of areas affected by growth

Area	Birth	Age 1 year	Age 5 years
A = ½ of head	5½	4½	3½
B = ½ of one thigh	4¼	4½	4¼
C = ½ of one leg	3	3¼	3½

Fig 33.7B: Estimation of distribution of burns in older children

Dehydration

Dehydration is due to loss of body water of more than 1 percent and is graded according to the percentage of weight loss.

mild—1 to 5 percent, moderate—5 to 10 percent, severe—15 percent.

Table 33.15: Management of life threatening burns

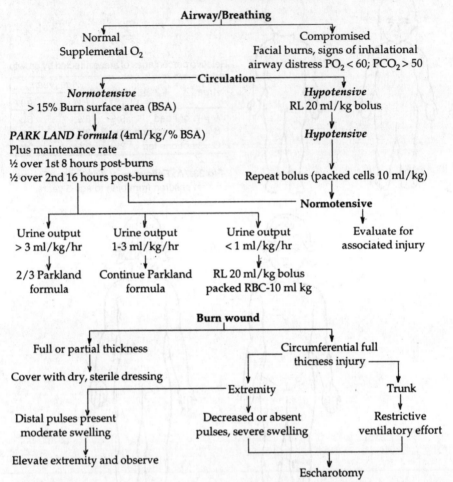

Airway/Breathing

Normal
Supplemental O$_2$

Compromised
Facial burns, signs of inhalational
airway distress PO$_2$ < 60; PCO$_2$ > 50

Circulation

Normotensive
> 15% Burn surface area (BSA)

Hypotensive
RL 20 ml/kg bolus

PARK LAND Formula (4ml/kg/% BSA)
Plus maintenance rate
½ over 1st 8 hours post-burns
½ over 2nd 16 hours post-burns

Hypotensive

Repeat bolus (packed cells 10 ml/kg)

Normotensive

Urine output
> 3 ml/kg/hr

Urine output
1-3 ml/kg/hr

Urine output
< 1 ml/kg/hr

Evaluate for
associated injury

2/3 Parkland
formula

Continue Parkland
formula

RL 20 ml/kg bolus
packed RBC-10 ml kg

Burn wound

Full or partial thickness

Cover with dry, sterile dressing

Circumferential full
thicness injury

Extremity

Trunk

Distal pulses present
moderate swelling

Decreased or absent
pulses, severe swelling

Restrictive
ventilatory effort

Elevate extremity and observe

Escharotomy

Table 33.16: Secondary survey in burns

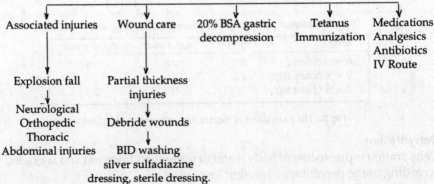

Associated injuries

Wound care

20% BSA gastric
decompression

Tetanus
Immunization

Medications
Analgesics
Antibiotics
IV Route

Explosion fall

Partial thickness
injuries

Neurological
Orthopedic
Thoracic
Abdominal injuries

Debride wounds

BID washing
silver sulfadiazine
dressing, sterile dressing.

Table 33.17: Assessment of dehydration

Look at	A	B	C
Condition	Well, alert	*Restless and irritable	*Lethargic unconsciouss or floppy
Eyes	Normal	Sunken	Very sunken or dry
Tears	Present	Absent	Absent
Mouth and Tongue	Moist	Dry	Very dry
Thirst	Drinks normally not thirsty.	*Thirsty, drinks eagerly.	*Drinks poorly not able to drink.
Feel			
Skin pinch	Goes back quickly	*Goes back slowly	*Goes back very slowly
Decide			
	The patient has no signs of dehydration.	If the patient has 2 or more signs including atleast one *sign there is severe dehydration.	If the patient has 2 or more signs, including at least one *sigh there is severe dehydration.
Treat	**Use Plan-A** *Three basics rules* - More fluids than usual to prevent dehydration - Plenty of nutritious food to prevent malnutrition - Take to health care centre if diarrhea worsens or signs of other disease develop.	Weigh the child **Use Plan B** - 75 ml/kg of ORS to be given after every loose stool. - Continue breast feeding. - If improves under observation-shift to A if not shift to C.	Weigh the child **Use Plan-C Urgently** Start IV Access and give RL or NS

* 3 Key signs

1. General condition
2. Thirst
3. Skin pinch

Age	30 ml/kg in	70 ml/kg in
< 12 month	1 hour	5 hours
Older	30 minutes	2½ hours

Reassess patient and shift to Plan-B if improves or continue similar treatment till condition improves.

But unfortunately in many circumstances the weight of the child prior to the onset of illness is not known. Hence, WHO has suggested the following grading of dehydration based on clinical parameters. The dehydration is graded as (1) no dehydration (2) some dehydration and (3) severe dehydration.

Plans of treatment administered vary according to severity of dehydration. Plans A, B, and C are utilized in no, some and severe dehydration respectively (Table 33.17).

34 Examination of the Child in Different Situations

DIFFERENT SITUATIONS OF EXAMINATION

a. Examination of playing child
b. Examination of crying child
c. Examination of child in parent's lap and on shoulder
d. Examination of sleeping child
e. Examination of standing child
f. Examination of feeding child
g. Special methods of distracting the child
h. General inspection of the child
i. Special techniques in special situations

Examination of Playing Child

1. You may assess musculoskeletal system, grips and psychological aspects.
2. Gait, jumping, hopping, range of motion, types of gait.
3. Muscle strength.
   a. Standing one leg—to assess differential strength and co-ordination.
   b. Hopping for strength in lower limbs and for identifying minimal difference on the two sides.
4. Tip toe walking for strength in extensors of lower limb.
5. Heel walking for strength in flexors of lower limbs.
6. Tandem gait for co-ordination in lower limbs.
7. Climbing chair and cot to assess pelvic girdle muscles
8. Jumping from chair and cot to assess pelvic girdle muscles.
9. Crawling in infants to assess flexors and extensors of hip, knee and foot.
10. Drawing, building, coloring for developmental assessment.

Examination of Crying Child

- While child is crying one should look for seventh cranial nerve asymmetry (facial palsy), observe the tongue for twitchings, fibrillations and for the strength of the tongue.
- Throat examination can be performed when the child is crying. Voice can be assessed when child is crying.
- Check for vocal fremitus, when child is crying.
- Respiratory cyanosis decreases during crying whereas cardiac cyanosis increases.

- When the child takes deep breath during crying check for inspiratory lung sounds and for crepitations and also palpate for liver and spleen.

Examination of Child in Parent's Lap and on Shoulders
General : Sickness, dehydration, toxicity, playfulness, color, anomalies, face, behavior, cry, posture, size and shape of the hand.

Upper limbs	:	Fingers, creases,
		Palpate radial arteries bilaterally
		Elicit biceps/triceps reflexes
		Record blood pressure, if cooperative.
Lower-limb	:	See muscles for their size, shape, and associated lesions.
		Feet, toes, arch and alignment.
		Palpate dorsalis pedis pulse
		Elicit plantar response with scratch.
		Elicit DTR (ankles, knee with figner tap)
Head and neck	:	Shape, hairline, auricular position
		Palpate sutures, hair, measure HC
		See neck for webs and movements
		Palpate glands and thyroid, trachea,
		Muscle tone and clavicle.
Chest and heart	:	Inspect respiratory movements, shape of the chest, respiratory rate, deformities.
		Nipple, breast, retractions.
		Palpate chest, apex, VF, VR, breath sounds,
		Auscultation of chest and heart.
Abdomen	:	Inspect for distention, movements of abodmen, umbilical hernia, look for visible peristalisis. Palpate abdominal organs light and then deep.
		Palpate femorals and glands in the inguinal region.
		See external genitalia and anus.

Examination of Sleeping Child
- Auscultate the heart for sounds and murmurs.
- Palpation of abdominal organs specially for details regarding masses.
- Position at rest can be observed.

Examination of Standing Child
Ask child to bend and see spine, observe gait, observe posture from front, back and sides.

In standing position of the child, one can look for the following things:
1. Neck movements
2. Spine while patient is bending—for scoliosis
3. Movements of spine
4. Gait
5. Romberg sign
6. Heel toe walking (Tandem)

7. Stands on one foot
8. Hop on each leg
9. Heel walking
10. Upper limb lift
11. Hernial orifices after coughing

Examination of Feeding Child

Good sucking and swallowing indicates intactness of V, VII, IX and X cranial nerves. Putting the child to feed is one of the best ways of relaxing the child for cardiac auscultation, abdominal palpation and elicitation of DTR and superficial reflexes.

Distracting the Child

a. Inspecting eyes for corneal, light reflex, red reflex, extraocular movements, mass and fundoscopic examination.
b. Otoscopic examination
c. Nasal mucosa
d. Mouth and throat

Special Methods of Distracting the Child for Palpation

1. Palpation on doll and then the child.
2. Palpation over child's hand.
4. Auscultation with chest piece held on child's body by the mother but tubings in examiner's ears.
5. Palpation of abdomen with chest piece.
6. Palpation and auscultation after sedation with trichloryl syrup.
7. Palpation while feeding.
8. Exam when the child is on mother's shoulder.

General Inspection of the Child

1. Color
2. Facial expression
3. Gait
4. Posture
5. Deformity
6. Eye contact with examiner
7. Nutrition
8. Respiratory distress
9. Vision/hearing
10. Speech
11. Dress
12. Apathy, playfulness, alertness, apprehension.

SPECIAL TECHNIQUES IN SPECIAL SITUATIONS

In the following situations few demonstration techniques and special examination may have to be done.

1. In situation where history is suggestive of a fit, ask the patient as the well as the attender to demonstrate the attack. If patient demonstrates in an accurate fashion it is most likely a hysterical conversion. If the attender demonstrates, it will give you an idea about the nature of the episode.
2. In episodic complaints like suspected epilepsies, fainting spells, numbness, etc. ask the patient to hyperventilate for 3 minutes. Petit mal epilepsy will be brought out by hyperventilation.
3. In cases of difficulty in swallowing, give the patients liquids and solids and observe the patient's act of swallowing.
4. If the patient complaints of weakness in climbing ask him to climb and observe.
5. If the patients complaint is specially facial muscle weakness, ask him to do 100 repetitive movements or do neostigmine test for myasthenia gravis.
6. In certain types of cough, a doctor has to show himself to the patient by making sounds.
7. In syndrome and malformation diagnosis, sometimes you may have to show your own album or standard album to the patient.
8. In the modern era, show short video clippings in certain clinical situations, e.g epilepsy (may be shown to patient to verify the type of episode).
9. If patient complains of dizziness on standing, test for orthostatic hypotension.
10. Observe children during play, this is not only to observe the physical activities but also about their emotional status.
11. Observing the act of micturition may help in assessing obstructive uropathy.

CHAPTER
35 Examination of Unconscious Patient

Assess Level of Consciousness

Consciousness is the awareness of self and environment. Consciousness is assessed by 3 methods: (1) By observing patient's response to ongoing visual, auditory and tactile stimuli (2) By conversation with the patient and noting the response. (3) By giving painful stimuli and noting the response.

Levels of Depressed Consciousness

Somnolence (drowsy) Arouses spontaneously at time or after normal stimuli but lapses back to drowsy state. When aroused responds normally.

Stupor Appears asleep but wakes up after loud verbal stimuli, sensorium is clouded and restlessness and spontaneous movements are common.

Semicoma (light coma) No response to verbal stimuli, withdraws limbs to painful stimuli. Reflexes (Corneal, pupillary) intact and breaths adequate.

Coma (deep coma) No spontaneous movements or arousal. Reflexes absent (Corneal, pupillary) breathing impaired.

Assess Glasgow Coma Scale (EMV Scale)

I Eye opening		II Best verbal response		III Best motor response	
• Spontaneous	4	• Oriented	5	• Obeying	6
• To speech	3	• Confused	4	• Localizing	5
• To pain	2	• Inappropriate	3	• Withdrawal	4
• None	1	• Incomprehensible	2	• Flexion (decorticate)	3
		• None	1	• Extension (decerebrate)	2
				• None	1

(A scale of 3-8 implies poor prognosis)
Table 35.1 shows GCS graphically.

Table 35.1: The scale can be put graphically

Condition	Score	Condition	Score	Condition	Score
				Best motor response	6
		Best verbal response	5		5
Eye opening	4		4		4
	3		3		3
	2		2		2
	1		1		1
			Time		

Posture

a. *Decerebrate rigidity* Extensive midbrain lesions, either intrinsic, or from unilateral or bilateral transientorial herniation, disconnects the cerebrum from the rest of the brainstem ie. decerebrate the individual. Decerebration can also be due to toxic, metabolic cause and increased ICP.

Decerebrate posture causes rigid extension of head, trunk and arms and legs with wrist pronation and wrist and finger flexion and ankle and toe flexion with internal rotation of the feet.

b. *Decorticate posture* Results from extensive damage to cortex.

The patient lies with upper limbs flexed and lower limbs extended.

c. *Opisthotanus* Body is bowed backward or hyperextended. It occurs in meningeal irritation (meningitis, SAH, encephalitis) dececrebrate rigidity, tetanus, strychnine poisoning, phenothiazine reaction and sometimes in hysteria.

d. *Detection of hemiplegia*

1. Flaccidity of cheek
2. Eyelid release test (gently pull eyelids up with your both thumbs and release them simultaneously. The eyelid on hemiplegic side glide down slowly (Fig. 35.1).
3. Observe Naso labial fold - less prominent on hemiplegic side
4. Limb dropping test - demonstrate flaccid weakness of limbs they depend on asymmetry of muscle tone. The tests are unreliable in deep coma and in LMN paralysis.
   - The wrist dropping test (Fig. 35.2)
   - The arm dropping test (Fig. 35.3)
   - The leg dropping test (Fig. 35.4).

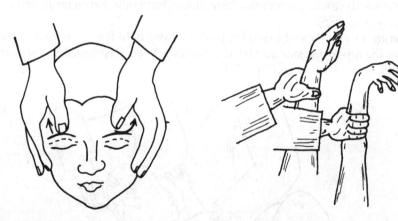

Fig. 35.1: Eyelid release test   **Fig. 35.2:** Wrist dropping test

Meningeal Signs

a. *Neck Rigidity* Resistance felt when attempt is made to flex the neck of the patient, with one of your hand under the patient's occipit. Other than meningeal irritation, neck rigidity is caused by phenothiazine reaction,

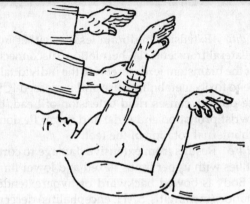

Fig. 35.3: The arm dropping test

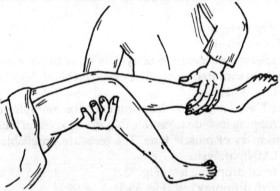

Fig. 35.4: The leg dropping test

tetanus, dystonia, postcranial fossa tumor, torticollis, kernicterus, cerebral palsy (Fig. 35.5).

b. *Kernig's signs* Patient in supine postion. Keep both legs straight and then flex the hip of one side and try to extend the knee. Resistance and wincing indicates positive sign (Fig. 35.6).

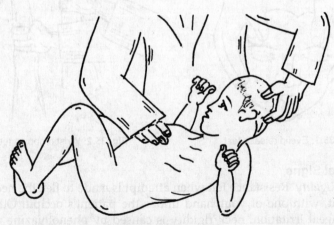

Fig. 35.5: Neck rigidity

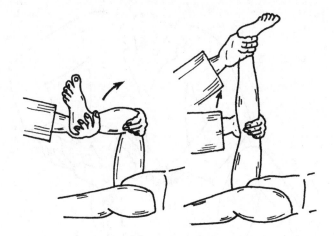

Fig. 35.6: Kernig's signs

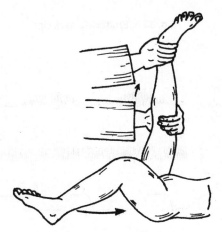

Fig. 35.7: Brudzinski leg sign

c. *Brudzinski leg sign* While eliciting Kernig's sign the opposite lower limb flexes and adducts (Fig. 35.7).

d. *Brudzinski's neck sign* When testing neck rigidity the lower limbs flex and adduct (Fig. 35.8).

e. *Head rolling test* In supine position to note neck rigidity.

f. *True and false neck rigidity* Bring the head to the edge of the table and try to flex the neck.

True neck rigidity persists, while voluntary rigidity disappears.

Meningeal signs may be absent in newborns, infants and in deep coma even in presence of meningeal irritation.

While doing movements of neck be careful in injured or suspected injured patient with cervical injury.

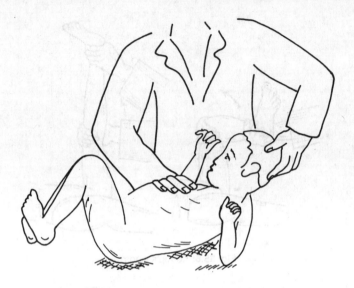

Fig. 35.8: Brudziski's neck sign

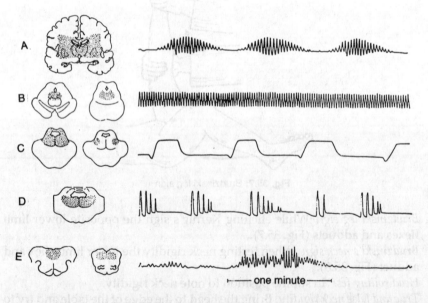

Fig. 35.9: Correlation of intra-axial brainstem lesions at successive levels, with the type of respiratory dysrhythmia caused. (A) Cheyne-Stokes respiration, (B) Central neurogenic hyperventilation, (C) Apneustic breathing, (D) Cluster breathing, (E) Ataxic breathing, *(Redrawn from F. Plum and J. Posner: The Diagnosis of Stupor and Coma. Philadelphia, F.A. Davis Company, 1966)*

Vital Signs

Pulse, BP respiration rate

Type of respiration Cheyne-Stokes, Biots breauthing, Kussmaul's breathing, apneustic breathing, ataxic breating, Cluster's breathing, central neurological hyperventilation (Fig. 35.9).

Signs of Raised ICP

Infants	*Older children*
Bulging anterior fontanelle	Papilloedema
Enlarging head	Macewan's sign positive
Sutural separation	Altered vital signs
Tachycerebrae	Palmar erythema
Altered vital signs	False localizing signs
	Extensor plantar response

      – Bounding pulse
      – Increased systolic pressure
      – Shallow, slow respiration

Palmar erythema
False localizing signs
      – Decerebrate posture
      – Cranial nerves III, VI, VII palsy.
      – Pyramidal and cerebellar signs

Signs of Systemic Disorders

a. Renal (Uremia)—edema, hypertension, skin rash (Scabies, pyoderma, SLE, HSP, drug rash), uremic breath, anemia, acidotic breathing.
b. Hepatic (Hepaticcoma)—jaundice, plamar erythema, ascites, edema of limbs, hepatosplenomegaly, spider naevi, flapping tremor, fetor hepaticus.
c. Childhood infections—skin rash (measles, chickenpox, coxsackie, EHCO, herpes) parotid enlargement (mumps), TB (Phlyctenular conjunctivitis, gland, erythema nodosum).
d. Metabolic—Diabetic breath, Kussmauls's breathing, Rye's syndrome (hepatomegaly)
e. Skin—neurocutaneous syndromes
f. Vascular—vasculitis syndrome
g. Hematological—bleeding, gland, HSM, pallor.
h. Iatrogenic probelms—*look for* exposure keratitis, oral hygiene, bed sores. Infection at the venipuncture site, distended bladder, loaded colon. Hypostatic pneumonia, dehydration, malnutrition, drug induced illness, position of Ryle's tube, bladder catheter and other connection of medical gadgets.

Cranial Nerve Examination in Unconscious Patients

Cranial Nerve II

Test for vision – Blink response to hand movements. Test separately in both eyes.
           – Positive blink not only indicates presence of vision but also intactness of cranial nerve VII.

- Perception of light and perception of rays also tests vision in unconscious patient.
- Opticokinetic nystagmus produced by rotation of a cylinder with black and white straps, in front of eyes indicates vision.
- Visual evoked potential is an advanced method of testing vision in unconscious patient.

Pupillary Response
Presence of pupillary response indicates that afferent path (II Cranial nerve) and efferent path (III Cranial Nerve) are intact.

Fundal Examination
Look for papilloedema, choroid tubercle, hemorrhage, vascular anomalies, phacomas, Roth's spots.

Cranial Nerve III, IV and VI
Note pupillary size and reaction

Following description gives types of pupils in unconsicous patient and their interpretation.

PUPILS IN UNCONSCIOUS PATIENT

Pupils Equal
Pinpoint pupils ⟶ Opiate poisoning or pontine lesion
Small ⟶ Reactive ⟶ Metabolic encephalopathy
Midsized ⟶ Fixed ⟶ Midbrain lesion
Reactive ⟶ Metabolic lesion

Pupils Unequal
Dilated ⟶ Unreactive ⟶ III Palsy
Small ⟶ Reactive ⟶ Horner's syndrome

Testing Motor Function of III, IV and VI Nerves
It is done by doll's eye maneuver. Where in head is turned side to side and then flexion and extension of head is done. Normally when head is turned to one side, both eyes move to the opposite side. When the head is flexed, both eye balls roll up together and when the head is extended, both eyeballs roll down.

Random slow conjugate movements of eyes to the side indicates intactness of III, IV and VI cranial nerves and the fronto pontine pathway for conjugate movement.

Focal seizures cause deviation of head and eyes to the side of irritative focus. Deviation of eyes to one side in absence of convulsion, indicates a destructive lesion in the ipsilateral frontal conjugate gaze center or contralateral half of the pons (Fig. 35.10).

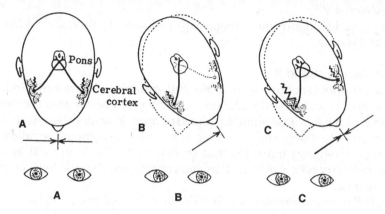

Fig. 35.10: The head and eye turning center (conjugate gaze center) in the posterior part of the frontal lobe. The arrows beneath the figures represent the strength of the vector originating on one side, acting to turn the head and eyes to the opposite side. Below each head is shown the position of the eyes. Notice the corticobulbar pathway to the pons and that it decussates. (A) Normal resting condition. The vectors are equal and the head and eyes are straight ahead. (B) A lesion has destroyed the conjugate gave center onthe left. The right center acts unopposed. The head and eyes deviate to the left. (C) An epileptogenic lesion has caused an excessive discharge of impulses from the right conjuctive gaze center. The vector from the right hemisphere overpowers the one from the left. The head and eyes deviate to the left

Doll's Eye Maneuver

1. Eyes move in the opposite direction to head movement as if trying to look straight—is normal
2. Eyes move to one side but not the other: lateral gaze palsy—brainstem lesion
3. Limitation of abduction of one eye—VI N palsy
4. Limitation of movement other than abduction in one eye with dilated pupil
   – III N Palsy
5. Eyes fail to move in any direction—Bilateral brainstem lesion.

Cranial Nerves V and VII

Test for cranial reflex with wisp of cotton. Positive test indicates intactness of both afferent (V) and efferent (VII) cranial nerves.

Supraorbital compression test for V and VII Nerve:

Press your thumb nail strongly into the patients eyebrows over the superciliary notch, the exit site of ophthalmic division of V cranial nerve. Note ipsilateral grimacing. In facial nerve palsy and in hemiplegia, grimace will be weaker.

Spontaneous or induced blinking or tonic closure of the eyelids indicate intactness of V and VII cranial nerves and hence that of pontine tegmentum.

Presence of rooting reflex indicates intactness of V cranial nerve.

Presence of sucking and swallowing reflex indicates intactness of V, VII, IX and X cranial nerves.

In VII nerve palsy palpebral fissure willl be wider and nasolabial fold less prominent on the paralyzed side.

Cranial Nerve VIII

Test by a sudden loud sound (e.g., clap) and note startle response (Audio-palpebral reflex).

Cranial Nerves IX and X

Watch for spontaneous swallowing and groaning. If present—indicate normality of IX and X nerves. Eliciting gag reflex may be dangerous or testing IX nerve, as it may cause vomiting and aspiration in an unconscious patiant.

Normal breathing and oro pharyngeal reflexes (cough, swallowing, hiccough, yawning) indicates that cranial nerve IX, X and XII and the pontomedullary reticular formation and cervical and thoracic level of spinal cord are intact.

Note the tongue for wasting, fibrillation, to test XII cranial nerve.

36 Examination of Disabled Child

- Physical disability
- Mental disability
- Learning disability
- Visual disability and
- Hearing disability

Disability refers to the inability to perform normal functions of daily living appropriate for that age. A disability could be physical, intellectual, visual or auditory. These could either be isolated or multiple. It is important to identify the specific disabilities as early as possible on their visit to the health centre or a clinic for any problem. The identification is necessary because they are likely to interfere with the child's normal growth, development and capacity to learn. Early identification minimizes these sequelae by the institution of early and appropriate therapy.

Examination of Disabled Person: Few Principles
1. Speak directly to the child but not to the attender.
2. Gentleness and patience.
3. Complete undressing may be difficult, do piece meal examination and comprehend.

Assessment of Disability
The objective of assessing a disabled child is to evaluate his abilities to perform daily activities appropriate for the child's age. This assessment is performed by obtaining a detailed history and clinical examination (Table 36.1).

Take History Pertaining to
- Abilities and disabilities
- Problems and their progress
- Impact of disability on child and family
- Secondary problem
- Resources of family
- Expectation of family from child
- Adjustment of child's family with disability.

Clinical Evaluation
- Examination to be conducted in a very friendly manner for good co-operation from the child

- Observe the posture of the limb
- Check the tone by feeling the muscles
- Check the range of movement at the joints
- Test the muscle power
- Check for the child's vision, hearing and speech
- Mental function.

Physical Disabilities

Physical disabilities may result from damage to the brain (as in cerebral palsy), from loss of function in the spinal cord (as in poliomyelitis), loss of function in the motor pathways in the brain/spinal cord (as in hemiplegia/paraplegia), injury to peripheral nerves, disease of the muscles (as in myopathies or muscular dystrophies) or of the joints (as in rheumatoid arthritis).

Some of the common causes of physical disabilities are:

Poliomyelitis

Paralytic poliomyelitis is the most common cause of physical disability in developing countries. Paralytic poliomyelitis may be divided in three stages:

Acute poliomyelitis	–	from onset up to 6 weeks.
Recovery stage	–	After 6 weeks to 2 years
Chronic stage	–	Residual paralysis beyond 2 years

The child should be evaluated for the extent of involvement of muscle groups and contractures. The deformities result from weight bearing on weak joints seen commonly at the knee, ankle, back and spine.

Cerebral Palsy

Definition and extent of problem Cerebral palsy is a disability that affects movements and body position due to damage to the motor parts of the brain. Once damaged, these parts of the brain neither recover nor worsen. It is often accompanied by other CNS impairments like mental retardation, speech, hearing and visual defects and seizure disorders.

It is one of the leading causes of chronic disability in children. The incidence is 2/1000 live births. In spite of improved obstetric and neonatal care, the incidence has not changed over the years.

Causes The factors which are likely to lead to cerebral palsy are prematurity, low birth weight birth, asphyxia, birth injuries, intracranial hemorrhages. If the mother has toxemia of pregnancy or any infection during the 1st trimester, the child may have cerebral palsy. It may also result from hypoglycemia, neonatal jaundice, infections (like meningitis and encephalitis), electrolyte imbalance, hyperpyrexia, intractable convulsions, head injury or drowning. In 30 percent cases no cause may be found.

Clinical profile About 50 percent of children are likely to have associated mental retardation. Visual deficits include squint, visual error, field defects, nystagmus. Speech and hearing may be impaired. About one-third of children have seizures. Behavior problems like attention deficit, hyperactivity and emotional lability may also be seen.

Table 36.1: Identification of disabilities

The child has this	And also this	He may have
I. • LIMP, weakness in part or whole body • No loss of feeling in affected parts • Normal intelligence	• Usually begins with fever, cold, diarrhea before 3 years • Irregular pattern of weakness most often one or both legs sometimes arms and back • The child limps, i.e., one leg is shorter • The lower limb is bent at hip, knee or ankle with contractures • The spine is curved • History of injection is present but no injury	Poliomyelitis
II. • LIMP, weakness of any body • No loss of feelings in affected parts • Slow development • Low-intelligence	• May be normal at birth • Usually present at 4-8 years • Progressive worsening • Other in the family may have it • Difficulty in walking, running, climbing stairs or walk on tip toe • Difficulty in sitting up from ground and typically climbs up supporting the hand on the legs and the thighs • Weakness first affects shoulders and hips (proximal) and then distal • Spine may be curved • Contractures at hip, foot, etc.	Muscular dystrophy
III. • Floppy at birth • Slow developmental milestones • Feeding problem like vomiting, choking • Abnormal stiffness of limbs • Abnormal position of body • Stiff/weak limbs	• Difficult delivery • Delayed breathing • Born premature • Scissoring/crossing of legs • Arching of back • Thumb clenched inside a fist • Jerky steps and uncontrolled movements • Poor balance • Abnormal movements of limbs • Does not respond to visual, auditory or other environmental stimuli	Cerebral palsy

Contd...

Contd...

	The child has this	And also this	He may have
IV.	• Weakness of limbs involving both lower limbs or all 4 limbs • Some loss of feeling • Loss of bladder or bowel control	• Injury to the back • Hump at the back • Sac at the back over spine • Normal back	• Spinal cord injury • Tuberculosis of spine • Spina bifida • Guillian-Barré syndrome
V.	• Large head at birth or increase in size later • Sac at the back	• Sun setting sign • Slow mental development • Weakness of limbs • Poor bladder and bowel control	Hydrocephalus Spina bifida
VI.	• Small head size • Slow development	• No or poor response to visual, auditory and environmental stimuli • Low-birth weight • Abnormal movements/convulsions	Microcephaly
VII.	• Slow to develop body functions or other basic skills	• Difficult delivery • Delayed cry after birth • Born premature • Abnormal facial features round face, slanting eyes, thick tongue • Does not fix eyes at an image or light • Behavior problems • Convulsions	Mental retardation Down's syndrome Cretinism
VIII.	• Slow to learn certain things	• May be otherwise of normal intelligence • Often overactive • May have behavior problem • May have seizures • May have visual or hearing problems	Learning disabilities

Contd...

Contd...

	The child has this	And also this	He may have
IX.	• Does not respond to sound	• Look for squint • Slow in using hands or moving around • Pupils may look grey • Eyes are red, swollen and watering • Eyes look dull, wrinkled • Difficulty in seeing at night • Child is slow school, difficulty in reading	• Cerebral palsy • Mental retardation • Cataract • Trachoma • Vitamin A deficiency
X.	• Does not respond to sound or voice • Does not begin to speak by 2 years of age	• Did not cry soonafter birth • Had fits after birth • Had neonatal jaundice • Had meningitis/encephalitis • Mother had infection during pregnancy • Abnormal facial features • Does not follow simple instructions • Does not respond in the classroom	Deafness

Limb Paralysis

At times a child may present with weakness of one-half of body, i.e. hemiplegia or of both lower limbs, i.e. paraplegia. The common causes for these disorders are vascular phenomena like thrombosis or hemorrhage, infective like meningitis or encephalitis or trauma (especially to the spinal cord) or tuberculosis of the spine.

Common Orthopedic Handicaps

There are several orthopedic deformities that may be seen either as a result of primary bony malformations or secondary to neurologic disorders. For example, club feet and spinal bifida.

Club feet Many children are born with their feet somewhat bent or crooked. This may run in families. It may be a result of intrauterine posture of the fetus or secondary to spinal cord problems like meningomyelocele or poliomyelitis.

Spina bifida In spinal bifida the vertebrae are not developed so as to close the spinal cord. There may be a sac containing cerebrospinal fluid with nerve fibers which is covered by the skin.

In spina bifida occulta there is no sac, and the skin covers the defect. However, overlying the defect may be found a thick tuft of hair or a hyper-pigmented area. There are generally no problems in early childhood. Later it may present with loss of urinary or bowel control, weakness of lower limbs or associated club feet.

Spina bifida cystica, also called as meningomyelocele or myelocele is detected soonafter birth. Those who survive into infancy may have paraplegia with usually an associated hydrocephalus.

Problems encountered in these children include:
1. Lack of urine control resulting in-frequent urinary infections
2. Pressure sores
3. Difficulty in sitting, standing or walking
4. Contractures

Mental Disabilities

Mental handicaps with or without physical disability results in severe dysadaptation of the human being in society. It results in a social stigma and ostracization of the child from family and society in which they live. It may be worth remembering that early detection of most mental handicaps and rehabilitation can result in a great deal of self sufficiency in most children.

Mental Retardation

Definition: Mental retardation is subaverage general intelligence resulting in diminished learning capacity and social adaptability manifesting during early childhood. These children learn things more slowly because the brain has suffered damage, the causes of which are enlisted below.
1. Chromosomal defects
2. Genetic defects
3. Chronic intrauterine infections in the mother

4. Cerebral malformations
5. Birth asphyxia, birth injury, intracranial hemorrhage
6. Prematurity and fetal growth retardations.
7. Metabolic problems in the first month of life
8. Infections of the CNS
9. Severe childhood malnutrition
10. Environmental deprivation.

Recognizing a child with mental retardation
1. Delayed achievement of developmental milestones is the cardinal symptom of mental retardation.
2. The child's behavior often consists of hyperactivity, short attention span, poor concentration, poor memory, awkward clumsy movements, disturbed sleep and emotional instability.
3. Their ability to care for themselves and interact with other is poor.

Mental retardation may be isolated or a part of multiple handicaps in the child.

Learning Disabilities

Definition Learning disability is a group of disorders manifesting as significant difficulties in the form of imperfect utility of listen, think, speak, write, spell or to do mathematical calculation. These are due to central nervous dysfunction. They may be associated with conditions like mental retardation, sensory impairments like visual and hearing, moto handicaps, emotional disturbances, environmental, cultural or economic disadvantages but are not the result of these conditions or influences.

Learning disabilities are diagnosed in about 10 percent of school going children and is twice as common in boys than in girls. The prevalence may be underestimated on account of failure of identification.

Identification of children with learning disability:
1. These children show evidence of early developmental delays.
2. Problems of reading are one of the earliest manifestations since they confuse letters of alphabets.
3. They have difficulty in discriminating between right and left.
4. They have difficulty in tying shoe laces or buttoning their clothes.
5. They cannot execute a function requiring organized sequence because they are unable to follow instructions and have poor memory. An example being a school aged child's inability to repeat the sequence of a story after it has been read out by the instructor.
6. They may have inability to draw figures and poor writing skills.
7. They are poor in mathematical skills.
8. They may have behavioral disturbances such as hyperactivity, poor attention span, easy distractibility, impulsive and aggressive behavior and throw temper tantrums.
9. These children may have delayed language development.
10. The physical examination may not reveal any abnormality.

Sensory Handicaps

Sensory handicaps include visual, speech and hearing defects. They may be isolated or associated with mental or physical handicaps.

Visual Disabilities

The severity of visual handicaps vary from complete blindness to not being able to see clearly. Some children are born blind while others become blind during early or late childhood. Visual problems are more common in children with other physical handicaps especially those with a neurological basis like cerebral palsy.

How to recognise with visual handicap:

1. The infant may have a white or a grey pupil.
2. If by 3 months the child does not focus on mother's face or object or light and does not follow them, suspect a visual handicap.
3. The child does not reach for an object held in front of them unless it makes a sound.
4. Child is slow to begin using hands, move about and may bump into objects while moving around.
5. The child has a squint.
6. The child has difficulty in seeing after sunset (night blindness).
7. In school the child cannot read clearly from the blackboard or complains of headache while reading.

Causes of Visual Problem

1. Vitamin A deficiency
2. Trachoma
3. Cerebral palsy
4. Children with hydrocephalus, brain tumors, meningitis and encephalitis may develop visual loss and paralysis of nerves supplying the muscles of eyes.
5. Cataracts (example being congenital rubella syndrome).
6. Eye injuries caused by playing with sharp objects or fireworks.

Speech and Hearing Handicaps

A child's inability to speak properly or a speech that is not easily understood or draws attention, is a speech defect. The most common cause is hearing impairment.

Causes of Speech and Hearing Defects

1. Speech
   a. Deafness
   b. Mental retardation
   c. Cleft palate
   d. Voice disorders
2. Hearing
   a. Hereditary deafness is the most common, seen in 50 percent of deaf children.

   b. Birth asphyxia and hyperbilirubinemia.

   c. Maternal intrauterine infections like German measles or cytomegalovirus.

   d. Medications to the mother like streptomycin, gentamycin, frusemide, etc.

   e. Infections in childhood like meningitis, encephalitis and chronic ear infections.

How to Recognize a Child with Hearing Disorder

If a child's hearing problem is not recognised early, it can result in serious learning and communication problems.

1. 0 to 6 months	: When an infant does not startle in response to a loud clap within 3 feet or does not turn towards the source of sound suspect a hearing defect.
2. 6 months to 2 years	: Does not respond to name, voice or a sound, does not understand phrases like 'no-no' or 'bye-bye'; does not initiate simple sounds and words; does not follow simple directions; child uses gestures for needs and desires rather than speaking.
3. 2 to 5 years	: Cannot understand and use simple words like go, come etc., cannot carry on a simple conversation and speech is difficult to understand.
4. School going child	: Has trouble paying attention, does not answer when called, gets confused about directions or questions, appears slow and does not do well in school, has poor speech, substitutes or omits sound.

CHAPTER 37 Evaluation of a Child or Adolescent with Sports Injury

Sports are becoming more and more popular in these days. Many children, adolescents are involved in competitive sports with their attendant risks. Some sports are associated with specific injuries, e.g.
- Gymnastics–spondylosis, bursitis (Impingement syndrome)
- Baseball–medial epicondylitis (Little league elbow)
- Ballet–snapping hip syndrome
- Wrestling–brachial plexus neuropraxias (Stingers or burners)
- Foot ball–concussion, contusion, ligament tears
- Running–stress fractures, patello-femoral pain syndrome, various tendinitis, including iliotibial band syndrome.
- Skiing–ulnar collateral ligament springs and tibia fractures, knee ligament sprains.

Evaluation for Sports
1. Hypertrophic cardiomyopathy is associated with risk of sudden death in heavy exercisers and competitive sports.
2. Hypertensive patients should avoid weight lifting and isometric exercises.
3. Patients with bronchial asthma may have exercise induced asthma, however it can be prevented with prior medications.
4. Improperly rehabilitated fractures put the patients at risk during sports.

Types of Disorders and Risks in Sports
1. Atlantoaxial instability (children with Down's syndrome)–neck injury can cause spinal cord damage.
2. Bleeding disorders, e.g. hemophilia–avoid contact games.
3. Carditis–sudden death
4. Hypertrophic cardiomyopathy–sudden death.
5. Hypertension–avoid weight lifting, body building and strength training.
6. Pulmonary stenosis and Aortic stenosis (severe)–can cause sudden death.
7. Congenital heart block–may be dangerous.
8. Heart murmurs–evolves.
9. Enlarged liver–avoid contact games it may lead to rupture.
10. Absent kidney (one)–evaluate for injury
11. Convulsions • Well controlled no risk
    • Poorly controlled-risk in swimming, weight lifting
12. Asthma–exercise induced asthma.
13. Enlarged spleen—rupture.

    Tables 37.1 and 37.3 illustrate medical conditions and sports participation and classification of sports by contact, respectively. Table 37.2 classifies sports by degree of strenuousness.

Table 37.1: Medical conditions and sports participation*

Conditions	May participate
Atlantoaxial instability (instability of the joint between cervical vertebrae 1 and 2)	Qualified yes
Explanation: Athlete needs evaluation to assess risk of spinal cord injury during sports participation.	
Bleeding disorder	Qualified yes
Explanation: Athlete needs evaluation.	
Cardiovascular disease	
Carditis (inflammation of the heart)	No
Explanation: Carditis may result in sudden death with exertion.	
Hypertension (high blood pressure)	Qualified yes
Explanation: Those with significant essential (unexplained) hypertension should avoid weight and power lifting, body building, and strength training. Those with secondary hypertension (hypertension caused by a previously identified disease) or severe essential hypertension need evaluation. The National High Blood Pressure Education Working group defined significant and severe hypertension.	
Congenital heart disease (structural heart defects present at birth)	Qualified yes
Explanation: Those with mild forms may participate fully; those with moderate or severe forms or who have undergone surgery need evaluation. The twenty-six Bethesda Conference defined mild, moderate, and severe disease for common cardiac lesions.	
Dysrhythmia (irregular heart rhythm)	Qualified yes
Explanation: Those with symptoms (chest pain, synocope, dizziness, shortness of breath, or other symptoms of possible dysrhythmia) or evidence of mitral regurgitation (leaking) on physical examination need evaluation. All others may participate fully.	
Heart murmur	Qualified yes
Explanation: If the murmur is innocent (does not indicate heart disease), full participation is permitted. Otherwise the athlete needs evaluation (see congenital heart disease and mitral valve prolapse).	
Cerebral palsy	Qualified yes
Explanation: Athlete need evaluation.	

Contd...

Contd...

Conditions	May participate
Diabetes mellitus	Yes
Explanation: All sports can be played with proper attention to diet, blood glucose concentration, hydration, and insulin therapy. Blood glucose concentration, hydration, and insulin therapy. Blood glucose concentration should be monitored every 30 minutes during continuous exercise and 15 minutes after completion of exercise.	
Diarrhea	Qualified no
Explanation: Unless disease is mild, no participation is permitted, because diarrhea may incarease the risk of dehydration and heat illness (See fever.)	
Eating disorders	Qualified yes
Anorexia nervosa	
Bulimia nervosa	
Explanation: Patients with these disorders need medical and psychiatric assessment before participation.	
Eyes	Qualified yes
Functionally one-eyed athlete	
Loss of an eye	
Detached retina	
Previous eye surgery or serious eye injury	
Explanation: A functionally one-eyed athlete has a best-corrected visual acuity of less than 20/40 in the eye with worse acuity. These athletes would suffer significant disability if the better eye were seriously injured, as would those with loss of an eye. Some athletes who previously have undergone eye surgery or had a serious eye injury may have an increased risk of injury because of weakened eye tissue. Availability of eye guards approved by the American society for testing and materials and other protective equipment may allow participation in most sports, but this must be judged on an individual basis.	
Fever	No
Explanation: Fever can increase cardiopulmonary effort, reduce maximum exercise capacity, make heat illness more likely, and increase orthostatic hypertension during exercise. Fever may rarely accompany myocarditis or other infections that may make exercise dangerous.	

Contd...

Contd....

Conditions	May participate
Heat illness, history of	Qualified yes
Explanation: Because of the increased likelihood of recurrence, the athlete needs individual assessment to determine the presence of predisposing conditions and to arrange a prevention stategy.	
Hepatitis	Yes
Explanation: Because of the apparent minimal risk to others, all sports may be played that the athlete's state of health allows. In all athletes, skin lesions should be covered properly, and athletic personnel should use universal precautions when handling blood or body fluids with visible blood.	
Human immunodeficiency virus infection	Yes
Explanation: Because of the apparent minimal risk to others, all sports may be played that the athlete's state of health allows. In all athletes, skin lesions should be covered properly, and athletic personnel should use universal precautions when handling blood or body fluids with visible blood.	
Kidney, absence of one	Qualified yes
Explanation: Athlete needs individual assessment for contact, collision, and limited-contact sports.	
Liver, enlarged	Qualified yes
Explanation: If the liver is acutely enlarged, participation should be acoided because of risk of rupture. If the liver is chronically enlarged, individual assessment is needed before collision, contact, or limited-contact sports are played.	
Malignant neoplasm	Qualified yes
Explanation: Athlete needs individual assessment.	
Musculoskeletal disorders	Qualified yes
Explanation: Athlete needs individual assessment.	
Neurologic disorders	
History of serious head or spine trauma, severe or repeated concussions, or crainotomy	Qualified yes
Explanation: Athlete needs individual assessment for collision, contact, or limited-contact sports and also for noncontact sports if deficits in judgment or cognition are present. Research supports a conservative approach to management of concussion.	

Contd....

Contd...

Conditions	May participate
Seizure disorder, well-controlled	Yes
Explanation: Risk of seizure during participation is minimal.	
Seizure disorder, poorly controlled	Qualified yes
Explanation: Athlete needs individual assessment for collision, contact, or limited-contact sports. The following non-contact sports should be avoided: archery, riflery, swimming, weight or power lifting, strength training, or sports involving heights. In these sports, occurrence of a seizure may pose a risk to self or others.	
Obesity	Qualified yes
Explanation: Because of the risk of heat illness, obese persons need careful acclimatization and hydration.	
Organ transplant recipient	Qualified yes
Explanation: Athlete needs individual assessment.	
Ovary, absence of one	Yes
Explanation: Risk of severe injury to the remaining ovary is minimal.	
Respiratory conditions	
Pulmonary compromise, including cystic fibrosis	Qualified yes
Explanation: Athlete needs individual assessment, but generally, all sports may be played if oxygenation remains satisfactory during a graded exercise test. Patients with cystic fibrosis need acclimatization and good hydration to reduce the risk of heat illness.	
Asthma	Yes
Explanation: With proper medication and education, only athletes with the most severe asthma will need to modify their participation.	
Acute upper respiratory infection	Qualified yes
Explanation: Upper respiratory obstruction may affect pulmonary function. Athlete needs individual assessment for all but mild disease (See fever).	
Sickle cell disease	Qualified yes
Explanation: Athlete needs individual assessment. In general, if status of the illness permits, all but high exertion, collision, and contact sports may be played. Overheating, dehydration, and chilling must be avoided.	

Contd...

Contd...

Conditions	May participate
Sickle cell trait	Yes
Explanation: It is unlikely that persons with sickle cell trait have an increased risk of sudden death or other medical problems during athletic participation, except under the most extreme conditions of heat, humidity, and possibly increased altitude;[11] These persons, like all athletes, should be carefully conditioned, acclimatized, and hydrated to reduce any possible risk.	
Skin disorders (boils, herpes simplex, impetigo, scabies, molluscum contagiosum)	Qualified yes
Explanation: While the patient is contagious, participation in gymnastics with mats; martial arts; wrestling; or other collision, contact, or limited-contact sports is not allowed.	
Spleen, enlarged	Qualified yes
Explanation: A patient with an acutely enlarged spleen should avoid all sports because of risk of rupture. A patient with a chronically enlarged spleen needs individual assessment before playing collision, contact, or limited-contact sports.	
Testicle, undescended or absence of one	Yes
Explanation: Certain sports may require a protective cup.	

* This table is designed for use by medical and nonmedical personnel. "Needs evaluation" means that a physician with appropriate knowledge and experience should assess the safety of a given sport for an athlete with the listed medical condition. Unless otherwise noted, this is because of variability of the severity of the disease, the risk of injury for the specific sports listed in table.

Table 37.2: Classification of sports by strenuousness

High to moderate dynamic amd static demands	High to moderate dynamic and low-static demands	High to moderate static and low-dynamic demands
Boxing	Badminton	Archery
Crew or rowing	Baseball	Auto racing
Cross-country skiing	Basketball	Diving
Cycling	Field hockey	Horseback riding (jumping)
Downhill skiing	Lacrosse	Field events (throwing)
Fencing	Orienteering	Gymnastics
Football	Race walking	Karate or judo
Ice hockey	Racquetball	Motorcycling
Rugby	Soccer	Rodeo
Running (sprint)	Squash	Sailing
Speed skating	Swimming	Ski jumping
Water polo	Table tennis	Water skiing
Wrestling	Tennis	Weight lifting
	Vollyball	

Low-Intensity (Low-Dynamic and Low-Static Demands)

Bowling
Cricket
Curling
Golf
Riflery

* Participation not recommended by the American Academy of Pediatrics

Table 37.3: Classification of sports by contact

Contact/collision	Limited contact	Noncontact
Basketball	Baseball	Archery
Boxing*	Bicycling	Badminton
Diving	Cheerleading	Body building
Field hockey	Canoeing/kayaking (white water)	Bowling
Football	Fencing	Canoeing/kayaking (flat water)
Flag	Field	Crew/rowing
Tackle	High jump	Curling
Ice hockey	Pole vault	Dancing
Lacrosse	Floor hockey	Field
Martial arts	Gymnastics	Discus
Rodeo	Handball	Javelin
Rugby	Horseback riding	Shot put
Ski jumping	Racquetball	Golf
Soccer	Skating	Orienteering
Team handball	Ice	Power lifting
Water polo	Inline	Race walking
Wrestling	Roller	Riflery

Contd...

Contd...

Contact/collision	Limited contact	Noncontact
	Skiing	Rope jumping
	Cross-country	Running
	Downhill	Sailing
	Water	SCUBA diving
	Softabll	Strength training
	Squash	Swimming
	Ultimate Frisbee	Table tennis
	Volleyball	Tennis
	Windsurfing/surfing	Track
		Weight lifting

38 OPD Evaluation

Out Patient Department (OPD) Evaluation

Out patient examination should be quick but comprehensive because of constraint of time. Following is an example of scheme of examination of children in out patient clinic.

Scheme of Examination of Children

General Observations
- Observe child's spontaneous activities
- See skills like throwing ball and drawing
- Evaluate gait, jumping, hopping, range of movements, muscle strength, climbing, stooping and recovering.

Upper Extremities
Observe arm movements, size, shape, use of hands and creases.

Lower Extremities
- Observe for movements, size, shape, alignment, length, feet, toes and arch of feet.
- Palpate anterior fontanelle and sutures.
- Observe neck for webbing, voluntary movements.
- Measure head circumference.
- Palpate neck for trachea, thyroid, muscletone and lymph nodes.

Chest, Heart, Lungs
Inspect chest movements, size, shape, precordial movement, deformity, nipples and breast development.
- Palpate anterior chest, apex, vocal fremitus (during talking and crying)
- Auscultate anterior, lateral and posterior chest for breath sounds and count respiration.
- Auscultate all cardiac areas for S1, S2, splits and murmur and locate apical impulse.

Abdomen
- Inspect abdomen
- Auscultate bowel sounds
- Palate liver, spleen and other masses

- Percuss
- Palpate femorals and compare with radial
- Palpate lymph nodes
- Inspect external genitalia
- Palpate scrotum for testis and other masses
- Inspect spine and then inspect spine on bending
- Inspect posture from all sides and see gait.

Last Examination

Eyes : Light reflex, eye movements, fundus

Ear, mouth, throat and otoscopic examination and nasal mucosal examination.

39 Examination during a Survey in a Community

The following are the few signs to be of value in community nutrition surveys and their interpretations (Table 39.1).

Table 39.1: Signs known to be of value in nutrition surveys and their interpretation

	Signs	*Associated disorder or nutrient*
1. Hair	Lack of lustre	
	Thinness and sparseness	
	Straightness	
	Dyspigmentation	Kwashiokor, less commonly marasmus
	Flag sign	
	Easy pluckability	
2. Face	Nasolabial dyssebacca	Riboflavin
	Moon face	Kwashiorkor
3. Eyes	Pale conjunctiva	Anemia (e.g. iron)
	Bitot's spots	
	Conjunctival xerosis	Vitamin A
	Corneal xerosis	
	Keratomalacia	
	Angular palpebritis	Riboflavin, pyridoxine
4. Lips	Angular stomatitis	
	Angular scars	Riboflavin
	Cheilosis	
5. Tongue	Scarlet and raw tongue	Nicotinic acid
	Magenta tongue	Riboflavin
6. Teeth	Mottled enamel	Fluorosis
7. Gums	Spongy bleeding gums	Ascorbic acid
8. Glands	Thyroid enlargement	Iodine
	Parotid enlargement	Starvation
9. Skin	Xerosis	
	Perifollicular hyperkeratosis	Vitamin A
	Petechiae	Ascorbic acid
	Pellagrous dermatosis	Nicotinic acid
	Flaky paint dermatosis	Kwashiorkor
	Scrotal and vulval dermatosis	Riboflavin
10. Nails	Koilonychia	Iron
11. Subcutaneous tissue	Edema	Kwashiorkor
	Fat decreased	Starvation, marasmus
	Fat increased	Obesity

Contd...

Contd...

	Signs	Associated disorder or nutrient
12. Muscular and skeletal systems	Muscle wasting	Starvation, marasmus, kwashiorkor
	Craniotabes	
	Frontal and pariental bossing ⎫	
	Epiphyseal enlargement ⎪	
	Persistently open anterior fontanelle ⎬ Vitamin D	
	Knock knees or bow legs ⎪	
	Thoracic rosary ⎭	Vitamin D, ascorbic acid
	Musculoskeletal hemorrhages	Ascorbic acid
13. Internal system		
a. Gastrointestinal	Hepatomegaly	Kwashiorkor
b. Nervous	Psychomotor changes	Kwashiorkor
	Mental confusion	Thiamin, nicotinic acid
	Sensory loss ⎫	
	Motor weakness ⎪	
	Loss of position sense ⎪	
	Loss of vibration ⎬ Thiamin	
	Loss of ankle and knee jerks ⎪	
	Calf tenderness ⎭	
c. Cardiac	Cardiac enlargement	
	Trachycardia	

CHAPTER

40 Screening or Periodic Examination

This is done on apparently healthy asymptomatic children.

Purpose
1. To Detect anomalies in newborns and early infancy.
2. To form a base line.
3. To assess physical growth, growth velocity, mental development and to mark on the road to health card for record and evaluation.
4. To detect early malnutrition, anemia, undescended testis, hearing and vision problems, early signs of cerebral palsy and dental development.
5. To establish good rapport, supervise feeding, immunization and development.
6. To assess periodically habits, diet, exercise which influence health of children.

Periodicity
In infancy every month and later every year.

What to Examine
Record weight, height, mid arm circumference, head circumference and chest circumference.

Assessment of hearing, vision.

Development of speech, adaptive, social and motor mile stones and teeth development. Frequent recording of blood pressure and sexual maturity assessment in adolescents.

The American Academy of Pediatrics recommend the following outline for examining children at different ages for preventive pediatric health care in the Tables 40.1 and 40.2.

Table 40.1: Preventive evaluation at specific ages*

Activity	1st week	1 mon	2 mon	4 mon	6 mon	9 mon	12 mon	15 mon	18 mon	2 yr	3 yr	4 yr	5 yr	6 yr	8 yr	10 yr	11-14 yr	15-17 yr	18-21 yr
Interview (for special attention)	✓	✓	✓	✓	✓	✓	✓	✓	✓	✓	✓	✓	✓	✓	✓	✓	✓	✓	✓
Family history	✓	✓	✓	✓	✓	✓	✓	✓	✓	✓	✓	✓	✓	✓	✓	✓	✓	✓	✓
Pregnancy and delivery	✓		✓																
Neonatal course	✓	✓	✓	✓															
Developmental evaluation/milestones	✓	✓	✓	✓	✓	✓	✓	✓	✓	✓	✓	✓	✓	✓	✓	✓	✓	✓	✓
Body systems (for special attention)																			
Hearing/vision	✓	✓	✓	✓	✓	✓	✓	✓	✓	✓	✓	✓	✓	✓	✓	✓	✓	✓	
CNS (including sleep)	✓	✓	✓	✓	✓	✓	✓	✓	✓	✓	✓	✓	✓	✓	✓	✓	✓	✓	
Gastrointestinal/feeding	✓	✓	✓	✓	✓	✓	✓	✓	✓	✓	✓				✓	✓	✓	✓	
Urinary	✓					✓	✓	✓	✓	✓	✓	✓	✓						
Dental care							✓	✓	✓	✓	✓	✓	✓	✓	✓	✓	✓	✓	
Drugs, alcohol, tobacco																	✓	✓	✓
Pica						✓	✓	✓	✓	✓	✓	✓							
Sexual behavior																			
Observations of parent-child interaction	✓	✓	✓	✓	✓	✓	✓	✓	✓	✓	✓	✓	✓	✓	✓	✓	✓	✓	✓
Physical examination (complete) (for special attention)	✓	✓	✓	✓	✓	✓	✓	✓	✓	✓	✓	✓	✓	✓	✓	✓	✓	✓	✓
Height and weight	✓	✓	✓	✓	✓	✓	✓	✓	✓	✓	✓	✓	✓	✓	✓	✓	✓	✓	✓
Head circumference	✓	✓	✓	✓	✓	✓	✓	✓	✓										
Blood pressure											✓	✓	✓	✓	✓	✓	✓	✓	
Skin	✓	✓	✓	✓	✓	✓	✓	✓	✓	✓	✓	✓	✓	✓	✓	✓	✓	✓	✓
Vision																			
Tear ducts	✓	✓	✓	✓															
Fixed eyes	✓	✓																	

Contd...

Contd...

Activity	1st week	1 mon	2 mon	4 mon	6 mon	9 mon	12 mon	15 mon	18 mon	2 yr	3 yr	4 yr	5 yr	6 yr	8 yr	10 yr	11-14 yr	15-17 yr	18-21 yr
Red reflex	✓	✓	✓	✓	✓	✓	✓												
Fundi	✓	✓	✓	✓	✓	✓	✓			✓		✓	✓	✓	✓	✓	✓	✓	✓
Stabismus/eye movements	✓																		
Hearing	✓	✓	✓	✓	✓	✓	✓	✓	✓	✓	✓	✓	✓	✓	✓	✓	✓	✓	✓
Speech	✓	✓	✓	✓	✓	✓	✓	✓	✓	✓		✓	✓	✓					
Neurologic problems	✓	✓	✓	✓	✓	✓	✓	✓	✓	✓	✓	✓	✓		✓	✓	✓	✓	✓
Cardiac murmurs	✓	✓	✓	✓	✓	✓	✓	✓	✓	✓	✓	✓	✓	✓	✓	✓	✓	✓	✓
Abdominal masses	✓	✓	✓	✓	✓	✓	✓	✓	✓	✓	✓	✓	✓	✓	✓	✓	✓	✓	✓
External genitalia	✓	✓	✓	✓	✓	✓	✓	✓	✓	✓	✓	✓	✓						
Hip dysplasia/dislocation	✓	✓	✓	✓	✓	✓		✓	✓										
Gait	✓																		
Deformities (metatarsus adductus)	✓	✓	✓	✓	✓	✓	✓	✓	✓	✓	✓	✓	✓	✓	✓	✓	✓	✓	✓
Sexual development																✓	✓	✓	✓
Scoliosis																✓	✓	✓	✓
Evidence of neglect/abuse						✓												✓	
Laboratory testing and screening																			
Hgb/Hct					✓or	✓or	✓								✓		✓		
Urinalysis					✓or	✓or	✓						✓		✓				
Urine culture (girls)					✓or	✓or	✓								✓	✓	✓		
Tuberculin						✓or				✓	or	✓or	✓or			✓	✓or	or	✓
Lipids										✓		✓	✓	✓	✓	✓	✓	✓	✓
Metabolic	✓	✓																	

Contd...

Contd...

Activity	1st week	1 mon	2 mon	4 mon	6 mon	9 mon	12 mon	15 mon	18 mon	2 yr	3 yr	4 yr	5 yr	6 yr	8 yr	10 yr	11-14 yr	15-17 yr	18-21 yr
Lead						✓													
Hearing screening	✓(Prior to 3 mo)											✓	✓	✓	✓	✓	✓	✓	✓
Vision screening											✓	✓	✓	✓	✓	✓	✓	✓	✓
STD																	✓	✓	✓
Immunizations	✓	✓	✓	✓	✓		✓	✓	✓			✓or	✓				✓	✓	✓
Anticipatory guidance and counseling (for special attention)	✓	✓	✓	✓	✓	✓	✓	✓	✓	✓	✓	✓	✓	✓	✓	✓	✓	✓	✓
Parent and child interaction	✓	✓	✓	✓	✓	✓	✓	✓	✓	✓	✓	✓	✓						
Diet/nutrition	✓	✓	✓	✓	✓	✓	✓	✓	✓	✓	✓	✓	✓	✓	✓	✓	✓	✓	✓
Sleep	✓	✓	✓	✓	✓	✓	✓	✓	✓	✓	✓								
Toilet training									✓	✓	✓								
Injury prevention	✓	✓	✓	✓	✓	✓	✓	✓	✓	✓	✓	✓	✓	✓	✓	✓	✓	✓	✓
Infant/child care (includes oral health)	✓	✓	✓	✓	✓	✓	✓	✓	✓	✓	✓	✓	✓	✓	✓	✓	✓	✓	✓
School problems											✓	✓	✓	✓	✓	✓	✓	✓	✓
Puberty and sexuality																✓	✓	✓	✓
Substance abuse																	✓	✓	✓
Family and social relationships	✓	✓	✓	✓	✓	✓	✓	✓	✓	✓	✓	✓	✓	✓	✓	✓	✓	✓	✓

* These suggestions or guidelines represent an analysis of recommendations by the American Academy of Pediatrics and Bright Futures. They are not intended to be all inclusive but rather to serve as reminders for some of the important preventive and health promotion activities that should be considered at various ages when physician–patient encounters may occur. The content and timing of visits will need to be altered according to special needs and the presence or absence of risk factors for the child and his or her family.

Table 40.2: Suggested schedule of health supervision visits

Infancy 0-1 year	Early childhood 1-4 year	Middle childhood 5-10 year	Adolescence 11-21 year
Prenatal	15 month	5 year	11 year
Neonatal	18 month	6 year	12 year
First week	2 year	8 year	13 year
1 month	3 year	10 year	14 year
2 month	4 year		15 year
4 month			16 year
6 month			17 year
9 month			18 year
12 month			19 year
			20 year
			21 year

41 Follow-up Examination

The initial examination is always a detailed one. But follow-up examination should be precise and relevent to the organ or system involved because of time constraint. The aim is to know the progress of the disease and its complications. Many residents and junior doctors may not know what to examine during daily follow-up of patients. These records help assessment of the illness and are important for medicolegal purposes as well, if need arises. Some of the examples are illustrated in Table 41.1.

Table 41.1: Assessment of illness with respect to signs and symptoms

Conditions	Signs	Symptoms

PEM	Weight
	Smile
	Edema
	Signs of systemic illness
	  (infection and associated
	  deficiencies)
		Appetite
		Activity
		Symptoms of systemic illness
		Food intake

Acute nephritis	Weight
	Blood pressure
	Edema
	Cardiac sounds, murmurs,
	  size, gallop
	Liver size
	Pulmonary congestion
	Fundus
	CNS
		Fluid intake
		Urine output
		Symptoms of complications
		— CNS
		Headache
		Vomiting
		Blurred vision
		— CVS
		Breathlessness— cough
		Renal failure–
		  Decreased urine
		Nausea/vomiting/
		  Drowsiness

Nephrotic syndrome	Weight BP Edema Abdominal and pleural fluid Signs of infection Chest–TB/Non TB Peritonitis Skin lesions Urinary protein.	Urine output Fluid intake Symptoms of systemic illness (infection) Appetite Abdominal pain Steroid toxicity.

Contd...

Contd...

Conditions	Signs	Symptoms

CCF	Cyanosis, decubitus,
	 Respiratory rate
	 Pulse
	 BP
	 Signs of shock, edema,
	     weight
	 Liver size
	 Cardiac signs
	 Pulmonary congestion
		Urine
		 Dyspnea
		 Sleep, feeding.
		 Nausea, vomiting,
		 Diarrhea (digoxin)
		 Abdominal pain in liver enlarge-
		     ment

Acute bronchiolitis and bronchopnemonia	Respiratory rate Signs of distress Cyanosis, toxemia and its complications Pulse rate Hydration Liver and spleen size Pulmonary signs Airleak/empyema Percussion of chest Cardiac auscultation	Feeding Fever Cough Sleep Urine output Playfulness

Asthma	RR, posture, alertness
	 Pulsus paradoxus
	 Cyanosis
	 Respiratory distress
	 Lung signs–
	     Rhonchi
	     Absent sounds (dangerous)
	 Liver size
	 Air leak features
	 Hydration
		Dyspnea
		 Cough
		 Wheeze
		 Sleep
		 Fluid intake
		 Urine output

Unconscious patient
   (TBM, encephalitis,
   meningitis, diabetic
   coma, hepatic coma,
   tetanus, uremia)
	Coma scale
	 Posture
	 Eyes
	 Oral cavity
	 Skin, bowel
	 Bladder, bedsores
	 Hydration,
	 Position of
	     Ryle's tube and aspiration
	     TPR, signs of increase ICP
	     Drug toxicity
	     Jaundice
	     Injection site,
	     IV lines
	     Neurological deficits
		Fluid intake
		 Urine output
		 Fits
		 Vomiting
		 Fever
		 Cross infection (diarrhea)
		 Feeding schedule

Contd...

Contd...

Conditions	Signs	Symptoms

Poliomyelitis	Muscle chart (attach a chart)
	Muscle tenderness
	Fever
	Bladder, bowel
	Deep tendon reflexes
	Bedsores
	Aspiration pnemonia
	Signs of incease ICP
	Progress of muscle involve-
	ment
		Muscle pain
		Feeding
		Fits
		Urine output
		Fluid intake
		Symptoms of increase ICP
		Stool samples for viral culture
		Reporting to authorities for
		    surveillance. (District immu-
		    nisation officer)
		Filling the AFP
		surveillance chart

Scorpion bite	Pulse
	BP
	Respiratory rate
	Temperature
	Peripheral signs
	Level of consciousness
	Focal neurological deficits
	Cardiac signs
	    First heart sound
	    Gallop rythm
	    Murmurs
	Evidence of acute pancreatitis
		Drowsiness
		Nausea
		Vomiting
		Urine
		Coldness
		Fits
		Altered sensorium
		Stroke
		Acute abdominal pain refering
		    to back (acute pancreatitis)

Snake bite	Gum bleeding and other bleeding sites Ptosis Respiratory pattern Blood pressure Urine Local signs	Urine output Sensorium Bleeding Pain
Hepatic coma	Jaundice Coma scale Signs of hepatocellular failure Aspiration pnemonia Vital signs Hydration Renal failure Care of unconscious patient	Fits Bleeding Urine output and color
Chronic renal failure	Anemia Weight Blood pressure Cardiomegaly Sensorium Pericardial rub. Peripheral neuropathy	Urine output Nausea Vomiting Fits Bleeding tendencies

Contd...

Contd...

Conditions	Signs	Symptoms
Acute gastroenteritis	Dehydration signs	**Diarrhea**
		Bloody stools
	Abdominal distention	– Amebiasis
	– Lactose intolerance	– Giardiasis
	– Hypokalemia	– Shigella
	– Drugs	– Viral
	– Sepsis	– Bacteria
	– Uraemia	Bloody stools
	– Surgical complication	Vomiting
		Urine output
	Fever	
	– Infection	**Fits**
	– Hypernatremia	– Drugs
	– Incidental	– Dehydration
		– Increased or decreased
	Associated infections	sodium
	– Lungs	– Rota virus
	– Measles	– Associated CNS involvement
	– Otitis media	– decreased calcium levels
	Perianal excoriation	– decreased glucose levels
	Associated deficiencies	– Febrile fit
	– Sepsis	– Shigella encephalopathy
	– PEM	– Uremia
	– Vit. A deficiency	– Cortical vein thrombosis
	Weight	– Subdural effusion assessment
	Nutrition	– Superior sagittal sinus thrombosis
		Feeding
		Drugs
Gram-negative shock (newborn)	Vital signs	
	Pupils, organs,	
	Weight, jaundice,	
	urine, stool, skin	
	Injection site,	
	Feeding, fits	
	Sleep	
Tetanus	Hydration	Spasm
	Muscle spasms (abdominal, jaw)	Fever
		Bowel
	Lungs	Bladder
	Unconsciousness	
	Temperature, pulse	
	Bladder, bowel	
Diabetic ketoacidosis	Weight	Fluid chart
	Hydration	Urine output
	Abdominal distention	Abdominal pain
	Vital signs	Appetite
	Sensorium, urine and blood sugar.	Stomach aspirate

Contd...

Contd...

Conditions	Signs	Symptoms
Kerosene poisoning	Lung signs,	Cough
	Pleural effusion	Vomiting
	Respiratory rate,	Feeding
	Respiratory distress,	
	Cyanosis	
OP poisoning	Pulse/Pupils	Vomiting
	Respiratory rate	Diarrhea
	Blood pressure	Urine
	Respiratory distress	Fits
	Lung signs	Twitching
	Signs of atropinisation	
Head injury	Pupil	Fits
	Sensorium (coma scale)	Vomiting
	Localized signs	Bleeding from ear, nose, throat
	TPR	Urine
	BP	
	Unconsciousness.	

CHAPTER

42 Healthy Baby Contest

Healthy child contests are the most attractive activities organized by many Govt and non-Govt. organisations all over the country. Over the last twenty years we have participated in innumerable healthy baby contests as judges. A standard proforma has been used by us in the field over the last twenty years to introduce objectivity in the contest and at the same time to educate the parents about the child.

A sample copy of the proforma is given in Table 42.1. The main highlights of the proforma are:

1. In most healthy baby contests children are aged between 0-2 years and we find it convenient to divide them in to three groups because of obvious child rearing practices.
   a. 0 - 6 months
   b. 6 - 12 months
   c. 12 months to 24 months.
2. A special emphasis is placed on feeding practices. Due importance is given for preventable health problems with lesser emphasis on nonpreventable health problems.
3. Mother's knowledge regarding management of common childhood problems like, fever and diarrhea are given importance in the evaluation, along with the family planning methods adopted by parents.

In each category appropriate points are given based on the proforma and totalling is done.

At the end of each session we always make it a point to address the mothers of the babies regarding the criteria on which babies are assessed and briefly discuss about various childrearing practices. This will not only act as health educative session but also the transparency and objectivity of the assessment are kept before the mothers.

We always make it a point to see that every child is given some appreciation, so that no mother is disappointed.

For every mother *"There is only one beautiful and healthy child in this world!"*

Table 42.1: Healthy baby show proforma

Name	:	Group-I	0-6 months		
		Group-II	6-12 months		
		Group-III	12-24 months		

Age   :

Father's name   :

Mother's name   :

1. **Growth** (Weight)	:	* Normal weight for age	:	4
		* Grade-I malnutrition	:	2
		* Grade-II malnutrition	:	1
		* Grade-III and IV malnutrition	:	0
2. **Development** (milestones)		* Appropriate	:	4
		* Delayed	:	2
3. **Feeding**	:			
a. Breastfeeding		* Exclusive 4-6 months	:	5
		* Breastfeeding into 2nd years	:	4
		* Breastfeeding + top milk in 6 months	:	2
		* Only top milk	:	0
b. Weaning time		* 4-6 months	:	5
		* Before 4 months	:	3
		* After 8 months	:	2
c. Food		* Home made	:	4
		* Proprietary	:	2
d. Bottle feeding		* Yes	:	2
4. **Immunisation**	:	* Age appropriate	:	5
		* Not appropriate	:	2
		* Not immunization	:	0
5. **Systemic illness**	:	* Yes	:	0
		* No	:	2
6. **Malformation**	:	* Yes	:	0
		* No	:	2
7. **Deficiency diseases**	:	* Yes	:	0
(Rickets, nutritional anemia)		* No	:	2
8. **Maternal knowledge about childhood illness** :				
a. Diarrhea (ORS)		* Yes	:	2
		* No	:	0
b. Fever (PCT, sponging)		* Yes	:	2
		* No	:	0
9. **Family planning** (Spacing)	:	* Yes	:	3
		* No	:	1
10. **Looks**	:	* Maximum	:	5
		* Minimum	:	2

Maximum Marks

1. Growth (Weight) — 4
2. Developmental milestones — 4
3. Appropriate feeding — 14
4. Appropriate immunization — 5
5. No systemic illness — 2
6. No malformation — 2
7. No deficiency states — 2
8. Adequate maternal knowledge about management of
   diarrhea/fever — 4
9. Proper family planning — 3
10. Appearance (looks) — 5

Total   45

43 School Health Survey

Objectives of School Health Services
- The promotion of positive health
- The prevention of diseases
- Early diagnosis, treatment and follow-up of diseases
- Awakening health consciousness in children
- Provision of healthful environment.

Aspects of School Health Services
- Health appraisal of school children and school personel
- Remedial measures and follow-up
- Prevention of communicable diseases
- Healthful school environment
- Nutritional services
- First aid and emergency care
- Mental health
- Dental health
- Eye health
- Education about health
- Education of handicapped child.

The School Health Community started in 1961 has recommended medical examination of children at the time of entry and there after every 4 years.

Examination Should Include
- Careful history
- Physical examination
- Tests for vision, hearing, speech, dental caries
- Routine examination of blood/urine should also be done.
  Table 43.1 illustrates a careful school health check-up.

Table 43.1: School health check-up proforma

Name of child :

Date of birth/Place :

Religion :

Name of the Father :

Address :

History :

        Fever

        Cough

        Cold

        Otitis, ear discharge

        Wheeze

        Itching skin lesions

        Dyspnea on exertion

        Palpitation

        Fainting

        Bleeding tendency

        Nausea/vomiting

        Diarrhea/constipation

        Passing of worms

        Pediculosis, joint pains

        Difficulty in passing urine

        Any allergy to drugs

        Any episodes of convulsions

Examination :   Check the vital signs

                  HR   —   BP   —

                  RR   —   Pulse —

    Check for—cyanosis, clubbing, pallor, jaundice, lymphadenopathy, edema.

Physical examination :

    Assessment of skin   – Dry

                           Scaly

                           Rash

                           Bleeding spots

                           Itching

    Assessment of eyes   – Pallor

                           Conjunctivitis

                           Vision, color vision

                           Other vit. deficiency signs (xerophthalmia)

    Assessment of ears   – Hearing

                           Discharge

    Assessment of throat   – Infection

    Assessment of oral cavity

                      – Hygiene

                      – Number of teeth

                      – Number of caries

                      – Discoloration of teeth

    Assessment of spine   – Scoliosis (after bending forwards)

    Assessment of immunization status

Contd...

Contd...

UIP Schedule   :

At birth	–	BCG + OPV
6 weeks	–	DPT + OPV
10 weeks	–	DPT + OPV
14 weeks	–	DPT + OPV
9 months	–	Measles
18 months	–	DPT + OPV
5 years	–	DT
10 years	–	TT

IAP schedule   :

Vaccine	–	*Age recommende*
BCG	–	Birth-2 weeks
OPV	–	Birth, 6, 10, 14 weeks, 9 months
		15-18 months, 5 years
HB	–	Birth, 6 weeks, 6-9 months, 10 years
DPT	–	6, 10, 14 weeks
		15-18 months, 5 years
Measles	–	9 months plus
MMR	–	15-18 months
TT	–	10, 16 years

Assessment of nutrition   :

Check
- Weight for the age
- Height for the age
- Head circumference for the age
- Chest circumference for the age
- Skin fold thickness.
- Chest expansion

Assessment of sexual maturity rating (SMR) :
(By Tanner's scale) for both boys and girls separately.

Systemic examination   :

Respiratory system
Cardiovascular system
Gastrointestinal tract
Central nervous system

Investigations   :

Urine analysis
Hemoglobin
Blood counts

Treatment advice :

Follow-up   :

SCHOOL HEALTH CARD

All information regarding the well being of the children is to be entered into a health card. This card should be handy in the clinic and should be periodically updated. Given below is a sample:

HEALTH CARD

A. General Information   **Reg. No.**

Name of School   :

Name of Student   :

Age   :

Class and Section   :

Address   :

Father's Name   :

Education of Father   :

Education of Mother   :

Father's Name   :

Land Holdings   :

Income   :

No. of Siblings—Total
        – Brother   :
        – Sisters   :

Immunization Status of Student

B. History

Present History of Illness

Past History of Illness

C. General Physical Examination

Height_____ Weight_____ Built_____
Hair_____ Color_____ Condition_____
Eyes-conjunctiva_____ Sclera_____
Nose_____ Any Septal Defect_____
Teeth_____
Oral hygiene_____
Caries_____
Dental fluorosis_____
Tongue_____
Thyroid_____

Lymph nodes Neck_____
    Axilla_____
    Inguinal_____
Nails_____
Color_____
Skin_____
Texture_____
Rash_____
Boils_____
Patches_____
Sensation_____

Speech   Normal/Lisp/Stammer/Stutter

D. Skeletal System

Bony structure_____
Rib cage_____
Joints_____
Knees_____
Shape of legs_____
Remarks

E. Cardiovascular System

JVP_____ Pulse/min._____
Respiratory Rate/min._____
Breath sounds_____
Movement of ribcage_____
Auscultation of chest_____

Contd...

Rhonchi _____

Crepts _____

Heart sounds _____

Murmur, if any _____

Remarks

_____

_____

F. Abdominal Examination

Palpation _____

Mention, if tenderness or lump _____

_____

Liver _____

Spleen _____

Kidneys _____

G. Eyes   RE   LE

Eyelids _____   _____   _____

Discharge, if any _____   _____   _____

Eyelashes _____   _____   _____

Conjunctiva _____   _____   _____

Sclera _____   _____   _____

Cornea _____   _____   _____

Pupil _____   _____   _____

Movement of Eyeball _____   _____   _____

Follicles_____   _____   _____

Squinting _____   _____   _____

Vision

    Distance _____

    Near _____

Colour Blindness _____

H. ENT Examination

Ears _____

Shape _____

Wax _____

Ear drum _____

Discharge _____

Contd...

Tenderness _____

Swelling _____

Audiometry test _____

Nose _____

Throat _____

_____

Tonsils _____

Lymph nodes _____

Remark on Eyes, Ears, Nose and Throat

Laboratory Investigations

Routine Blood

        HB%

        TLC

        DLC

        ESR

Urine

        Micro-Puscells/RBC

        Albumin

        Sugar

Stool

        Ova/Cyst/RBCs

Special Investigations if required:

Test for IQ of child:

Remarks:

Remarks by Psychologist:

Doctor's Notes:

Date   I Visit   II Visit   III Visit   IV visit

Treatment Advised:

Contd...

Teacher's Remarks:

Signature of Class-teacher

Signature of Doctor

Date   :

Equipments Required for Organising School Health Services

Equipment for Setting up Clinic

Writing table	:	One
Chairs	:	Three
Stool (revolving)	:	One
Bench	:	One
Cot-	:	One
Mattres for cot	:	One
Pillow for cot	:	One
Examination table	:	One
Foot stool	:	One
Mattress for examination table	:	One
Mackintosh	:	One + One
Bucket	:	One
Mug–	:	One
Towels	:	Three
Soaps dish	:	One
Sheets	:	Four
Soaps	:	Two (to be replaced)
Basin and Kidney tray	:	Two each

Equipment Required for Medical Examination

BP instrument	:	One
Stethoscope	:	One
Snellen's chart	:	One
Color blindness chart	:	One
Torch	:	One
Reflex hammer	:	One
Weighing machine	:	One
Height measuring scale	:	One
Thermometer	:	One
Health Cards	:	Five hundred at least

First Aid Kit
Bandages
Cotton roll
ORS Packets
Antacids
Antispasmodics
Eye drops
Anti allergens
Wax melting drops
Splints
Local anesthesia
Mercurochrome
Tincture iodine/Betadine
Savlon
Spirit (Methylated)
Chittle's forceps
Sterilizer
Drum (small)
Vaccine carrier with tetanus
Toxoid (also available at nearest subcentre)
Syringes, needles
Gentian violet
Carbolic acid
Soaps

Logistics and Transport
a. Publicity material
b. Health education material
c. Referral units and establish network with them
d. Vehicle (Jeep) and POL.

CHAPTER 44 Gynecological Examination of an Adolescent*

Over the past few years, many pediatricians, obstetrician-gynecologists, family practitioners, have expressed an interest in a simplified approach to the common gynecologic problems of children and adolescents. Problems such as the differential diagnosis of ambiguous genitalia, vulvovaginitis, precocious development, and sexual abuse arise in the care of infants and children. Dysmenorrhea, irregular periods, sexually transmitted diseases, and pregnancy represent common presenting complaints of adolescents.

Many gynecologic problems can be diagnosed on the basis of the history and the physical examination, including rectoabdominal palpation. A step-by-step description of the routine examination of the child and adolescent is covered in this chapter.

In general, the discussion focuses on the most common diagnosis rather than rare conditions that the generalist is less likely to encounter.

The traditional avoidance of the female external genitalia has sometimes prevented parents and physicians from dealing with the total health care of the young girl. Although gynecologic problems are not common among young girls, the pediatrician should always include inspection of the external genitalia and palpation of the breast as part of the routine physical examination. If the child accepts a brief look at her genitalia as part of the normal physical examination, she is less likely to feel embarrassed or upset by the same examination when she reaches adolescence. In addition, the physician may note smegma or feces in the labial folds, indicating inadequate perineal hygiene. Careful instruction to the parents and child during the examination may prevent the later occurrence of a nonspecific vulvovaginitis. The presence of a cyst, clitoromegaly, early signs of puberty, *Candida* vulvitis, or an abnormality of the hymen may be a clue to other problems.

A healthy dialogue between parents and children on issues of sexuality should begin during the prepubertal years. Parents should be encouraged to answer the questions of their young children with simple facts and correct terminology.

Vaginal discharge or bleeding, pruritus, signs of sexual development, or an allegation of sexual abuse should prompt a more thorough evaluation. The

---

*Adapted from *Pediatric and Adolescent Gynaecology*, 4th Edition, 1998, by S. Jean Ewans, Marc R. Laufer, Donald Peter Goldstein. Lippincott-Raven Publishers.

nature of the history obviously depends on the presenting complaint. If the problem is vaginitis, questions should focus on perineal hygiene, antibiotic therapy, recent infections in the patient or other members of the family, and the possibility of sexual molestation. Behavioral changes and somatic symptoms such as abdominal pain, headaches, and enuresis may suggest abuse. Information on the caretaker should always be elicited. If the problem is vaginal bleeding, the history should include recent growth and development, signs of puberty, use of hormone creams or tablets (including maternal exposure), trauma, and a previous finding of foreign bodies in the vagina. Although the history is usually obtained chiefly from a parent, the child should be asked questions not only about genital complaints but also about toys or school to put her at ease. Eye contact should be maintained with the child, and it should be stressed that she is an important part of the team. Questions focusing on what has bothered the child (such as itching or discharge) can help the child understand why the examination is important. She should be given the opportunity to ask questions.

The gynecologic examination should be carefully explained in advance to the parent and the child. It is extremely important to tell the parent that the size of the vaginal opening is quite variable and that the examination will in no way alter the hymen. Often a diagram showing the introitus is helpful because many parents still believe that the virginal introitus is totally covered by the hymen.

Both parent and child should be told that instruments will be used that are specially designed for little girls. The otoscope or hand lens to be used for external examination should be shown to the child with an emphasis that the physician will use these instruments "to look". If a colposcope will be used for a sexual abuse evaluation, the child should have a chance to look at the instrument, turn on and off the light, and view fingers or jewellery through the binocular eyepieces to feel comfortable with the examination.

The child can then be offered the choice of gown color and whether she wishes to have her parent lift her onto the table or climb "up the big stairs". The mother most commonly plays an active role during the examination. The older child should be asked whom she prefers in or out during the examination. Most children and many young adolescents prefer their mothers in the room; almost all mid to late adolescents prefer their mothers out of the examining room.

The majority of children are comfortable on the examining tables with mother (or father) sitting close by or holding a hand. Some girls are quite fearful, especially if they have been previously sexually abused or had a painful genital examination. In this case, the mother (or the caretaker bringing the child) can sit on the table in a semireclined position with her feet in stirrups and have the child's legs straddle her thighs. The use of a hand mirror has been found helpful in relaxing the child and become an active participant in the examination. If the pediatrician is confident and relaxed, the patient usually responds with cooperation. An abrupt or hurried approach will precipitate anxiety and resistance in the child. Sometimes it is necessary to leave the room and return when the patient feels ready.

The examination of any child having gynecologic complaints should include a general pediatric assessment of the child's weight, height, head and neck, heart, lungs, and abdomen. The abdominal examination is often easier if the child places her hands on the examiner's hand; she is then less likely to tense her muscles or complain of being "tickled". The inguinal areas should be carefully palpated for a hernia or gonad; occasionally, an inguinal gonad is the testis of an undiagnosed male pseudohermaphrodite. The breasts should be carefully inspected and palpated. The increasing diameter of the areola or a unilateral tender breast bud is often the first sign of puberty.

The gynecologic examination of the child includes inspection of the external genitalia, visualization of the vagina and cervix, and rectoabdominal palpation. This examination is usually possible without anesthesia if the child has not been traumatized by previous examinations and if the pediatrician proceeds slowly. The child should be explicitly told that "the exam will not hurt". The young child should be examined supine with her knees apart and feet touching in the frog-leg position or in the lithotomy position with the use of adjustable stirrups. As the external genitalia are inspected the young child may be less anxious if she assists the pediatrician by holding the labia apart. The pediatrician should note the presence of pubic hair, size of the clitoris, type of hymen, signs of estrogenization of the vaginal introitus, and perineal hygiene. Friability of the posterior forchette as the labia are separated can occur in children with vulvitis and/or history of sexual abuse. If the hymenal orifice is still not visible, the labia can be gently gripped and pulled forward (traction maneuver) to view the anterior vagina. The average size of the normal clitoral glans in the premenarcheal child is 3 mm in length and 3 mm in transverse diameter. The vaginal mucosa of the prepubertal child appears thin and red in contrast with the moist, dull pink, estrogenized mucosa of the pubertal child. Frequently, the perihymenal tissue is erythematous. The vaginal introitus will often gape open if the child is asked to take a deep breath or cough; if not, the labia should be gently pulled downward and laterally.

The type of hymen should be noted using a hand lens or the light and magnification of an otoscope (without a speculum) (Fig. 44.1). Hymens can be classified as posterior rim (or crescent), annular, or redundant. The edges of the redundant hymen and the orifice are often difficult to visualize. Congenital abnormalities of the hymen are not uncommon, especially microperforate and septate hymens. The presence of an opening in a microperforate hymen may be difficult to establish. Congenital absence of the hymen has not been documented to occur. Acquired abnormalities of the hymen usually result from sexual abuse and rarely from accidental trauma. Pediatrician seeing girls for annual physical examinations should be encouraged to visualize the genitalia and the hymen and the make a drawing in the office notes of its type. Knowledge of a change from previously noted anatomy could provide an important clue to ongoing sexual abuse.

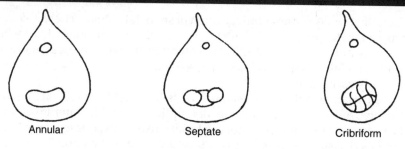

Annular   Septate   Cribriform

Fig. 44.1: Types of hymen

The significance of measurements of the diameter of the hymenal orifice is controversial. The transverse and anterior-posterior measurements are influenced by age, relaxation of the child, method of examination and measurement, and type of hymen. The older the child and the more relaxed, the larger the opening. The opening is larger with retraction on the labia and in the knee-chest position than with gentle separation alone in the supine position. The orifice of a posterior rim hymen will appear larger than the opening of a redundant hymen. Because the hymen is distensible, vaginal penetration can have occurred even though the measurement is only 5 mm. In cases of sexual abuse, measure both anterior-posterior and transverse dimensions using a Tine test 5 cm ruler. Some colposcopes have the markings in the eyepiece, and direct measurement can be done during the examination. A good rule of thumb is 1 mm for each year of age as the upper limits of normal (i.e. 8 mm for an 8 year old), remembering all the caveats of changes with relaxation and position. Abnormal measurements in the prepubertal child are often 10 to 15 mm. The finding of a large hymenal orifice may be consistent with a history of sexual abuse but should only be considered a part of the evaluation, not the absolute criteria.

The anus and labia should always be examined for cleanliness, excoriations, and erythema. Perianal excoriation is often a clue to the presence of pinworm infestation.

Once the external genitalia have been carefully examined, the physician should proceed with visualization of the vagina. In girls more than 2 years old, knee-chest position provides a particularly good view of the vagina and cervix without instrumentation. The patient is told that she should "lie on her tummy with her bottom in the air". She is reassured that the examiner plans to "take a look at her bottom" but "will not put anything inside her". In the knee-chest position (also used for sigmoidscopy in older patients), the child rests her head to one side on her folded arms and supports her weight on bent knees (6-8 inches apart). With her buttocks held up in the air, she is encouraged to let her spine and stomach "sag downward." A pillow can be placed under her abdomen. As the child takes deep breaths, the vaginal orifice falls open for examination. In 80 to 90 percent of prepubertal girls, an ordinary otoscope head (without a speculum) provides the magnification and light necessary to visualize the cervix. Clearly the child's anxiety will be allayed if she is again shown the otoscope light and her full confidence is gained before this part of the examination. A running conversation of small talk about school, toys, and siblings often diverts the child's attention and helps her maintain this position for several minutes without moving or objecting. Since the vagina of the prepubertal child is quite short, the presence of a foreign body or a lesion is often easily ascertained.

An alternative method of visualization is the use of a small vaginoscope, cystoscope, hysteroscope, or flexible fiberoptic scope with water insufflation of the vagina. Application of viscous xylocaine to the introitus makes insertion easier. Good visualization of the cervix and vagina is thus possible without general anesthesia. Vaginal speculum can only rarely be useful in examining the older child if insertion does not cause pain or trauma. For anesthesia examinations, a nasal speculum with light source can be used.

If vaginal discharge is present, samples should be obtained for culture, Gram stain, and saline and potassium hydroxide (KOH) preparations. Usually, the child prefers to lie on her back with her knees apart with feet together or in stirrups so that she can watch the procedure without becoming excessively anxious.

Evaluation of the Adolescent

The evaluation of the adolescent requires additional technical skills, including speculum examination of the vagina (Figs 44.2A and B) and rectal-vaginal abdominal palpation. More importantly, the physician needs the interpersonal skills, sensitivity, and time to establish a primary relationship with the adolescent herself. The doctor must be willing to see the teenager alone and listen to her concerns. For example, the patient with oligomenorrhea may return each visit with the same question, "Why am I not normal"? Listening to her describe her feelings is just as important as drawing diagrams of the

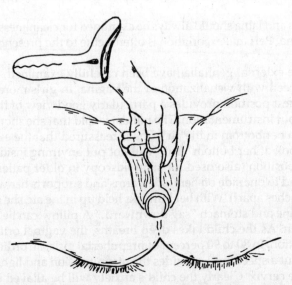

Fig. 44.2A: Vaginal speculum examination speculum in inset

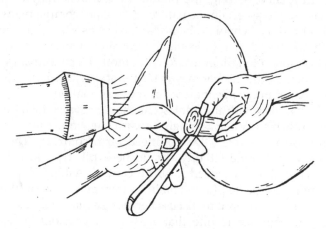

Fig. 44.2B: Speculum examination of vagina

hypothalamic-ovarian axis. The statement, "Your pelvic exam is normal," answers few questions for the adolescent.

It is helpful to discuss the special needs of adolescents with the pubescent girls when she reaches her eleventh or twelfth birthday. The parents also need to hear that adolescents require special time to discuss concerns about pee relations, school, family, drugs, and sexuality.

Parents should be included as much as possible in important medical decisions, but the need for the adolescent to have medical privacy should be respected. Parents should be encouraged to call in advance of an appointment if they have special concerns since an adolescent may sometimes be strikingly nonverbal about troubling issues at home or in school. At the same time, parents may need help communicating more effectively with their adolescent.

Consider the body changes involved in the development of the prepubertal latency-age girls of 10 years as she changes into the sexually mature woman of 20. These changes underscore the many issues that arise in the medical care of adolescent girls. The appearance of pubic hair and breast development, over which the girl has no control, can be quite distressing. The fact that these changes occur at the same rate within her peer group may offer some reassurance; to be early or late can provoke considerable anxiety. A 12 year-old girl who looks 16 may be confronted with heterosexual demands that she is unable to cope with; a 16-year-old girl who looks 10 may be embarrassed to undress in physical education class or to interact with her peer group. Since the young adolescent has many fantasies about her body and its changes, she may ask the same questions at each visit. The older teenager is intellectually more capable of coping with a diagnosis and the physical examination. The pediatrician must, therefore, be sensitive to the different needs of each patient.

Obtaining the History

The source of the medical history depends on the medical setting and the age of the patient. The older adolescent tends to seek gynecologic care on her own initiative. In a clinic setting, the mother (and father) may be seen by the pediatrician first to ascertain the nature of the chief complaint, as well as the past medical history, school problems, and psychosocial adjustment. Most of the visit should be devoted to seeing the teenager alone, since her presenting complaint is quite often different from her mother's concerns. In the seeking of private practice, the mother may make the appointment by telephone, and then the teenager may appear alone for the examination.

The routine visit with the adolescent should always include a carefully taken menstrual history and a straightforward question about sexual relations and birth control, such as, "Do you need birth control?" The physician's approach toward confidentiality should be explicitly stated because few teenagers will volunteer a need for birth control. Asking about peer group behaviors may also be helpful in obtaining information about the adolescent patient seemingly reluctant to discuss her own sexual behavior.

It is not uncommon to find that a 13- or 14 year old girls with school problems, mother-daughter conflict, and a history of running away.

Gynecologic Examination

Once the history is obtained and the problems identified, the patient should be given a thorough explanation of a pelvic examination. The use of diagrams or a pelvic plastic model is helpful. For first examination, the feelings of the adolescent should be acknowledged. A statement such as "some girls I see are worried about pain or embarrassment" helps establish good patient-doctor communication. Adequate drapes and gowns and allowing the adolescent to control the tempo of the examination will alleviate her concerns. The patient should then be given a gown and asked to remove all her clothes, including brassiere and underpants. If she is covered appropriately and approached in a relaxed manner, resistance is unlikely. The presence of a female nurse in the room is often reassuring, especially if the pediatrician is a man. The young adolescent may request that her mother stay with her during a pelvic examination. Most patients prefer the mother to stay in the waiting room. The patient's wishes should be respected. The general physical examination of a teenage girl should always include a breast examination, inspection of the genitalia, and a careful notation of the Tanner stages of breast and pubic hair development. Demonstrating self-examination of the breast of the patient as one actually performs the breast examination often puts the young woman at ease. Pediatric patients occasionally ask why it is necessary to look at the genitalia. There are a number of reasons: *Candida* vulvitis may be the first sign of diabetes; an imperforate hymen may be the cause of adominal pain or primary amenorrhea; a cyst or clitoromegaly may be found unexpectedly. The actual examination frequently initiates questions that the teenager was embarrassed to ask, such as queries about a vaginal discharge, a lump, or irregular periods.

When is a pelvic examination indicated? A bimanual rectoabdominal examination (in the lithotomy position) should be performed on any teenager with gynecologic complaints or unexplained abdominal pain. A vaginal examination is important to assess irregular bleeding, severe dysmenorrhea, vaginal discharge, *in utero* exposure to DES, sexually transmitted diseases, and amenorrhea, sexually active patients, sexually transmitted diseases, and amenorrhea. Sexually active patients should have a routine vaginal examination every 6 to 12 months; a patient who is not sexually active can begin routine annual examination at any age that she feels comfortable with initiating gynecologic care, hopefully at least by the age of 17 or 18 years. Contrary to popular belief, rarely is a patient unable to be fully cooperative during a pelvic examination if she has received a careful explanation about the procedure and its importance in evaluating her individual problem.

The pelvic examination is done with the patient in the lithotomy position with the use of stirrups. A mirror can be offered to the patient. The external genitalia are inspected first; type of hymenal opening, estrogenization of the vaginal mucosa, distribution of the pubic hair, and the size of the clitoris are assessed. The pubic hair should be inspected for pediculosis pubis if itching is present. The inguinal areas should be palpated for evidence of lymphadenopathy. The estrogenized vagina has a moist or thickened, dull pink mucosa in contrast to the thin, red mucosa of the prepubertal child. The normal clitoral glans is 2 to 4 mm in width; a width of 10 mm is considered significant virilization. The hymen in the adolescent girls is estrogenized and thickened. Minor changes due to sexual abuse or minor trauma that might have been easily seen in the thin unestrogenized hymen of the prepubertal child may be impossible to visualize in the estrogenized adolescent. Because the hymen is elastic, tampons can be inserted by most adolescents without tearing the hymen. The hymenal opening in the virginal adolescent is usually large enough to allow insertion of a finger for palpation or a small speculum. An adolescent who has been sexually active may have a hymen without any obvious trauma or may have old or new lacerations of the hymen (down to the base of the hymen) or myrtiform caruncles (small bumps of residual hymen along the lower edge). In the examination of the sexually abused adolescent, the hymenal ring can be carefully examined by running a saline-moistened cotton-tipped applicator around the edges.

The stratified squamous epithelium of the cervix usually a homogeneous dull pink color; however, in many adolescents an erythematous area surrounding the os is noted. The so-called ectropion is the presence of endocervical columnar epithelium on the cervix. The squamocolumnar junction, instead of being inside the endocervical canal, is visible on the portion of the cervix; it does not represent a disease process.

After visualization of the vagina and cervix, the speculum is removed, the uterus and adnexa are carefully palpated with one or two fingers in the vagina and the other hand on the abdomen. Normal ovaries are usually less than 3 cm and are rubbery. The adolescent may complain of discomfort with palpation.

A rectal-vaginal abdominal examination performed with the index finger in the vagina, the middle finger in the rectum, and the other hand on the abdomen permits palpation of a retroverted uterus and assessment of mobility of the adnexa and uterus. The uterosacral ligaments should be palpated carefully in patients with pain or dysmenorrhea since tenderness is often found in patients with endometriosis. The patient is usually less anxious if she is told in advance that the rectal examination may seem disturbing because of the sensation that she is "moving her bowels" or "going to the bathroom". Allaying this fear usually elicits better relaxation and cooperation.

In patients with a tight hymen, a simple bimanual rectoabdominal examination with the index finger pushing the cervix upward allows palpation of the uterus and adnexa. In a relaxed patient, a negative examination rules out the possibility that are large ovarian masses or uterine enlargement.

After the examination is concluded and the patient has dressed, the pediatrician should sit down and discuss in detail the patient's complaint and what was found on examination. It is essential that the adolescent be treated as an adult capable of understanding the explanation. If her parent has accompanied her, the patient should be asked whether she would like to tell her parent the findings herself or whether she would prefer to have the pediatrician discuss the diagnosis in her presence. It is extremely important for the patient to know that the doctor and her parent will not have a "secret" about her and that confidential information will not be divulged to her parent.

Examination of an Adolescent

For a detailed examination of an adolescent kindly refer to the following Chapters:
1. Vol-II; Sec. 3; Chapter 29—Developmental Assessment: (Growth and Development of Early, Middle and Late Adolescence).
2. Vol-II; Sec. 2; Chapter 22—Examination of Genitalia and Anus).
3. Vol-II; Sec. 3; Chapter 30—Psychiatric Evaluation of an Adolescent.

CHAPTER 45 Examination of Sexually Abused Child/Rape Victim

SEXUALLY ABUSED CHILD EXAMINATION CHECKLIST

Checklist for Sexual Abuse (Collected within 72 hours of the Offense)

1. Consent for evidence collected from the parent/guardian
2. Collection of clothing
3. Skin samples (suspected semenstrain swabed with moistened cotton swab)
4. Oropharyngeal swab for gram stain, gonococcal throat culture, *Chlamydia* throat culture.
5. Vaginal and cervical sample, rectal sample, combed pubic hair, clipped pubic hair, gonococcal vaginal and cervical culture, *Chlamydia* rectal culture
6. Head hair collected.
7. Blood for HIV (after consent) HBsAg
8. Paper works
   - Police information
   - Office record
   - Social worker informed
   - Signature

Proforma for Suspected Sexual Abuse

Patient name   :

Date of birth   :

Age   :

Date of visit   :

Time of visit   :

Patient current address   :

Legal guardian/Primary caretaker   :

Relationship to child   :

Normal development   :

Allied Perpetrator name   :   Age :   Sex :

                                      Relationship to child :

                                      Current address :

Family demographics   :
(Other members of household/
site of abuse/age/relationship)   :

History of assault given by adult
(Identify relationship of adult)   :

History of assault given by child
(Use exact words)   :

Medical history   :

Current medications   :

Allergies   :

Immunisations   :

Review of the systems   :

Abdominal pain, perineal pain, discharge, dysuria, vaginal bleeding, rectal bleeding, incontinence, nausea, vomiting, behavioral changes.

Age at menarche   :

LMP   :

Sexually active   :

Contraceptive use   :   Yes/No   What type :

                             Date and Time of last intercourse

History of sexually transmitted diseases :   Yes/No

                                  When :

                                  Treatment received :

Did penetration occur vaginally or rectally ?   Yes/No

Did digital penetration or fondling occur ?   Yes/No

Did ejaculation occur ?   Yes/No

What oral sex peformed on/by the child ?   Yes/No

Since the assault has the child :   Changed clothes   :   Yes/No

                             Eaten/brushed teeth :   Yes/No

                             Urinated/defecated   :   Yes/No

Physical examination   :   Vital signs   :

                             Heart rate   :

                             Blood pressure :

                             Respiratory rate :

                             Temperature   :

                             Weight   :

                             Height   :

General appearance   :

Skin   :

Head, eye, ear, nose and throat :

Neck :

Chest :

Cardiovascular system :

Abdomen :

Extremities :

Central nervous system :

Tanner stage :

Genitourinary examination :

Presence of blood : Yes/No

Presence of semen : Yes/No

Vulvar/labia majora/minora :

Appearance of hymen :

Cervix :

Appearance of vagina :

Anus :

Appearance of penis/scrotum :

Suspected Sexual Abuse Form

Results of Evidence collected :	Check off those tests performed and note results : Rape Kit done :	
Photographs taken : Yes/No	Urine analysis :	Urine Pregnancy Test
Urine toxicology :	Blood alcohol Level :	RPR :
Gonococcal culture : Throat,	Rectum, vagina	
Chlamydia cultures : Rectum, Vagina, Gram stain		
HIV (with consent)	Wet preparation :	Herpes simplex culture

Signature of Medical Officer

46 Quick Examinations

- Two-minute orthopedic examination
- Quick neurological examination
- Soft neurological signs
- Coma scale
- Evaluation of a case of acute respiratory infection (ARI)
- Evaluation of a case of diarrhea with dehydration
- Evaluation of a case of asthma
- Evaluation of a case of snake bite
- Evaluation of a case of diabetic ketoacidosis (Diabetic coma)

TWO-MINUTE ORTHOPEDIC EXAMINATION (Table 46.1)

Table 46.1: A two-minute orthopedic examination

Instructions	Observations
Stand facing examiner	Acromioclavicular joints and general habitus of the child
Look at ceiling floor over both shoulders	Motion of cervical spine
Shrug shoulders (while examiner resists)	Strength of trapezius muscle
Abduct shoulders 90°	Deltoid strength
Full external rotation of arms	Shoulder motion
Flex and extend elbow	Elbow motion
Arms at sides, elbow 90° flexed, pronate and supinate wrist	Elbow/wrist motion
Spread fingers, make fist	Hand or finger motions and deformities relaxation
Tightening and of quadriceps	Symmetry, knee effusion and ankle effusion
Duck walk (4 steps)	Hip, knee and ankle motion
Turnback to examiner	Shoulder symmetry and scoliosis
Keep knee straight, touch toes	Scoliosis, hip motion and hamstring tightness.
Raise upon toes, raise heels	Calf symmetry, leg strength

(This quick orthopedic examination is recommended by American Academy of Pediatrics—Sports Medicine Branch)

QUICK NEUROLOGICAL EXAMINATIONS

Quick neurological examinations depicts various maneuvers to be performed for assessment of different neurological conditions in infants (Table 46.2).

Table 46.2: Quick neurological examination in infant

Maneuver		Assess for
1. See posture	–	Hypotonia, hypertonia, opisthotonus
2. Talk, smile to infant or make mother to talk to infant and see respose.	–	Level of consciousness Orientation to person, hearing.
3. Show bright object and make him follow in different directions and then offer or make mother go around and see his visual pathway.	–	Vision III, IV, VI Nerve function Hand function, co-ordination
4. Put the patient to breast and observe feeding or offer him a biscuit and observe	–	V cranial nerve (rooting, sucking) IX, X cranial nerve (Swallowing)
5. Stimulate limbs and other parts with a blunt pin and see response.	–	Motor function and pain sensation
6. Observe posture, neck movements	–	XI cranial nerve and meningeal signs
7. Observe infant playing	–	Motor function
8. Make child cry (Do it at the end of examiantion)	–	VII cranial nerve, tongue, IX cranial nerve, voice, X cranial nerve

QUICK NEUROLOGICAL EXAMINATION IN AN OLDER CHILD (Table 46.3)

Table 46.3: Maneuvers for corresponding functions test in a quick neurological examination of an older child

Maneuver		Function tested
1. Ask him to walk	–	Gait
	–	Coordination
2. Walk on tip toes	–	Strength of antigravity muscles in lower limbs (tibialis anterior, quadriceps)
3. Walk on heels	–	Strength of calf muscles, hamstrings
4. Tandem gait	–	Coordination Cerebellar function Soft neurological sign
5. Stand on one leg	–	Strength of lower limb on that side
6. Hop on alternate legs	–	Comparison of strength of two lower limbs (It is a test that detects minimal weakness)
7. Sit down and get up	–	Pelvic girdle muscles
8. Climb on a stool with each legs separately	–	Pelvic girdle muscles
9. Straight leg raising in supine	–	Meningeal sign
10. Stand up from supine	–	Gover sign in DMD (Duschenne muscular dystrophy)
11. Stretch the arm infront and hold	–	Differential weakness of upper limbs
12. Throw ball, comb hair	–	Shoulder girdle

Contd...

Contd...

Maneuver		Function tested
13. Bend forward and to side	–	Spinal muscle
14. Grip examiners finger milkmaid sign in	–	Small muscles of hand, rheumatic chorea
15. Spread fingers against resistance	–	Interossii muscles
16. Pull-paper held between fingers	–	Lumbricoid muscles
17. Alternate pronation supination, finger nose, finger finger test	–	Cerebellar sings
18. Bend head turn side to side, shrug shoulders	–	Meningeal signs and XI cranial nerve
19. Show tongue and Say 'Aha'	–	X cranial nerve, XII cranial nerve
20. Clench teeth	–	V cranial nerve
21. Show teeth, raise eye brows, whistle	–	VII cranial nerve
22. Look in different direction	–	III, IV and VI cranial nerves

QUICK EXAMINATION FOR SPINAL CORD LEVEL INVOLVEMENT (Table 46.4)

Table 46.4: Indications for respective tests for spinal cord level involvement

Test	Indicates
1. Elevation at shoulder joint	C5 and above intact
2. Normal breathing and cough	C4 and C5 intact Diaphragm)
3. Flex elbow	C6 intact
4. Extend elbow	C7 intact
5. Able to grasp	C8-T1 intact
6. Hip flexion	L1-L2 intact
7. Knee extension	L3 intact
8. Adduct thigh	L4 intact
9. Dorsiflex foot	L5 intact
10. Plantar flexion	S1 intact
11. Roll toe into ball	S2 intact
12. Rectal sphincter tone present	S2-S3 intact

QUICK SCREENING FOR MOTOR FUNCTION AND CRANIAL NERVES (Table 46.5)

Table 46.5: Illustrates a quick screening for motor function and cranial nerves

Motor function and cranial nerves		Screening
III, IV, VI 'Follow the finger'	–	Test for ocular movements in all direction
	–	Nystagmus (finger to side)
	–	Convergence (Finger brought from distance to near)
VII 'Close your eyes tight'	–	Strength of closure of orbicularis oris
'Whistle', 'blow'	–	Buccinator strength

Contd...

Contd...

	Motor function and cranial nerves		Screening
	'Show your teeth'	–	Orbicularis oris look for nasolabial folds, deviation of angle of mouth
	'Look up' or 'frown'	–	Frontal belly, of occipitofrontalis muscle
V	'Bite your jaws hard'	–	Palpate masseter
	'Open your jaw'	–	Temporalis muscle
	'Move your jaw side to side'	–	Pterygoid muscles
XII	'Put out your tongue'	–	Look for weakness
	'Move your tongue	–	Strength, wasting and fibrillation side to side
IX and X	'Say Ah'	–	Look for palatal elevation, deviation of Uvula, do gag reflex
XI	'Turn your head side to side'	–	To test sternocleidomastoid muscle
	'Shrug your shoulder'	–	To test trapezius muscle

EVALUATION OF SOFT NEUROLOGICAL SIGNS

ACTIVITIES FOR EVALUATING NEUROLOGIC SOFT SIGNS IN CHILDREN (Table 46.6)

Table 46.6: Represents soft sign findings in children, with respect to their activities and latest age of disappearance

Activity	Soft sign findings	Latest expected age of disappearance (years)
Walking, running gait	Stiff-legged with a foot slapping quality, unusual posturing of the arms	3
Heel walking	Difficulty remaining on heels for a distance of 10 ft	7
Tip toe walking	Difficulty remaining on toes for a distance of 10 ft	7
Tandem gait	Difficulty walking heel to-toe, unusual posturing of arms	7
One-foot standing	Unable to remain standing on one foot longer than 5-10 sec	5
Hopping in place	Unable to rhythmically hop on each foot	6
Motor-stance	Difficulty maintaining stance (arms extended in front, feet together, and eyes closed), drifting of arms, mild writhing movements of hands or fingers	3
Visual tracking	Difficulty following object with eyes when keeping the head still; nystagmus	5
Rapid thumb-to finger test	Rapid touching thumb to fingers in sequence is uncoordinated; unable to suppress mirror movements in contralateral hand	8
Rapid alternating movements of hands	Irregular speed and rhythm with pronation and supinations of hands patting the knees	10

Contd...

Contd...

Activity	Soft sign findings	Latest expected age of disappearance (years)
Finger-nose test	Unable to alternately touch examiner's finger and own nose consecutively	7
Right-left discrimination	Unable to identify right and left sides of own body	5
Two-point discrimination	Difficulty in localizing and discriminating when touched in one or two places	6
Graphesthesia	Unable to identify geometric shapes you draw in child's open hand	8
Stereognosis	Unable to identify common objects placed in own hand	5

COMA SCALE

The Glasgow Coma Scale (GCS) is the most widely used and thoroughly tested measure of acute injury severity and it can be applied quite well to adolescents and older children. However, its strong reliance on fully developed language skills and the underlying presumptions of willingness or ability of the patient to co-operate with the examiner, limit its applicability to young children and infants. Therefore, alternative scales have been developed, such as children's coma scale (CCS) and the Adelaide Pediatric coma scale. Although modifications of GCS are used in practice, there is as yet no universally accepted pediatric coma scale in widespread clinical use.

Glasgow Coma Scale

When a patient has an altered level of consciousness because of head trauma, another hypoxic event the Glasgow coma scale is often used to quantify consciousness. This instrument assesses the function of the cerebral cortex and brainstem through the patient's verbal response, motor response and eye opening to specific stimuli. This assessment can be repeated at intervals to detect improvement or deterioration in patient's level of consciousness.

The patient's best response in each category is matched to the criteria for scoring. Appropriate verbal stimuli are questions eliciting the patient's level of orientation to person, place and time. Painful stimuli are used when necessary to obtain eye, opening and motor responses. Begin with less painful stimuli such as Pincing, the skin and progress to squeezing the muscle mass or tendons if there is no response.

Scores

Maximum score of 14 indicates optimum level of consciousness. The lowest score possible is 3 indicating deepest coma.

Given below are the GCS and the modified coma scales for children (Table 46.7).

Table 46.7: Modified coma scales for infants: Glasgow coma scale (GCS), childrens coma scale (CCS), and modified version of the GCS

GCS	CCS	Modified GCS
Eyes		
4-spontaneous	4 (same)	4 (same)
3-to speech	3	3
2-to pain	2	2
1-none	1	1
Motor		
6-obeys	6 (same)	6 (reaches)
5-localizes	5	5
4-withdraws	4	4
3-abnormal flexion	3	3
2-abnormal extension	2	2
1-flaccid	1	1
Verbal		
5-oriented	5-smiles, interacts	5-babbles/gestures
4-cibfysed	4-cries, interacts	4-cries of nees
3-words	3-+/- consolable,	3-cries, nonspecific
2-sounds	2-irritable, restless	2-sounds
1-none	1-none	1-none

Adelaide Pediatric Coma Scale

Eyes Open

Spontaneously	4
To speech	3
To pain	2
None	1

Best Motor Response

Obeys commands	5
Localizes pain	4
Flexion to pain	3
Extension to pain	2
None	1

Best Verbal Response

Oriented	5
Words	4
Verbal sounds	3
Cries	2
None	1

EVALUATION OF A CASE OF ACUTE RESPIRATORY INFECTION (ARI)

ARI ASSESSMENT

The term Acute Respiratory Infections (ARI) encompasses a spectrum of diseases involving the upper (AURI) and lower respiratory tract (ALRI). AURI includes common cold, otitis media and pharyngitis, whereas ALRI comprises croup, bronchitis, bronchiolitis and pneumonia. ARI includes the above said conditions if their duration is less than 30 days except, acute otitis media, which is an ear infection of less than 14 days duration.

ARI constitutes one of the principal causes of morbidity and mortality in children under five years of age in developing countries. The total number of episodes of ARI in young children in the world is estimated to be over 2 thousand million a year. Further, nearly 50-60 percent of pediatric outpatient consultations are due to ARI in the developing countries. The latest extrapolation suggests that ARI accounts for one-third of the deaths in developing countries in this age group. In India, roughly 15-30% under five deaths are ARI related.

Pneumonia is the leading cause of deaths due to ARI and pneumonia associated with measles accounts for 70 percent of ARI deaths, followed by postmeasles bronchopneumonia (15%) pertussis (10%), and bronchiolitis and croup (5%). Hence, pneumonia can be taken as the practical equivalent of ARI for interventional purposes. Strategies for control of ARI are therefore, primarily focused on the effective management of pneumonia in the primary care setting in the developing countries.

Categorization and Recommendations for Treatment of Pneumonia

For the child aged 2 months upto 5 years with cough or difficult breathing (who does not have stridor, severe undernutrition, or signs suggesting meningitis) (Table 46.8).

Table 46.8: Categorization and treatment recommendations for pneumonia

Clinical signs	Classify as	Summary of treatment instructions
• Central cyanosis or • Not able to drink	Very severe pneumonia	**Admit** Give oxygen Give an antibiotic chloramphenicol Treat fever, if present Treat wheezing, if present Give supportive care Reassess twice daily.
• Chest indrawing and • No central cyanosis and • Able to drink	Severe pneumonia If child is wheezing, assess further before classifying	**Admit** Give an antibiotic benzylpenicillin Treat fever, if present Treat wheezing, if present Give supportive care Reassess daily.

Contd...

Contd...

Clinical signs	Classify as	Summary of treatment instructions
• No chest indrawing and • Fast breathing	Pneumonia	**Advice Mother to give Home Care** Give an antibiotic (at home) cotri- moxazole, amoxycillin or procaine penicillin. Treat fever, if present Treat wheezing, if present Advise the mother to return in 2 days for reassessment, or earlier if the child is getting worse. If coughing more than 30 days assess for causes of chronic cough. Assess and treat ear problem or sore throat, if present. Assess and treat other problems.
• No chest indrawing and • No fast breathing	No pneumonia cough or cold	**Advice Mother to give Home Care** Treat fever, if present. Treat wheezing, if present.

a. If the child has stridor, follow the treatment guidelines.
   If the child has severe undernutrition, admit for nutritional rehabilitation and medical therapy.
   Treat pneumonia with chloramphenicol.
b. These classifications include some children with bronchiolitis and asthma.
c. If oxygen supply is ample, also give oxygen to a child with:
   restlessness (if oxygen improves the condition),
   severe chest indrawing, or
   breathing rate if 70 breaths per minute or more.
d. Fast breathing is: 50 breaths per minute or more in a child age 2 months upto 12 months; 40 breaths per minute or more in a child age 12 months upto 5 years.

Summary of Categorisation and Management of Young Infant (< 2 months) with pneumonia (Table 46.9)

Table 46.9: Treatment instruction for infant infected with pheunonia with age less than two months

Clinical signs	Classify as	Summary of treatment instructions

• Stopped feeding well
• Convulsions
• Abnormally sleepy or
  difficult to wake,
• Stridor in calm child
• Wheezing
• Fever (38° C or more)
  or low body tempe-
  rature (below 35.5°C),
• Fast breathing,
	Severe pneumonia
	or very severe
	disease
		Admit
		• Give oxygen
		
		• Give antibiotics:
		benzylpenicillin and gentamicin.
		• Careful fluid management
		• Maintain a good thermal environment

Contd...

Contd...

Clinical signs	Classify as	Summary of treatment instructions
• Severe chest indrawing • Central cyanosis • Grunting • Apneic episodes, or • Distended and tense abdomen		• Specific management of wheezing or stridor
• No fast breathing and • No signs of pneumonia or very severe disease.	No pneumonia: cough or cold	**Advise Mother to give the following Care** Keep young infant warm. Breastfeed frequently. Clear nose if it interferes with feeding Return quickly if: Breathing becomes difficult Breathing becomes fast Feeding becomes a problem The young infant becomes sicker.

a. Fast breathing is 60 breaths per minute or more in the young infant (age less than 2 months) repeat the count.

b. If oxygen supply is ample, also give oxygen to a young infant with:
   • restlessness (if oxygen improves the condition)
   • severe chest indrawing, or
   • grunting.

Treatment of a Wheezing Child (Table 46.10)

Table 46.10: Summary of treatment instructions for children with wheezing

Clinical signs	Summary of treatment instructions
• Central cyanosis or • Not able to drink	**Admit** Give oxygen Give rapid-acting bronchodilators Give an antibiotic: chloramphenicol Treat fever, if present Supportive care.
Respiratory distress persists with: • No central cyanosis and • Able to drink	**Admit** Give rapid-acting bronchodilator Give an antibiotic benzylpenicillin Treat fever, it present Supportive care.
No respiratory distress and: • Fast breathing	**Advise Mother to give Home Care** Give oral salbutamol at home Give an antibiotic (at home): cotrimoxazole, amoxycillin, ampicillin or procaine penicillin
• No fast breathing	**Advise Mother to give Home Care** Give oral salbutamol at home.

a. An antibiotic is usually not necessary if the child has asthma.
b. If oxygen supply is ample, also give oxygen to a child with restlessness (if oxygen improves the condition), or severe chest indrawing, or a breathing rate of 70 breaths per minute or more.
c. Fast breathing is: 50 breaths per minute or more in a child age 2 months up to 12 months; 40 breaths per minute or more in a child age 12 months upto 5 years.

If no relief with 2 doses of salbutamol by nebulizer or metered dose inhaler, give an addition steroids, orally, or IV. May add IV aminophylline also.

ARI Syndroms, their Clinical Features and Recommended Treatment (Table 46.11)

Table 46.11: Treatment recommendation for ARI syndromes and their corresponding symptoms

Conditions	Clinical signs and symptoms	Treatment
1. Nasopharyngitis (Common cold)	• Fever • Nasal discharge	• Treat at home • No antibiotics • Treat fever • Normal saline drops for nasal block • No cough/cold remedies • Rule out ASOM, pneumonia
2. Sinusitis	• Persistent purulent nasal discharge plus sinus tenderness, swelling or persistent fever • Cough	• Treat at home • Continue feeding • Antibiotics (cotrimoxazole, ampicillin or amoxicillin) only if suggestive of bacterial sinusitis, i.e. sinus tenderness, facial or periorbital swelling, persistent fever. However, this is uncommon in children less than 5 years of age.
3. Acute otitis media (ASOM)	• Sudden persistent earache • Pus discharge less than 2 week duration • Ear rubbing is not a reliable sign in infants	• Treat at home • Treat fever • Keep ear dry • Start antibiotics—cotrimoxazole, ampicillin or amoxycillin • Reassess after 5 days. If pain, fever, pus discharge are present, antibiotics are continued for another 5 days. Refer if no response after 10 days.
4. Mastoiditis	• Painful swelling behind the ear or above the ear in infants	• Admit • Start antibiotics—chloramphenicol for 10 days. • If the child has signs of brain involvement, refer for neurosurgical evaluation.
5. Pharyngitis	• Fever • Throatache	• Treat at home • Treat fever • Antibiotics only if streptococcal pharyngitis suspected,

Contd...

Contd...

Conditions	Clinical signs and symptoms	Treatment
		a. Tender enlarged cervical lymph nodes
		b. White pharyngeal exudate
		c. Absence of signs suggestive of viral infection.
		Give benzylpenicillin single dose in children more than five years of age or ampicillin, amoxicillin or penicillin.
		Not cotrimoxazole.
6. Acute epigloititis	• Fever	• Admit
	• Drooling of saliva	• Antibiotics—chloramphenicol
	• Stridor	• Watch for signs of obstruction (severe chest indrawing, restlessness, cyanosis) to decide for tracheostomy.
		• If tracheostomy available, avoid oxygen as it may mask signs of obstruction.

Adapted from: Acute Respiratory Infectious in children : Case management in small hospitals in developing countries. A manual for doctors and senior health workers. Geneva, WHO, Document WHO/ARI/90.5, 1990

ARI Assessment Chart

Learn to recognize the clinical signs of ARI so that you may classify and manage them. You have to take histories of at least 5 children in your workplace. Record the 5 cases in the format given.

ARI Cases Record Form

Registration No .... Admission Date .... Time...............

Discharge Date .... Time ....

Name ....

Address ....

Father's Name ....

Age .... Years .... Months .... Sex ....

History

Cough/Difficult Breathing .... Yes/No Duration .... days

Fever .... Yes/No   Refusal to feed/drink .... Yes/No

Convulsions .... Yes/No

Any episode of turning blue or no breathing .... Yes/No

Any other complaints ....

Assessment

General Condition .... Child .... Alert/excessively sleepy/
unconcious

Contd...

AIR Cases Record Form Contd...

Malnutrition .... Yes/No Weight ....

Fast breathing .... Yes/No

Chest Indrawing .... Yes/No

Wheezing .... Yes/No

Stridor .... Yes/No

Cyanosis .... Yes/No

Any other relevant findings ....

Diagnosis .... No pneumonia/Pneumonia/Severe pneumonia/Very severe illness.

With ....

Practical Manual

Treatment

Sent home with advise/Admit or refer for admission.

Sent home with advise (No pneumonia/pneumonia):

Feeding/Breastfeeding

Fluids

Cleaning of nasal passage

Treat for fever if present

Advice for antibiotics ....

Advice on repeat visit ....

Treatment for admitted cases

Progress of the Patient

Discharge Advice to Mother on Home Management of ARI

Home fluids ....

Foods to offer ....

Early signs of referral
(when should she come back) ....

Any other advice ....

....

Immunisation status/advice ....

....

Spacing for the next child ....

EVALUATION OF A CASE OF SEVERE ASTHMA

Quick assessment and therapeutic decision making is very essential in managing patients with acute severe asthma.

Ask and record	Examine for
1. Duration of present episode.	1. Sensorium, the length of sentences being spoken.
2. Medications already being used.	
3. Time of last aminophylline dose (if taking).	2. Respiratory rate, heart rate, color, and use of accessory muscles. Breath sounds intensity, wheeze
4. Precipitating factors—infections, exercise, drugs, stress, seasonal, etc.	3. Saturation PaO_2 if pulse oxymeter is available.
5. Severity of previous episodes and of treatment required.	4. Peak expiratory flow rate.
6. Any previous ICU admissions.	5. Make a severity assessment according to the guideliness given in Table (46.12). However, the basic steps of management be started early like oxygen inhalation and inhaled short acting beta-2 agonists.

Table 46.12: Assessment of severity of asthma exacerbations

	Mild	Moderate	Severe	Imminent respiratory arrest
Symptoms:				
Breathlessness	While walking	While talking (infant: softer, shorter cry; difficulty feeding)	While at rest (infant stops feeding)	
	Can lie down	Prefers sitting	Sits upright	
Talks in	Sentences	Phrases	Words	
Alertness	May be agitated	Usually agitated	Usually agitated	Drowsy or confused
Signs:				
Respiratory rate	Increased	Increased	Often increased but may be decreased	
Use of accessory muscles; suprasternal retractions	Usually not	Commonly	Usually	Paradoxical thoraco-abdominal movement
Wheeze	Moderate, often only and expiratory	Loud; throughout exhalation	Usually loud; throughout inhalation and exhalation	Absence of wheeze
Pulse min	Increased by 10%	Increased by 10-20%	Increased by more than 20%	Bradycardia
Pulsus paradoxus	Absent < 10 mmHg	May be present 10-25 mmHg	Often present> 25 mm Hg (adult) 20-40 mm hg (child)	Absence suggest respiratory muscle fatigue

Reference: 1. Sly. RM New guidelines for diagnosis and management of asthma. Am Allergy. Asthma Immunol. 1997, 78: 427-37.

2. Singh M Kumar L, Ramanatham RMPL. (Writing Group). Consensus guidelines on management of childhood asthma in India. *Indian Pediatrics* 1999, 26, 157-65.

QUICK EVALUATION OF A CASE OF DIARRHEA WITH DEHYDRATION

QUICK ASSESSMENT OF DEHYDRATED PATIENT (Table 46.13)

Table 46.13: Elicits a quick assessment of dehydrated patient

First assess your patient for dehydration			
	A	**B**	**C**
1. **Look at condition**	Well, alert	• Restless, irritable	• Lethargic or unconsciousness;
Eyes	Normal	Sunken	Very sunken and dry
Tears	Present	Absent	Absent
Mouth and Tongue	Moist	Dry	Very dry
Thirst	Drinks normally, not thirsty	• Thirsty, drinks eagerly	• Drinks poorly or not able to drink
2. **Feel:**			
Skin pinch	Goes back quickly	• Goes back slowly	• Goes back very slowly
3. **Decide:**	The patient has No Signs of dehydration	If the patient has two or more signs including at least one sign*, there is some dehydration	If the patient has two or more signs, including at least one sign, there is severe dehydration
4. **Treat:**	Use treatment Plan A	Weigh the patient, if possible, and use treatment Plan B	Weigh the patient and use treatment Plan C, urgently

Diarrhea Case Record Form and Dehydration Assessment Chart

Learn to recognise clinical signs of dehydration and classification of diarrhea patients accordingly. You must also inculcate skills of counseling mother on feeding and recognition of danger signs and preparation of ORS. You are required to take case histories of at least 5 children in your workplace record the 5 cases in the format given.

Diarrhea Case Record Form

Registration No .... Admission Date .... Time ....

Discharge Date .... Time ....

Name .... Father's Name ....

Address ....

....

Age ....Years .... Months ....Sex ....

Check for Signs of Dehydration

Child Restless/irritable   Yes/No

Increased thirst	Yes/No
Decreased skin turgor	Yes/No
Mouth and tongue dry	Yes/No
Tears absent	Yes/No
Sunken eyes	Yes/No
Child floppy, lethargic or unconscious	Yes/No
Unable to drink	Yes/No

Decide the degree of dehydration—No dehydration/dehydration/ severe dehydration

Signs of severe malnutrition	Yes/No
Any associated illness	Yes/No
Diagnosis with Degree of dehydration	Yes/No

Weight of the child .... kg.

Before the assessment of the child take a brief history of the diarrhea episode including its duration and whether blood has been in the feces. Also about pre-illness feeding pattern; as well as food and fluids taken since the onset of diarrhea. Immunization status and drugs taken. Now carry out physical examination of the child to assess the degree of dehydration. Nutritional status of the child and presence of infections like pneumonia, otitis media or other associated infections.

Treatment
1. ORS/I.V. fluids:
   - Quantity of ORS in the first 4 hours .... ml
   - Quantity of IV solution:.
     Infant : in first 1 hour IV Solution:
     Infant : in first 1 hour .... next 5 hours ....

   Older children in first 30 min. .... next 2½ hours ....

2. Other children in first 30 min. .... next 2½ hours ....

3. Foods to be given during treatment (including breast milk)?

Progress of the Patient
After 4 hours

Quantity of ORS consumed

No. of stools passed

Episodes of vomiting

Assess for hydration status

Decision taken :
- Child well and sent home ....
- Still dehydrated. degree ....
- Treatment continued with ORS ....
- IV infusion ....
- Others ....

Discharge Advise to the Mother on Home Management of Diarrhea and Dehydration

Fluid .... Foods to other .... Early signs of referral ....

Prevention of diarrhea ....

Immunization status/advise ....

Spacing of next child ....

EVALUATION OF A CASE OF SNAKE BITE

Name .... Age/Sex .... IP No. .... DOA: ....

1. Confirm whether bitten by snake   Yes/No
2. Date and time of bite ....
3. Date and time of reporting to hospital ....
4. First aid measures if any :...
5. Any prior treatment native/PHC ....
6. Any other person bitten by the snake   Yes/No
   If yes the outcome of the bite ....

History (Table 46.14)

Table 46.14: Illustrates history of victim of enable bite

The snake	The bite	The victim
Brought killed snake?	Provoked/unprovoked	Consciousness
Length	Site of bite	Convulsion
Color	Fang marks	Fainting
Hood	Local swelling	Headache
Marks over head and body	Rapid progression of swelling	Vomiting
Species	Pain at the site of bite	Diplopia
Poisonous/non-poisonous	Bleeding at the site of bite	Dysphagia
Circumstantial evidence		Epistaxis
Available snakes in locality		Bleeding gums
Unknown		Hematuria
		Melena
		Hemoptysis
		Pain abdomen
		Jaundice
		Rash
		Muscle cramps

Vitals

1. Temperature
2. PR
3. RR
4. BP   HESS TEST

Local Examination

1. Site of bite
2. Fang marks – No
   Description
3. Bleeding
4. Cellulitis – Level
   Extent
   Progression
5. Gangrene – Extent
   Sloughing

6. Ecchymosis/Petechiae/blebs
7. Temperature
8. Tenderness
9. Numbness
10. Distal pulse
11. Regional LN

Grade:

Systemic Examination

CNS
1. Sensorium
2. Convulsion
3. Orientation
4. Irritability
5. Ptosis
6. Pupils, palatal palsy dysphagia
7. Fasciculation
8. Other neurologic deficit

PA
1. Distention
2. Tenderness
3. Gaurding
4. Bowel sounds

CVS
1. Anemia
2. Heart sounds
3. Arrhythmia

Lungs
1. Pulmonary edema
2. Aspiration

Grade:

Investigations

1. Urine – Macro
         – Alb.
         – Micro (RBC)
2. Stool – Occult blood
3. Blood and serum – Hb%
                   – Blood group
                   – Clotting time
                   – Bleeding time
                   – Urea
                   – Creatinine
                   – Electrolytes
                   – SGOT/SGPT/LDH
                   – PTT
                   – FDP
4. ECG – Bradycardia
       – T-wave inversion
       – Prolonged QTC interval
       – Arrhythmia
5. Chest X-ray

Absolute Indications of ASV
1. Neurotoxic features
2. Bleeding systemic symptoms
3. Unconscious patients
4. Rapidly spreading swelling
5. Hemoglobinuria/myoglobinuria
6. Defective clot quality/prolonged clotting time

Grading of a Case of Snake Bite

Importance
1. To ascertain the clinical stage of envenomation
2. To study the course of venom effect
3. To assess the value of therapeutic agents
4. For the prognosis of the case.

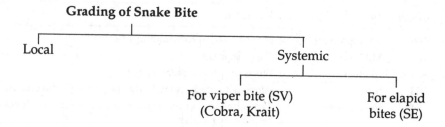

Grading of Local Features
– According to criteria of *Reid et al* Table 46.15.

Table 46.15: Clinical examination of different grades of snake bite

	Grade	Clinical examination
L1	Mild	No local swelling only Fang marks present
L2	Negligible	Final local swelling 1 cm or less
L3	Slight	Final local swelling 1 to 4 cm no necrosis
L4	Moderate	Final local swelling 4 cm and above no necrosis
L5	Severe	Any degree of final local swelling necrosis present

Final Local Swelling
Measure the circumference of bitten limb, at the thinnest part of (1) Foot/hand and (2) Ankle/wrist and also at the thickest part of (3) Calf/forearm and (4) Thigh arm. Record corresponding four measurements in the unbitten limb. The sum of the four figures of bitten limb minus such figures of the unbitten limb gives the final local swelling.

Final local features develop by 48-72 hours in viper bites, hence local grading should be done at admission and subsequently daily (Tables 46.16 and 46.17).

Table 46.16: Viper bite systemic grading (SV)

Grades	Type	Clinical features
SV0	Asymptomatic	No systemic manifestation, no abnormality in lab tests
SV1	Asymptomatic	No hemorrhagic manifestation, hemoptysis on forced cough or positive Hess test
		Microscopic hematuria.
SV2	Mild	Frank hemorrhagic manifestation
		Blood pressure normal.
SV3	Severe	Along with ptosis, palatal palsy, respiratory failure
		Delirium.
SV4	Very severe	Severe hemorrhage and fatal complications like subarachnoid hemorrhage which develops within short period, i.e. 3-6 hours.

Table 46.17: Elapid bite systemic grading (SE)

Grades	Type	Clinical features
SE0	Asymptomatic	No systemic signs vomiting +/−
SE1	Mild	Ptosis is present
SE2	Moderate	Ptosis dysphagia palatal palsy
SE3	Severe	Along with ptosis, palatal palsy, respiratory failure delirium
SE4	Very severe	Temporal sequence very rapid (< 3 hours) to develop respiratory paralysis.
		Deliruim and coma

E.g.: A cobra bite can be graded as follows:

L1	SE0	—	No local no systemic
L2	SE2	—	Mild local no systemic
L5	SE2	—	Severe local moderate systemic
L2	SE4	—	Mild local severe systemic

How Can You Differentiate Poisonous from Non-poisonous Snakes (Fig. 46.1 and Table 46.18)

Table 46.18: Comparative account of poisonous and non-poisonous snakes

Non-venomous		Venomous
Oval	Head	Large and triangular (pit vipers); small and narrow (coral snake)
Round	Pupils	Vertically elliptical (pit vipers); round (coral snake)
Absent	Pit organs	present in all pit vipers (copperhead, cottonmouth, rattlesnakes); absent in coral snake
Absent	Fangs	Present in all venomous species. Large, long, recurved teeth. Long and movable in pit vipers. Short, erect, and fixed in coral snake. Usually 2 (1 on each side upper jaw) unless shed or reserve fangs also in use.

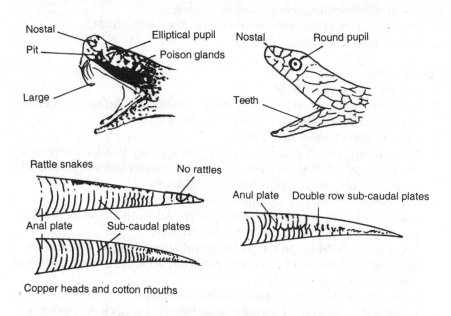

Poisonous (pit vipers)   Harmless

Nostal — Elliptical pupil   Nostal   Round pupil
Pit — Poison glands
Large   Teeth

Rattle snakes   No rattles
Anul plate   Double row sub-caudal plates
Anal plate   Sub-caudal plates

Copper heads and cotton mouths

Fig. 46.1: Ways to differentiate poisonous from non-poisonous snakes

EVALUATION OF A CASE OF DIABETIC KETOACIDOSIS
(Diabetic coma)

PRESENTING COMPLAINTS AND HISTORY OF PRESENTING ILLNESS

1. Classic triad—polyuria, polyphagia, polydypsia.
2. Weight loss despite polyphagia
3. Symptoms suggestive of infections:
   Pulmonary tuberculosis
   Skin infections, UTI
   Recent viral infection e.g. mumps, rubella, etc.
4. Symptoms suggestive of ketoacidosis—vomiting, abdominal pain.
5. Symptoms suggestive and pancreatitis—acute abdominal pain.
6. Symptoms suggestive of hypoglycemia—sweating, pallor tremors, hunger, headache, bad temper, dizziness and fits.
7. Symptoms suggestive of complications.
   a. Eye—Cataract-vision
      Refractive errors—reading problems
      Retinopathy—usually after 15-20 years after onset- vision failure.
   b. Nephropathy—rare in children
   c. Neuropathy (rare in children)—Paresthesia (distal), autonomic, carpal tunnel syndrome, mononeuropathy (cranial nerves)
   d. Limited joint mobility.
8. Ask about treatment and its response, complications of treatment, fat atrophy, insulin allergy, degree of control, frequency of hypoglycemia.

9. Diet followed
10. Social effect—child, siblings, family, coping.
11. Family history of diabetes, autoimmune disease (thyroid).
12. Immunization, mumps.

Examination

1. Growth assessment/SMR
2. Syndromes associated with diabetes-DIDMOD, Turner, Klinefelter, Pradder Willi, Friedreich's ataxia, Cushing's syndrome.
3. Signs of dehydration-Ketoacidosis
4. Eyes-squint, visual acuity, cataract, neuropathy (ocular movements, pupillary reflex), fundus (retinopathy-background lesions, proliferative lesion, maculopathy, optic atrophy-DIDMOD),
5. Oral cavity-dry tongue, candidiasis, ketone breath.
6. Associated autoimmune disease-goiter, Addison's disease (knuckle pigmentation, pigmentation of palmar creases).
7. Hepatomegaly-Mauriac syndrome (short stature, hepatomegaly, round face and diabetes mellitus), protruberant abdomen, truncal obesity, associated with poor control.
8. Look for associated infections-TB, ENT, UTI, skin.
9. Limited joint mobility-'Namaste' or cathedral sign (lack of apposition).
10. Therapy related-fat atrophy and hypertrophy
11. Peripheral neuropathy evidence, trophic changes.
12. Neurobiosis lipoidica diabeticorum
13. BP-increased blood pressure, nephropathy, postural hypotension in autonomic neuropathy, hypotension in Addison's disease.
14. Signs often seen in malnutrition related diabetes-bilateral parotid swelling, abdominal distention and pancreatic calcifications.

Evaluation of Diabetic Ketoacidosis

It comprises of two types of evaluation—clinical and diagnostic.

Clinical Evaluation
– Conscious
– Semiconscious
– Comatose

Symptoms to be asked for
– Polyuria
– Polydypsia
– Weakness
– Lethargy
– Myalgia
– Headache
– Nausea
– Others

– Vomiting
– Abdominal pain
– Dyspnea
– Look for infection
  • Skin and chest infection
  • Fungal candidiasis
  • Urinary tract infection

Signs of Diabetic Ketoacidosis
1. Respiratory system
   - Kussmaul's respiration
   - Smell of breath
2. Gastro-intestinal system
   - Acute abdomen
   - Distention of abdomen

Assess the Amount of Dehydration (Table 46.19)

Table 46.19: Illustrates assessment of mild, moderate and severe dehydration

Dehydration	Mild	Moderate	Severe
Volume deficit			
> 2 years	30 ml/kg	60 ml/kg	90 ml/kg
< 2 years	50 ml/kg	100 ml/kg	150 ml/kg
Clinical features			
Peripheral pulses	Normal	Normal or decreased	Decreased or absent
Capillary filling time	< 2 second	< 2-3 seconds	< 3 seconds
Skin temperature	Normal	Normal or cold	Cold
Heart rate	Normal or Mild increase	Moderately increased	Moderate to severely increased

Central Nervous System
- Hyporeflexia
- Hypotonia
- Stupor-coma
- Uncoordinated occular movements
- Fixed dilated pupils

Laboratory Parameters for Diabetic Ketoacidosis
- Blood glucose > 300 mg/dl
- Ketonuria/ketonemia
- pH < 7.3
- Serum bicarbonates
- Serum Na and K
- Blood urea
- Serum creatinine
- ECG
- Anion gap
- Chest X-ray
- Blood counts
- PPD
- Urine routine and culture

Assessment Base on Osmolar Value of Plasma
324 mOsmol/kg .... Drowsy
340 mOsmol/kg .... Semicoma
370 mOsmol/kg .... Coma

Diabetic Ketoacidosis Follow-up Chart

Hours after Admission	0	½	1	1½	2	2½	3	3½	4	4.½	5
Dextrostix											
Blood glucose											
Ketostix											
Na/K											
Ca/PO$_4$											
ABG											
BUN											
Creatinine											
Urine glucose											
Urine ketones											
Insulin/U/kg											
Fluid in											
Fluid out											
BP											
HR											
RR											
ECG											

SECTION 6

Pediatric Records
&
Appendices

47 Pediatric Records

- Out patient records (OP)
- Inpatient records (IP)
- Pediatric intensive care records
- Discharge summary sheet
- Referral sheet
- — Growth charts (Refer Charts 31.1, 31.2, 31.3A and B, 31.4)
  — Road to health IAP (Refer Chart 31.6)
  — NCHS (Refer Tables 31.12 and 31.13)
  — Agarwal, etc. (Refer Appendix 47.1 to 47.15).
- Genetic charts
- Nutritional and survey charts

OUTPATIENT RECORD SHEET

Name :   OP no :

Age :   Date :

Sex :

Address :

Chief complaints :

H/o presenting illness :

Relevant past history :

Relevant family history :

Relevant antenatal, natal and postnatal history :

Immunization history :

Developmental history :

Dietic history :

Comprehensive summary :

General observations :

Vital signs :

Anthropometry :

Relevant head to foot examination   (in relation to symptoms or suspected disease) :

Systemic examination (Brief and quick in relation to the disease and its complication) :

R/S

CVS

CNS

P/A

Impression/provisional diagnosis :

Investigation :

Follow up :

INPATIENT RECORDS

Name of the child :   OP/IP no :

Age :   Unit :

Sex :   Date of birth :

Address :   Date of admission :

                                       Time of admission :

Telephone No :   Date of discharge :

Family names : Father/mother/grand parents :

Informant :

Chief complaints (In chronological order) :

History of presenting illness :

Important negative history :

Past history :

Family history (Pedigree—three generation chart) :

Antenatal/natal/postnatal history :

Immunization history :

Developmental history :

Dietic/feeding history :

Socioeconomic status :

Summary of the history :

General physical examination :
  a. General appearance of child :
  b. Vital signs :
  c. Anthropometry
  d. Head to foot examination (Regional) :

Systemic examination :

Central nervous system :

  Higher mental functions :

  Cranial nerves :

  Motor system :

  Sensory system :

  Cerebellar signs :

  Meningeal signs :

  Autonomic nervous system :

  Superficial and deep reflexes

  Primitive and somatic reflexes :

  Skull and spine :

Cardiovascular system :

  Inspection :

  Palpation :

  Percussion :

  Auscultation :

Respiratory system :
    Inspection :
    Palpation :
    Percussion :
    Auscultation :

Per abdomen :
    Inspection :
    Palpation :
    Percussion :
    Auscultation :

Other systemic examination :
Case oriented examination :
Summary of examination findings :
Provisional diagnosis :
Investigations :
Final diagnosis :
Treatment :
Advise on discharge :
Follow up :

MONITORING IN PICU SET UP

Name : .... I.P. No : ....

Age : .... Unit : ....

Sex : .... Diagnosis : ....

                                                       Dates : ....

Neurological Monitoring :
Level of Consciousness :

Coma scale :

Respiratory Monitoring :

Respiratory Rate

Oral/Tracheal Secretions

Air Way Patency

Retraction

Grunting

Color

Air Entry

Chest

Breath Sounds

RDS Grading

Stridor

Wheeze

Chest X-ray

Blood Gas Analysis

PaO_2

PCO_2

PH

HCO_3

Cardiac Monitoring :   Dates

Heart Rate

Pulse

BP

CVP

Peripheral Pulses

Capillary Filling Time

Skin Temperature

Skin Color

Cardiac Size

Peripheral Signs of Shock

Signs of CCF

Renal Monitoring

Urine Output

Fluid Intake

Weight

Sp. Gravity of Urine

Albumin in Urine

Serum Na
Serum K
Serum   Creatinine
               BUN
               Glucose
               Calcium

GIT Monitoring :

Abdomen Girth
Stool Blood
Gastric Content
Feeding

Hematological Monitoring :

Hematocrit

Platelets

Bleeding Time

Clotting Time

PT/APTT

Biochemical Monitoring :

Blood Glucose

Serum Calcium

Serum Sodium

Serum Potassium

Septic Screening

Absolute Neutrophilic Count

Band Forms

C-Reactive Protein

Blood Culture and Sensitivity

Pharmacological Monitoring

Drugs—Dose Frequency

Drug Toxicity

DISCHARGE SUMMARY SHEET

Name : .... Age .... Sex ....

Date of birth .... Date of discharge .... Hospital No. ....

Birth weight .... Wt. at discharge .... Length ....

Suggested diet ....

....

Medications ....

....

....

....

....

....

....

Return visit: Date .... Time ....

Place .... Phone ....

Pediatrician's name: ....

Relevant antenatal history: ....

....

....

....

....

....

Complete diagnosis of all problems in chronological order: ....

....

....

....

....

Details of each diagnosis : ....

....

....

....

....

Course in the hospital : ....
....
....
....

Special instructions: ....
....
....
....
....

Other instructions : ....
....
....
....
....
....

REFERRAL SHEET

Name of the Hospital : .... Name of the child : ....
                                                     OP/IP No.: ....
Address of the Hospital : .... Date of birth : ....
                .... Time of birth : ....
                .... Age of the child : ....

Address of the patient : ....
....

Telephone: .... Unit : .... Date of discharge : ....
Family names: Mother .... Father ....
Grand parents ....
Diagnosis :...
....
....

Information given to family regarding prognosis : ....
Reasons for referral : ....
....
....
....

Problems	Plan
....	....
....	....
....	....
....	....
....	....
....	....
....	....
....	....

Patients discharge information including procedures, medications, treatments, referrals and individualized care plan   ☐ is attached

(please tick right in the box)   ☐ will be sent later

Name of the referring Doctor : ....

Signature :..

Additional refferals made to: ....

Report to be sent back to : ....

Referral given to : ....

Name of the Hospital : .... Address: ....

Name of the Doctor : .... Telephone number: ....

APPENDIX 47.1

WEIGHT (KG) OF INDIAN CHILDREN FROM BIRTH TO 6 YEARS (BOYS AND GIRLS)

Boys Percentiles							Age (Months)	Girls Percentiles						
3rd	10th	25th	50th	75th	90th	97th		3rd	10th	25th	50th	75th	90th	97th
2.54	2.69	3.01	3.14	3.49	3.72	4.04	0	2.53	2.66	2.95	3.15	3.41	3.76	3.93
4.78	4.95	5.29	5.65	6.04	6.41	6.71	3	4.50	4.79	5.04	5.44	5.91	6.25	6.63
6.24	6.50	6.86	7.35	7.77	8.24	8.64	6	5.86	6.25	6.54	7.03	7.59	7.94	8.44
7.17	7.56	7.95	8.49	8.94	9.49	10.06	9	6.79	7.24	7.62	8.13	8.70	9.10	9.64
7.80	8.32	8.75	9.32	9.80	10.42	11.17	12	7.47	7.96	8.45	8.96	9.55	9.96	10.5
8.86	9.58	10.08	10.71	11.26	12.02	13.06	18	8.57	9.10	9.81	10.36	10.91	11.49	12.17
9.77	10.59	11.18	11.89	12.53	13.43	14.66	24	9.44	10.08	10.91	11.55	12.18	12.87	13.73
10.56	11.43	12.11	12.90	13.65	14.69	16.02	30	10.14	10.87	11.80	12.57	13.33	14.15	15.23
11.25	12.14	12.91	13.78	14.66	15.83	17.20	36	10.75	11.56	12.42	13.48	14.40	15.32	16.66
11.89	12.78	13.64	14.60	15.60	16.88	18.28	42	11.31	12.22	13.23	14.31	15.40	16.44	18.03
12.51	13.41	14.36	15.39	16.51	17.89	19.30	48	11.90	12.89	13.90	15.12	16.37	17.50	19.35
13.12	14.09	15.11	16.19	17.43	18.88	20.34	54	12.58	13.64	14.63	15.94	17.31	18.53	20.64
13.77	14.88	15.96	17.07	18.40	19.90	21.46	60	13.40	14.53	15.47	16.82	18.26	19.55	21.89
14.48	15.82	16.95	18.05	19.46	20.97	22.71	66	14.43	15.62	16.50	17.80	19.25	20.59	23.10
15.28	16.98	18.10	19.19	20.65	22.14	24.16	72	15.73	16.96	17.78	18.94	20.28	21.67	24.30

Data from: Physical and sexual growth of affluent Indian children from Birth to 6 yrs. Agarwal DK, Indian pediatrics. 1992;29:1203-84.

APPENDIX 47.2

WEIGHT (KG) OF MEAN AND PERCENTILES OF INDIAN BOYS AND GIRLS (5 TO 18 YEARS)[*]

| Boys (Percentiles) | | | | | | | Age | Girls (Percentiles) | | | | | | |
Mean	3rd	10th	25th	50th	75th	97th	(Year)	Mean	3rd	10th	25th	50th	75th	97th
17.4	13.8	14.9	16.0	17.1	18.4	21.5	5.0	17.0	13.6	14.6	15.6	16.8	18.2	21.1
18.4	14.5	15.8	17.0	18.1	19.5	22.7	5.5	17.9	14.0	15.2	16.0	17.4	18.8	22.2
19.2	15.2	16.2	18.0	19.0	20.7	25.4	6.0	18.7	14.1	15.7	16.4	17.8	19.2	23.7
20.6	15.7	17.4	18.6	20.0	21.9	27.7	6.5	19.6	14.4	16.1	16.9	18.3	19.9	25.4
21.0	16.2	18.2	19.4	21.0	22.9	29.7	7.0	20.5	14.8	16.4	17.3	19.0	20.9	27.5
22.4	16.8	18.7	20.0	22.0	23.9	31.6	7.5	21.7	15.3	16.9	18.0	19.9	22.2	29.8
23.5	17.5	19.1	20.7	22.6	25.0	33.5	8.0	23.0	15.9	17.2	18.7	20.8	23.6	32.3
24.5	18.2	19.7	21.3	23.5	26.3	35.5	8.5	24.9	16.4	17.8	19.6	22.0	25.3	34.9
26.5	19.2	20.3	22.0	24.4	27.7	37.7	9.0	25.8	17.1	18.7	20.7	23.5	27.2	37.7
26.8	19.9	21.2	22.9	25.6	29.4	40.1	9.5	27.5	18.3	19.7	22.1	25.1	29.3	40.5
28.7	20.9	22.3	24.1	27.0	31.3	42.7	10.0	29.6	19.5	21.0	23.6	26.9	31.4	43.4
30.8	21.9	23.5	25.5	28.7	33.4	45.4	10.5	31.9	20.9	22.4	25.3	28.9	33.7	46.4
31.9	22.9	24.9	27.1	30.6	35.6	48.2	11.0	34.3	22.3	24.0	27.1	30.9	36.0	49.3
33.8	24.1	26.3	28.9	32.7	37.9	51.1	11.5	36.8	23.7	25.6	28.9	32.9	38.4	52.2
35.4	25.3	27.9	30.7	34.8	40.3	54.1	12.0	38.7	25.1	27.3	30.8	35.0	40.7	55.1
37.9	26.7	29.6	32.7	37.1	42.7	57.1	12.5	41.9	26.5	29.0	32.6	37.1	42.9	57.9
39.4	28.1	31.3	34.7	39.4	45.1	60.0	13.0	42.6	27.9	30.7	34.5	39.1	45.1	60.7
43.2	29.6	33.1	36.8	41.8	47.6	63.0	13.5	45.2	29.3	32.4	36.2	41.0	47.1	63.2
44.7	31.2	34.9	38.8	44.1	50.0	65.9	14.0	45.7	30.7	34.0	37.8	42.7	48.9	65.7
48.1	32.9	36.7	40.9	46.3	52.4	68.7	14.5	46.6	32.1	35.5	39.3	44.3	50.5	67.9
51.0	34.6	38.6	42.8	48.5	54.6	71.4	15.0	48.0	33.4	36.9	40.6	45.7	51.8	70.0
52.4	36.5	40.3	44.7	50.5	56.8	73.9	15.5	48.9	34.6	38.2	41.7	46.8	52.9	71.8
54.0	38.5	42.1	46.5	52.4	58.8	76.3	16.0	49.2	35.7	39.3	42.5	47.7	53.6	73.3
55.0	40.6	43.8	48.1	54.0	60.6	78.5	16.5	49.4	36.7	40.1	43.0	48.2	54.0	74.6
56.6	42.8	45.9	50.0	55.5	62.3	80.5	17.0	50.0	37.6	40.7	43.3	48.4	53.9	75.9
56.9	45.2	46.9	52.0	57.2	63.7	82.2	17.5							
59.7	47.6	48.3	54.0	58.6	64.9	83.6	18.0							

Data from: Physical and sexual growth of affluent Indian children from 5 to 18 years. Agarwal DK, Agarwal KN, Upadhyay SK, *et al.*, Indian pediatrics. 1992;29:1203-84.

APPENDIX 47.3

LENGTH OR HEIGHT (CM) OF INDIAN CHILDREN FROM BIRTH TO 6 YEARS

| | Boys | | | | | | | Age | Girls | | | | | | |
| | Percentiles | | | | | | | (Months) | Percentiles | | | | | | |
3rd	10th	25th	50th	75th	90th	97th			3rd	10th	25th	50th	75th	90th	97th
47.55	48.20	49.25	50.38	51.18	52.23	53.28		0	47.46	48.39	49.26	50.27	51.25	52.06	53.10
56.34	57.36	58.20	59.36	60.57	61.99	63.75		3	55.75	57.12	58.06	59.10	60.32	61.47	62.90
62.49	63.70	64.64	65.86	67.24	68.74	70.76		6	61.55	63.62	64.31	65.45	66.77	68.13	69.70
56.80	68.08	69.30	70.60	71.99	73.42	75.40		9	65.59	67.48	68.78	70.04	71.48	72.27	74.43
70.06	71.37	72.92	74.32	75.67	76.98	78.82		12	68.64	70.70	72.23	73.49	74.98	76.54	78.04
75.55	77.00	79.02	80.67	82.01	83.25	84.94		18	73.82	76.18	78.08	79.77	81.20	82.90	84.42
80.14	81.83	84.09	86.00	87.46	88.86	90.33		24	78.22	80.86	83.03	84.97	86.58	88.42	90.16
84.01	85.99	88.33	90.51	92.18	93.90	95.90		30	81.99	84.88	87.24	89.93	91.26	93.23	95.30
87.30	89.60	91.93	94.35	96.32	98.46	100.77		36	86.00	88.39	90.88	93.26	95.37	97.45	99.82
90.17	92.77	95.09	97.73	100.01	102.60	105.24		42	88.32	91.54	94.12	96.68	99.04	101.20	103.98
92.79	95.64	98.00	100.80	103.41	106.41	109.33		48	91.19	94.47	97.13	99.82	102.41	104.61	107.63
95.32	98.32	100.85	103.74	106.67	110.97	113.06		54	94.08	97.34	100.08	102.87	105.51	107.51	110.87
97.90	100.94	103.85	106.74	109.93	113.36	116.43		60	97.15	100.30	103.13	105.99	108.78	110.91	113.87
100.71	103.62	107.18	109.95	113.33	116.67	119.46		66	100.56	103.49	106.45	109.34	112.04	114.05	116.38
103.89	106.47	111.04	113.59	117.04	119.06	122.16		72	104.46	107.06	110.22	113.09	115.53	117.35	118.73

Data from: Agarwal DK et al., Indian pediatrics. 1992;29:1203-04.

APPENDIX 47.4

HEIGHT (CM) MEAN AND PERCENTILES ON INDIAN BOYS AND GIRLS (5 TO 18 YEARS)*

Boys (Percentiles)							Age	Girls (Percentiles)						
Mean	3rd	10th	25th	50th	75th	97th	(Year)	Mean	3rd	10th	25th	50th	75th	97th
107.1	97.9	100.4	103.8	106.7	109.9	116.4	5.0	106.0	97.2	100.3	103.1	106.0	108.8	113.8
110.4	100.7	103.6	107.2	109.9	113.3	119.5	5.5	109.4	99.6	103.5	105.0	108.1	112.2	116.4
113.7	103.7	106.9	112.0	114.2	118.0	125.9	6.0	113.0	102.1	106.1	108.8	112.5	115.9	123.3
117.5	106.1	109.6	113.5	117.3	120.7	128.4	6.5	115.4	104.5	108.4	111.1	114.9	118.4	126.0
118.6	108.5	112.0	115.9	119.7	23.0	130.8	7.0	118.2	107.1	110.7	113.7	117.4	121.3	129.3
121.6	110.9	114.2	117.8	121.6	125.2	133.2	7.5	120.2	109.7	113.1	116.4	120.3	124.4	132.8
124.1	113.3	116.3	119.7	123.6	127.4	135.8	8.0	122.7	112.3	115.5	119.3	123.2	127.5	136.4
126.4	115.2	118.6	121.9	125.7	129.8	138.5	8.5	126.2	115.0	118.1	122.2	126.2	130.7	139.8
130.4	118.0	120.9	124.2	128.2	132.5	141.4	9.0	128.6	117.8	120.9	125.1	129.2	133.8	143.1
131.5	120.3	123.4	126.7	130.8	135.3	144.5	9.5	131.9	120.6	123.6	128.0	132.3	136.9	146.2
134.7	122.7	125.9	129.4	133.6	138.3	147.7	10.0	134.8	123.4	126.5	130.8	135.2	139.8	149.0
137.6	125.1	128.6	132.2	136.6	141.5	151.0	10.5	137.9	126.1	129.3	133.7	138.1	142.7	151.7
139.6	127.5	131.2	135.6	139.6	144.7	154.3	11.0	141.3	128.8	132.1	136.4	140.9	145.4	154.2
142.3	129.9	133.9	138.0	142.7	147.9	157.5	11.5	144.3	131.4	134.8	139.0	143.5	147.9	156.5
144.7	132.4	136.6	141.0	145.8	151.1	160.8	12.0	146.7	133.9	137.4	141.5	146.0	150.3	158.5
147.9	134.9	139.3	143.9	148.9	154.2	163.9	12.5	149.9	136.3	139.8	143.8	148.3	152.5	160.4
150.3	137.4	142.0	146.8	152.0	157.3	166.9	13.0	151.4	138.5	142.1	145.9	150.4	154.4	162.1
154.9	140.0	144.7	149.7	154.9	160.2	169.7	13.5	153.2	140.6	144.1	147.8	152.2	156.2	163.5
158.0	142.6	147.4	152.4	157.6	162.9	172.3	14.0	153.6	142.4	145.9	149.4	153.8	157.6	164.7
161.4	145.2	149.9	155.0	160.2	165.4	174.7	14.5	154.8	144.1	147.4	150.8	155.1	158.8	165.8
164.3	148.0	152.4	157.4	162.5	167.7	176.8	15.0	155.0	145.5	148.6	151.8	156.0	159.7	166.5
165.5	150.8	154.9	159.6	164.6	169.6	178.5	15.5	155.4	146.6	149.3	152.6	156.6	160.4	167.1
167.1	153.6	157.9	161.6	166.3	171.2	179.8	16.0	155.8	147.5	149.7	152.9	156.8	160.4	167.4
167.9	156.6	159.4	163.3	167.7	172.4	180.7	16.5	156.0	148.0	149.7	152.9	156.5	160.5	167.6
168.6	159.6	161.5	165.0	168.7	173.1	181.2	17.0	157.1	148.3	149.8	153.0	157.0	160.5	168.0
169.4	162.7	163.4	167.5	169.3	173.4	181.1	17.5							
169.8	161.0	164.0	168.8	169.8	173.4	181.6	18.0							

*Data from: Physical and sexual growth of affluent Indian children from 5 to 18 years of age. Agarwal DK, Agarwal KN, Upadhyay SK, et al. Indian Pediatrics, 1992;29: 1203-1284.

APPENDIX 47.5

MEANS OF SITTING HEIGHT (CM) AND LEG LENGTH (CM) ACCORDING TO SEX AT DIFFERENT AGE POINTS

Age (year)	Boys		Girls	
	Sitting height	Leg length	Sitting height	Leg length
6.0	61.7	55.1	60.6	53.5
6.5	62.3	56.1	61.5	55.3
7.0	63.1	57.3	62.4	57.1
7.5	64.1	58.6	63.4	58.7
8.0	65.4	60.1	64.4	60.2
8.5	65.8	61.5	65.9	62.4
9.0	66.9	63.1	67.2	64.1
9.5	68.1	64.8	68.9	65.6
10.0	69.3	66.5	69.8	67.2
10.5	70.6	68.2	71.2	68.6
11.0	71.9	70.0	72.5	69.9
11.5	73.2	71.7	73.8	71.1
12.0	74.6	73.4	75.1	72.2
12.5	75.9	75.0	76.2	73.2
13.0	77.2	76.5	77.3	74.0
13.5	78.5	77.9	78.3	74.7
14.0	79.8	79.2	79.2	75.2
14.5	81.0	80.4	79.9	75.5
15.0	82.2	81.4	80.4	75.7
15.5	83.3	82.2	80.8	75.7
16.0	84.3	82.8	81.0	75.8
16.5	85.2	83.2	81.0	75.8
17.0	86.0	83.3	81.0	75.8
17.5	86.7	83.3		
18.0	87.2	83.3		

Data from Physical and sexual growth of affluent Indian children from *Indian Pediatrics 1992;29:1203-1284.*

APPENDIX 47.6

MEAN BIACROMIAL AND BICRISTAL DIAMETER (CM) FOR BOYS AND GIRLS AT DIFFERENT AGE POINTS

Age (year)	Boys		Girls	
	Biacromial	Bicristal	Biacromial	Bicristal
6.0	25.1	17.6	24.4	17.3
6.5	25.4	17.7	24.8	17.4
7.0	25.8	18.0	25.3	17.7
7.5	26.2	18.3	25.8	18.0
8.0	26.7	18.8	26.3	18.4
8.5	27.0	18.9	27.0	18.9
9.0	27.5	19.3	27.6	19.4
9.5	28.0	19.7	28.2	20.0
10.0	28.6	20.1	28.8	20.5
10.5	29.2	20.5	29.4	21.5
11.0	29.8	21.0	30.0	21.7
11.5	30.4	21.4	30.0	22.3
12.0	31.0	21.9	31.2	22.8
12.5	31.6	22.3	31.7	23.4
13.0	32.3	22.8	32.2	23.9
13.5	32.9	23.2	32.6	24.3
14.0	33.5	23.6	33.0	24.7
14.5	34.1	24.0	33.3	25.1
15.0	34.7	24.4	33.6	25.3
15.5	35.3	24.8	33.7	25.5
16.0	35.9	25.1	33.8	25.5
16.5	36.4	25.4	33.8	25.5
17.0	36.9	25.6	33.8	25.5
17.5	37.4	25.8		
18.0	37.9	26.0		

Agarwal DK, Agarwal KN, Upadhyay SK, *et al., Indian Pediatrics 1992.*

APPENDIX 47.7

WEIGHT (KG) BY AGE OF
BOYS AGED 0 TO 36 MONTHS (NCHS STANDARDS)

Age (Months)	Percentiles													Standard Deviations							Age (Months)
	3rd	5th	10th	20th	30th	40th	50th	60th	70th	80th	90th	95th	97th	-3S.D.	-2S.D.	-1S.D.	Median	+1S.D.	+2S.D.	+3S.D.	
0	2.5	2.6	2.7	2.9	3.1	3.2	3.3	3.4	3.5	3.7	3.9	4.1	4.2	2.0	2.4	2.9	3.3	3.8	4.3	4.8	0
1	3.0	3.2	3.4	3.7	3.9	4.1	4.3	4.5	4.6	4.9	5.1	5.4	5.6	2.2	2.9	3.6	4.3	5.0	5.6	6.3	1
2	3.6	3.8	4.1	4.5	4.7	5.0	5.2	5.4	5.6	5.9	6.2	6.5	6.7	2.6	3.5	4.3	5.2	6.0	6.8	7.6	2
3	4.2	4.4	4.8	5.2	5.5	5.7	6.0	6.2	6.4	6.7	7.1	7.4	7.6	3.1	4.1	5.0	6.0	6.9	7.7	8.6	3
4	4.8	5.1	5.4	5.8	6.2	6.4	6.7	6.9	7.2	7.5	7.9	8.2	8.4	3.7	4.7	5.7	6.7	7.6	8.5	9.4	4
5	5.4	5.7	6.0	6.5	6.8	7.0	7.3	7.5	7.8	8.1	8.5	8.9	9.1	4.3	5.3	6.3	7.3	8.2	9.2	10.1	5
6	6.0	6.2	6.6	7.0	7.3	7.6	7.8	8.1	8.4	8.7	9.1	9.4	9.7	4.9	5.9	6.9	7.8	8.8	9.8	10.8	6
7	6.5	6.7	7.1	7.5	7.8	8.1	8.3	8.6	8.9	9.2	9.6	10.0	10.2	5.4	6.4	7.4	8.3	9.3	10.3	11.3	7
8	7.0	7.2	7.5	8.0	8.3	8.5	8.8	9.0	9.3	9.6	10.1	10.5	10.7	5.9	6.9	7.8	8.8	9.8	10.8	11.8	8
9	7.4	7.6	7.9	8.4	8.7	8.9	9.2	9.4	9.7	10.1	10.5	10.9	11.1	6.3	7.2	8.2	9.2	10.2	11.3	12.3	9
10	7.7	7.9	8.3	8.7	9.0	9.3	9.5	9.8	10.1	10.4	10.9	11.3	11.5	6.6	7.6	8.6	9.5	10.6	11.7	12.7	10
11	8.0	8.2	8.6	9.0	9.3	9.6	9.9	10.1	10.4	10.8	11.3	11.6	11.9	6.9	7.9	8.9	9.9	10.9	12.0	13.1	11
12	8.2	8.5	8.8	9.3	9.6	9.9	10.2	10.4	10.7	11.1	11.6	12.0	12.2	7.1	8.1	9.1	10.2	11.3	12.4	13.5	12
13	8.5	8.7	9.1	9.5	9.9	10.1	10.4	10.7	11.0	11.4	11.9	12.3	12.5	7.3	8.3	9.4	10.4	11.5	12.7	13.8	13
14	8.7	8.9	9.3	9.8	10.1	10.4	10.7	10.9	11.3	11.6	12.1	12.6	12.8	7.5	8.5	9.6	10.7	11.8	13.0	14.1	14
15	8.8	9.1	9.5	10.0	10.3	10.6	10.9	11.2	11.5	11.9	12.4	12.8	13.1	7.6	8.7	9.8	10.9	12.0	13.2	14.4	15
16	9.0	9.2	9.6	10.1	10.5	10.8	11.1	11.4	11.7	12.1	12.6	13.0	13.3	7.7	8.8	10.0	11.1	12.3	13.5	14.7	16
17	9.1	9.4	9.8	10.3	10.7	11.0	11.3	11.6	11.9	12.3	12.8	13.3	13.6	7.8	9.0	10.1	11.3	12.5	13.7	14.9	17
18	9.3	9.5	10.0	10.5	10.9	11.2	11.5	11.8	12.1	12.5	13.0	13.5	13.8	7.9	9.1	10.3	11.5	12.7	13.9	15.2	18

Contd...

Contd....

Age (Months)	Percentiles													Standard Deviations							Age (Months)
	3rd	5th	10th	20th	30th	40th	50th	60th	70th	80th	90th	95th	97th	-3S.D.	-2S.D.	-1S.D.	Median	+1S.D.	+2S.D.	+3S.D.	
19	9.4	9.7	10.1	10.6	11.0	11.4	11.7	12.0	12.3	12.7	13.3	13.7	14.0	8.0	9.2	10.5	11.7	12.9	14.1	15.4	19
20	9.5	9.8	10.3	10.8	11.2	11.5	11.8	12.2	12.5	12.9	13.5	13.9	14.2	8.1	9.4	10.6	11.8	13.1	14.4	15.6	20
21	9.7	10.0	10.4	11.0	11.4	11.7	12.0	12.4	12.7	13.1	13.7	14.1	14.4	8.3	9.5	10.8	12.0	13.3	14.6	15.8	21
22	9.8	10.1	10.6	11.1	11.5	11.9	12.2	12.5	12.9	13.3	13.9	14.3	14.6	8.4	9.7	10.9	12.2	13.5	14.8	16.0	22
23	9.9	10.3	10.7	11.3	11.7	12.1	12.4	12.7	13.1	13.5	14.1	14.5	14.8	8.5	9.8	11.1	12.4	13.7	15.0	16.3	23
24	10.1	10.4	10.9	11.5	11.9	12.3	12.6	12.9	13.3	13.7	14.2	14.7	15.0	8.6	9.9	11.3	12.6	13.9	15.2	16.5	24
25	10.2	10.5	11.0	11.6	12.1	12.4	12.8	13.1	13.5	13.9	14.4	14.9	15.2	8.7	10.1	11.4	12.8	14.1	15.4	16.7	25
26	10.4	10.7	11.2	11.8	12.2	12.6	13.0	13.3	13.6	14.1	14.6	15.1	15.4	8.8	10.2	11.6	13.0	14.3	15.6	16.9	26
27	10.5	10.8	11.3	12.0	12.4	12.8	13.1	13.5	13.8	14.2	14.8	15.3	15.6	8.9	10.3	11.7	13.1	14.5	15.8	17.1	27
28	10.6	11.0	11.5	12.1	12.6	13.0	13.3	13.7	14.0	14.4	15.0	15.5	15.8	9.1	10.5	11.9	13.3	14.6	16.0	17.3	28
29	10.8	11.1	11.7	12.3	12.7	13.1	13.5	13.8	14.2	14.6	15.2	15.7	16.0	9.2	10.6	12.1	13.5	14.8	16.2	17.5	29
30	10.9	11.3	11.8	12.4	12.9	13.3	13.7	14.0	14.4	14.8	15.4	15.9	16.2	9.3	10.8	12.2	13.7	15.0	16.4	17.7	30
31	11.1	11.4	12.0	12.6	13.1	13.5	13.8	14.2	14.6	15.0	15.6	16.1	16.4	9.4	10.9	12.4	13.8	15.2	16.6	17.9	31
32	11.2	11.6	12.1	12.8	13.2	13.6	14.0	14.4	14.7	15.2	15.8	16.3	16.6	9.5	11.0	12.5	14.0	15.4	16.8	18.2	32
33	11.3	11.7	12.3	12.9	13.4	13.8	14.2	14.5	14.9	15.4	16.0	16.5	16.8	9.7	11.2	12.7	14.2	15.6	17.0	18.4	33
34	11.5	11.8	12.4	13.1	13.6	14.0	14.4	14.7	15.1	15.6	16.2	16.7	17.0	9.8	11.3	12.8	14.4	15.8	17.2	18.6	34
35	11.6	12.0	12.5	13.2	13.7	14.1	14.5	14.9	15.3	15.7	16.4	16.9	17.3	9.9	11.4	13.0	14.5	16.0	17.4	18.9	35
36	11.8	12.1	12.7	13.4	13.9	14.3	14.7	15.1	15.5	15.9	16.6	17.1	17.5	10.0	11.6	13.1	14.7	16.2	17.7	19.1	36

APPENDIX 47.8

WEIGHT (KG) BY AGE OF BOYS AGED 2 TO 18 YEARS (NCHS STANDARDS)

Age Yrs Mths	Percentiles													Standard Deviations							Age Yrs Mths
	3rd	5th	10th	20th	30th	40th	50th	60th	70th	80th	90th	95th	97th	-3S.D.	-2S.D.	-1S.D.	Median	+1S.D.	+2S.D.	+3S.D.	
2 0	10.2	10.5	10.9	11.4	11.8	12.1	12.3	12.8	13.2	13.8	14.5	15.1	15.5	9.0	10.1	11.2	12.3	14.0	15.7	17.4	2 0
2 1	10.3	10.6	11.0	11.6	11.9	12.2	12.5	13.0	13.4	14.0	14.7	15.3	15.7	9.0	10.2	11.4	12.5	14.2	15.9	17.6	2 1
2 2	10.4	10.7	11.2	11.7	12.1	12.4	12.7	13.2	13.6	14.2	14.9	15.5	15.9	9.1	10.3	11.5	12.7	14.4	16.1	17.8	2 2
2 3	10.6	10.9	11.3	11.9	12.3	12.6	12.9	13.4	13.8	14.4	15.1	15.7	16.1	9.1	10.4	11.7	12.9	14.6	16.3	18.0	2 3
2 4	10.7	11.0	11.5	12.0	12.4	12.8	13.1	13.6	14.0	14.6	15.3	16.0	16.4	9.2	10.5	11.8	13.1	14.8	16.6	18.3	2 4
2 5	10.8	11.1	11.6	12.2	12.6	13.0	13.3	13.8	14.2	14.8	15.5	16.2	16.6	9.3	10.6	12.0	13.3	15.1	16.8	18.5	2 5
2 6	10.9	11.2	11.7	12.3	12.8	13.2	13.5	14.0	14.4	15.0	15.7	16.4	16.8	9.4	10.7	12.1	13.5	15.3	17.0	18.7	2 6
2 7	11.0	11.4	11.9	12.5	13.0	13.3	13.7	14.1	14.6	15.2	15.9	16.6	17.0	9.4	10.9	12.3	13.7	15.5	17.2	19.0	2 7
2 8	11.1	11.5	12.0	12.7	13.1	13.5	13.9	14.3	14.8	15.4	16.1	16.8	17.2	9.5	11.0	12.4	13.9	15.7	17.4	19.2	2 8
2 9	11.3	11.6	12.2	12.8	13.3	13.7	14.1	14.5	15.0	15.6	16.4	17.0	17.4	9.6	11.1	12.6	14.1	15.9	17.6	19.4	2 9
2 10	11.4	11.7	12.3	13.0	13.5	13.9	14.3	14.7	15.2	15.8	16.6	17.2	17.6	9.7	11.2	12.7	14.3	16.0	17.8	19.6	2 10
2 11	11.5	11.9	12.4	13.1	13.6	14.0	14.4	14.9	15.4	16.0	16.8	17.4	17.8	9.7	11.3	12.9	14.4	16.2	18.0	19.8	2 11
3 0	11.6	12.0	12.6	13.3	13.8	14.2	14.6	15.1	15.6	16.2	17.0	17.6	18.0	9.8	11.4	13.0	14.6	16.4	18.3	20.1	3 0
3 1	11.7	12.1	12.7	13.4	13.9	14.4	14.8	15.3	15.8	16.3	17.2	17.8	18.2	9.9	11.5	13.2	14.8	16.6	18.5	20.3	3 1
3 2	11.9	12.3	12.9	13.6	14.1	14.6	15.0	15.4	15.9	16.5	17.3	18.0	18.5	10.0	11.7	13.3	15.0	16.8	18.7	20.5	3 2
3 3	12.0	12.4	13.0	13.7	14.3	14.7	15.2	15.6	16.1	16.7	17.5	18.2	18.7	10.1	11.8	13.5	15.2	17.0	18.9	20.7	3 3
3 4	12.1	12.5	13.1	13.9	14.4	14.9	15.3	15.8	16.3	16.9	17.7	18.4	18.9	10.2	11.9	13.6	15.3	17.2	19.1	21.0	3 4
3 5	12.2	12.6	13.3	14.0	14.6	15.1	15.5	16.0	16.5	17.1	17.9	18.6	19.1	10.3	12.0	13.8	15.5	17.4	19.3	21.2	3 5
3 6	12.4	12.8	13.4	14.2	14.8	15.2	15.7	16.2	16.7	17.3	18.1	18.8	19.3	10.4	12.1	13.9	15.7	17.6	19.5	21.4	3 6
3 7	12.5	12.9	13.6	14.3	14.9	15.4	15.8	16.3	16.9	17.5	18.3	19.0	19.5	10.5	12.3	14.1	15.8	17.8	19.7	21.7	3 7
3 8	12.6	13.0	13.7	14.5	15.1	15.6	16.0	16.5	17.0	17.7	18.5	19.2	19.7	10.6	12.4	14.2	16.0	18.0	19.9	21.9	3 8
3 9	12.7	13.2	13.8	14.6	15.2	15.7	16.2	16.7	17.2	17.9	18.7	19.4	19.9	10.7	12.5	14.4	16.2	18.2	20.1	22.1	3 9
3 10	12.9	13.3	14.0	14.8	15.4	15.9	16.4	16.9	17.4	18.0	18.9	19.7	20.1	10.8	12.6	14.5	16.4	18.4	20.4	22.4	3 10
3 11	13.0	13.4	14.1	14.9	15.5	16.1	16.5	17.0	17.6	18.2	19.1	19.9	20.3	10.9	12.8	14.6	16.5	18.6	20.6	22.6	3 11

Contd...

Contd...

Age Yrs Mths		Percentiles													Standard Deviations							Age Yrs Mths	
		3rd	5th	10th	20th	30th	40th	50th	60th	70th	80th	90th	95th	97th	-3S.D.	-2S.D.	-1S.D.	Median	+1S.D.	+2S.D.	+3S.D.		
4	0	13.1	13.6	14.3	15.1	15.7	16.2	16.7	17.2	17.8	18.4	19.3	20.1	20.5	11.0	12.9	14.8	16.7	18.7	20.8	22.8	4	0
4	1	13.2	13.7	14.4	15.2	15.9	16.4	16.9	17.4	17.9	18.6	19.5	20.3	20.8	11.1	13.0	14.9	16.9	18.9	21.0	23.1	4	1
4	2	13.4	13.8	14.5	15.4	16.0	16.5	17.0	17.6	18.1	18.8	19.7	20.5	21.0	11.2	13.1	15.1	17.0	19.1	21.2	23.3	4	2
4	3	13.5	14.0	14.7	15.5	16.2	16.7	17.2	17.7	18.3	19.0	19.9	20.7	21.2	11.3	13.3	15.2	17.2	19.3	21.4	23.6	4	3
4	4	13.6	14.1	14.8	15.7	16.3	16.9	17.4	17.9	18.5	19.2	20.1	20.9	21.4	11.4	13.4	15.4	17.4	19.5	21.7	23.8	4	4
4	5	13.8	14.2	15.0	15.8	16.5	17.0	17.5	18.1	18.7	19.4	20.3	21.1	21.6	11.5	13.5	15.5	17.5	19.7	21.9	24.1	4	5
4	6	13.9	14.4	15.1	16.0	16.6	17.2	17.7	18.2	18.8	19.5	20.5	21.3	21.8	11.6	13.7	15.7	17.7	19.9	22.1	24.3	4	6
4	7	14.0	14.5	15.2	16.1	16.8	17.3	17.9	18.4	19.0	19.7	20.7	21.5	22.1	11.8	13.8	15.8	17.9	20.1	22.3	24.6	4	7
4	8	14.2	14.6	15.4	16.3	16.9	17.5	18.0	18.6	19.2	19.9	20.9	21.8	22.3	11.9	13.9	16.0	18.0	20.3	22.6	24.8	4	8
4	9	14.3	14.8	15.5	16.4	17.1	17.7	18.2	18.8	19.4	20.1	21.1	22.0	22.5	12.0	14.0	16.1	18.2	20.5	22.8	25.1	4	9
4	10	14.4	14.9	15.7	16.6	17.3	17.8	18.3	18.9	19.6	20.3	21.3	22.2	22.7	12.1	14.2	16.3	18.3	20.7	23.0	25.4	4	10
4	11	14.6	15.0	15.8	16.7	17.4	18.0	18.5	19.1	19.8	20.5	21.6	22.4	23.0	12.2	14.3	16.4	18.5	20.9	23.3	25.6	4	11
5	0	14.7	15.2	16.0	16.9	17.6	18.1	18.7	19.3	19.9	20.7	21.8	22.6	23.2	12.3	14.4	16.6	18.7	21.1	23.5	25.9	5	0
5	1	14.8	15.3	16.1	17.0	17.7	18.3	18.8	19.5	20.1	20.9	22.0	22.9	23.4	12.4	14.6	16.7	18.8	21.3	23.7	26.2	5	1
5	2	15.0	15.5	16.2	17.2	17.9	18.5	19.0	19.6	20.3	21.1	22.2	23.1	23.7	12.6	14.7	16.9	19.0	21.5	24.0	26.5	5	2
5	3	15.1	15.6	16.4	17.3	18.0	18.6	19.2	19.8	20.5	21.3	22.4	23.3	23.9	12.7	14.8	17.0	19.2	21.7	24.2	26.7	5	3
5	4	15.2	15.7	16.5	17.5	18.2	18.8	19.3	20.0	20.7	21.5	22.6	23.6	24.2	12.8	15.0	17.1	19.3	21.9	24.5	27.0	5	4
5	5	15.4	15.9	16.7	17.6	18.3	18.9	19.5	20.2	20.9	21.7	22.8	23.8	24.4	12.9	15.1	17.3	19.5	22.1	24.7	27.3	5	5
5	6	15.5	16.0	16.8	17.8	18.5	19.1	19.7	20.3	21.1	21.9	23.1	24.0	24.7	13.0	15.2	17.4	19.7	22.3	25.0	27.6	5	6
5	7	15.6	16.2	17.0	18.0	18.7	19.3	19.8	20.5	21.2	22.1	23.3	24.3	24.9	13.1	15.4	17.6	19.8	22.5	25.2	27.9	5	7
5	8	15.8	16.3	17.1	18.1	18.8	19.4	20.0	20.7	21.4	22.3	23.5	24.5	25.2	13.2	15.5	17.7	20.0	22.7	25.5	28.2	5	8
5	9	15.9	16.4	17.3	18.3	19.0	19.6	20.2	20.9	21.6	22.5	23.7	24.8	25.4	13.4	15.6	17.9	20.2	23.0	25.7	28.5	5	9
5	10	16.0	16.6	17.4	18.4	19.1	19.8	20.3	21.1	21.8	22.7	24.0	25.0	25.7	13.5	15.8	18.0	20.3	23.2	26.0	28.9	5	10
5	11	16.2	16.7	17.5	18.6	19.3	19.9	20.5	21.2	22.0	22.9	24.2	25.3	25.9	13.6	15.9	18.2	20.5	23.4	26.3	29.2	5	11

Contd...

Contd...

Age Yrs	Mths	Percentiles													Standard Deviations							Age Yrs	Mths
		3rd	5th	10th	20th	30th	40th	50th	60th	70th	80th	90th	95th	97th	-3S.D.	-2S.D.	-1S.D.	Median	+1S.D.	+2S.D.	+3S.D.		
6	0	16.3	16.8	17.7	18.7	19.5	20.1	20.7	21.4	22.2	23.2	24.5	25.5	26.2	13.7	16.0	18.4	20.7	23.6	26.6	29.5	6	0
6	1	16.4	17.0	17.8	18.9	19.6	20.3	20.9	21.6	22.4	23.4	24.7	25.8	26.5	13.8	16.2	18.5	20.9	23.8	26.8	29.8	6	1
6	2	16.6	17.1	18.0	19.0	19.8	20.4	21.0	21.8	22.6	23.6	24.9	26.0	26.8	13.9	16.3	18.7	21.0	24.1	27.1	30.2	6	2
6	3	16.7	17.3	18.1	19.2	20.0	20.6	21.2	22.0	22.8	23.8	25.2	26.3	27.0	14.0	16.4	18.8	21.2	24.3	27.4	30.5	6	3
6	4	16.8	17.4	18.3	19.3	20.1	20.8	21.4	22.2	23.0	24.0	25.4	26.6	27.3	14.1	16.5	19.0	21.4	24.5	27.7	30.9	6	4
6	5	17.0	17.5	18.4	19.5	20.3	20.9	21.6	22.4	23.2	24.3	25.7	26.9	27.6	14.2	16.7	19.1	21.6	24.8	28.0	31.2	6	5
6	6	17.1	17.7	18.6	19.7	20.4	21.1	21.7	22.6	23.5	24.5	25.9	27.1	27.9	14.3	16.8	19.3	21.7	25.0	28.3	31.6	6	6
6	7	17.2	17.8	18.7	19.8	20.6	21.3	21.9	22.8	23.7	24.7	26.2	27.4	28.2	14.4	16.9	19.4	21.9	25.3	28.6	31.9	6	7
6	8	17.4	18.0	18.9	20.0	20.8	21.5	22.1	23.0	23.9	25.0	26.5	27.7	28.5	14.6	17.1	19.6	22.1	25.5	28.9	32.3	6	8
6	9	17.5	18.1	19.0	20.1	21.0	21.6	22.3	23.2	24.1	25.2	26.7	28.0	28.8	14.7	17.2	19.7	22.3	25.8	29.2	32.7	6	9
6	10	17.6	18.2	19.2	20.3	21.1	21.8	22.5	23.4	24.3	25.5	27.0	28.3	29.1	14.8	17.3	19.9	22.5	26.0	29.5	33.1	6	10
6	11	17.8	18.4	19.3	20.5	21.3	22.0	22.7	23.6	24.6	25.7	27.3	28.6	29.4	14.9	17.5	20.1	22.7	26.3	29.9	33.5	6	11
7	0	17.9	18.5	19.5	20.6	21.5	22.2	22.9	23.8	24.8	25.9	27.6	28.9	29.8	15.0	17.6	20.2	22.9	26.5	30.2	33.9	7	0
7	1	18.0	18.7	19.6	20.8	21.6	22.4	23.0	24.0	25.0	26.2	27.8	29.2	30.1	15.1	17.7	20.4	23.0	26.8	30.5	34.3	7	1
7	2	18.2	18.8	19.8	21.0	21.8	22.6	23.2	24.2	25.2	26.5	28.1	29.5	30.4	15.1	17.8	20.5	23.2	27.1	30.9	34.7	7	2
7	3	18.3	18.9	19.9	21.1	22.0	22.7	23.4	24.4	25.5	26.7	28.4	29.8	30.8	15.2	18.0	20.7	23.4	27.3	31.2	35.1	7	3
7	4	18.4	19.1	20.1	21.3	22.2	22.9	23.6	24.6	25.7	27.0	28.7	30.2	31.1	15.3	18.1	20.9	23.6	27.6	31.6	35.5	7	4
7	5	18.6	19.2	20.2	21.5	22.4	23.1	23.8	24.9	26.0	27.2	29.0	30.5	31.5	15.4	18.2	21.0	23.8	27.9	31.9	36.0	7	5
7	6	18.7	19.4	20.4	21.6	22.5	23.3	24.0	25.1	26.2	27.5	29.3	30.8	31.8	15.5	18.4	21.2	24.0	28.2	32.3	36.4	7	6
7	7	18.8	19.5	20.5	21.8	22.7	23.5	24.2	25.3	26.4	27.8	29.6	31.2	32.2	15.6	18.5	21.4	24.2	28.5	32.7	36.9	7	7
7	8	18.9	19.6	20.7	22.0	22.9	23.7	24.4	25.5	26.7	28.1	30.0	31.5	32.5	15.7	18.6	21.5	24.4	28.7	33.0	37.3	7	8
7	9	19.1	19.8	20.9	22.2	23.1	23.9	24.7	25.8	27.0	28.3	30.3	31.9	32.9	15.8	18.7	21.7	24.7	29.0	33.4	37.8	7	9
7	10	19.2	19.9	21.0	22.3	23.3	24.1	24.9	26.0	27.2	28.6	30.6	32.2	33.3	15.8	18.9	21.9	24.9	29.3	33.8	38.3	7	10
7	11	19.3	20.1	21.2	22.5	23.5	24.3	25.1	26.2	27.5	28.9	30.9	32.6	33.7	15.9	19.0	22.0	25.1	29.6	34.2	38.8	7	11

Contd...

Contd...

Age Yrs	Mths	3rd	5th	10th	20th	30th	40th	50th	60th	70th	80th	90th	95th	97th	-3S.D.	-2S.D.	-1S.D.	Median	+1S.D.	+2S.D.	+3S.D.	Age Yrs	Mths
							Percentiles										Standard Deviations						
8	0	19.5	20.2	21.3	22.7	23.7	24.5	25.3	26.5	27.7	29.2	31.3	33.0	34.1	16.0	19.1	22.2	25.3	30.0	34.6	39.3	8	0
8	1	19.6	20.3	21.5	22.9	23.9	24.7	25.5	26.7	28.0	29.5	31.6	33.3	34.5	16.1	19.2	22.4	25.5	30.3	35.0	39.8	8	1
8	2	19.7	20.5	21.6	23.0	24.1	24.9	25.7	27.0	28.3	29.8	32.0	33.7	34.9	16.1	19.3	22.5	25.7	30.6	35.4	40.3	8	2
8	3	19.8	20.6	21.8	23.2	24.3	25.1	26.0	27.2	28.6	30.1	32.3	34.1	35.3	16.2	19.5	22.7	26.0	30.9	35.9	40.8	8	3
8	4	20.0	20.8	22.0	23.4	24.5	25.4	26.2	27.5	28.8	30.4	32.7	34.5	35.7	16.3	19.6	22.9	26.2	31.2	36.3	41.3	8	4
8	5	20.1	20.9	22.1	23.6	24.7	25.6	26.4	27.7	29.1	30.8	33.0	34.9	36.1	16.3	19.7	23.1	26.4	31.6	36.7	41.9	8	5
8	6	20.2	21.0	22.3	23.8	24.9	25.8	26.7	28.0	29.4	31.1	33.4	35.3	36.5	16.4	19.8	23.2	26.7	31.9	37.2	42.4	8	6
8	7	20.4	21.2	22.4	24.0	25.1	26.0	26.9	28.3	29.7	31.4	33.8	35.7	37.0	16.5	19.9	23.4	26.9	32.3	37.6	43.0	8	7
8	8	20.5	21.3	22.6	24.2	25.3	26.2	27.1	28.5	30.0	31.7	34.1	36.1	37.4	16.5	20.1	23.6	27.1	32.6	38.1	43.5	8	8
8	9	20.6	21.5	22.8	24.4	25.5	26.5	27.4	28.8	30.3	32.1	34.5	36.5	37.9	16.6	20.2	23.8	27.4	32.9	38.5	44.1	8	9
8	10	20.7	21.6	22.9	24.5	25.7	26.7	27.6	29.1	30.6	32.4	34.9	37.0	38.3	16.6	20.3	24.0	27.6	33.3	39.0	44.7	8	10
8	11	20.9	21.7	23.1	24.7	25.9	26.9	27.9	29.3	30.9	32.8	35.3	37.4	38.8	16.7	20.4	24.2	27.9	33.7	39.5	45.2	8	11
9	0	21.0	21.9	23.3	24.9	26.1	27.2	28.1	29.6	31.2	33.1	35.7	37.8	39.2	16.8	20.5	24.3	28.1	34.0	39.9	45.8	9	0
9	1	21.1	22.0	23.4	25.1	26.4	27.4	28.4	29.9	31.5	33.4	36.1	38.3	39.7	16.8	20.7	24.5	28.4	34.4	40.4	46.4	9	1
9	2	21.3	22.2	23.6	25.3	26.6	27.7	28.6	30.2	31.9	33.8	36.5	38.7	40.2	16.9	20.8	24.7	28.6	34.8	40.9	47.0	9	2
9	3	21.4	22.3	23.8	25.5	26.8	27.9	28.9	30.5	32.2	34.2	36.9	39.2	40.6	16.9	20.9	24.9	28.9	35.2	41.4	47.6	9	3
9	4	21.5	22.5	24.0	25.8	27.0	28.2	29.2	30.8	32.5	34.5	37.3	39.6	41.1	17.0	21.0	25.1	29.2	35.5	41.9	48.2	9	4
9	5	21.7	22.6	24.1	26.0	27.3	28.4	29.5	31.1	32.8	34.9	37.7	40.1	41.6	17.0	21.2	25.3	29.5	35.9	42.4	48.9	9	5
9	6	21.8	22.8	24.3	26.2	27.5	28.7	29.7	31.4	33.2	35.3	38.2	40.6	42.1	17.1	21.3	25.5	29.7	36.3	42.9	49.5	9	6
9	7	22.0	23.0	24.5	26.4	27.8	28.9	30.0	31.7	33.5	35.6	38.6	41.0	42.6	17.2	21.4	25.7	30.0	36.7	43.4	50.1	9	7
9	8	22.1	23.1	24.7	26.6	28.0	29.2	30.3	32.0	33.9	36.0	39.0	41.5	43.1	17.2	21.6	25.9	30.3	37.1	43.9	50.7	9	8
9	9	22.2	23.3	24.9	26.8	28.2	29.4	30.6	32.3	34.2	36.4	39.5	42.0	43.6	17.3	21.7	26.1	30.6	37.5	44.4	51.4	9	9
9	10	22.4	23.5	25.1	27.1	28.5	29.7	30.9	32.6	34.6	36.8	39.9	42.5	44.1	17.4	21.9	26.4	30.9	37.9	45.0	52.0	9	10
9	11	22.5	23.6	25.3	27.3	28.7	30.0	31.1	33.0	34.9	37.2	40.3	43.0	44.6	17.4	22.0	26.6	31.1	38.3	45.5	52.7	9	11

Contd...

Contd....

Age						Percentiles										Standard Deviations						Age	
Yrd	Mths	3rd	5th	10th	20th	30th	40th	50th	60th	70th	80th	90th	95th	97th	-3S.D.	-2S.D.	-1S.D.	Median	+1S.D.	+2S.D.	+3S.D.	Yrs	Mths
10	0	22.7	23.8	25.5	27.5	29.0	30.3	31.4	33.3	35.3	37.6	40.8	43.4	45.2	17.5	22.1	26.8	31.4	38.7	46.0	53.3	10	0
10	1	22.9	24.0	25.7	27.8	29.3	30.5	31.7	33.6	35.6	38.0	41.2	43.9	45.7	17.6	22.3	27.0	31.7	39.2	46.6	54.0	10	1
10	2	23.0	24.1	25.9	28.0	29.5	30.8	32.0	34.0	36.0	38.4	41.7	44.4	46.2	17.6	22.4	27.2	32.0	39.6	47.1	54.6	10	2
10	3	23.2	24.3	26.1	28.2	29.8	31.1	32.4	34.3	36.4	38.8	42.2	44.9	46.8	17.7	22.6	27.5	32.4	40.0	47.7	55.3	10	3
10	4	23.3	24.5	26.3	28.5	30.1	31.4	32.7	34.6	36.7	39.2	42.6	45.5	47.3	17.8	22.8	27.7	32.7	40.4	48.2	56.0	10	4
10	5	23.5	24.7	26.5	28.7	30.3	31.7	33.0	35.0	37.1	39.6	43.1	46.0	47.8	17.9	22.9	27.9	33.0	40.9	48.8	56.7	10	5
10	6	23.7	24.9	26.7	29.0	30.6	32.0	33.3	35.3	37.5	40.0	43.6	46.5	48.4	18.0	23.1	28.2	33.3	41.3	49.3	57.3	10	6
10	7	23.9	25.1	27.0	29.3	30.9	32.3	33.6	35.7	37.9	40.5	43.0	47.0	48.9	18.1	23.2	28.4	33.6	41.8	49.9	58.0	10	7
10	8	24.0	25.3	27.2	29.5	31.2	32.6	33.9	36.0	38.3	40.9	44.5	47.5	49.5	18.1	23.4	28.7	33.9	42.2	50.4	58.7	10	8
10	9	24.2	25.5	27.4	29.8	31.5	32.9	34.3	36.4	38.7	41.3	45.0	48.0	50.0	18.2	23.6	28.9	34.3	42.6	51.0	59.4	10	9
10	10	24.4	25.7	27.7	30.1	31.8	33.2	34.6	36.8	39.1	41.8	45.5	48.6	50.6	18.3	23.8	29.2	34.6	43.1	51.6	60.1	10	10
10	11	24.6	25.9	27.9	30.3	32.1	33.6	35.0	37.1	39.5	42.2	46.0	49.1	51.1	18.5	24.0	29.5	35.0	43.6	52.2	60.8	10	11
11	0	24.8	26.1	28.1	30.6	32.4	33.9	35.3	37.5	39.9	42.6	46.5	49.6	51.7	18.6	24.1	29.7	35.3	44.0	52.7	61.5	11	0
11	1	25.0	26.3	28.4	30.9	32.7	34.2	35.6	37.9	40.3	43.1	47.0	50.2	52.3	18.7	24.3	30.0	35.6	44.5	53.3	62.2	11	1
11	2	25.2	26.6	28.7	31.2	33.0	34.5	36.0	38.3	40.7	43.5	47.5	50.7	52.8	18.8	24.5	30.3	36.0	45.0	53.9	62.9	11	2
11	3	25.4	26.8	28.9	31.5	33.3	34.9	36.4	38.7	41.1	44.0	48.0	51.3	53.4	18.9	24.7	30.5	36.4	45.4	54.5	63.6	11	3
11	4	25.6	27.0	29.2	31.8	33.6	35.2	36.7	39.0	41.5	44.4	48.5	51.8	54.0	19.0	24.9	30.8	36.7	45.9	55.1	64.3	11	4
11	5	25.9	27.3	29.4	32.1	34.0	35.6	37.1	39.4	42.0	44.9	49.0	52.4	54.6	19.2	25.2	31.1	37.1	46.4	55.7	65.0	11	5
11	6	26.1	27.5	29.7	32.4	34.3	35.9	37.5	39.8	42.4	45.4	49.5	52.9	55.1	19.3	25.4	31.4	37.5	46.9	56.3	65.7	11	6
11	7	26.3	27.8	30.0	32.7	34.6	36.3	37.8	40.2	42.8	45.8	50.0	53.5	55.7	19.5	25.6	31.7	37.8	47.3	56.9	66.4	11	7
11	8	26.6	28.0	30.3	33.0	35.0	36.6	38.2	40.6	43.3	46.3	50.5	54.0	56.3	19.6	25.8	32.0	38.2	47.8	57.5	67.1	11	8
11	9	26.8	28.3	30.6	33.3	35.3	37.0	38.6	41.1	43.7	46.8	51.1	54.6	56.9	19.8	26.1	32.3	38.6	48.3	58.1	67.8	11	9
11	10	27.0	28.5	30.9	33.6	35.7	37.4	39.0	41.5	44.1	47.3	51.6	55.2	57.5	19.9	26.3	32.6	39.0	48.8	58.7	68.5	11	10
11	11	27.3	28.8	31.2	34.0	36.0	37.8	39.4	41.9	44.6	47.7	52.1	55.7	58.1	20.1	26.5	33.0	39.4	49.3	59.3	69.2	11	11

Contd....

Contd...

Age							Percentiles								Standard Deviations							Age	
Yrs	Mths	3rd	5th	10th	20th	30th	40th	50th	60th	70th	80th	90th	95th	97th	-3S.D.	-2S.D.	-1S.D.	Median	+1S.D.	+2S.D.	+3S.D.	Yrs	Mths
12	0	27.6	29.1	31.5	34.3	36.4	38.1	39.8	42.3	45.0	48.2	52.6	56.3	58.7	20.3	26.8	33.3	39.8	49.8	59.9	69.9	12	0
12	1	27.8	29.4	31.8	34.7	36.7	38.5	40.2	42.8	45.5	48.7	53.2	56.9	59.3	20.5	27.1	33.6	40.2	50.3	60.5	70.6	12	1
12	2	28.1	29.7	32.1	35.0	37.1	38.9	40.6	43.2	46.0	49.2	53.7	57.4	59.9	20.7	27.3	34.0	40.6	50.8	61.1	71.3	12	2
12	3	28.4	30.0	32.4	35.4	37.5	39.3	41.0	43.6	46.4	49.7	54.3	58.0	60.5	20.9	27.6	34.3	41.0	51.3	61.7	72.0	12	3
12	4	28.7	30.3	32.7	35.7	37.9	39.7	41.4	44.1	46.9	50.2	54.8	58.6	61.1	21.1	27.9	34.6	41.4	51.9	62.3	72.7	12	4
12	5	29.0	30.6	33.1	36.1	38.3	40.1	41.8	44.5	47.4	50.7	55.3	59.2	61.7	21.3	28.2	35.0	41.8	52.4	62.9	73.4	12	5
12	6	29.3	30.9	33.4	36.5	38.6	40.5	42.3	45.0	47.8	51.2	55.9	59.8	62.3	21.5	28.4	35.4	42.3	52.9	63.5	74.1	12	6
12	7	29.6	31.2	33.8	36.8	39.0	40.9	42.7	45.4	48.3	51.7	56.4	60.3	62.9	21.8	28.7	35.7	42.7	53.4	64.1	74.9	12	7
12	8	29.9	31.6	34.1	37.2	39.4	41.4	43.1	45.9	48.8	52.2	57.0	60.9	63.5	22.0	29.0	36.1	43.1	53.9	64.8	75.6	12	8
12	9	30.2	31.9	34.5	37.6	39.9	41.8	43.6	46.3	49.3	52.8	57.5	61.5	64.1	22.3	29.4	36.5	43.6	54.5	65.4	76.3	12	9
12	10	30.5	32.2	34.8	38.0	40.3	42.2	44.0	46.8	49.8	53.3	58.1	62.1	64.7	22.5	29.7	36.9	44.0	55.0	66.0	77.0	12	10
12	11	30.9	32.6	35.2	38.4	40.7	42.7	44.5	47.3	50.3	53.8	58.7	62.7	65.3	22.8	30.0	37.3	44.5	55.5	66.6	77.7	12	11
13	0	31.2	32.9	35.6	38.8	41.1	43.1	45.0	47.8	50.8	54.3	59.2	63.3	65.9	23.1	30.4	37.7	45.0	56.1	67.2	78.3	13	0
13	1	31.6	33.3	36.0	39.2	41.6	43.6	45.4	48.3	51.3	54.9	59.8	63.9	66.5	23.3	30.7	38.1	45.4	56.6	67.8	79.0	13	1
13	2	31.9	33.7	36.4	39.6	42.0	44.0	45.9	48.7	51.8	55.4	60.3	64.4	67.1	23.6	31.1	38.5	45.9	57.2	68.5	79.7	13	2
13	3	32.3	34.1	36.8	40.1	42.4	44.5	46.4	49.2	52.3	55.9	60.9	65.0	67.7	23.9	31.4	38.9	46.4	57.7	69.1	80.4	13	3
13	4	32.7	34.5	37.2	40.5	42.9	44.9	46.8	49.7	52.8	56.5	61.5	65.6	68.3	24.2	31.8	39.3	46.8	58.3	69.7	81.1	13	4
13	5	33.1	34.8	37.6	40.9	43.3	45.4	47.3	50.2	53.3	57.0	62.0	66.2	68.9	24.6	32.2	39.7	47.3	58.8	70.3	81.8	13	5
13	6	33.4	35.2	38.0	41.4	43.8	45.9	47.8	50.7	53.9	57.5	62.6	66.8	69.5	24.9	32.5	40.2	47.8	59.4	70.9	82.5	13	6
13	7	33.8	35.6	38.4	41.8	44.3	46.3	48.3	51.2	54.4	58.1	63.2	67.4	70.2	25.2	32.9	40.6	48.3	59.9	71.5	83.2	13	7
13	8	34.2	36.1	38.9	42.3	44.7	46.8	48.8	51.7	54.9	58.6	63.8	68.0	70.8	25.6	33.3	41.0	48.8	60.5	72.1	83.8	13	8
13	9	34.6	36.5	39.3	42.7	45.2	47.3	49.3	52.3	55.4	59.2	64.3	68.6	71.4	25.9	33.7	41.5	49.3	61.0	72.8	84.5	13	9
13	10	35.0	36.9	39.7	43.2	45.7	47.8	49.8	52.8	56.0	59.7	64.9	69.2	72.0	26.3	34.1	41.9	49.8	61.6	73.4	85.2	13	10
13	11	35.4	37.3	40.2	43.6	46.1	48.3	50.3	53.3	56.5	60.2	65.5	69.8	72.6	26.6	34.5	42.4	50.3	62.1	74.0	85.8	13	11

Contd...

Contd...

Age Yrs Mths	Percentiles													Standard Deviations							Age Yrs Mths
	3rd	5th	10th	20th	30th	40th	50th	60th	70th	80th	90th	95th	97th	-3S.D.	-2S.D.	-1S.D.	Median	+1S.D.	+2S.D.	+3S.D.	
14 0	35.9	37.7	40.6	44.1	46.6	48.8	50.8	53.8	57.0	60.8	66.0	70.4	73.2	27.0	34.9	42.8	50.8	62.7	74.6	86.5	14 0
14 1	36.3	38.2	41.1	44.6	47.1	49.3	51.3	54.3	57.5	61.3	66.6	70.9	73.8	27.4	35.3	43.3	51.3	63.2	75.2	87.1	14 1
14 2	36.7	38.6	41.5	45.0	47.6	49.7	51.8	54.8	58.1	61.9	67.2	71.5	74.4	27.7	35.7	43.8	51.8	63.8	75.8	87.8	14 2
14 3	37.1	39.0	41.9	45.5	48.0	50.2	52.3	55.3	58.6	62.4	67.7	72.1	75.0	28.1	36.2	44.2	52.3	64.3	76.4	88.4	14 3
14 4	37.5	39.4	42.4	46.0	48.5	50.7	52.8	55.8	59.1	63.0	68.3	72.7	75.5	28.5	36.6	44.7	52.8	64.9	77.0	89.1	14 4
14 5	38.0	39.9	42.8	46.4	49.0	51.2	53.3	56.3	59.6	63.5	68.8	73.3	76.1	28.9	37.0	45.1	53.3	65.4	77.6	89.7	14 5
14 6	38.4	40.3	43.3	46.9	49.5	51.7	53.8	56.9	60.2	64.0	69.4	73.8	76.7	29.2	37.4	45.6	53.8	66.0	78.2	90.4	14 6
14 7	38.8	40.7	43.7	47.3	50.0	52.2	54.3	57.4	60.7	64.6	70.0	74.4	77.3	29.6	37.8	46.0	54.3	66.5	78.8	91.0	14 7
14 8	39.2	41.2	44.2	47.8	50.4	52.7	54.8	57.9	61.2	65.1	70.5	75.0	77.9	30.0	38.3	46.5	54.8	67.0	79.3	91.6	14 8
14 9	39.7	41.6	44.6	48.3	50.9	53.1	55.2	58.4	61.7	65.6	71.1	75.5	78.4	30.4	38.7	47.0	55.2	67.6	79.9	92.2	14 9
14 10	40.1	42.1	45.1	48.7	51.4	53.6	55.7	58.9	62.2	66.2	71.6	76.1	79.0	30.8	39.1	47.4	55.7	68.1	80.5	92.9	14 10
14 11	40.5	42.5	45.5	49.2	51.8	54.1	56.2	59.4	62.7	66.7	72.1	76.6	79.6	31.2	39.5	47.9	56.2	68.6	81.1	93.5	14 11
15 0	40.9	42.9	46.0	49.6	52.3	54.6	56.7	59.9	63.2	67.2	72.7	77.2	80.1	31.6	39.9	48.3	56.7	69.2	81.6	94.1	15 0
15 1	41.4	43.3	46.4	50.1	52.8	55.1	57.2	60.4	63.7	67.7	73.2	77.7	80.7	31.9	40.4	48.8	57.2	69.7	82.2	94.7	15 1
15 2	41.8	43.8	46.8	50.6	53.2	55.5	57.7	60.8	64.2	68.2	73.7	78.3	81.2	32.3	40.8	49.2	57.7	70.2	82.7	95.3	15 2
15 3	42.2	44.2	47.3	51.0	53.7	56.0	58.1	61.3	64.7	68.7	74.2	78.8	81.8	32.7	41.2	49.7	58.1	70.7	83.3	95.9	15 3
15 4	42.6	44.6	47.7	51.4	54.1	56.4	58.6	61.8	65.2	69.2	74.8	79.3	82.3	33.1	41.6	50.1	58.6	71.2	83.8	96.4	15 4
15 5	43.0	45.0	48.1	51.9	54.6	56.9	59.1	62.3	65.7	69.7	75.3	79.9	82.9	33.5	42.0	50.5	59.1	71.7	84.4	97.0	15 5
15 6	43.4	45.4	48.5	52.3	55.0	57.3	59.5	62.7	66.2	70.2	75.8	80.4	83.4	33.8	42.4	51.0	59.5	72.2	84.9	97.6	15 6
15 7	43.8	45.8	49.0	52.7	55.5	57.8	60.0	63.2	66.6	70.7	76.3	80.9	83.9	34.2	42.8	51.4	60.0	72.7	85.4	98.2	15 7
15 8	44.2	46.2	49.4	53.2	55.9	58.2	60.4	63.6	67.1	71.2	76.8	81.4	84.4	34.6	43.2	51.8	60.4	73.2	85.9	98.7	15 8
15 9	44.6	46.6	49.8	53.6	56.3	58.7	60.8	64.1	67.6	71.6	77.3	81.9	84.9	35.0	43.6	52.2	60.8	73.6	86.5	99.3	15 9
15 10	45.0	47.0	50.2	54.0	56.7	59.1	61.3	64.5	68.0	72.1	77.7	82.4	85.4	35.3	44.0	52.6	61.3	74.1	87.0	99.8	15 10
15 11	45.4	47.4	50.6	54.4	57.1	59.5	61.7	65.0	68.4	72.5	78.2	82.9	85.9	35.7	44.3	53.0	61.7	74.6	87.5	100.3	15 11

Contd...

Contd...

Age Yrs	Mths	Percentiles													Standard Deviations						
		3rd	5th	10th	20th	30th	40th	50th	60th	70th	80th	90th	95th	97th	-3S.D.	-2S.D.	-1S.D.	Median	+1S.D.	+2S.D.	+3S.D.
16	0	45.7	47.8	51.0	54.8	57.5	59.9	62.1	65.4	68.9	73.0	78.7	83.4	86.4	36.0	44.7	53.4	62.1	75.0	87.9	100.9
16	1	46.1	48.2	51.3	55.2	57.9	60.3	62.5	65.8	69.3	73.4	79.1	83.8	86.9	36.4	45.1	53.8	62.5	75.5	88.4	101.4
16	2	46.5	48.5	51.7	55.6	58.3	60.7	62.9	66.2	69.7	73.8	79.6	84.3	87.4	36.7	45.4	54.2	62.9	75.9	88.9	101.9
16	3	46.8	48.9	52.1	55.9	58.7	61.1	63.3	66.6	70.1	74.3	80.0	84.7	87.8	37.0	45.8	54.5	63.3	76.3	89.4	102.4
16	4	47.2	49.2	52.4	56.3	59.1	61.4	63.7	67.0	70.5	74.7	80.4	85.2	88.3	37.4	46.1	54.9	63.7	76.8	89.8	102.9
16	5	47.5	49.6	52.8	56.6	59.4	61.8	64.0	67.4	70.9	75.1	80.9	85.6	88.7	37.7	46.5	55.3	64.0	77.2	90.3	103.4
16	6	47.8	49.9	53.1	57.0	59.8	62.2	64.4	67.7	71.3	75.5	81.3	86.1	89.2	38.0	46.8	55.6	64.4	77.6	90.7	103.9
16	7	48.2	50.2	53.4	57.3	60.1	62.5	64.7	68.1	71.7	75.9	81.7	86.5	89.6	38.3	47.1	55.9	64.7	78.0	91.2	104.4
16	8	48.5	50.6	53.8	57.6	60.4	62.8	65.1	68.4	72.0	76.2	82.1	86.9	90.0	38.6	47.4	56.2	65.1	78.3	91.6	104.8
16	9	48.8	50.9	54.1	58.0	60.8	63.2	65.4	68.8	72.4	76.6	82.5	87.3	90.4	38.9	47.7	56.6	65.4	78.7	92.0	105.3
16	10	49.1	51.2	54.4	58.3	61.1	63.5	65.7	69.1	72.7	77.0	82.8	87.7	90.8	39.2	48.0	56.9	65.7	79.1	92.4	105.8
16	11	49.3	51.4	54.7	58.6	61.4	63.8	66.0	69.4	73.0	77.3	83.2	88.1	91.2	39.4	48.3	57.2	66.0	79.4	92.8	106.2
17	0	49.6	51.7	54.9	58.8	61.7	64.1	66.3	69.7	73.4	77.6	83.5	88.4	91.6	39.7	48.6	57.4	66.3	79.8	93.2	106.6
17	1	49.9	52.0	55.2	59.1	61.9	64.3	66.6	70.0	73.7	77.9	83.9	88.8	92.0	39.9	48.8	57.7	66.6	80.1	93.6	107.1
17	2	50.1	52.2	55.4	59.4	62.2	64.6	66.8	70.3	74.0	78.3	84.2	89.1	92.3	40.2	49.1	57.9	66.8	80.4	93.9	107.5
17	3	50.3	52.4	55.7	59.6	62.4	64.8	67.1	70.5	74.2	78.5	84.5	89.5	92.7	40.4	49.3	58.2	67.1	80.7	94.3	107.9
17	4	50.6	52.7	55.9	59.8	62.7	65.1	67.3	70.8	74.5	78.8	84.8	89.8	93.0	40.6	49.5	58.4	67.3	81.0	94.6	108.3
17	5	50.8	52.9	56.1	60.1	62.9	65.3	67.6	71.0	74.8	79.1	85.1	90.1	93.4	40.8	49.7	58.6	67.6	81.3	95.0	108.7
17	6	51.0	53.1	56.3	60.3	63.1	65.5	67.8	71.3	75.0	79.4	85.4	90.4	93.7	41.0	49.9	58.9	67.8	81.5	95.3	109.1
17	7	51.2	53.3	56.5	60.5	63.3	65.7	68.0	71.5	75.2	79.6	85.7	90.7	94.0	41.2	50.1	59.0	68.0	81.8	95.6	109.4
17	8	51.3	53.5	56.7	60.7	63.5	65.9	68.2	71.7	75.5	79.9	86.0	91.0	94.3	41.3	50.3	59.2	68.2	82.1	95.9	109.8
17	9	51.5	53.6	56.9	60.8	63.7	66.1	68.4	71.9	75.7	80.1	86.2	91.3	94.6	41.5	50.5	59.4	68.4	82.3	96.2	110.1
17	10	51.7	53.8	57.1	61.0	63.9	66.3	68.6	72.1	75.9	80.3	86.5	91.5	94.8	41.6	50.6	59.6	68.6	82.5	96.5	110.5
17	11	51.8	54.0	57.2	61.2	64.0	66.4	68.7	72.3	76.1	80.5	86.7	91.8	95.1	41.8	50.8	59.7	68.7	82.7	96.8	110.8
18	0	52.0	54.1	57.4	61.3	64.2	66.6	68.9	72.4	76.3	80.7	86.9	92.0	95.3	41.9	50.9	59.9	68.9	82.9	97.0	111.1

APPENDIX 47.9

WEIGHT (KG) BY AGE OF
GIRLS AGED 0 TO 36 MONTHS (NCHS STANDARDS)

Age Mths	Percentiles													Standard Deviations							Age Yrs	Mths
	3rd	5th	10th	20th	30th	40th	50th	60th	70th	80th	90th	95th	97th	-3S.D.	-2S.D.	-1S.D.	Median	+1S.D.	+2S.D.	+3S.D.		
0	2.3	2.4	2.6	2.8	3.0	3.1	3.2	3.3	3.4	3.5	3.7	3.8	3.9	1.8	2.2	2.7	3.2	3.6	4.0	4.3	0	0
1	2.9	3.0	3.2	3.5	3.7	3.8	4.0	4.1	4.3	4.4	4.7	4.9	5.0	2.2	2.8	3.4	4.0	4.5	5.1	5.6		1
2	3.4	3.6	3.8	4.1	4.4	4.5	4.7	4.9	5.1	5.3	5.6	5.8	6.0	2.7	3.3	4.0	4.7	5.4	6.1	6.7		2
3	4.0	4.2	4.4	4.8	5.0	5.2	5.4	5.6	5.8	6.1	6.4	6.7	6.9	3.2	3.9	4.7	5.4	6.2	7.0	7.7		3
4	4.6	4.7	5.0	5.4	5.6	5.8	6.0	6.3	6.5	6.8	7.1	7.4	7.6	3.7	4.5	5.3	6.0	6.9	7.7	8.6		4
5	5.1	5.3	5.6	6.0	6.2	6.4	6.7	6.9	7.1	7.4	7.8	8.1	8.3	4.1	5.0	5.8	6.7	7.5	8.4	9.3		5
6	5.6	5.8	6.1	6.5	6.8	7.0	7.2	7.4	7.7	8.0	8.4	8.7	8.9	4.6	5.5	6.3	7.2	8.1	9.0	10.0		6
7	6.0	6.2	6.5	6.9	7.2	7.5	7.7	7.9	8.2	8.5	8.9	9.3	9.5	5.0	5.9	6.8	7.7	8.7	9.6	10.5		7
8	6.4	6.6	7.0	7.4	7.7	7.9	8.2	8.4	8.7	9.0	9.4	9.8	10.0	5.3	6.3	7.2	8.2	9.1	10.1	11.1		8
9	6.7	7.0	7.3	7.7	8.1	8.3	8.6	8.8	9.1	9.4	9.8	10.2	10.4	5.7	6.6	7.6	8.6	9.6	10.5	11.5		9
10	7.0	7.3	7.6	8.1	8.4	8.7	8.9	9.2	9.4	9.8	10.2	10.6	10.8	5.9	6.9	7.9	8.9	9.9	10.9	11.9		10
11	7.3	7.6	7.9	8.4	8.7	9.0	9.2	9.5	9.8	10.1	10.6	10.9	11.2	6.2	7.2	8.2	9.2	10.3	11.3	12.3		11
12	7.6	7.8	8.2	8.6	9.0	9.3	9.5	9.8	10.1	10.4	10.9	11.2	11.5	6.4	7.4	8.5	9.5	10.6	11.6	12.7		12
13	7.8	8.0	8.4	8.9	9.2	9.5	9.8	10.1	10.3	10.7	11.1	11.5	11.8	6.6	7.6	8.7	9.8	10.8	11.9	13.0		13
14	8.0	8.2	8.6	9.1	9.5	9.8	10.0	10.3	10.6	10.9	11.4	11.8	12.0	6.7	7.8	8.9	10.0	11.1	12.2	13.2		14
15	8.1	8.4	8.8	9.3	9.7	10.0	10.2	10.5	10.8	11.2	11.6	12.0	12.3	6.9	8.0	9.1	10.2	11.3	12.4	13.5		15
16	8.3	8.6	9.0	9.5	9.9	10.2	10.4	10.7	11.0	11.4	11.9	12.3	12.5	7.0	8.2	9.3	10.4	11.5	12.6	13.7		16
17	8.5	8.7	9.2	9.7	10.0	10.3	10.6	10.9	11.2	11.6	12.1	12.5	12.7	7.2	8.3	9.5	10.6	11.8	12.9	14.0		17
18	8.6	8.9	9.3	9.8	10.2	10.5	10.8	11.1	11.4	11.8	12.3	12.7	13.0	7.3	8.5	9.7	10.8	12.0	13.1	14.2		18

Contd....

Contd...

Age Mths	Percentiles													Standard Deviations							Age Yrs Mths
	3rd	5th	10th	20th	30th	40th	50th	60th	70th	80th	90th	95th	97th	-3S.D.	-2S.D.	-1S.D.	Median	+1S.D.	+2S.D.	+3S.D.	
19	8.8	9.1	9.5	10.0	10.4	10.7	11.0	11.3	11.6	12.0	12.5	12.9	13.2	7.5	8.6	9.8	11.0	12.2	13.3	14.5	19
20	8.9	9.2	9.7	10.2	10.6	10.9	11.2	11.5	11.8	12.2	12.7	13.1	13.4	7.6	8.8	10.0	11.2	12.4	13.5	14.7	20
21	9.1	9.4	9.8	10.4	10.7	11.1	11.4	11.7	12.0	12.4	12.9	13.3	13.6	7.7	9.0	10.2	11.4	12.6	13.8	15.0	21
22	9.3	9.5	10.0	10.5	10.9	11.2	11.5	11.9	12.2	12.6	13.1	13.6	13.9	7.9	9.1	10.3	11.5	12.8	14.0	15.2	22
23	9.4	9.7	10.2	10.7	11.1	11.4	11.7	12.0	12.4	12.8	13.3	13.8	14.1	8.0	9.3	10.5	11.7	13.0	14.2	15.5	23
24	9.6	9.9	10.3	10.9	11.3	11.6	11.9	12.2	12.6	13.0	13.6	14.0	14.3	8.2	9.4	10.7	11.9	13.2	14.5	15.8	24
25	9.7	10.0	10.5	11.0	11.4	11.8	12.1	12.4	12.8	13.2	13.8	14.2	14.6	8.3	9.6	10.8	12.1	13.4	14.7	16.0	25
26	9.9	10.2	10.6	11.2	11.6	11.9	12.3	12.6	13.0	13.4	14.0	14.5	14.8	8.5	9.7	11.0	12.3	13.6	14.9	16.3	26
27	10.1	10.3	10.8	11.4	11.8	12.1	12.4	12.8	13.1	13.6	14.2	14.7	15.0	8.6	9.9	11.2	12.4	13.8	15.2	16.6	27
28	10.2	10.5	11.0	11.5	11.9	12.3	12.6	13.0	13.3	13.8	14.4	14.9	15.2	8.8	10.1	11.3	12.6	14.0	15.4	16.8	28
29	10.4	10.7	11.1	11.7	12.1	12.4	12.8	13.1	13.5	14.0	14.6	15.1	15.5	8.9	10.2	11.5	12.8	14.2	15.6	17.1	29
30	10.5	10.8	11.3	11.8	12.3	12.6	12.9	13.3	13.7	14.2	14.8	15.3	15.7	9.1	10.3	11.6	12.9	14.4	15.9	17.3	30
31	10.6	11.0	11.4	12.0	12.4	12.8	13.1	13.5	13.9	14.4	15.0	15.6	15.9	9.2	10.5	11.8	13.1	14.6	16.1	17.6	31
32	10.8	11.1	11.6	12.2	12.6	12.9	13.3	13.7	14.1	14.6	15.2	15.8	16.1	9.3	10.6	11.9	13.3	14.8	16.3	17.8	32
33	10.9	11.2	11.7	12.3	12.7	13.1	13.4	13.8	14.2	14.7	15.4	16.0	16.3	9.4	10.7	12.1	13.4	15.0	16.5	18.1	33
34	11.0	11.4	11.9	12.5	12.9	13.3	13.6	14.0	14.4	14.9	15.6	16.2	16.6	9.5	10.9	12.2	13.6	15.2	16.7	18.3	34
35	11.2	11.5	12.0	12.6	13.0	13.4	13.8	14.2	14.6	15.1	15.8	16.4	16.8	9.6	11.0	12.4	13.8	15.4	16.9	18.5	35
36	11.3	11.6	12.1	12.7	13.2	13.6	13.9	14.3	14.8	15.3	16.0	16.6	17.0	9.7	11.1	12.5	13.9	15.5	17.1	18.8	36

APPENDIX 47.10

WEIGHT (KG) BY AGE OF

GIRLS AGED 2 TO 18 YEARS (NCHS STANDARDS)

Age Yrs Mths	Percentiles													Standard Deviations							Age Yrs Mths
	3rd	5th	10th	20th	30th	40th	50th	60th	70th	80th	90th	95th	97th	-3S.D.	-2S.D.	-1S.D.	Median	+1S.D.	+2S.D.	+3S.D.	
2 0	9.6	9.9	10.3	10.8	11.2	11.5	11.8	12.2	12.5	13.0	13.6	14.1	14.4	8.3	9.4	10.6	11.8	13.2	14.6	16.0	2 0
2 1	9.7	10.0	10.5	11.0	11.4	11.7	12.0	12.4	12.8	13.2	13.9	14.4	14.8	8.4	9.6	10.8	12.0	13.5	14.9	16.4	2 1
2 2	9.9	10.2	10.6	11.2	11.6	11.9	12.2	12.6	13.0	13.5	14.2	14.7	15.1	8.5	9.8	11.0	12.2	13.7	15.2	16.8	2 2
2 3	10.1	10.4	10.8	11.4	11.8	12.1	12.4	12.8	13.3	13.7	14.4	15.0	15.4	8.6	9.9	11.2	12.4	14.0	15.6	17.1	2 3
2 4	10.2	10.5	11.0	11.6	12.0	12.3	12.6	13.0	13.5	14.0	14.7	15.3	15.7	8.8	10.1	11.3	12.6	14.2	15.9	17.5	2 4
2 5	10.4	10.7	11.1	11.7	12.1	12.5	12.8	13.3	13.7	14.2	15.0	15.6	16.0	8.9	10.2	11.5	12.8	14.5	16.1	17.8	2 5
2 6	10.5	10.8	11.3	11.9	12.3	12.7	13.0	13.5	13.9	14.5	15.2	15.8	16.2	9.0	10.3	11.7	13.0	14.7	16.4	18.1	2 6
2 7	10.6	11.0	11.5	12.1	12.5	12.9	13.2	13.7	14.1	14.7	15.5	16.1	16.5	9.1	10.5	11.9	13.2	15.0	16.7	18.5	2 7
2 8	10.8	11.1	11.6	12.2	12.7	13.0	13.4	13.9	14.3	14.9	15.7	16.3	16.8	9.2	10.6	12.0	13.4	15.2	17.0	18.8	2 8
2 9	10.9	11.3	11.8	12.4	12.8	13.2	13.6	14.0	14.5	15.1	15.9	16.6	17.0	9.4	10.8	12.2	13.6	15.4	17.2	19.1	2 9
2 10	11.1	11.4	11.9	12.6	13.0	13.4	13.8	14.2	14.7	15.3	16.2	16.8	17.3	9.5	10.9	12.3	13.8	15.6	17.5	19.4	2 10
2 11	11.2	11.5	12.1	12.7	13.2	13.6	13.9	14.4	14.9	15.5	16.4	17.1	17.5	9.6	11.0	12.5	13.9	15.8	17.8	19.7	2 11
3 0	11.3	11.7	12.2	12.9	13.3	13.7	14.1	14.6	15.1	15.7	16.6	17.3	17.8	9.7	11.2	12.6	14.1	16.1	18.0	20.0	3 0
3 1	11.5	11.8	12.4	13.0	13.5	13.9	14.3	14.8	15.3	15.9	16.8	17.5	18.0	9.8	11.3	12.8	14.3	16.3	18.3	20.2	3 1
3 2	11.6	11.9	12.5	13.2	13.6	14.1	14.4	15.0	15.5	16.1	17.0	17.8	18.3	9.9	11.4	12.9	14.4	16.5	18.5	20.5	3 2
3 3	11.7	12.1	12.6	13.3	13.8	14.2	14.6	15.1	15.7	16.3	17.2	18.0	18.5	10.0	11.5	13.1	14.6	16.7	18.7	20.8	3 3
3 4	11.8	12.2	12.8	13.4	13.9	14.4	14.8	15.3	15.9	16.5	17.4	18.2	18.7	10.1	11.6	13.2	14.8	16.9	19.0	21.1	3 4
3 5	12.0	12.3	12.9	13.6	14.1	14.5	14.9	15.5	16.0	16.7	17.6	18.4	18.9	10.2	11.8	13.3	14.9	17.0	19.2	21.3	3 5
3 6	12.1	12.5	13.0	13.7	14.2	14.7	15.1	15.6	16.2	16.9	17.8	18.6	19.1	10.3	11.9	13.5	15.1	17.2	19.4	21.6	3 6
3 7	12.2	12.6	13.2	13.9	14.4	14.8	15.2	15.8	16.4	17.1	18.0	18.8	19.4	10.4	12.0	13.6	15.2	17.4	19.6	21.8	3 7
3 8	12.3	12.7	13.3	14.0	14.5	15.0	15.4	15.9	16.5	17.3	18.2	19.0	19.6	10.5	12.1	13.7	15.4	17.6	19.8	22.1	3 8
3 9	12.4	12.8	13.4	14.1	14.7	15.1	15.5	16.1	16.7	17.4	18.4	19.3	19.8	10.6	12.2	13.9	15.5	17.8	20.1	22.3	3 9
3 10	12.5	12.9	13.5	14.3	14.8	15.2	15.7	16.3	16.9	17.6	18.6	19.5	20.0	10.7	12.3	14.0	15.7	18.0	20.3	22.6	3 10
3 11	12.6	13.0	13.7	14.4	14.9	15.4	15.8	16.4	17.0	17.8	18.8	19.7	20.2	10.8	12.4	14.1	15.8	18.1	20.5	22.8	3 11

Contd...

Contd...

Age Yrs	Mths	3rd	5th	10th	20th	30th	40th	50th	60th	70th	80th	90th	95th	97th	-3S.D.	-2S.D.	-1S.D.	Median	+1S.D.	+2S.D.	+3S.D.	Age Yrs	Mths
4	0	12.8	13.2	13.8	14.5	15.1	15.5	16.0	16.6	17.2	18.0	19.0	19.9	20.4	10.9	12.6	14.3	16.0	18.3	20.7	23.1	4	0
4	1	12.9	13.3	13.9	14.7	15.2	15.7	16.1	16.7	17.4	18.1	19.2	20.0	20.6	10.9	12.7	14.4	16.1	18.5	20.9	23.3	4	1
4	2	13.0	13.4	14.0	14.8	15.3	15.8	16.2	16.9	17.5	18.3	19.4	20.2	20.8	11.0	12.8	14.5	16.2	18.7	21.1	23.5	4	2
4	3	13.1	13.5	14.1	14.9	15.5	15.9	16.4	17.0	17.7	18.5	19.5	20.4	21.0	11.1	12.9	14.6	16.4	18.9	21.3	23.8	4	3
4	4	13.2	13.6	14.3	15.0	15.6	16.1	16.5	17.2	17.8	18.6	19.7	20.6	21.2	11.2	13.0	14.8	16.5	19.0	21.5	24.0	4	4
4	5	13.3	13.7	14.4	15.2	15.7	16.2	16.7	17.3	18.0	18.8	19.9	20.8	21.4	11.3	13.1	14.9	16.7	19.2	21.7	24.3	4	5
4	6	13.4	13.8	14.5	15.3	15.9	16.4	16.8	17.5	18.2	19.0	20.1	21.0	21.6	11.4	13.2	15.0	16.8	19.4	21.9	24.5	4	6
4	7	13.5	13.9	14.6	15.4	16.0	16.5	17.0	17.6	18.3	19.1	20.3	21.2	21.8	11.5	13.3	15.1	17.0	19.6	22.2	24.8	4	7
4	8	13.6	14.1	14.7	15.5	16.1	16.6	17.1	17.8	18.5	19.3	20.5	21.4	22.1	11.5	13.4	15.2	17.1	19.7	22.4	25.0	4	8
4	9	13.7	14.2	14.8	15.7	16.3	16.8	17.2	17.9	18.6	19.5	20.7	21.6	22.3	11.6	13.5	15.4	17.2	19.9	22.6	25.3	4	9
4	10	13.8	14.3	15.0	15.8	16.4	16.9	17.4	18.1	18.8	19.7	20.8	21.8	22.5	11.7	13.6	15.5	17.4	20.1	22.8	25.5	4	10
4	11	13.9	14.4	15.1	15.9	16.5	17.0	17.5	18.2	19.0	19.8	21.0	22.0	22.7	11.8	13.7	15.6	17.5	20.3	23.0	25.8	4	11
5	0	14.0	14.5	15.2	16.0	16.7	17.2	17.7	18.4	19.1	20.0	21.2	22.2	22.9	11.9	13.8	15.7	17.7	20.4	23.2	26.0	5	0
5	1	14.1	14.6	15.3	16.2	16.8	17.3	17.8	18.5	19.3	20.2	21.4	22.5	23.1	11.9	13.9	15.9	17.8	20.6	23.5	26.3	5	1
5	2	14.2	14.7	15.4	16.3	16.9	17.5	18.0	18.7	19.5	20.4	21.6	22.7	23.3	12.0	14.0	16.0	18.0	20.8	23.7	26.5	5	2
5	3	14.3	14.8	15.5	16.4	17.1	17.6	18.1	18.8	19.6	20.5	21.8	22.9	23.6	12.1	14.1	16.1	18.1	21.0	23.9	26.8	5	3
5	4	14.4	14.9	15.7	16.5	17.2	17.7	18.3	19.0	19.8	20.7	22.0	23.1	23.8	12.2	14.2	16.2	18.3	21.2	24.1	27.1	5	4
5	5	14.5	15.0	15.8	16.7	17.3	17.9	18.4	19.2	20.0	20.9	22.2	23.3	24.0	12.2	14.3	16.4	18.4	21.4	24.4	27.4	5	5
5	6	14.6	15.1	15.9	16.8	17.5	18.0	18.6	19.3	20.1	21.1	22.4	23.6	24.3	12.3	14.4	16.5	18.6	21.6	24.6	27.7	5	6
5	7	14.7	15.2	16.0	16.9	17.6	18.2	18.7	19.5	20.3	21.3	22.7	23.8	24.5	12.4	14.5	16.6	18.7	21.8	24.9	28.0	5	7
5	8	14.9	15.4	16.1	17.1	17.7	18.3	18.9	19.7	20.5	21.5	22.9	24.0	24.8	12.5	14.6	16.7	18.9	22.0	25.1	28.3	5	8
5	9	15.0	15.5	16.3	17.2	17.9	18.5	19.0	19.8	20.7	21.7	23.1	24.3	25.0	12.5	14.7	16.9	19.0	22.2	25.4	28.6	5	9
5	10	15.1	15.6	16.4	17.3	18.0	18.6	19.2	20.0	20.9	21.9	23.3	24.5	25.3	12.6	14.8	17.0	19.2	22.4	25.7	28.9	5	10
5	11	15.2	15.7	16.5	17.5	18.2	18.8	19.4	20.2	21.1	22.1	23.6	24.8	25.5	12.7	14.9	17.1	19.4	22.6	25.9	29.2	5	11

Contd...

Contd...

Age Yrs Mths		Percentiles													Standard Deviations							Age Yrs Mths	
		3rd	5th	10th	20th	30th	40th	50th	60th	70th	80th	90th	95th	97th	-3S.D.	-2S.D.	-1S.D.	Median	+1S.D.	+2S.D.	+3S.D.		
6	0	15.3	15.8	16.6	17.6	18.3	19.0	19.5	20.4	21.3	22.3	23.8	25.0	25.8	12.8	15.0	17.3	19.5	22.9	26.2	29.6	6	0
6	1	15.4	15.9	16.8	17.8	18.5	19.1	19.7	20.6	21.5	22.6	24.1	25.3	26.1	12.8	15.1	17.4	19.7	23.1	26.5	29.9	6	1
6	2	15.5	16.0	16.9	17.9	18.7	19.3	19.9	20.7	21.7	22.8	24.3	25.6	26.4	12.9	15.2	17.5	19.9	23.3	26.8	30.2	6	2
6	3	15.6	16.2	17.0	18.1	18.8	19.5	20.0	20.9	21.9	23.0	24.6	25.8	26.7	13.0	15.3	17.7	20.0	23.6	27.1	30.6	6	3
6	4	15.7	16.3	17.2	18.2	19.0	19.6	20.2	21.1	22.1	23.2	24.8	26.1	27.0	13.0	15.4	17.8	20.2	23.8	27.4	31.0	6	4
6	5	15.8	16.4	17.3	18.4	19.1	19.8	20.4	21.3	22.3	23.5	25.1	26.4	27.3	13.1	15.5	18.0	20.4	24.1	27.7	31.4	6	5
6	6	15.9	16.5	17.4	18.5	19.3	20.0	20.6	21.5	22.6	23.7	25.4	26.7	27.6	13.2	15.7	18.1	20.6	24.3	28.0	31.8	6	6
6	7	16.1	16.7	17.6	18.7	19.5	20.2	20.8	21.8	22.8	24.0	25.7	27.0	27.9	13.2	15.8	18.3	20.8	24.6	28.4	32.2	6	7
6	8	16.2	16.8	17.7	18.8	19.7	20.3	21.0	22.0	23.0	24.2	25.9	27.3	28.3	13.3	15.9	18.4	21.0	24.9	28.7	32.6	6	8
6	9	16.3	16.9	17.9	19.0	19.8	20.5	21.2	22.2	23.3	24.5	26.2	27.7	28.6	13.4	16.0	18.6	21.2	25.1	29.1	33.0	6	9
6	10	16.4	17.0	18.0	19.2	20.0	20.7	21.4	22.4	23.5	24.8	26.6	28.0	29.0	13.4	16.1	18.8	21.4	25.4	29.4	33.5	6	10
6	11	16.5	17.2	18.2	19.3	20.2	20.9	21.6	22.7	23.8	25.1	26.9	28.4	29.3	13.5	16.2	18.9	21.6	25.7	29.8	33.9	6	11
7	0	16.7	17.3	18.3	19.5	20.4	21.1	21.8	22.9	24.0	25.4	27.2	28.7	29.7	13.6	16.3	19.1	21.8	26.0	30.2	34.4	7	0
7	1	16.8	17.4	18.5	19.7	20.6	21.4	22.1	23.1	24.3	25.7	27.5	29.1	30.1	13.6	16.5	19.3	22.1	26.3	30.6	34.9	7	1
7	2	16.9	17.6	18.6	19.9	20.8	21.6	22.3	23.4	24.6	26.0	27.9	29.5	30.5	13.7	16.6	19.4	22.3	26.6	31.0	35.4	7	2
7	3	17.0	17.7	18.8	20.1	21.0	21.8	22.5	23.7	24.9	26.3	28.2	29.8	30.9	13.8	16.7	19.6	22.5	27.0	31.4	35.9	7	3
7	4	17.2	17.9	19.0	20.3	21.2	22.0	22.8	23.9	25.1	26.6	28.6	30.2	31.3	13.9	16.8	19.8	22.8	27.3	31.8	36.4	7	4
7	5	17.3	18.0	19.1	20.5	21.4	22.2	23.0	24.2	25.4	26.9	28.9	30.6	31.7	13.9	16.9	20.0	23.0	27.6	32.3	36.9	7	5
7	6	17.4	18.2	19.3	20.7	21.6	22.5	23.3	24.5	25.7	27.2	29.3	31.0	32.2	14.0	17.1	20.2	23.3	28.0	32.7	37.5	7	6
7	7	17.6	18.3	19.5	20.9	21.9	22.7	23.5	24.7	26.0	27.6	29.7	31.5	32.6	14.1	17.2	20.4	23.5	28.3	33.2	38.0	7	7
7	8	17.7	18.5	19.6	21.1	22.1	23.0	23.8	25.0	26.4	27.9	30.1	31.9	33.1	14.1	17.3	20.6	23.8	28.7	33.6	38.6	7	8
7	9	17.9	18.6	19.8	21.3	22.3	23.2	24.0	25.3	26.7	28.3	30.5	32.3	33.5	14.2	17.5	20.8	24.0	29.1	34.1	39.2	7	9
7	10	18.0	18.8	20.0	21.5	22.5	23.4	24.3	25.6	27.0	28.6	30.9	32.8	34.0	14.3	17.6	21.0	24.3	29.5	34.6	39.8	7	10
7	11	18.2	19.0	20.2	21.7	22.8	23.7	24.6	25.9	27.3	29.0	31.3	33.2	34.5	14.3	17.7	21.2	24.6	29.8	35.1	40.4	7	11

Contd...

Contd...

Age Yrs Mths	3rd	5th	10th	20th	30th	40th	50th	60th	70th	80th	90th	95th	97th	-3S.D.	-2S.D.	-1S.D.	Median	+1S.D.	+2S.D.	+3S.D.	Age Yrs	Mths
8 0	18.3	19.1	20.4	21.9	23.0	24.0	24.8	26.2	27.7	29.4	31.7	33.7	35.0	14.4	17.9	21.4	24.8	30.2	35.6	41.0	8	0
8 1	18.4	19.3	20.6	22.1	23.3	24.2	25.1	26.5	28.0	29.7	32.2	34.2	35.4	14.5	18.0	21.6	25.1	30.6	36.1	41.6	8	1
8 2	18.6	19.5	20.8	22.4	23.5	24.5	25.4	26.8	28.3	30.1	32.6	34.6	35.9	14.6	18.2	21.8	25.4	31.0	36.6	42.2	8	2
8 3	18.8	19.6	21.0	22.6	23.8	24.8	25.7	27.1	28.7	30.5	33.0	35.1	36.5	14.6	18.3	22.0	25.7	31.4	37.1	42.9	8	3
8 4	18.9	19.8	21.2	22.8	24.0	25.0	26.0	27.5	29.0	30.9	33.5	35.6	37.0	14.7	18.5	22.2	26.0	31.8	37.7	43.5	8	4
8 5	19.1	20.0	21.4	23.1	24.3	25.3	26.3	27.8	29.4	31.3	33.9	36.1	37.5	14.8	18.6	22.5	26.3	32.2	38.2	44.1	8	5
8 6	19.2	20.2	21.6	23.3	24.5	25.6	26.6	28.1	29.8	31.7	34.4	36.6	38.0	14.9	18.8	22.7	26.6	32.7	38.7	44.8	8	6
8 7	19.4	20.3	21.8	23.5	24.8	25.9	26.9	28.5	30.1	32.1	34.8	37.1	38.5	14.9	18.9	22.9	26.9	33.1	39.3	45.5	8	7
8 8	19.6	20.5	22.0	23.8	25.1	26.2	27.2	28.8	30.5	32.5	35.3	37.6	39.1	15.0	19.1	23.1	27.2	33.5	39.8	46.1	8	8
8 9	19.7	20.7	22.2	24.0	25.3	26.5	27.5	29.1	30.9	32.9	35.8	38.1	39.6	15.1	19.2	23.4	27.5	33.9	40.4	46.8	8	9
8 10	19.9	20.9	22.4	24.3	25.6	26.8	27.8	29.5	31.3	33.3	36.2	38.6	40.2	15.2	19.4	23.6	27.8	34.4	41.0	47.5	8	10
8 11	20.1	21.1	22.6	24.5	25.9	27.1	28.1	29.8	31.6	33.8	36.7	39.1	40.7	15.3	19.6	23.9	28.1	34.8	41.5	48.2	8	11
9 0	20.2	21.3	22.9	24.8	26.2	27.4	28.5	30.2	32.0	34.2	37.2	39.7	41.3	15.4	19.7	24.1	28.5	35.3	42.1	48.9	9	0
9 1	20.4	21.5	23.1	25.0	26.5	27.7	28.8	30.5	32.4	34.6	37.7	40.2	41.8	15.5	19.9	24.3	28.8	35.7	42.7	49.6	9	1
9 2	20.6	21.7	23.3	25.3	26.7	28.0	29.1	30.9	32.8	35.1	38.2	40.7	42.4	15.5	20.1	24.6	29.1	36.2	43.2	50.3	9	2
9 3	20.8	21.9	23.5	25.6	27.0	28.3	29.4	31.3	33.2	35.5	38.7	41.3	43.0	15.6	20.2	24.8	29.4	36.6	43.8	51.0	9	3
9 4	21.0	22.1	23.8	25.8	27.3	28.6	29.8	31.6	33.6	35.9	39.2	41.8	43.5	15.7	20.4	25.1	29.8	37.1	44.4	51.7	9	4
9 5	21.2	22.3	24.0	26.1	27.6	28.9	30.1	32.0	34.0	36.4	39.7	42.4	44.1	15.8	20.6	25.4	30.1	37.6	45.0	52.5	9	5
9 6	21.3	22.5	24.3	26.4	27.9	29.2	30.5	32.4	34.4	36.8	40.2	42.9	44.7	15.9	20.8	25.6	30.5	38.0	45.6	53.2	9	6
9 7	21.5	22.7	24.5	26.7	28.2	29.6	30.8	32.7	34.8	37.3	40.7	43.5	45.3	16.0	21.0	25.9	30.8	38.5	46.2	53.9	9	7
9 8	21.7	22.9	24.7	26.9	28.5	29.9	31.1	33.1	35.2	37.7	41.2	44.0	45.9	16.1	21.1	26.1	31.1	39.0	46.8	54.6	9	8
9 9	21.9	23.1	25.0	27.2	28.8	30.2	31.5	33.5	35.7	38.2	41.7	44.6	46.5	16.2	21.3	26.4	31.5	39.4	47.4	55.3	9	9
9 10	22.1	23.4	25.2	27.5	29.1	30.5	31.8	33.9	36.1	38.6	42.2	45.1	47.0	16.4	21.5	26.7	31.8	39.9	48.0	56.1	9	10
9 11	22.3	23.6	25.5	27.8	29.4	30.9	32.2	34.3	36.5	39.1	42.7	45.7	47.6	16.5	21.7	27.0	32.2	40.4	48.6	56.8	9	11

Contd...

Contd....

Age		Percentiles													Standard Deviations							Age	
Yrs	Mths	3rd	5th	10th	20th	30th	40th	50th	60th	70th	80th	90th	95th	97th	-3S.D.	-2S.D.	-1S.D.	Median	+1S.D.	+2S.D.	+3S.D.	Yrs	Mths
10	0	22.5	23.8	25.7	28.1	29.8	31.2	32.5	34.7	36.9	39.6	43.2	46.2	48.2	16.6	21.9	27.2	32.5	40.9	49.2	57.5	10	0
10	1	22.7	24.0	26.0	28.4	30.1	31.5	32.9	35.0	37.3	40.0	43.7	46.8	48.8	16.7	22.1	27.5	32.9	41.4	49.8	58.3	10	1
10	2	23.0	24.2	26.2	28.7	30.4	31.9	33.3	35.4	37.8	40.5	44.3	47.4	49.4	16.8	22.3	27.8	33.3	41.8	50.4	59.0	10	2
10	3	23.2	24.5	26.5	28.9	30.7	32.2	33.6	35.8	38.2	40.9	44.8	47.9	50.0	16.9	22.5	28.1	33.6	42.3	51.0	59.7	10	3
10	4	23.4	24.7	26.8	29.2	31.0	32.6	34.0	36.2	38.6	41.4	45.3	48.5	50.6	17.1	22.7	28.3	34.0	42.8	51.6	60.4	10	4
10	5	23.6	25.0	27.0	29.5	31.4	32.9	34.4	36.6	39.0	41.9	45.8	49.1	51.2	17.2	22.9	28.6	34.4	43.3	52.2	61.2	10	5
10	6	23.8	25.2	27.3	29.8	31.7	33.3	34.7	37.0	39.5	42.3	46.3	49.6	51.8	17.3	23.1	28.9	34.7	43.8	52.8	61.9	10	6
10	7	24.0	25.4	27.6	30.1	32.0	33.6	35.1	37.4	39.9	42.8	46.9	50.2	52.4	17.5	23.3	29.2	35.1	44.3	53.4	62.6	10	7
10	8	24.3	25.7	27.8	30.5	32.3	34.0	35.5	37.8	40.3	43.3	47.4	50.7	52.9	17.6	23.6	29.5	35.5	44.8	54.0	63.3	10	8
10	9	24.5	25.9	28.1	30.8	32.7	34.3	35.8	38.2	40.8	43.8	47.9	51.3	53.5	17.8	23.8	29.8	35.8	45.2	54.6	64.1	10	9
10	10	24.7	26.2	28.4	31.1	33.0	34.7	36.2	38.6	41.2	44.2	48.4	51.9	54.1	17.9	24.0	30.1	36.2	45.7	55.2	64.8	10	10
10	11	25.0	26.4	28.7	31.4	33.3	35.0	36.6	39.0	41.6	44.7	48.9	52.4	54.7	18.1	24.2	30.4	36.6	46.2	55.8	65.5	10	11
11	0	25.2	26.7	28.9	31.7	33.7	35.4	37.0	39.4	42.1	45.2	49.4	53.0	55.3	18.2	24.5	30.7	37.0	46.7	56.4	66.2	11	0
11	1	25.4	26.9	29.2	32.0	34.0	35.7	37.3	39.8	42.5	45.6	50.0	53.5	55.9	18.4	24.7	31.0	37.3	47.2	57.0	66.9	11	1
11	2	25.7	27.2	29.5	32.3	34.3	36.1	37.7	40.2	42.9	46.1	50.5	54.1	56.4	18.5	24.9	31.3	37.7	47.7	57.6	67.6	11	2
11	3	25.9	27.5	29.8	32.6	34.7	36.4	38.1	40.6	43.4	46.6	51.0	54.6	57.0	18.7	25.2	31.6	38.1	48.2	58.2	68.3	11	3
11	4	26.2	27.7	30.1	33.0	35.0	36.8	38.5	41.0	43.8	47.0	51.5	55.2	57.6	18.9	25.4	31.9	38.5	48.6	58.8	69.0	11	4
11	5	26.4	28.0	30.4	33.3	35.4	37.2	38.8	41.4	44.2	47.5	52.0	55.7	58.2	19.0	25.6	32.2	38.8	49.1	59.4	69.7	11	5
11	6	26.7	28.3	30.7	33.6	35.7	37.5	39.2	41.9	44.7	48.0	52.5	56.3	58.7	19.2	25.9	32.6	39.2	49.6	60.0	70.3	11	6
11	7	26.9	28.5	31.0	33.9	36.1	37.9	39.6	42.3	45.1	48.4	53.0	56.8	59.3	19.4	26.1	32.9	39.6	50.1	60.5	71.0	11	7
11	8	27.2	28.8	31.3	34.3	36.4	38.3	40.0	42.7	45.5	48.9	53.5	57.4	59.9	19.6	26.4	33.2	40.0	50.5	61.1	71.7	11	8
11	9	27.5	29.1	31.6	34.6	36.8	38.6	40.4	43.1	46.0	49.3	54.0	57.9	60.4	19.8	26.6	33.5	40.4	51.0	61.7	72.3	11	9
11	10	27.7	29.4	31.9	34.9	37.1	39.0	40.8	43.5	46.4	49.8	54.5	58.4	61.0	20.0	26.9	33.8	40.8	51.5	62.2	73.0	11	10
11	11	28.0	29.6	32.2	35.3	37.5	39.4	41.1	43.9	46.8	50.3	55.0	58.9	61.5	20.2	27.2	34.2	41.1	52.0	62.8	73.6	11	11

Contd...

Contd...

Age Yrs	Mths	3rd	5th	10th	20th	30th	40th	50th	60th	70th	80th	90th	95th	97th	-3S.D.	-2S.D.	-1S.D.	Median	+1S.D.	+2S.D.	+3S.D.	Age Yrs	Mths
					Percentiles												Standard Deviations						
12	0	28.3	29.9	32.5	35.6	37.8	39.7	41.5	44.3	47.2	50.7	55.5	59.5	62.0	20.4	27.4	34.5	41.5	52.4	63.3	74.2	12	0
12	1	28.5	30.2	32.8	35.9	38.2	40.1	41.9	44.7	47.7	51.2	56.0	60.0	62.6	20.6	27.7	34.8	41.9	52.9	63.9	74.8	12	1
12	2	28.8	30.5	33.1	36.3	38.5	40.5	42.3	45.1	48.1	51.6	56.5	60.5	63.1	20.8	28.0	35.1	42.3	53.4	64.4	75.5	12	2
12	3	29.1	30.8	33.4	36.6	38.9	40.9	42.7	45.5	48.5	52.1	56.9	61.0	63.6	21.0	28.2	35.5	42.7	53.8	64.9	76.1	12	3
12	4	29.4	31.1	33.7	36.9	39.3	41.2	43.1	45.9	48.9	52.5	57.4	61.5	64.1	21.2	28.5	35.8	43.1	54.3	65.5	76.7	12	4
12	5	29.7	31.4	34.1	37.3	39.6	41.6	43.5	46.3	49.4	52.9	57.9	62.0	64.6	21.5	28.8	36.1	43.5	54.7	66.0	77.2	12	5
12	6	30.0	31.7	34.4	37.6	40.0	42.0	43.8	46.7	49.8	53.4	58.4	62.5	65.1	21.7	29.1	36.5	43.8	55.2	66.5	77.8	12	6
12	7	30.2	32.0	34.7	38.0	40.3	42.3	44.2	47.1	50.2	53.8	58.8	63.0	65.6	21.9	29.4	36.8	44.2	55.6	67.0	78.4	12	7
12	8	30.5	32.3	35.0	38.3	40.7	42.7	44.6	47.5	50.6	54.2	59.3	63.4	66.1	22.2	29.6	37.1	44.6	56.0	67.5	78.9	12	8
12	9	30.8	32.6	35.3	38.6	41.0	43.1	45.0	47.9	51.0	54.7	59.7	63.9	66.6	22.4	29.9	37.5	45.0	56.5	68.0	79.5	12	9
12	10	31.1	32.9	35.7	39.0	41.4	43.4	45.4	48.3	51.4	55.1	60.2	64.4	67.1	22.7	30.2	37.8	45.4	56.9	68.5	80.0	12	10
12	11	31.4	33.2	36.0	39.3	41.7	43.8	45.7	48.7	51.8	55.5	60.6	64.8	67.6	22.9	30.5	38.1	45.7	57.3	68.9	80.6	12	11
13	0	31.7	33.5	36.3	39.7	42.1	44.2	46.1	49.0	52.2	55.9	61.0	65.3	68.0	23.1	30.8	38.4	46.1	57.8	69.4	81.1	13	0
13	1	32.0	33.8	36.6	40.0	42.4	44.5	46.5	49.4	52.6	56.3	61.5	65.7	68.5	23.4	31.1	38.8	46.5	58.2	69.9	81.6	13	1
13	2	32.3	34.1	36.9	40.3	42.8	44.9	46.8	49.8	53.0	56.7	61.9	66.2	68.9	23.6	31.4	39.1	46.8	58.6	70.3	82.1	13	2
13	3	32.6	34.4	37.2	40.7	43.1	45.2	47.2	50.2	53.4	57.1	62.3	66.6	69.4	23.9	31.7	39.4	47.2	59.0	70.8	82.6	13	3
13	4	32.9	34.7	37.6	41.0	43.5	45.6	47.6	50.6	53.8	57.5	62.7	67.0	69.8	24.2	32.0	39.8	47.6	59.4	71.2	83.1	13	4
13	5	33.2	35.0	37.9	41.3	43.8	45.9	47.9	50.9	54.1	57.9	63.1	67.4	70.3	24.4	32.2	40.1	47.9	59.8	71.7	83.5	13	5
13	6	33.5	35.3	38.2	41.6	44.1	46.3	48.3	51.3	54.5	58.3	63.5	67.9	70.7	24.7	32.5	40.4	48.3	60.2	72.1	84.1	13	6
13	7	33.8	35.6	38.5	42.0	44.5	46.6	48.6	51.6	54.9	58.7	63.9	68.3	71.1	24.9	32.8	40.7	48.6	60.6	72.5	84.4	13	7
13	8	34.0	35.9	38.8	42.3	44.8	46.9	49.0	52.0	55.2	59.0	64.3	68.7	71.5	25.2	33.1	41.0	49.0	60.9	72.9	84.9	13	8
13	9	34.3	36.2	39.1	42.6	45.1	47.3	49.3	52.3	55.6	59.4	64.7	69.0	71.9	25.4	33.4	41.3	49.3	61.3	73.3	85.3	13	9
13	10	34.6	36.5	39.4	42.9	45.4	47.6	49.6	52.7	55.9	59.8	65.1	69.4	72.3	25.7	33.7	41.7	49.6	61.7	73.7	85.7	13	10
13	11	34.9	36.8	39.7	43.2	45.8	47.9	50.0	53.0	56.3	60.1	65.4	69.8	72.7	26.0	34.0	42.0	50.0	62.0	74.1	86.2	13	11

Contd...

Contd...

Age Yrs Mths	3rd	5th	10th	20th	30th	40th	50th	60th	70th	80th	90th	95th	97th	-3S.D.	-2S.D.	-1S.D.	Median	+1S.D.	+2S.D.	+3S.D.	Age Yrs Mths
							Percentiles										Standard Deviations				
14 0	35.2	37.1	40.0	43.5	46.1	48.2	50.3	53.3	56.6	60.5	65.8	70.2	73.0	26.2	34.2	42.3	50.3	62.4	74.5	86.6	14 0
14 1	35.5	37.4	40.3	43.8	46.4	48.6	50.6	53.7	57.0	60.8	66.1	70.5	73.4	26.5	34.5	42.6	50.6	62.7	74.8	86.9	14 1
14 2	35.8	37.7	40.6	44.1	46.7	48.9	50.9	54.0	57.3	61.1	66.5	70.9	73.7	26.7	34.8	42.9	50.9	63.0	75.2	87.3	14 2
14 3	36.0	37.9	40.9	44.4	47.0	49.2	51.2	54.3	57.6	61.5	66.8	71.2	74.1	27.0	35.1	43.1	51.2	63.4	75.5	87.7	14 3
14 4	36.3	38.2	41.2	44.7	47.3	49.5	51.5	54.6	57.9	61.8	67.1	71.6	74.4	27.3	35.3	43.4	51.5	63.7	75.9	88.1	14 4
14 5	36.6	38.5	41.4	45.0	47.6	49.8	51.8	54.9	58.2	62.1	67.4	71.9	74.8	27.5	35.6	43.7	51.8	64.0	76.2	88.4	14 5
14 6	36.8	38.8	41.7	45.3	47.8	50.0	52.1	55.2	58.5	62.4	67.8	72.2	75.1	27.8	35.9	44.0	52.1	64.3	76.5	88.7	14 6
14 7	37.1	39.0	42.0	45.5	48.1	50.3	52.4	55.5	58.8	62.7	68.1	72.5	75.4	28.0	36.1	44.3	52.4	64.6	76.8	89.1	14 7
14 8	37.4	39.3	42.2	45.8	48.4	50.6	52.7	55.8	59.1	63.0	68.4	72.8	75.7	28.3	36.4	44.5	52.7	64.9	77.1	89.4	14 8
14 9	37.6	39.5	42.5	46.1	48.7	50.9	52.9	56.0	59.4	63.2	68.6	73.1	76.0	28.5	36.6	44.8	52.9	65.2	77.4	89.7	14 9
14 10	37.9	39.8	42.7	46.3	48.9	51.1	53.2	56.3	59.6	63.5	68.9	73.4	76.3	28.8	36.9	45.0	53.2	65.5	77.7	90.0	14 10
14 11	38.1	40.0	43.0	46.6	49.2	51.4	53.4	56.5	59.9	63.8	69.2	73.6	76.5	29.0	37.1	45.3	53.4	65.7	78.0	90.3	14 11
15 0	38.3	40.3	43.2	46.8	49.4	51.6	53.7	56.8	60.1	64.0	69.4	73.9	76.8	29.2	37.4	45.5	53.7	66.0	78.3	90.6	15 0
15 1	38.6	40.5	43.5	47.1	49.6	51.9	53.9	57.0	60.4	64.3	69.7	74.1	77.1	29.5	37.6	45.8	53.9	66.2	78.5	90.8	15 1
15 2	38.8	40.7	43.7	47.3	49.9	52.1	54.1	57.3	60.6	64.5	69.9	74.4	77.3	29.7	37.9	46.0	54.1	66.4	78.8	91.1	15 2
15 3	39.0	41.0	43.9	47.5	50.1	52.3	54.4	57.5	60.8	64.7	70.1	74.6	77.5	29.9	38.1	46.2	54.4	66.7	79.0	91.3	15 3
15 4	39.3	41.2	44.1	47.7	50.3	52.5	54.6	57.7	61.0	64.9	70.4	74.8	77.8	30.2	38.3	46.4	54.6	66.9	79.2	91.5	15 4
15 5	39.5	41.4	44.4	47.9	50.5	52.7	54.8	57.9	61.2	65.1	70.6	75.1	78.0	30.4	38.5	46.6	54.8	67.1	79.4	91.8	15 5
15 6	39.7	41.6	44.6	48.1	50.7	52.9	55.0	58.1	61.4	65.3	70.8	75.3	78.2	30.6	38.7	46.8	55.0	67.3	79.6	92.0	15 6
15 7	39.9	41.8	44.7	48.3	50.9	53.1	55.1	58.3	61.6	65.5	71.0	75.4	78.4	30.8	38.9	47.0	55.1	67.5	79.8	92.2	15 7
15 8	40.1	42.0	44.9	48.5	51.1	53.3	55.3	58.4	61.8	65.7	71.1	75.6	78.5	31.0	39.1	47.2	55.3	67.7	80.0	92.3	15 8
15 9	40.3	42.2	45.1	48.7	51.2	53.4	55.5	58.6	61.9	65.9	71.3	75.8	78.7	31.2	39.3	47.4	55.5	67.8	80.2	92.5	15 9
15 10	40.5	42.4	45.3	48.8	51.4	53.6	55.6	58.7	62.1	66.0	71.5	75.9	78.9	31.4	39.5	47.6	55.6	68.0	80.3	92.7	15 10
15 11	40.6	42.5	45.4	49.0	51.5	53.7	55.8	58.9	62.2	66.2	71.6	76.1	79.0	31.6	39.7	47.7	55.8	68.1	80.5	92.8	15 11

Contd...

Contd...

Age Yrs Mths	3rd	5th	10th	20th	30th	40th	50th	60th	70th	80th	90th	95th	97th	-3S.D.	-2S.D.	-1S.D.	Median	+1S.D.	+2S.D.	+3S.D.	Age Yrs Mths
					Percentiles											Standard Deviations					
16 0	40.8	42.7	45.6	49.1	51.7	53.9	55.9	59.0	62.4	66.3	71.7	76.2	79.1	31.8	39.8	47.9	55.9	68.2	80.6	93.0	16 0
16 1	41.0	42.8	45.8	49.3	51.8	54.0	56.0	59.1	62.5	66.4	71.9	76.3	79.3	32.0	40.0	48.0	56.0	68.4	80.7	93.1	16 1
16 2	41.1	43.0	45.9	49.4	51.9	54.1	56.1	59.2	62.6	66.5	72.0	76.5	79.4	32.2	40.2	48.1	56.1	68.5	80.8	93.2	16 2
16 3	41.2	43.1	46.0	49.5	52.0	54.2	56.2	59.3	62.7	66.6	72.1	76.6	79.5	32.4	40.3	48.3	56.2	68.6	81.0	93.3	16 3
16 4	41.4	43.3	46.1	49.6	52.1	54.3	56.3	59.4	62.8	66.7	72.2	76.7	79.6	32.5	40.4	48.4	56.3	68.7	81.0	93.4	16 4
16 5	41.5	43.4	46.3	49.7	52.2	54.4	56.4	59.5	62.9	66.8	72.2	76.7	79.7	32.7	40.6	48.5	56.4	68.7	81.1	93.5	16 5
16 6	41.6	43.5	46.4	49.8	52.3	54.4	56.4	59.6	62.9	66.9	72.3	76.8	79.7	32.8	40.7	48.6	56.4	68.8	81.2	93.6	16 6
16 7	41.8	43.6	46.5	49.9	52.4	54.5	56.5	59.6	63.0	66.9	72.4	76.9	79.8	33.0	40.8	48.7	56.5	68.9	81.3	93.6	16 7
16 8	41.9	43.7	46.6	50.0	52.5	54.6	56.6	59.7	63.0	67.0	72.4	76.9	79.8	33.1	40.9	48.7	56.6	68.9	81.3	93.7	16 8
16 9	42.0	43.8	46.6	50.1	52.5	54.6	56.6	59.7	63.1	67.0	72.5	77.0	79.9	33.3	41.1	48.8	56.6	69.0	81.4	93.7	16 9
16 10	42.1	43.9	46.7	50.1	52.6	54.7	56.6	59.8	63.1	67.1	72.5	77.0	79.9	33.4	41.2	48.9	56.6	69.0	81.4	93.8	16 10
16 11	42.2	44.0	46.8	50.2	52.6	54.7	56.7	59.8	63.2	67.1	72.5	77.0	80.0	33.6	41.3	49.0	56.7	69.0	81.4	93.8	16 11
17 0	42.3	44.1	46.9	50.2	52.7	54.7	56.7	59.8	63.2	67.1	72.6	77.1	80.0	33.7	41.3	49.0	56.7	69.1	81.5	93.8	17 0
17 1	42.3	44.1	46.9	50.3	52.7	54.8	56.7	59.8	63.2	67.1	72.6	77.1	80.0	33.8	41.4	49.1	56.7	69.1	81.5	93.9	17 1
17 2	42.4	44.2	47.0	50.3	52.7	54.8	56.7	59.9	63.2	67.1	72.6	77.1	80.0	33.9	41.5	49.1	56.7	69.1	81.5	93.9	17 2
17 3	42.5	44.3	47.0	50.4	52.8	54.8	56.7	59.9	63.2	67.1	72.6	77.1	80.0	34.0	41.6	49.2	56.7	69.1	81.5	93.9	17 3
17 4	42.6	44.3	47.1	50.4	52.8	54.8	56.7	59.9	63.2	67.1	72.6	77.1	80.0	34.1	41.7	49.2	56.7	69.1	81.5	93.9	17 4
17 5	42.6	44.4	47.1	50.4	52.8	54.8	56.7	59.9	63.2	67.1	72.6	77.1	80.0	34.2	41.7	49.2	56.7	69.1	81.5	93.9	17 5
17 6	42.7	44.4	47.2	50.4	52.8	54.8	56.7	59.9	63.2	67.1	72.6	77.1	80.0	34.3	41.8	49.3	56.7	69.1	81.5	93.8	17 6
17 7	42.7	44.5	47.2	50.5	52.8	54.8	56.7	59.8	63.2	67.1	72.6	77.1	80.0	34.4	41.9	49.3	56.7	69.1	81.5	93.8	17 7
17 8	42.8	44.5	47.2	50.5	52.8	54.8	56.7	59.8	63.2	67.1	72.5	77.0	80.0	34.5	41.9	49.3	56.7	69.1	81.4	93.8	17 8
17 9	42.8	44.6	47.2	50.5	52.8	54.8	56.7	59.8	63.2	67.1	72.5	77.0	79.9	34.6	42.0	49.3	56.7	69.0	81.4	93.8	17 9
17 10	42.9	44.6	47.3	50.5	52.8	54.8	56.7	59.8	63.1	67.1	72.5	77.0	79.9	34.7	42.0	49.3	56.7	69.0	81.4	93.7	17 10
17 11	42.9	44.6	47.3	50.5	52.8	54.8	56.6	59.8	63.1	67.0	72.5	77.0	79.9	34.8	42.0	49.3	56.6	69.0	81.4	93.7	17 11
18 0	42.9	44.7	47.3	50.5	52.8	54.8	56.6	59.7	63.1	67.0	72.5	76.9	79.9	34.8	42.1	49.4	56.6	69.0	81.3	93.7	18 0

APPENDIX 47.11

LENGTH (CM) BY AGE OF
BOYS AGED 0 TO 36 MONTHS (NCHS STANDARDS)

Age Months	Percentiles													Standard Deviations							Age Months
	3rd	5th	10th	20th	30th	40th	50th	60th	70th	80th	90th	95th	97th	-3S.D.	-2S.D.	-1S.D.	Median	+1S.D.	+2S.D.	+3S.D.	
0	46.2	46.7	47.6	48.6	49.3	49.9	50.5	51.1	51.7	52.4	53.4	54.2	54.8	43.6	45.9	48.2	50.5	52.8	55.1	57.4	0
1	49.9	50.5	51.4	52.5	53.3	53.9	54.6	55.2	55.9	56.6	57.7	58.6	59.2	47.2	49.7	52.1	54.6	57.0	59.5	61.9	1
2	53.2	53.9	54.8	55.9	56.7	57.4	58.1	58.7	59.4	60.2	61.4	62.3	62.9	50.4	52.9	55.5	58.1	60.7	63.2	65.8	2
3	56.1	56.8	57.7	58.9	59.7	60.4	61.1	61.8	62.5	63.3	64.5	65.5	66.1	53.2	55.8	58.5	61.1	63.7	66.4	69.0	3
4	58.6	59.3	60.3	61.4	62.3	63.0	63.7	64.4	65.1	66.0	67.1	68.1	68.7	55.6	58.3	61.0	63.7	66.4	69.1	71.7	4
5	60.8	61.5	62.5	63.6	64.5	65.2	65.9	66.6	67.3	68.2	69.4	70.3	71.0	57.8	60.5	63.2	65.9	68.6	71.3	74.0	5
6	62.8	63.4	64.4	65.6	66.4	67.1	67.8	68.5	69.2	70.1	71.3	72.2	72.9	59.8	62.4	65.1	67.8	70.5	73.2	75.9	6
7	64.5	65.1	66.1	67.2	68.1	68.8	69.5	70.2	70.9	71.7	72.9	73.9	74.5	61.5	64.1	66.8	69.5	72.2	74.8	77.5	7
8	66.0	66.6	67.6	68.7	69.6	70.3	71.0	71.6	72.4	73.2	74.4	75.3	76.0	63.0	65.7	68.3	71.0	73.6	76.3	78.9	8
9	67.4	68.0	68.9	70.1	70.9	71.7	72.3	73.0	73.7	74.6	75.7	76.7	77.3	64.4	67.0	69.7	72.3	75.0	77.6	80.3	9
10	68.7	69.3	70.2	71.4	72.2	73.0	73.6	74.3	75.0	75.9	77.0	78.0	78.6	65.7	68.3	71.0	73.6	76.3	78.9	81.6	10
11	69.9	70.5	71.5	72.6	73.5	74.2	74.9	75.6	76.3	77.1	78.3	79.3	79.9	66.9	69.6	72.2	74.9	77.5	80.2	82.9	11
12	71.0	71.6	72.6	73.8	74.7	75.4	76.1	76.8	77.5	78.4	79.5	80.5	81.2	68.0	70.7	73.4	76.1	78.8	81.5	84.2	12
13	72.1	72.7	73.7	74.9	75.8	76.5	77.2	77.9	78.7	79.5	80.7	81.7	82.4	69.0	71.8	74.5	77.2	80.0	82.7	85.5	13
14	73.1	73.8	74.8	76.0	76.9	77.6	78.3	79.1	79.8	80.7	81.9	82.9	83.6	70.0	72.8	75.6	78.3	81.1	83.9	86.7	14
15	74.1	74.7	75.8	77.0	77.9	78.7	79.4	80.1	80.9	81.8	83.1	84.1	84.8	70.9	73.7	76.6	79.4	82.3	85.1	88.0	15
16	75.0	75.7	76.7	77.9	78.9	79.7	80.4	81.2	82.0	82.9	84.2	85.2	85.9	71.7	74.6	77.5	80.4	83.4	86.3	89.2	16
17	75.9	76.6	77.6	78.9	79.9	80.7	81.4	82.2	83.0	83.9	85.3	86.3	87.0	72.5	75.5	78.5	81.4	84.4	87.4	90.4	17
18	76.7	77.4	78.5	79.8	80.8	81.6	82.4	83.2	84.0	85.0	86.3	87.4	88.1	73.3	76.3	79.4	82.4	85.4	88.5	91.5	18

Contd...

Contd...

Age Months	Percentiles													Standard Deviations							Age Months
	3rd	5th	10th	20th	30th	40th	50th	60th	70th	80th	90th	95th	97th	-3S.D.	-2S.D.	-1S.D.	Median	+1S.D.	+2S.D.	+3S.D.	
19	77.5	78.2	79.4	80.7	81.7	82.6	83.3	84.1	85.0	86.0	87.3	88.4	89.2	74.0	77.1	80.2	83.3	86.4	89.5	92.7	19
20	78.3	79.0	80.2	81.6	82.6	83.4	84.2	85.0	85.9	86.9	88.3	89.5	90.2	74.7	77.9	81.1	84.2	87.4	90.6	93.8	20
21	79.1	79.8	81.0	82.4	83.4	84.3	85.1	85.9	86.8	87.8	89.3	90.4	91.2	75.4	78.7	81.9	85.1	88.4	91.6	94.8	21
22	79.8	80.6	81.8	83.2	84.3	85.2	86.0	86.8	87.7	88.7	90.2	91.4	92.2	76.1	79.4	82.7	86.0	89.3	92.5	95.8	22
23	80.6	81.3	82.6	84.0	85.1	86.0	86.8	87.7	88.6	89.6	91.1	92.3	93.1	76.8	80.2	83.5	86.8	90.2	93.5	96.8	23
24	81.3	82.1	83.3	84.8	85.9	86.8	87.6	88.5	89.4	90.5	92.0	93.2	94.0	77.5	80.9	84.3	87.6	91.0	94.4	97.7	24
25	82.1	82.9	84.1	85.6	86.7	87.6	88.5	89.3	90.2	91.3	92.8	94.0	94.8	78.3	81.7	85.1	88.5	91.8	95.2	98.6	25
26	82.8	83.6	84.9	86.4	87.5	88.4	89.2	90.1	91.0	92.1	93.6	94.9	95.7	79.0	82.4	85.8	89.2	92.7	96.1	99.5	26
27	83.6	84.4	85.6	87.1	88.2	89.2	90.0	90.9	91.8	92.9	94.4	95.7	96.5	79.8	83.2	86.6	90.0	93.4	96.9	100.3	27
28	84.4	85.2	86.4	87.9	89.0	89.9	90.8	91.7	92.6	93.7	95.2	96.4	97.2	80.5	83.9	87.4	90.8	94.2	97.6	101.1	28
29	85.1	85.9	87.2	88.7	89.8	90.7	91.6	92.4	93.3	94.4	95.9	97.2	98.0	81.3	84.7	88.1	91.6	95.0	98.4	101.8	29
30	85.8	86.7	87.9	89.4	90.5	91.4	92.3	93.2	94.1	95.2	96.7	97.9	98.7	82.0	85.4	88.9	92.3	95.7	99.2	102.6	30
31	86.6	87.4	88.6	90.1	91.2	92.2	93.0	93.9	94.8	95.9	97.4	98.7	99.5	82.7	86.2	89.6	93.0	96.5	99.9	103.3	31
32	87.3	88.1	89.3	90.9	91.9	92.9	93.7	94.6	95.5	96.6	98.2	99.4	100.2	83.4	86.9	90.3	93.7	97.2	100.6	104.1	32
33	88.0	88.8	90.0	91.6	92.6	93.6	94.5	95.3	96.3	97.4	98.9	100.1	100.9	84.1	87.6	91.0	94.5	97.9	101.4	104.8	33
34	88.6	89.4	90.7	92.2	93.3	94.3	95.2	96.0	97.0	98.1	99.6	100.9	101.7	84.7	88.2	91.7	95.2	98.6	102.1	105.6	34
35	89.3	90.1	91.4	92.9	94.0	95.0	95.8	96.7	97.7	98.8	100.3	101.6	102.4	85.4	88.8	92.3	95.8	99.3	102.8	106.3	35
36	89.9	90.7	92.0	93.5	94.7	95.6	96.5	97.4	98.4	99.5	101.0	102.3	103.2	85.9	89.4	93.0	96.5	100.1	103.6	107.1	36

APPENDIX 47.12

STATURE (CM) BY AGE OF BOYS AGED 2 TO 18 YEARS (NCHS STANDARDS)

Age Yrs Mths	Percentiles													Standard Deviations							Age Yrs Mths
	3rd	5th	10th	20th	30th	40th	50th	60th	70th	80th	90th	95th	97th	-3S.D.	-2S.D.	-1S.D.	Median	+1S.D.	+2S.D.	+3S.D.	
2 0	79.6	80.4	81.5	82.9	83.9	84.8	85.6	86.4	87.3	88.3	89.7	90.8	91.6	76.0	79.2	82.4	85.6	88.8	92.0	95.2	2 0
2 1	80.3	81.1	82.3	83.7	84.7	85.6	86.4	87.2	88.1	89.2	90.6	91.8	92.5	76.7	79.9	83.2	86.4	89.7	92.9	96.2	2 1
2 2	81.0	81.8	83.0	84.5	85.5	86.4	87.2	88.1	89.0	90.0	91.5	92.7	93.5	77.3	80.6	83.9	87.2	90.6	93.9	97.2	2 2
2 3	81.7	82.5	83.8	85.2	86.3	87.2	88.1	88.9	89.8	90.9	92.4	93.6	94.4	78.0	81.3	84.7	88.1	91.4	94.8	98.1	2 3
2 4	82.4	83.2	84.5	86.0	87.1	88.0	88.9	89.7	90.7	91.7	93.2	94.5	95.3	78.6	82.0	85.4	88.9	92.3	95.7	99.1	2 4
2 5	83.1	83.9	85.2	86.7	87.8	88.8	89.7	90.5	91.5	92.6	94.1	95.4	96.2	79.2	82.7	86.2	89.7	93.1	96.6	100.1	2 5
2 6	83.8	84.6	85.9	87.5	88.6	89.5	90.4	91.3	92.3	93.4	94.9	96.2	97.1	79.9	83.4	86.9	90.4	94.0	97.5	101.0	2 6
2 7	84.5	85.3	86.6	88.2	89.3	90.3	91.2	92.1	93.1	94.2	95.8	97.1	97.9	80.5	84.1	87.6	91.2	94.8	98.3	101.9	2 7
2 8	85.2	86.0	87.3	88.9	90.1	91.0	92.0	92.9	93.9	95.0	96.6	97.9	98.8	81.1	84.7	88.3	92.0	95.6	99.2	102.8	2 8
2 9	85.8	86.7	88.0	89.6	90.8	91.8	92.7	93.6	94.6	95.8	97.4	98.8	99.6	81.7	85.4	89.0	92.7	96.4	100.1	103.7	2 9
2 10	86.5	87.3	88.7	90.3	91.5	92.5	93.5	94.4	95.4	96.6	98.2	99.6	100.5	82.3	86.0	89.7	93.5	97.2	100.9	104.6	2 10
2 11	87.1	88.0	89.4	91.0	92.2	93.2	94.2	95.1	96.2	97.4	99.0	100.4	101.3	82.9	86.7	90.4	94.2	98.0	101.7	105.5	2 11
3 0	87.8	88.7	90.0	91.7	92.9	94.0	94.9	95.9	96.9	98.1	99.8	101.2	102.1	83.5	87.3	91.1	94.9	98.7	102.5	106.3	3 0
3 1	88.4	89.3	90.7	92.4	93.6	94.7	95.6	96.6	97.7	98.9	100.6	102.0	102.9	84.1	87.9	91.8	95.6	99.5	103.3	107.2	3 1
3 2	89.0	89.9	91.3	93.1	94.3	95.4	96.3	97.3	98.4	99.6	101.3	102.7	103.7	84.7	88.6	92.4	96.3	100.2	104.1	108.0	3 2
3 3	89.6	90.6	92.0	93.7	95.0	96.0	97.0	98.0	99.1	100.4	102.1	103.5	104.4	85.2	89.2	93.1	97.0	101.0	104.9	108.8	3 3
3 4	90.2	91.2	92.6	94.4	95.6	96.7	97.7	98.7	99.8	101.1	102.8	104.3	105.2	85.8	89.8	93.8	97.7	101.7	105.7	109.7	3 4
3 5	90.9	91.8	93.3	95.0	96.3	97.4	98.4	99.4	100.5	101.8	103.6	105.0	106.0	86.4	90.4	94.4	98.4	102.4	106.4	110.5	3 5
3 6	91.5	92.4	93.9	95.7	97.0	98.1	99.1	100.1	101.2	102.5	104.3	105.7	106.7	86.9	91.0	95.0	99.1	103.1	107.2	111.2	3 6
3 7	92.0	93.0	94.5	96.3	97.6	98.7	99.7	100.8	101.9	103.2	105.0	106.5	107.4	87.5	91.6	95.7	99.7	103.8	107.9	112.0	3 7
3 8	92.6	93.6	95.1	96.9	98.2	99.4	100.4	101.4	102.6	103.9	105.7	107.2	108.2	88.0	92.1	96.3	100.4	104.5	108.7	112.8	3 8
3 9	93.2	94.2	95.7	97.5	98.9	100.0	101.0	102.1	103.2	104.6	106.4	107.9	108.9	88.6	92.7	96.9	101.0	105.2	109.4	113.5	3 9
3 10	93.8	94.8	96.3	98.2	99.5	100.6	101.7	102.8	103.9	105.2	107.1	108.6	109.6	89.1	93.3	97.5	101.7	105.9	110.1	114.3	3 10
3 11	94.4	95.4	96.9	98.8	100.1	101.3	102.3	103.4	104.5	105.9	107.7	109.3	110.3	89.6	93.9	98.1	102.3	106.6	110.8	115.0	3 11

Contd...

Contd...

Age Yrs	Mths	Percentiles 3rd	5th	10th	20th	30th	40th	50th	60th	70th	80th	90th	95th	97th	Std Dev -3S.D.	-2S.D.	-1S.D.	Median	+1S.D.	+2S.D.	+3S.D.	Age Yrs	Mths
4	0	94.9	95.9	97.5	99.4	100.7	101.9	102.9	104.0	105.2	106.5	108.4	110.0	111.0	90.2	94.4	98.7	102.9	107.2	111.5	115.7	4	0
4	1	95.5	96.5	98.1	100.0	101.3	102.5	103.6	104.7	105.8	107.2	109.1	110.6	111.6	90.7	95.0	99.3	103.6	107.9	112.2	116.5	4	1
4	2	96.0	97.1	98.6	100.5	101.9	103.1	104.2	105.3	106.4	107.8	109.7	111.3	112.3	91.2	95.5	99.9	104.2	108.5	112.8	117.2	4	2
4	3	96.6	97.6	99.2	101.1	102.5	103.7	104.8	105.9	107.1	108.4	110.4	111.9	113.0	91.7	96.1	100.4	104.8	109.1	113.5	117.8	4	3
4	4	97.1	98.2	99.8	101.7	103.1	104.3	105.4	106.5	107.7	109.1	111.0	112.6	113.6	92.2	96.6	101.0	105.4	109.8	114.2	118.5	4	4
4	5	97.7	98.7	100.3	102.3	103.7	104.9	106.0	107.1	108.3	109.7	111.6	113.2	114.3	92.7	97.1	101.6	106.0	110.4	114.8	119.2	4	5
4	6	98.2	99.2	100.9	102.8	104.2	105.4	106.6	107.7	108.9	110.3	122.2	113.9	114.9	93.2	97.7	102.1	106.6	111.0	115.4	119.9	4	6
4	7	98.7	99.8	101.4	103.4	104.8	106.0	107.1	108.3	109.5	110.9	112.9	114.5	115.5	93.7	98.2	102.7	107.1	111.6	116.1	120.5	4	7
4	8	99.2	100.3	101.9	103.9	105.3	106.6	107.7	108.8	110.1	111.5	113.5	115.1	116.2	94.2	98.7	103.2	107.7	112.2	116.7	121.2	4	8
4	9	99.8	100.8	102.5	104.5	105.9	107.1	108.3	109.4	110.6	112.1	114.1	115.7	116.8	94.7	99.2	103.7	108.3	112.8	117.3	121.8	4	9
4	10	100.3	101.3	103.0	105.0	106.4	107.7	108.8	110.0	111.2	112.7	114.7	116.3	117.4	95.2	99.7	104.3	108.8	113.4	117.9	122.5	4	10
4	11	100.8	101.9	103.5	105.5	107.0	108.2	109.4	110.5	111.8	113.2	115.2	116.9	118.0	95.7	100.2	104.8	109.4	114.0	118.5	123.1	4	11
5	0	101.3	102.4	104.0	106.1	107.5	108.8	109.9	111.1	112.3	113.8	115.8	117.5	118.6	96.1	100.7	105.3	109.9	114.5	119.1	123.7	5	0
5	1	101.8	102.9	104.5	106.6	108.0	109.3	110.5	111.6	112.9	114.4	116.4	118.1	119.2	96.6	101.2	105.8	110.5	115.1	119.7	124.3	5	1
5	2	102.3	103.4	105.1	107.1	108.6	109.8	111.0	112.2	113.4	114.9	117.0	118.6	119.7	97.1	101.7	106.4	111.0	115.6	120.3	124.9	5	2
5	3	102.8	103.9	105.6	107.6	109.1	110.4	111.5	112.7	114.0	115.5	117.5	119.2	120.3	97.5	102.2	106.9	111.5	116.2	120.9	125.5	5	3
5	4	103.2	104.3	106.0	108.1	109.6	110.9	112.1	113.2	114.5	116.0	118.1	119.8	120.9	98.0	102.7	107.4	112.1	116.8	121.4	126.1	5	4
5	5	103.7	104.8	106.5	108.6	110.1	111.4	112.6	113.8	115.1	116.5	118.6	120.3	121.4	98.4	103.2	107.9	112.6	117.3	122.0	126.7	5	5
5	6	104.2	105.3	107.0	109.1	110.6	111.9	113.1	114.3	115.6	117.1	119.2	120.9	122.0	98.9	103.6	108.4	113.1	117.8	122.6	127.3	5	6
5	7	104.7	105.8	107.5	109.6	111.1	112.4	113.6	114.8	116.1	117.6	119.7	121.4	122.6	99.3	104.1	108.9	113.6	118.4	123.1	127.9	5	7
5	8	105.1	106.3	108.0	110.1	111.6	112.9	114.1	115.3	116.6	118.1	120.2	122.0	123.1	99.8	104.6	109.3	114.1	118.9	123.7	128.4	5	8
5	9	105.6	106.7	108.5	110.6	112.1	113.4	114.6	115.8	117.1	118.7	120.8	122.5	123.6	100.2	105.0	109.8	114.6	119.4	124.2	129.0	5	9
5	10	106.0	107.2	108.9	111.1	112.6	113.9	115.1	116.3	117.6	119.2	121.3	123.0	124.2	100.7	105.5	110.3	115.1	119.9	124.7	129.6	5	10
5	11	106.5	107.6	109.4	111.5	113.1	114.4	115.6	116.8	118.1	119.7	121.8	123.6	124.7	101.1	105.9	110.8	115.6	120.4	125.3	130.1	5	11

Contd...

Contd...

Age Yrs	Mths	Percentiles													Standard Deviations							Age Yrs	Mths
		3rd	5th	10th	20th	30th	40th	50th	60th	70th	80th	90th	95th	97th	-3S.D.	-2S.D.	-1S.D.	Median	+1S.D.	+2S.D.	+3S.D.		
6	0	107.0	108.1	109.9	112.0	113.5	114.9	116.1	117.3	118.6	120.2	122.3	124.1	125.2	101.5	106.4	111.2	116.1	121.0	125.8	130.7	6	0
6	1	107.4	108.6	110.3	112.5	114.0	115.3	116.6	117.8	119.1	120.7	122.8	124.6	125.8	101.9	106.8	111.7	116.6	121.5	126.3	131.2	6	1
6	2	107.8	109.0	110.8	112.9	114.5	115.8	117.1	118.3	119.6	121.2	123.3	125.1	126.3	102.4	107.3	112.2	117.1	122.0	126.9	131.8	6	2
6	3	108.3	109.4	111.2	113.4	115.0	116.3	117.5	118.8	120.1	121.7	123.8	125.6	126.8	102.8	107.7	112.6	117.5	122.5	127.4	132.3	6	3
6	4	108.7	109.9	111.7	113.9	115.4	116.8	118.0	119.3	120.6	122.2	124.3	126.1	127.3	103.2	108.1	113.1	118.0	123.0	127.9	132.8	6	4
6	5	109.2	110.3	112.1	114.3	115.9	117.2	118.5	119.7	121.1	122.7	124.8	126.6	127.8	103.6	108.6	113.5	118.5	123.4	128.4	133.4	6	5
6	6	109.6	110.8	112.6	114.8	116.3	117.7	119.0	120.2	121.6	123.1	125.3	127.1	128.3	104.0	109.0	114.0	119.0	123.9	128.9	133.9	6	6
6	7	110.0	111.2	113.0	115.2	116.8	118.1	119.4	120.7	122.0	123.6	125.8	127.6	128.8	104.4	109.4	114.4	119.4	124.4	129.4	134.4	6	7
6	8	110.4	111.6	113.4	115.7	117.2	118.6	119.9	121.1	122.5	124.1	126.3	128.1	129.3	104.8	109.8	114.9	119.9	124.9	129.9	134.9	6	8
6	9	110.9	112.1	113.9	116.1	117.7	119.1	120.3	121.6	123.0	124.6	126.8	128.6	129.8	105.2	110.3	115.3	120.3	125.4	130.4	135.4	6	9
6	10	111.3	112.5	114.3	116.5	118.1	119.5	120.8	122.1	123.4	125.0	127.3	129.1	130.3	105.6	110.7	115.7	120.8	125.8	130.9	136.0	6	10
6	11	111.7	112.9	114.7	117.0	118.6	120.0	121.2	122.5	123.9	125.5	127.7	129.6	130.8	106.0	111.1	116.2	121.2	126.3	131.4	136.5	6	11
7	0	112.1	113.3	115.2	117.4	119.0	120.4	121.7	123.0	124.4	126.0	128.2	130.1	131.3	106.4	111.5	116.6	121.7	126.8	131.9	137.0	7	0
7	1	112.5	113.7	115.6	117.8	119.5	120.8	122.1	123.4	124.8	126.4	128.7	130.6	131.8	106.8	111.9	117.0	122.1	127.3	132.4	137.5	7	1
7	2	112.9	114.1	116.0	118.3	119.9	121.3	122.6	123.9	125.3	126.9	129.2	131.0	132.3	107.2	112.3	117.5	122.6	127.7	132.9	138.0	7	2
7	3	113.3	114.6	116.4	118.7	120.3	121.7	123.0	124.3	125.7	127.4	129.6	131.5	132.7	107.6	112.7	117.9	123.0	128.2	133.3	138.5	7	3
7	4	113.7	115.0	116.8	119.1	120.8	122.2	123.5	124.8	126.2	127.8	130.1	132.0	133.2	108.0	113.1	118.3	123.5	128.7	133.8	139.0	7	4
7	5	114.1	115.4	117.3	119.5	121.2	122.6	123.9	125.2	126.6	128.3	130.6	132.5	133.7	108.3	113.5	118.7	123.9	129.1	134.3	139.5	7	5
7	6	114.5	115.8	117.7	120.0	121.6	123.0	124.4	125.7	127.1	128.8	131.0	132.9	134.2	108.7	113.9	119.1	124.4	129.6	134.8	140.0	7	6
7	7	114.9	116.2	118.1	120.4	122.0	123.5	124.8	126.1	127.5	129.2	131.5	133.4	134.7	109.1	114.3	119.6	124.8	130.0	135.3	140.5	7	7
7	8	115.3	116.6	118.5	120.8	122.5	123.9	125.2	126.6	128.0	129.7	132.0	133.9	135.1	109.5	114.7	120.0	125.2	130.5	135.8	141.0	7	8
7	9	115.7	117.0	118.9	121.2	122.9	124.3	125.7	127.0	128.4	130.1	132.4	134.4	135.6	109.8	115.1	120.4	125.7	131.0	136.2	141.5	7	9
7	10	116.1	117.4	119.3	121.6	123.3	124.8	126.1	127.4	128.9	130.6	132.9	134.8	136.1	110.2	115.5	120.8	126.1	131.4	136.7	142.0	7	10
7	11	116.5	117.8	119.7	122.1	123.7	125.2	126.5	127.9	129.3	131.0	133.4	135.3	136.6	110.6	115.9	121.2	126.5	131.9	137.2	142.5	7	11

Contd...

Contd...

Age Yrs	Mths	3rd	5th	10th	20th	30th	40th	50th	60th	70th	80th	90th	95th	97th	-3S.D.	-2S.D.	-1S.D.	Median	+1S.D.	+2S.D.	+3S.D.	Age Yrs	Mths
								Percentiles									Standard Deviations						
8	0	116.9	118.2	120.1	122.5	124.2	125.6	127.0	128.3	129.8	131.5	133.8	135.8	137.0	110.9	116.3	121.6	127.0	132.3	137.7	143.0	8	0
8	1	117.3	118.6	120.5	122.9	124.6	126.0	127.4	128.8	130.2	131.9	134.3	136.2	137.5	111.3	116.7	122.0	127.4	132.8	138.2	143.5	8	1
8	2	117.7	119.0	120.9	123.3	125.0	126.5	127.8	129.2	130.7	132.4	134.8	136.7	138.0	111.6	117.0	122.4	127.8	133.2	138.6	144.0	8	2
8	3	118.1	119.3	121.3	123.7	125.4	126.9	128.3	129.6	131.1	132.8	135.2	137.2	138.5	112.0	117.4	122.8	128.3	133.7	139.1	144.5	8	3
8	4	118.4	119.7	121.7	124.1	125.8	127.3	128.7	130.1	131.6	133.3	135.7	137.7	139.0	112.4	117.8	123.2	128.7	134.1	139.6	145.0	8	4
8	5	118.8	120.1	122.1	124.5	126.3	127.7	129.1	130.5	132.0	133.7	136.1	138.1	139.4	112.7	118.2	123.7	129.1	134.6	140.1	145.6	8	5
8	6	119.2	120.5	122.5	124.9	126.7	128.2	129.6	131.0	132.4	134.2	136.6	138.6	139.9	113.1	118.6	124.1	129.6	135.1	140.6	146.1	8	6
8	7	119.6	120.9	122.9	125.3	127.1	128.6	130.0	131.4	132.9	134.6	137.1	139.1	140.4	113.4	118.9	124.5	130.0	135.5	141.1	146.6	8	7
8	8	120.0	121.3	123.3	125.7	127.5	129.0	130.4	131.8	133.3	135.1	137.5	139.6	140.9	113.8	119.3	124.9	130.4	136.0	141.5	147.1	8	8
8	9	120.4	121.7	123.7	126.2	127.9	129.4	130.9	132.3	133.8	135.6	138.0	140.0	141.4	114.1	119.7	125.3	130.9	136.4	142.0	147.6	8	9
8	10	120.7	122.1	124.1	126.6	128.3	129.9	131.3	132.7	134.2	136.0	138.5	140.5	141.9	114.5	120.1	125.7	131.3	136.9	142.5	148.1	8	10
8	11	121.1	122.4	124.5	127.0	128.8	130.3	131.7	133.2	134.7	136.5	139.0	141.0	142.3	114.8	120.4	126.1	131.7	137.4	143.0	148.7	8	11
9	0	121.5	122.8	124.9	127.4	129.2	130.7	132.2	133.6	135.1	136.9	139.4	141.5	142.8	115.1	120.8	126.5	132.2	137.8	143.5	149.2	9	0
9	1	121.9	123.2	125.3	127.8	129.6	131.2	132.6	134.0	135.6	137.4	139.9	142.0	143.3	115.5	121.2	126.9	132.6	138.3	144.0	149.7	9	1
9	2	122.2	123.6	125.7	128.2	130.0	131.6	133.0	134.5	136.0	137.9	140.4	142.5	143.8	115.8	121.6	127.3	133.0	138.8	144.5	150.3	9	2
9	3	122.6	124.0	126.1	128.6	130.5	132.0	133.5	134.9	136.5	138.3	140.9	143.0	144.3	116.2	121.9	127.7	133.5	139.2	145.0	150.8	9	3
9	4	123.0	124.4	126.5	129.0	130.9	132.4	133.9	135.4	137.0	138.8	141.4	143.5	144.8	116.5	122.3	128.1	133.9	139.7	145.5	151.3	9	4
9	5	123.4	124.8	126.9	129.4	131.3	132.9	134.4	135.8	137.4	139.3	141.8	144.0	145.3	116.8	122.7	128.5	134.4	140.2	146.0	151.9	9	5
9	6	123.7	125.1	127.3	129.9	131.7	133.3	134.8	136.3	137.9	139.8	142.3	144.5	145.9	117.2	123.1	128.9	134.8	140.7	146.6	152.4	9	6
9	7	124.1	125.5	127.7	130.3	132.1	133.8	135.3	136.7	138.4	140.2	142.8	145.0	146.4	117.5	123.4	129.3	135.3	141.2	147.1	153.0	9	7
9	8	124.5	125.9	128.1	130.7	132.6	134.2	135.7	137.2	138.8	140.7	143.3	145.5	146.9	117.8	123.8	129.7	135.7	141.6	147.6	153.5	9	8
9	9	124.9	126.3	128.5	131.1	133.0	134.6	136.1	137.7	139.3	141.2	143.8	146.0	147.4	118.2	124.2	130.2	136.1	142.1	148.1	154.1	9	9
9	10	125.3	126.7	128.9	131.5	133.4	135.1	136.6	138.1	139.8	141.7	144.3	146.5	147.9	118.5	124.5	130.6	136.6	142.6	148.7	154.7	9	10
9	11	125.6	127.1	129.3	131.9	133.9	135.5	137.1	138.6	140.2	142.2	144.8	147.0	148.5	118.8	124.9	131.0	137.1	143.1	149.2	155.3	9	11

Contd...

Contd...

Age Yrs	Mths	Percentiles													Standard Deviations							Age Yrs	Mths
		3rd	5th	10th	20th	30th	40th	50th	60th	70th	80th	90th	95th	97th	-3S.D.	-2S.D.	-1S.D.	Median	+1S.D.	+2S.D.	+3S.D.		
10	0	126.0	127.5	129.7	132.4	134.3	136.0	137.5	139.1	140.7	142.7	145.3	147.6	149.0	119.2	125.3	131.4	137.5	143.6	149.7	155.9	10	0
10	1	126.4	127.9	130.1	132.8	134.7	136.4	138.0	139.5	141.2	143.2	145.9	148.1	149.6	119.5	125.7	131.8	138.0	144.1	150.3	156.4	10	1
10	2	126.8	128.2	130.5	133.2	135.2	136.9	138.4	140.0	141.7	143.7	146.4	148.6	150.1	119.8	126.0	132.2	138.4	144.6	150.8	157.0	10	2
10	3	127.2	128.6	130.9	133.7	135.6	137.3	138.9	140.5	142.2	144.2	146.9	149.2	150.7	120.2	126.4	132.7	138.9	145.2	151.4	157.6	10	3
10	4	127.5	129.0	131.3	134.1	136.1	137.8	139.4	141.0	142.7	144.7	147.4	149.7	151.2	120.5	126.8	133.1	139.4	145.7	152.0	158.3	10	4
10	5	127.9	129.4	131.7	134.5	136.5	138.2	139.9	141.5	143.2	145.2	148.0	150.3	151.8	120.8	127.2	133.5	139.9	146.2	152.5	158.9	10	5
10	6	128.3	129.8	132.1	135.0	137.0	138.7	140.3	141.9	143.7	145.7	148.5	150.8	152.3	121.2	127.6	133.9	140.3	146.7	153.1	159.5	10	6
10	7	128.7	130.2	132.6	135.4	137.4	139.2	140.8	142.4	144.2	146.2	149.1	151.4	152.9	121.5	127.9	134.4	140.8	147.2	153.7	160.1	10	7
10	8	129.1	130.6	133.0	135.8	137.9	139.6	141.3	142.9	144.7	146.8	149.6	152.0	153.5	121.8	128.3	134.8	141.3	147.8	154.3	160.8	10	8
10	9	129.5	131.0	133.4	136.3	138.3	140.1	141.8	143.4	145.2	147.3	150.2	152.5	154.1	122.2	128.7	135.2	141.8	148.3	154.9	161.4	10	9
10	10	129.9	131.4	133.8	136.7	138.8	140.6	142.3	143.9	145.7	147.8	150.7	153.1	154.7	122.5	129.1	135.7	142.3	148.9	155.5	162.1	10	10
10	11	130.3	131.8	134.2	137.2	139.3	141.1	142.8	144.5	146.3	148.4	151.3	153.7	155.3	122.8	129.5	136.1	142.8	149.4	156.1	162.7	10	11
11	0	130.6	132.2	134.7	137.6	139.8	141.6	143.3	145.0	146.8	148.9	151.9	154.3	155.9	123.1	129.9	136.6	143.3	150.0	156.7	163.4	11	0
11	1	131.0	132.6	135.1	138.1	140.2	142.1	143.8	145.5	147.3	149.5	152.5	154.9	156.5	123.5	130.2	137.0	143.8	150.5	157.3	164.1	11	1
11	2	131.4	133.1	135.5	138.5	140.7	142.6	144.3	146.0	147.9	150.0	153.0	155.5	157.1	123.8	130.6	137.5	144.3	151.1	157.9	164.8	11	2
11	3	131.8	133.5	136.0	139.0	141.2	143.1	144.8	146.5	148.4	150.6	153.6	156.1	157.8	124.1	131.0	137.9	144.8	151.7	158.6	165.5	11	3
11	4	132.2	133.9	136.4	139.5	141.7	143.6	145.3	147.1	149.0	151.2	154.2	156.8	158.4	124.5	131.4	138.4	145.3	152.3	159.2	166.2	11	4
11	5	132.6	134.3	136.8	139.9	142.2	144.1	145.8	147.6	149.5	151.8	154.8	157.4	159.0	124.8	131.8	138.8	145.8	152.9	159.9	166.9	11	5
11	6	133.0	134.7	137.3	140.4	142.7	144.6	146.4	148.2	150.1	152.3	155.5	158.0	159.7	125.1	132.2	139.3	146.4	153.5	160.5	167.6	11	6
11	7	133.5	135.1	137.7	140.9	143.2	145.1	146.9	148.7	150.7	152.9	156.1	158.7	160.4	125.5	132.6	139.8	146.9	154.1	161.2	168.4	11	7
11	8	133.9	135.6	138.2	141.4	143.7	145.6	147.4	149.3	151.2	153.5	156.7	159.3	161.0	125.8	133.0	140.2	147.4	154.7	161.9	169.1	11	8
11	9	134.3	136.0	138.6	141.9	144.2	146.1	148.0	149.8	151.8	154.1	157.3	160.0	161.7	126.1	133.4	140.7	148.0	155.3	162.6	169.9	11	9
11	10	134.7	136.4	139.1	142.3	144.7	146.7	148.5	150.4	152.4	154.7	158.0	160.7	162.4	126.5	133.8	141.2	148.5	155.9	163.3	170.6	11	10
11	11	135.1	136.9	139.6	142.8	145.2	147.2	149.1	151.0	153.0	155.4	158.6	161.3	163.1	126.8	134.2	141.7	149.1	156.5	164.0	171.4	11	11

Contd....

Contd...

Age			Percentiles													Standard Deviations							Age	
Yrs	Mths	3rd	5th	10th	20th	30th	40th	50th	60th	70th	80th	90th	95th	97th	-3S.D.	-2S.D.	-1S.D.	Median	+1S.D.	+2S.D.	+3S.D.	Yrs	Mths
12	0	135.5	137.3	140.0	143.3	145.7	147.8	149.7	151.6	153.6	156.0	159.3	162.0	163.8	127.1	134.6	142.1	149.7	157.2	164.7	172.2	12	0
12	1	136.0	137.7	140.5	143.8	146.2	148.3	150.2	152.1	154.2	156.6	159.9	162.7	164.5	127.5	135.1	142.6	150.2	157.8	165.4	172.9	12	1
12	2	136.4	138.2	141.0	144.3	146.8	148.8	150.8	152.7	154.8	157.2	160.6	163.4	165.2	127.8	135.5	143.1	150.8	158.4	166.1	173.7	12	2
12	3	136.8	138.6	141.4	144.8	147.3	149.4	151.3	153.3	155.4	157.8	161.2	164.0	165.9	128.2	135.9	143.6	151.3	159.1	166.8	174.5	12	3
12	4	137.3	139.1	141.9	145.3	147.8	149.9	151.9	153.9	156.0	158.5	161.9	164.7	166.6	128.5	136.3	144.1	151.9	159.7	167.5	175.3	12	4
12	5	137.7	139.5	142.4	145.9	148.4	150.5	152.5	154.5	156.6	159.1	162.5	165.4	167.3	128.9	136.8	144.6	152.5	160.3	168.2	176.0	12	5
12	6	138.1	140.0	142.9	146.4	148.9	151.0	153.0	155.0	157.2	159.7	163.2	166.1	167.9	129.3	137.2	145.1	153.0	161.0	168.9	176.8	12	6
12	7	138.6	140.5	143.4	146.9	149.4	151.6	153.6	155.6	157.8	160.3	163.9	166.8	168.6	129.6	137.6	145.6	153.6	161.6	169.6	177.6	12	7
12	8	139.0	140.9	143.9	147.4	150.0	152.1	154.2	156.2	158.4	161.0	164.5	167.4	169.3	130.0	138.1	146.1	154.2	162.2	170.3	178.3	12	8
12	9	139.5	141.4	144.4	147.9	150.5	152.7	154.8	156.8	159.0	161.6	165.2	168.1	170.0	130.4	138.5	146.6	154.8	162.9	171.0	179.1	12	9
12	10	140.0	141.9	144.9	148.4	151.0	153.3	155.3	157.4	159.6	162.2	165.8	168.8	170.7	130.8	139.0	147.2	155.3	163.5	171.7	179.8	12	10
12	11	140.4	142.4	145.4	149.0	151.6	153.8	155.9	158.0	160.2	162.8	166.4	169.4	171.4	131.2	139.4	147.7	155.9	164.1	172.4	180.6	12	11
13	0	140.9	142.9	145.9	149.5	152.1	154.4	156.5	158.6	160.8	163.4	167.1	170.1	172.0	131.6	139.9	148.2	156.5	164.7	173.0	181.3	13	0
13	1	141.4	143.3	146.4	150.0	152.7	154.9	157.0	159.1	161.4	164.0	167.7	170.7	172.7	132.1	140.4	148.7	157.0	165.4	173.7	182.0	13	1
13	2	141.9	143.8	146.9	150.6	153.2	155.5	157.6	159.7	162.0	164.7	168.3	171.4	173.4	132.5	140.9	149.2	157.6	166.0	174.4	182.7	13	2
13	3	142.3	144.3	147.4	151.1	153.8	156.0	158.2	160.3	162.6	165.3	169.0	172.0	174.0	132.9	141.3	149.8	158.2	166.6	175.0	183.4	13	3
13	4	142.8	144.8	147.9	151.6	154.3	156.6	158.7	160.9	163.2	165.9	169.6	172.6	174.6	133.4	141.8	150.3	158.7	167.2	175.6	184.1	13	4
13	5	143.3	145.3	148.4	152.2	154.8	157.1	159.3	161.4	163.7	166.4	170.2	173.3	175.3	133.8	142.3	150.8	159.3	167.8	176.3	184.8	13	5
13	6	143.8	145.9	148.9	152.7	155.4	157.7	159.9	162.0	164.3	167.0	170.8	173.9	175.9	134.3	142.8	151.3	159.9	168.4	176.9	185.4	13	6
13	7	144.4	146.4	149.5	153.2	155.9	158.2	160.4	162.6	164.9	167.6	171.4	174.5	176.5	134.8	143.3	151.9	160.4	168.9	177.5	186.0	13	7
13	8	144.9	146.9	150.0	153.8	156.5	158.8	161.0	163.1	165.4	168.2	171.9	175.0	177.1	135.3	143.9	152.4	161.0	169.5	178.1	186.6	13	8
13	9	145.4	147.4	150.5	154.3	157.0	159.3	161.5	163.7	166.0	168.7	172.5	175.6	177.6	135.8	144.4	152.9	161.5	170.1	178.6	187.2	13	9
13	10	145.9	148.0	151.1	154.8	157.6	159.9	162.1	164.2	166.5	169.3	173.0	176.1	178.2	136.3	144.9	153.5	162.1	170.6	179.2	187.8	13	10
13	11	146.5	148.5	151.6	155.4	158.1	160.4	162.6	164.8	167.1	169.8	173.6	176.7	178.7	136.9	145.4	154.0	162.6	171.2	179.7	188.3	13	11

Contd...

Contd...

Age Yrs Mths	3rd	5th	10th	20th	30th	40th	50th	60th	70th	80th	90th	95th	97th	-3S.D.	-2S.D.	-1S.D.	Median	+1S.D.	+2S.D.	+3S.D.	Age Yrs Mths
14 0	147.0	149.0	152.1	155.9	158.6	161.0	163.1	165.3	167.6	170.3	174.1	177.2	179.2	137.4	146.0	154.6	163.1	171.7	180.2	188.8	14 0
14 1	147.6	149.6	152.7	156.5	159.2	161.5	163.6	165.8	168.1	170.8	174.6	177.7	179.7	138.0	146.5	155.1	163.6	172.2	180.8	189.3	14 1
14 2	148.1	150.1	153.2	157.0	159.7	162.0	164.2	166.3	168.6	171.4	175.1	178.2	180.2	138.6	147.1	155.6	164.2	172.7	181.2	189.8	14 2
14 3	148.7	150.7	153.8	157.5	160.2	162.5	164.7	166.8	169.1	171.8	175.6	178.7	180.7	139.2	147.7	156.2	164.7	173.2	181.7	190.2	14 3
14 4	149.3	151.3	154.3	158.1	160.8	163.0	165.2	167.3	169.6	172.3	176.1	179.1	181.1	139.8	148.2	156.7	165.2	173.7	182.1	190.6	14 4
14 5	149.8	151.8	154.9	158.6	161.3	163.6	165.7	167.8	170.1	172.8	176.5	179.6	181.6	140.4	148.8	157.3	165.7	174.1	182.6	191.0	14 5
14 6	150.4	152.4	155.4	159.1	161.8	164.1	166.2	168.3	170.6	173.3	177.0	180.0	182.0	141.0	149.4	157.8	166.2	174.6	183.0	191.4	14 6
14 7	151.0	152.9	156.0	159.7	162.3	164.6	166.7	168.8	171.1	173.7	177.4	180.4	182.4	141.6	150.0	158.3	166.7	175.0	183.4	191.7	14 7
14 8	151.6	153.5	156.5	160.2	162.8	165.1	167.2	169.3	171.5	174.1	177.8	180.8	182.8	142.3	150.6	158.9	167.2	175.5	183.8	192.1	14 8
14 9	152.1	154.1	157.1	160.7	163.3	165.5	167.6	169.7	172.0	174.6	178.2	181.2	183.1	142.9	151.1	159.4	167.6	175.9	184.1	192.4	14 9
14 10	152.7	154.6	157.6	161.2	163.8	166.0	168.1	170.2	172.4	175.0	178.6	181.6	183.5	143.5	151.7	159.9	168.1	176.3	184.5	192.7	14 10
14 11	153.3	155.2	158.1	161.7	164.3	166.5	168.6	170.6	172.8	175.4	179.0	181.9	183.8	144.2	152.3	160.4	168.6	176.7	184.8	192.9	14 11
15 0	153.8	155.7	158.7	162.2	164.8	167.0	169.0	171.0	173.2	175.8	179.3	182.3	184.2	144.8	152.9	160.9	169.0	177.1	185.1	193.2	15 0
15 1	154.4	156.3	159.2	162.7	165.2	167.4	169.4	171.5	173.6	176.2	179.7	182.6	184.5	145.5	153.5	161.4	169.4	177.4	185.4	193.4	15 1
15 2	155.0	156.8	159.7	163.2	165.7	167.9	169.9	171.9	174.0	176.5	180.0	182.9	184.8	146.1	154.0	161.9	169.9	177.8	185.7	193.6	15 2
15 3	155.5	157.4	160.2	163.7	166.2	168.3	170.3	172.3	174.4	176.9	180.3	183.2	185.1	146.7	154.6	162.4	170.3	178.1	186.0	193.8	15 3
15 4	156.1	157.9	160.7	164.1	166.6	168.7	170.7	172.7	174.8	177.2	180.7	183.5	185.3	147.3	155.1	162.9	170.7	178.5	186.2	194.0	15 4
15 5	156.6	158.4	161.2	164.6	167.0	169.1	171.1	173.0	175.1	177.6	181.0	183.8	185.6	148.0	155.7	163.4	171.1	178.8	186.5	194.2	15 5
15 6	157.1	158.9	161.7	165.0	167.5	169.5	171.5	173.4	175.5	177.9	181.3	184.0	185.8	148.6	156.2	163.8	171.5	179.1	186.7	194.4	15 6
15 7	157.6	159.4	162.2	165.5	167.9	169.9	171.8	173.8	175.8	178.2	181.5	184.3	186.1	149.2	156.7	164.3	171.8	179.4	187.0	194.5	15 7
15 8	158.1	159.9	162.6	165.9	168.3	170.3	172.2	174.1	176.1	178.5	181.8	184.5	186.3	149.8	157.2	164.7	172.2	179.7	187.2	194.7	15 8
15 9	158.6	160.4	163.1	166.3	168.7	170.7	172.6	174.4	176.4	178.8	182.1	184.8	186.5	150.3	157.7	165.2	172.6	180.0	187.4	194.8	15 9
15 10	159.1	160.8	163.5	166.7	169.1	171.0	172.9	174.8	176.8	179.1	182.3	185.0	186.7	150.9	158.2	165.6	172.9	180.2	187.6	194.9	15 10
15 11	159.6	161.3	163.9	167.1	169.4	171.4	173.2	175.1	177.0	179.3	182.5	185.2	186.9	151.4	158.7	166.0	173.2	180.5	187.8	195.0	15 11

Percentiles | Standard Deviations

Contd...

Contd...

Age Yrs	Age Mths	Percentiles 3rd	5th	10th	20th	30th	40th	50th	60th	70th	80th	90th	95th	97th	Standard Deviations -3S.D.	-2S.D.	-1S.D.	Median	+1S.D.	+2S.D.	+3S.D.	Age Yrs	Age Mths
16	0	160.0	161.7	164.3	167.5	169.8	171.7	173.5	175.4	177.3	179.6	182.8	185.4	187.1	152.0	159.2	166.4	173.5	180.7	187.9	195.1	16	0
16	1	160.4	162.1	164.7	167.9	170.1	172.0	173.8	175.7	177.6	179.8	183.0	185.6	187.2	152.5	159.6	166.7	173.8	181.0	188.1	195.2	16	1
16	2	160.9	162.5	165.1	168.2	170.4	172.4	174.1	175.9	177.8	180.1	183.2	185.7	187.4	153.0	160.0	167.1	174.1	181.2	188.2	195.3	16	2
16	3	161.3	162.9	165.5	168.5	170.7	172.6	174.4	176.2	178.1	180.3	183.4	185.9	187.6	153.4	160.4	167.4	174.4	181.4	188.4	195.4	16	3
16	4	161.6	163.3	165.8	168.8	171.0	172.9	174.7	176.4	178.3	180.5	183.6	186.1	187.7	153.9	160.8	167.7	174.7	181.6	188.5	195.5	16	4
16	5	162.0	163.6	166.1	169.1	171.3	173.2	174.9	176.7	178.5	180.7	183.7	186.2	187.8	154.3	161.2	168.1	174.9	181.8	188.7	195.5	16	5
16	6	162.3	163.9	166.4	169.4	171.6	173.4	175.2	176.9	178.7	180.9	183.9	186.4	188.0	154.7	161.5	168.3	175.2	182.0	188.8	195.6	16	6
16	7	162.7	164.2	166.7	169.7	171.8	173.7	175.4	177.1	178.9	181.1	184.0	186.5	188.1	155.1	161.8	168.6	175.4	182.1	188.9	195.7	16	7
16	8	162.9	164.5	167.0	169.9	172.1	173.9	175.6	177.3	179.1	181.2	184.2	186.6	188.2	155.4	162.1	168.9	175.6	182.3	189.0	195.7	16	8
16	9	163.2	164.8	167.2	170.1	172.3	174.1	175.8	177.4	179.3	181.4	184.3	186.7	188.3	155.8	162.4	169.1	175.8	182.4	189.1	195.8	16	9
16	10	163.5	165.0	167.4	170.3	172.5	174.2	175.9	177.6	179.4	181.5	184.4	186.8	188.4	156.0	162.7	169.3	175.9	182.6	189.2	195.8	16	10
16	11	163.7	165.2	167.6	170.5	172.6	174.4	176.1	177.8	179.5	181.6	184.5	186.9	188.5	156.3	162.9	169.5	176.1	182.7	189.3	195.9	16	11
17	0	163.9	165.4	167.8	170.7	172.8	174.6	176.2	177.9	179.7	181.8	184.6	187.0	188.6	156.5	163.1	169.7	176.2	182.8	189.4	195.9	17	0
17	1	164.0	165.6	168.0	170.8	172.9	174.7	176.3	178.0	179.8	181.9	184.7	187.1	188.7	156.7	163.2	169.8	176.3	182.9	189.4	196.0	17	1
17	2	164.2	165.7	168.1	171.0	173.0	174.8	176.4	178.1	179.9	181.9	184.8	187.2	188.7	156.9	163.4	169.9	176.4	183.0	189.5	196.0	17	2
17	3	164.3	165.8	168.2	171.1	173.1	174.9	176.5	178.2	180.0	182.0	184.9	187.3	188.8	157.0	163.5	170.0	176.5	183.1	189.6	196.1	17	3
17	4	164.4	165.9	168.3	171.1	173.2	175.0	176.6	178.3	180.0	182.1	185.0	187.3	188.9	157.1	163.6	170.1	176.6	183.1	189.6	196.2	17	4
17	5	164.4	166.0	168.3	171.2	173.3	175.0	176.7	178.3	180.1	182.2	185.0	187.4	188.9	157.1	163.7	170.2	176.7	183.2	189.7	196.2	17	5
17	6	164.5	166.0	168.4	171.2	173.3	175.1	176.7	178.4	180.1	182.2	185.1	187.5	189.0	157.2	163.7	170.2	176.7	183.2	189.8	196.3	17	6
17	7	164.5	166.1	168.4	171.3	173.3	175.1	176.8	178.4	180.2	182.3	185.1	187.5	189.0	157.2	163.7	170.2	176.8	183.3	189.8	196.3	17	7
17	8	164.5	166.1	168.4	171.3	173.4	175.1	176.8	178.5	180.2	182.3	185.2	187.5	189.1	157.2	163.7	170.3	176.8	183.3	189.9	196.4	17	8
17	9	164.5	166.1	168.4	171.3	173.4	175.2	176.8	178.5	180.2	182.3	185.2	187.6	189.1	157.2	163.7	170.3	176.8	183.4	189.9	196.5	17	9
17	10	164.5	166.0	168.4	171.3	173.4	175.2	176.8	178.5	180.3	182.3	185.2	187.6	189.2	157.1	163.7	170.3	176.8	183.4	189.9	196.5	17	10
17	11	164.5	166.0	168.4	171.3	173.4	175.2	176.8	178.5	180.3	182.4	185.3	187.6	189.2	157.1	163.7	170.2	176.8	183.4	190.0	196.6	17	11
18	0	164.4	166.0	168.4	171.3	173.4	175.2	176.8	178.5	180.3	182.4	185.3	187.7	189.2	157.0	163.6	170.2	176.8	183.4	190.0	196.6	18	0

APPENDIX 47.13

LENGTH (CM) BY AGE OF
GIRLS AGED 0 TO 36 MONTHS (NCHS STANDARDS)

Age Months	Percentiles													Standard Deviations							Age Months
	3rd	5th	10th	20th	30th	40th	50th	60th	70th	80th	90th	95th	97th	-3S.D.	-2S.D.	-1S.D.	Median	+1S.D.	+2S.D.	+3S.D.	
0	45.8	46.3	47.1	48.0	48.7	49.3	49.9	50.4	51.0	51.7	52.6	53.4	53.9	43.4	45.5	47.7	49.9	52.0	54.2	56.4	0
1	49.2	49.8	50.6	51.6	52.3	53.0	53.5	54.1	54.8	55.5	56.5	57.3	57.9	46.7	49.0	51.2	53.5	55.8	58.1	60.4	1
2	52.2	52.8	53.7	54.7	55.5	56.1	56.8	57.4	58.0	58.8	59.8	60.7	61.3	49.6	52.0	54.4	56.8	59.2	61.6	64.0	2
3	54.9	55.5	56.4	57.5	58.2	58.9	59.5	60.2	60.9	61.6	62.7	63.6	64.2	52.1	54.6	57.1	59.5	62.0	64.5	67.0	3
4	57.2	57.8	58.7	59.8	60.6	61.3	62.0	62.6	63.3	64.1	65.2	66.2	66.8	54.3	56.9	59.4	62.0	64.5	67.1	69.6	4
5	59.2	59.8	60.7	61.9	62.7	63.4	64.1	64.7	65.4	66.3	67.4	68.4	69.0	56.3	58.9	61.5	64.1	66.7	69.3	71.9	5
6	61.0	61.6	62.5	63.7	64.5	65.3	65.9	66.6	67.3	68.2	69.3	70.3	70.9	58.0	60.6	63.3	65.9	68.6	71.2	73.9	6
7	62.5	63.2	64.1	65.3	66.2	66.9	67.6	68.3	69.0	69.8	71.0	72.0	72.6	59.5	62.2	64.9	67.6	70.2	72.9	75.6	7
8	64.0	64.6	65.6	66.8	67.6	68.4	69.1	69.7	70.5	71.3	72.5	73.5	74.2	60.9	63.7	66.4	69.1	71.8	74.5	77.2	8
9	65.3	66.0	66.9	68.1	69.0	69.8	70.4	71.1	71.9	72.8	74.0	74.9	75.6	62.2	65.0	67.7	70.4	73.2	75.9	78.7	9
10	66.6	67.2	68.2	69.5	70.3	71.1	71.8	72.5	73.2	74.1	75.3	76.3	77.0	63.5	66.2	69.0	71.8	74.5	77.3	80.1	10
11	67.8	68.5	69.5	70.7	71.6	72.4	73.1	73.8	74.5	75.4	76.6	77.7	78.3	64.7	67.5	70.3	73.1	75.9	78.7	81.5	11
12	69.0	69.6	70.7	71.9	72.8	73.6	74.3	75.0	75.8	76.7	77.9	79.0	79.6	65.8	68.6	71.5	74.3	77.1	80.0	82.8	12
13	70.1	70.8	71.8	73.1	74.0	74.8	75.5	76.2	77.0	77.9	79.2	80.2	80.9	66.9	69.8	72.6	75.5	78.4	81.2	84.1	13
14	71.2	71.9	72.9	74.2	75.1	75.9	76.7	77.4	78.2	79.1	80.4	81.4	82.1	67.9	70.8	73.7	76.7	79.6	82.5	85.4	14
15	72.2	72.9	74.0	75.3	76.2	77.0	77.8	78.5	79.3	80.3	81.6	82.6	83.3	68.9	71.9	74.8	77.8	80.7	83.7	86.6	15
16	73.2	73.9	75.0	76.3	77.3	78.1	78.9	79.6	80.4	81.4	82.7	83.8	84.5	69.9	72.9	75.9	78.9	81.8	84.8	87.8	16
17	74.2	74.9	76.0	77.4	78.3	79.1	79.9	80.7	81.5	82.5	83.8	84.9	85.6	70.8	73.8	76.9	79.9	82.9	86.0	89.0	17
18	75.1	75.9	77.0	78.3	79.3	80.1	80.9	81.7	82.5	83.5	84.9	86.0	86.7	71.7	74.8	77.9	80.9	84.0	87.1	90.1	18

Contd....

Contd...

Age Months	Percentiles													Standard Deviations							Age Months
	3rd	5th	10th	20th	30th	40th	50th	60th	70th	80th	90th	95th	97th	-3S.D.	-2S.D.	-1S.D.	Median	+1S.D.	+2S.D.	+3S.D.	
19	76.1	76.8	77.9	79.3	80.3	81.1	81.9	82.7	83.5	84.5	85.9	87.0	87.8	72.6	75.7	78.8	81.9	85.0	88.1	91.2	19
20	77.0	77.7	78.8	80.2	81.2	82.1	82.9	83.7	84.5	85.5	86.9	88.0	88.8	73.4	76.6	79.7	82.9	86.0	89.2	92.3	20
21	77.8	78.6	79.7	81.1	82.1	83.0	83.8	84.6	85.5	86.5	87.9	89.0	89.8	74.3	77.4	80.6	83.8	87.0	90.2	93.4	21
22	78.7	79.4	80.6	82.0	83.0	83.9	84.7	85.5	86.4	87.4	88.8	90.0	90.8	75.1	78.3	81.5	84.7	87.9	91.1	94.4	22
23	79.5	80.3	81.4	82.9	83.9	84.8	85.6	86.4	87.3	88.3	89.8	90.9	91.7	75.9	79.1	82.4	85.6	88.9	92.1	95.3	23
24	80.3	81.1	82.3	83.7	84.8	85.6	86.5	87.3	88.2	89.2	90.7	91.9	92.6	76.6	79.9	83.2	86.5	89.8	93.0	96.3	24
25	81.1	81.9	83.1	84.5	85.6	86.5	87.3	88.2	89.1	90.1	91.6	92.8	93.5	77.4	80.7	84.0	87.3	90.6	93.9	97.2	25
26	81.9	82.7	83.9	85.4	86.4	87.3	88.2	89.0	89.9	91.0	92.4	93.6	94.4	78.2	81.5	84.8	88.2	91.5	94.8	98.1	26
27	82.7	83.5	84.7	86.2	87.2	88.1	89.0	89.8	90.7	91.8	93.3	94.5	95.3	78.9	82.3	85.6	89.0	92.3	95.7	99.0	27
28	83.4	84.2	85.5	86.9	88.0	88.9	89.8	90.6	91.5	92.6	94.1	95.3	96.1	79.7	83.0	86.4	89.8	93.1	96.5	99.9	28
29	84.2	85.0	86.2	87.7	88.8	89.7	90.6	91.4	92.3	93.4	94.9	96.1	96.9	80.4	83.8	87.2	90.6	93.9	97.3	100.7	29
30	84.9	85.7	86.9	88.4	89.5	90.5	91.3	92.2	93.1	94.2	95.7	96.9	97.7	81.1	84.5	87.9	91.3	94.7	98.1	101.5	30
31	85.6	86.4	87.7	89.2	90.3	91.2	92.1	92.9	93.9	95.0	96.5	97.7	98.5	81.8	85.2	88.6	92.1	95.5	98.9	102.4	31
32	86.3	87.1	88.4	89.9	91.0	91.9	92.8	93.7	94.6	95.7	97.2	98.5	99.3	82.4	85.9	89.3	92.8	96.3	99.7	103.2	32
33	87.0	87.8	89.1	90.6	91.7	92.6	93.5	94.4	95.3	96.4	98.0	99.2	100.1	83.1	86.6	90.0	93.5	97.0	100.5	104.0	33
34	87.6	88.4	89.7	91.3	92.4	93.3	94.2	95.1	96.1	97.2	98.7	100.0	100.8	83.7	87.2	90.7	94.2	97.7	101.2	104.7	34
35	88.2	89.1	90.4	91.9	93.0	94.0	94.9	95.8	96.8	97.9	99.4	100.7	101.6	84.3	87.8	91.4	94.9	98.4	102.0	105.5	35
36	88.8	89.7	91.0	92.6	93.7	94.7	95.6	96.5	97.4	98.6	100.2	101.5	102.3	84.8	88.4	92.0	95.6	99.1	102.7	106.3	36

APPENDIX 47.14

STATURE (CM) BY AGE OF GIRLS AGED 2 TO 18 YEARS (NCHS STANDARDS)

Age Yrs Mths	3rd	5th	10th	20th	30th	40th	50th	60th	70th	80th	90th	95th	97th	-3S.D.	-2S.D.	-1S.D.	Median	+1S.D.	+2S.D.	+3S.D.	Yrs	Mths
2 0	78.5	79.2	80.4	81.8	82.8	83.7	84.5	85.3	86.2	87.2	88.6	89.8	90.5	74.9	78.1	81.3	84.5	87.7	90.9	94.1	2	0
2 1	79.2	80.0	81.2	82.6	83.6	84.5	85.4	86.2	87.1	88.1	89.5	90.7	91.5	75.6	78.8	82.1	85.4	88.6	91.9	95.1	2	1
2 2	80.0	80.8	82.0	83.4	84.5	85.4	86.2	87.0	87.9	89.0	90.5	91.7	92.4	76.3	79.6	82.9	86.2	89.5	92.8	96.2	2	2
2 3	80.7	81.5	82.7	84.2	85.3	86.2	87.0	87.9	88.8	89.9	91.4	92.6	93.4	77.0	80.3	83.7	87.0	90.4	93.8	97.1	2	3
2 4	81.4	82.3	83.5	85.0	86.1	87.0	87.9	88.7	89.7	90.7	92.2	93.5	94.3	77.6	81.0	84.5	87.9	91.3	94.7	98.1	2	4
2 5	82.2	83.0	84.2	85.8	86.9	87.8	88.7	89.5	90.5	91.6	93.1	94.4	95.2	78.8	81.8	85.2	88.7	92.1	95.6	99.0	2	5
2 6	82.9	83.7	85.0	86.5	87.6	88.6	89.5	90.3	91.3	92.4	93.9	95.2	96.0	79.0	82.5	86.0	89.5	93.0	96.5	100.0	2	6
2 7	83.6	84.4	85.7	87.3	88.4	89.3	90.2	91.1	92.1	93.2	94.8	96.1	96.9	79.6	83.2	86.7	90.2	93.8	97.3	100.9	2	7
2 8	84.3	85.1	86.4	88.0	89.1	90.1	91.0	91.9	92.9	94.0	95.6	96.9	97.7	80.3	83.8	87.4	91.0	94.6	98.2	101.7	2	8
2 9	84.9	85.8	87.1	88.7	89.8	90.8	91.7	92.7	93.6	94.8	96.4	97.7	98.6	80.9	84.5	88.1	91.7	95.4	99.0	102.6	2	9
2 10	85.6	86.5	87.8	89.4	90.6	91.6	92.5	93.4	94.4	95.6	97.2	98.5	99.4	81.5	85.2	88.8	92.5	96.1	99.8	103.4	2	10
2 11	86.3	87.1	88.5	90.1	91.3	92.3	93.2	94.1	95.1	96.3	97.9	99.3	100.1	82.1	85.8	89.5	93.2	96.9	100.6	104.3	2	11
3 0	86.9	87.8	89.1	90.8	92.0	93.0	93.9	94.9	95.9	97.0	98.7	100.0	100.9	82.8	86.5	90.2	93.9	97.6	101.4	105.1	3	0
3 1	87.6	88.4	89.8	91.5	92.6	93.7	94.6	95.6	96.6	97.8	99.4	100.8	101.7	83.4	87.1	90.9	94.6	98.4	102.1	105.9	3	1
3 2	88.2	89.1	90.4	92.1	93.3	94.3	95.3	96.3	97.3	98.5	100.1	101.5	102.4	84.0	87.7	91.5	95.3	99.1	102.9	106.6	3	2
3 3	88.8	89.7	91.1	92.8	94.0	95.0	96.0	96.9	98.0	99.2	100.9	102.2	103.1	84.5	88.4	92.2	96.0	99.8	103.6	107.4	3	3
3 4	89.4	90.3	91.7	93.4	94.6	95.7	96.6	97.6	98.6	99.9	101.6	103.0	103.9	85.1	89.0	92.8	96.6	100.5	104.3	108.2	3	4
3 5	90.0	90.9	92.3	94.0	95.3	96.3	97.3	98.3	99.3	100.5	102.2	103.6	104.6	85.7	89.6	93.4	97.3	101.2	105.0	108.9	3	5
3 6	90.6	91.5	92.9	94.7	95.9	97.0	97.9	98.9	100.0	101.2	102.9	104.3	105.3	86.3	90.2	94.0	97.9	101.8	105.7	109.6	3	6
3 7	91.2	92.1	93.5	95.3	96.5	97.6	98.6	99.6	100.6	101.9	103.6	105.0	105.9	86.8	90.7	94.7	98.6	102.5	106.4	110.3	3	7
3 8	91.8	92.7	94.1	95.9	97.1	98.2	99.2	100.2	101.3	102.5	104.3	105.7	106.6	87.4	91.3	95.3	99.2	103.1	107.1	111.0	3	8
3 9	92.3	93.3	94.7	96.5	97.7	98.8	99.8	100.8	101.9	103.2	104.9	106.3	107.2	87.9	91.9	95.8	99.8	103.8	107.8	111.7	3	9
3 10	92.9	93.9	95.3	97.1	98.3	99.4	100.4	101.4	102.5	103.8	105.6	107.0	107.9	88.4	92.4	96.4	100.4	104.4	108.4	112.4	3	10
3 11	93.5	94.4	95.9	97.6	98.9	100.0	101.0	102.1	103.1	104.4	106.2	107.6	108.6	89.0	93.0	97.0	101.0	105.1	109.1	113.1	3	11

Contd...

Contd...

Age Yrs	Mths	3rd	5th	10th	20th	30th	40th	50th	60th	70th	80th	90th	95th	97th	-3S.D.	-2S.D.	-1S.D.	Median	+1S.D.	+2S.D.	+3S.D.	Age Yrs	Mths
							Percentiles											Standard Deviations					
4	0	94.0	95.0	96.4	98.2	99.5	100.6	101.6	102.7	103.8	105.0	106.8	108.3	109.2	89.5	93.5	97.6	101.6	105.7	109.7	113.8	4	0
4	1	94.6	95.5	97.0	98.8	100.1	101.2	102.2	103.3	104.4	105.6	107.4	108.9	109.9	90.0	94.1	98.1	102.2	106.3	110.4	114.4	4	1
4	2	95.1	96.1	97.5	99.3	100.7	101.8	102.8	103.8	105.0	106.3	108.1	109.5	110.5	90.5	94.6	98.7	102.8	106.9	111.0	115.1	4	2
4	3	95.6	96.6	98.1	99.9	101.2	102.3	103.4	104.4	105.5	106.9	108.7	110.2	111.1	91.0	95.1	99.3	103.4	107.5	111.6	115.8	4	3
4	4	96.1	97.1	98.6	100.5	101.8	102.9	104.0	105.0	106.1	107.5	109.3	110.8	111.8	91.5	95.6	99.8	104.0	108.1	112.3	116.4	4	4
4	5	96.6	97.6	99.2	101.0	102.3	103.5	104.5	105.6	106.7	108.0	109.9	111.4	112.4	92.0	96.1	100.3	104.5	108.7	112.9	117.1	4	5
4	6	97.2	98.1	99.7	101.5	102.9	104.0	105.1	106.2	107.3	108.6	110.5	112.0	113.0	92.4	96.7	100.9	105.1	109.3	113.5	117.7	4	6
4	7	97.7	98.7	100.2	102.1	103.4	104.6	105.6	106.7	107.9	109.2	111.1	112.6	113.6	92.9	97.1	101.4	105.6	109.9	114.1	118.4	4	7
4	8	98.1	99.2	100.7	102.6	104.0	105.1	106.2	107.3	108.4	109.8	111.7	113.2	114.2	93.4	97.6	101.9	106.2	110.5	114.8	119.0	4	8
4	9	98.6	99.7	101.2	103.1	104.5	105.7	106.7	107.8	109.0	110.4	112.3	113.8	114.9	93.8	98.1	102.4	106.7	111.1	115.4	119.7	4	9
4	10	99.1	100.1	101.7	103.6	105.0	106.2	107.3	108.4	109.6	111.0	112.9	114.4	115.5	94.3	98.6	102.9	107.3	111.6	116.0	120.3	4	10
4	11	99.6	100.6	102.2	104.2	105.5	106.7	107.8	109.0	110.1	111.5	113.5	115.1	116.1	94.7	99.1	103.5	107.8	112.2	116.6	121.0	4	11
5	0	100.1	101.1	102.7	104.7	106.1	107.3	108.4	109.5	110.7	112.1	114.0	115.7	116.7	95.1	99.5	104.0	108.4	112.8	117.2	121.6	5	0
5	1	100.5	101.6	103.2	105.2	106.6	107.8	108.9	110.0	111.3	112.7	114.6	116.3	117.3	95.5	100.0	104.5	108.9	113.4	117.8	122.3	5	1
5	2	101.0	102.1	103.7	105.7	107.1	108.3	109.5	110.6	111.8	113.2	115.2	116.8	117.9	96.0	100.5	105.0	109.5	113.9	118.4	122.9	5	2
5	3	101.5	102.5	104.2	106.2	107.6	108.8	110.0	111.1	112.4	113.8	115.8	117.4	118.5	96.4	100.9	105.4	110.0	114.5	119.1	123.6	5	3
5	4	101.9	103.0	104.6	106.7	108.1	109.4	110.5	111.7	112.9	114.4	116.4	118.0	119.1	96.8	101.4	105.9	110.5	115.1	119.7	124.2	5	4
5	5	102.4	103.4	105.1	107.1	108.6	109.9	111.0	112.2	113.5	114.9	117.0	118.6	119.7	97.2	101.8	106.4	111.0	115.7	120.3	124.9	5	5
5	6	102.8	103.9	105.6	107.6	109.1	110.4	111.6	112.7	114.0	115.5	117.5	119.2	120.3	97.6	102.2	106.9	111.6	116.2	120.9	125.5	5	6
5	7	103.2	104.3	106.1	108.1	109.6	110.9	112.1	113.3	114.5	116.0	118.1	119.8	120.9	98.0	102.7	107.4	112.1	116.8	121.5	126.2	5	7
5	8	103.7	104.8	106.5	108.6	110.1	111.4	112.5	113.8	115.1	116.6	118.7	120.4	121.5	98.4	103.1	107.9	112.6	117.3	122.1	126.8	5	8
5	9	104.1	105.2	107.0	109.1	110.6	111.9	113.1	114.3	115.6	117.1	119.2	121.0	122.1	98.8	103.5	108.3	113.1	117.9	122.7	127.5	5	9
5	10	104.5	105.7	107.4	109.6	111.1	112.4	113.6	114.8	116.1	117.7	119.8	121.6	122.7	99.1	104.0	108.8	113.6	118.4	123.3	128.1	5	10
5	11	105.0	106.1	107.9	110.0	111.6	112.9	114.1	115.4	116.7	118.2	120.4	122.1	123.3	99.5	104.4	109.3	114.1	119.0	123.9	128.7	5	11

Contd...

Contd...

Age Yrs	Mths	Percentiles													Standard Deviations							Age Yrs	Mths
		3rd	5th	10th	20th	30th	40th	50th	60th	70th	80th	90th	95th	97th	-3S.D.	-2S.D.	-1S.D.	Median	+1S.D.	+2S.D.	+3S.D.		
6	0	105.4	106.5	108.3	110.5	112.1	113.4	114.6	115.9	117.2	118.8	120.9	122.7	123.9	99.9	104.8	109.7	114.6	119.6	124.5	129.4	6	0
6	1	105.8	107.0	108.8	111.0	112.5	113.9	115.1	116.4	117.7	119.3	121.5	123.3	124.5	100.2	105.2	110.2	115.1	120.1	125.1	130.0	6	1
6	2	106.2	107.4	109.2	111.4	113.0	114.4	115.6	116.9	118.3	119.9	122.1	123.9	125.1	100.6	105.6	110.6	115.6	120.6	125.7	130.7	6	2
6	3	106.6	107.8	109.7	111.9	113.5	114.9	116.1	117.4	118.8	120.4	122.6	124.5	125.7	101.0	106.0	111.1	116.1	121.2	126.3	131.3	6	3
6	4	107.0	108.2	110.1	112.3	114.0	115.3	116.6	117.9	119.3	120.9	123.2	125.0	126.2	101.3	106.4	111.5	116.6	121.7	126.8	131.9	6	4
6	5	107.4	108.7	110.5	112.8	114.4	115.8	117.1	118.4	119.8	121.5	123.7	125.6	126.8	101.7	106.8	112.0	117.1	122.3	127.4	132.6	6	5
6	6	107.9	109.1	111.0	113.3	114.9	116.3	117.6	118.9	120.4	122.0	124.3	126.2	127.4	102.0	107.2	112.4	117.6	122.8	128.0	133.2	6	6
6	7	108.3	109.5	111.4	113.7	115.4	116.8	118.1	119.5	120.9	122.5	124.8	126.7	128.0	102.4	107.6	112.9	118.1	123.4	128.6	133.9	6	7
6	8	108.7	109.9	111.8	114.2	115.8	117.3	118.6	120.0	121.4	123.1	125.4	127.3	128.6	102.7	108.0	113.3	118.6	123.9	129.2	134.5	6	8
6	9	109.1	110.3	112.3	114.6	116.3	117.8	119.1	120.5	121.9	123.6	125.9	127.9	129.1	103.1	108.4	113.8	119.1	124.4	129.8	135.1	6	9
6	10	109.5	110.7	112.7	115.1	116.8	118.2	119.6	121.0	122.4	124.1	126.5	128.5	129.7	103.4	108.8	114.2	119.6	125.0	130.4	135.8	6	10
6	11	109.9	111.2	113.1	115.5	117.2	118.7	120.1	121.5	122.9	124.7	127.0	129.0	130.3	103.8	109.2	114.7	120.1	125.5	131.0	136.4	6	11
7	0	110.3	111.6	113.6	116.0	117.7	119.2	120.6	122.0	123.4	125.2	127.6	129.6	130.9	104.1	109.6	115.1	120.6	126.1	131.5	137.0	7	0
7	1	110.7	112.0	114.0	116.4	118.2	119.7	121.1	122.5	124.0	125.7	128.1	130.2	131.5	104.5	110.0	115.5	121.1	126.6	132.1	137.6	7	1
7	2	111.1	112.4	114.4	116.9	118.6	120.1	121.5	123.0	124.5	126.2	128.7	130.7	132.0	104.8	110.4	116.0	121.5	127.1	132.7	138.3	7	2
7	3	111.5	112.8	114.8	117.3	119.1	120.6	122.0	123.5	125.0	126.8	129.2	131.3	132.6	105.2	110.8	116.4	122.0	127.7	133.3	138.9	7	3
7	4	111.9	113.2	115.3	117.7	119.5	121.1	122.5	124.0	125.5	127.3	129.8	131.8	133.2	105.5	111.2	116.8	122.5	128.2	133.9	139.5	7	4
7	5	112.2	113.6	115.7	118.2	120.0	121.6	123.0	124.4	126.0	127.8	130.3	132.4	133.8	105.9	111.6	117.3	123.0	128.7	134.4	140.1	7	5
7	6	112.6	114.0	116.1	118.6	120.5	122.0	123.5	124.9	126.5	128.3	130.9	133.0	134.3	106.2	112.0	117.7	123.5	129.2	135.0	140.8	7	6
7	7	113.0	114.4	116.5	119.1	120.9	122.5	124.0	125.4	127.0	128.9	131.4	133.5	134.9	106.5	112.4	118.2	124.0	129.8	135.6	141.4	7	7
7	8	113.4	114.8	116.9	119.5	121.4	123.0	124.5	125.9	127.5	129.4	132.0	134.1	135.5	106.9	112.7	118.6	124.5	130.3	136.2	142.0	7	8
7	9	113.8	115.2	117.4	120.0	121.8	123.4	124.9	126.4	128.0	129.9	132.5	134.6	136.0	107.2	113.1	119.0	124.9	130.8	136.7	142.6	7	9
7	10	114.2	115.6	117.8	120.4	122.3	123.9	125.4	126.9	128.5	130.4	133.0	135.2	136.6	107.6	113.5	119.5	125.4	131.4	137.3	143.2	7	10
7	11	114.6	116.0	118.2	120.9	122.8	124.4	125.9	127.4	129.0	130.9	133.6	135.8	137.2	107.9	113.9	119.9	125.9	131.9	137.9	143.9	7	11

Contd...

Contd...

Age Yrs	Mths	3rd	5th	10th	20th	30th	40th	50th	60th	70th	80th	90th	95th	97th	-3S.D.	-2S.D.	-1S.D.	Median	+1S.D.	+2S.D.	+3S.D.	Age Yrs	Mths
8	0	115.0	116.5	118.7	121.3	123.2	124.9	126.4	127.9	129.5	131.5	134.1	136.3	137.7	108.3	114.3	120.4	126.4	132.4	138.4	144.5	8	0
8	1	115.4	116.9	119.1	121.8	123.7	125.3	126.9	128.4	130.1	132.0	134.7	136.9	138.3	108.6	114.7	120.8	126.9	132.9	139.0	145.1	8	1
8	2	115.8	117.3	119.5	122.2	124.1	125.8	127.4	128.9	130.6	132.5	135.2	137.4	138.9	109.0	115.1	121.2	127.4	133.5	139.6	145.7	8	2
8	3	116.2	117.7	119.9	122.6	124.6	126.3	127.8	129.4	131.1	133.0	135.7	138.0	139.4	109.4	115.5	121.7	127.8	134.0	140.2	146.3	8	3
8	4	116.7	118.1	120.4	123.1	125.1	126.7	128.3	129.9	131.6	133.5	136.3	138.5	140.0	109.7	115.9	122.1	128.3	134.5	140.7	146.9	8	4
8	5	117.1	118.5	120.8	123.6	125.5	127.2	128.8	130.4	132.1	134.1	136.8	139.1	140.6	110.1	116.3	122.6	128.8	135.0	141.3	147.5	8	5
8	6	117.5	119.0	121.2	124.0	126.0	127.7	129.3	130.9	132.6	134.6	137.3	139.6	141.1	110.4	116.7	123.0	129.3	135.6	141.9	148.1	8	6
8	7	117.9	119.4	121.7	124.5	126.5	128.2	129.8	131.4	133.1	135.1	137.9	140.2	141.7	110.8	117.1	123.5	129.8	136.1	142.4	148.8	8	7
8	8	118.3	119.8	122.1	124.9	126.9	128.7	130.3	131.9	133.6	135.6	138.4	140.7	142.2	111.2	117.5	123.9	130.3	136.6	143.0	149.4	8	8
8	9	118.7	120.2	122.6	125.4	127.4	129.1	130.8	132.4	134.1	136.1	139.0	141.3	142.8	111.6	118.0	124.4	130.8	137.2	143.6	150.0	8	9
8	10	119.1	120.7	123.0	125.8	127.9	129.6	131.2	132.9	134.6	136.7	139.5	141.8	143.4	111.9	118.4	124.8	131.2	137.7	144.1	150.6	8	10
8	11	119.6	121.1	123.4	126.3	128.3	130.1	131.7	133.4	135.1	137.2	140.0	142.4	143.9	112.3	118.8	125.3	131.7	138.2	144.7	151.2	8	11
9	0	120.0	121.5	123.9	126.8	128.8	130.6	132.2	133.9	135.6	137.7	140.6	142.9	144.5	112.7	119.2	125.7	132.2	138.7	145.3	151.8	9	0
9	1	120.4	122.0	124.3	127.2	129.3	131.1	132.7	134.4	136.2	138.2	141.1	143.5	145.0	113.1	119.6	126.2	132.7	139.3	145.8	152.4	9	1
9	2	120.9	122.4	124.8	127.7	129.8	131.6	133.2	134.9	136.7	138.8	141.7	144.0	145.6	113.5	120.1	126.7	133.2	139.8	146.4	153.0	9	2
9	3	121.3	122.9	125.3	128.2	130.3	132.1	133.7	135.4	137.2	139.3	142.2	144.6	146.2	113.9	120.5	127.1	133.7	140.3	146.9	153.5	9	3
9	4	121.7	123.3	125.7	128.6	130.7	132.5	134.2	135.9	137.7	139.8	142.7	145.1	146.7	114.3	121.0	127.6	134.2	140.9	147.5	154.1	9	4
9	5	122.2	123.8	126.2	129.1	131.2	133.0	134.7	136.4	138.2	140.3	143.3	145.7	147.3	114.7	121.4	128.1	134.7	141.4	148.1	154.7	9	5
9	6	122.6	124.2	126.7	129.5	131.7	133.5	135.2	136.9	138.7	140.9	143.8	146.2	147.8	115.2	121.8	128.5	135.2	141.9	148.6	155.3	9	6
9	7	123.1	124.7	127.1	130.1	132.2	134.0	135.7	137.4	139.3	141.4	144.4	146.8	148.4	115.6	122.3	129.0	135.7	142.5	149.2	155.9	9	7
9	8	123.6	125.2	127.6	130.6	132.7	134.5	136.2	138.0	139.8	141.9	144.9	147.3	148.9	116.0	122.8	129.5	136.2	143.0	149.7	156.5	9	8
9	9	124.0	125.6	128.1	131.1	133.2	135.0	136.8	138.5	140.3	142.5	145.4	147.9	149.5	116.4	123.2	130.0	136.8	143.5	150.3	157.1	9	9
9	10	124.5	126.1	128.6	131.6	133.7	135.6	137.3	139.0	140.8	143.0	146.0	148.5	150.1	116.9	123.7	130.5	137.3	144.1	150.9	157.7	9	10
9	11	125.0	126.6	129.1	132.1	134.2	136.1	137.8	139.5	141.4	143.5	146.5	149.0	150.6	117.3	124.2	131.0	137.8	144.6	151.4	158.2	9	11

Contd..

Contd...

Age (Yrs Mths)	Percentiles													Standard Deviations							Age (Yrs Mths)
	3rd	5th	10th	20th	30th	40th	50th	60th	70th	80th	90th	95th	97th	-3S.D.	-2S.D.	-1S.D.	Median	+1S.D.	+2S.D.	+3S.D.	
10 0	125.4	127.1	129.5	132.6	134.7	136.6	138.3	140.0	141.9	144.1	147.1	149.6	151.2	117.8	124.6	131.5	138.3	145.1	152.0	158.8	10 0
10 1	125.9	127.6	130.0	133.1	135.2	137.1	138.8	140.6	142.4	144.6	147.6	150.1	151.1	118.3	125.1	132.0	138.8	145.7	152.5	159.4	10 1
10 2	126.4	128.1	130.6	133.6	135.8	137.6	139.4	141.1	143.0	145.1	148.2	150.7	152.3	118.7	125.6	132.5	139.4	146.2	153.1	160.0	10 2
10 3	126.9	128.6	131.1	134.1	136.3	138.1	139.9	141.6	143.5	145.7	148.7	151.2	152.8	119.2	126.1	133.0	139.9	146.8	153.7	160.5	10 3
10 4	127.4	129.1	131.6	134.6	136.8	138.7	140.4	142.2	144.0	146.2	149.3	151.8	153.4	119.7	126.6	133.5	140.4	147.3	154.2	161.1	10 4
10 5	127.9	129.6	132.1	135.1	137.3	139.2	140.9	142.7	144.6	146.8	149.8	152.3	154.0	120.2	127.1	134.0	140.9	147.9	154.8	161.7	10 5
10 6	128.5	130.1	132.6	135.7	137.9	139.7	141.5	143.2	145.1	147.3	150.4	152.9	154.5	120.7	127.6	134.6	141.5	148.4	155.3	162.3	10 6
10 7	129.0	130.6	133.1	136.2	138.4	140.3	142.0	143.8	145.7	147.9	150.9	153.4	155.1	121.2	128.2	135.1	142.0	149.0	155.9	162.8	10 7
10 8	129.5	131.2	133.7	136.7	138.9	140.8	142.6	144.3	146.2	148.4	151.5	153.9	155.6	121.8	128.7	135.6	142.6	149.5	156.4	163.4	10 8
10 9	130.1	131.7	134.2	137.3	139.5	141.4	143.1	144.9	146.8	149.0	152.0	154.5	156.2	122.3	129.2	136.2	143.1	150.1	157.0	163.9	10 9
10 10	130.6	132.2	134.8	137.8	140.0	141.9	143.7	145.4	147.3	149.5	152.6	155.1	156.7	122.8	129.8	136.7	143.7	150.6	157.6	164.5	10 10
10 11	131.2	132.8	135.3	138.4	140.6	142.5	144.2	146.0	147.9	150.1	153.1	155.6	157.3	123.4	130.3	137.3	144.2	151.2	158.1	165.1	10 11
11 0	131.7	133.4	135.9	138.9	141.1	143.0	144.8	146.5	148.4	150.6	153.7	156.2	157.8	123.9	130.9	137.8	144.8	151.7	158.7	165.6	11 0
11 1	132.3	133.9	136.4	139.5	141.7	143.6	145.3	147.1	149.0	151.2	154.2	156.8	158.4	124.5	131.5	138.4	145.3	152.3	159.2	166.2	11 1
11 2	132.9	134.5	137.0	140.1	142.3	144.2	145.9	147.7	149.5	151.8	154.8	157.3	159.0	125.1	132.0	139.0	145.9	152.8	159.8	166.7	11 2
11 3	133.4	135.1	137.6	140.6	142.8	144.7	146.5	148.2	150.1	152.3	155.4	157.9	159.5	125.7	132.6	139.5	146.5	153.4	160.3	167.3	11 3
11 4	134.0	135.7	138.2	141.2	143.4	145.3	147.0	148.8	150.7	152.9	155.9	158.4	160.1	126.3	133.2	140.1	147.0	154.0	160.9	167.8	11 4
11 5	134.6	136.2	138.8	141.8	144.0	145.9	147.6	149.4	151.2	153.4	156.5	159.0	160.6	126.9	133.8	140.7	147.6	154.5	161.4	168.4	11 5
11 6	135.2	136.8	139.3	142.4	144.6	146.4	148.2	149.9	151.8	154.0	157.0	159.5	161.2	127.5	134.4	141.3	148.2	155.1	162.0	168.9	11 6
11 7	135.8	137.4	139.9	142.9	145.1	147.0	148.8	150.5	152.4	154.6	157.6	160.1	161.7	128.1	135.0	141.9	148.8	155.6	162.5	169.4	11 7
11 8	136.4	138.0	140.5	143.5	145.7	147.6	149.3	151.1	152.9	155.1	158.1	160.6	162.3	128.7	135.6	142.4	149.3	156.2	163.1	170.0	11 8
11 9	137.0	138.6	141.1	144.1	146.3	148.1	149.9	151.6	153.5	155.7	158.7	161.2	162.8	129.3	136.1	143.0	149.9	156.7	163.6	170.5	11 9
11 10	137.5	139.2	141.6	144.7	146.8	148.7	150.4	152.2	154.0	156.2	159.2	161.7	163.3	129.9	136.7	143.6	150.4	157.3	164.1	171.0	11 10
11 11	138.1	139.7	142.2	145.2	147.4	149.2	151.0	152.7	154.6	156.7	159.7	162.2	163.8	130.5	137.3	144.1	151.0	157.8	164.7	171.5	11 11

Contd...

Contd...

Age Yrs	Mths	3rd	5th	10th	20th	30th	40th	50th	60th	70th	80th	90th	95th	97th	-3S.D.	-2S.D.	-1S.D.	Median	+1S.D.	+2S.D.	+3S.D.	Age Yrs	Mths
						Percentiles											Standard Deviations						
12	0	138.7	140.3	142.8	145.8	147.9	149.8	151.5	153.2	155.1	157.3	160.3	162.7	164.4	131.1	137.9	144.7	151.5	158.3	165.2	172.0	12	0
12	1	139.2	140.9	143.3	146.3	148.5	150.3	152.1	153.8	155.6	157.8	160.8	163.3	164.9	131.6	138.4	145.2	152.1	158.9	165.7	172.5	12	1
12	2	139.8	141.4	143.9	146.9	149.0	150.9	152.6	154.3	156.1	158.3	161.3	163.8	165.4	132.2	139.0	145.8	152.6	159.4	166.2	173.0	12	2
12	3	140.3	141.9	144.4	147.4	149.5	151.4	153.1	154.8	156.6	158.8	161.8	164.2	165.8	132.8	139.5	146.3	153.1	159.9	166.6	173.4	12	3
12	4	140.9	142.5	144.9	147.9	150.1	151.9	153.6	155.3	157.1	159.3	162.3	164.7	166.3	133.3	140.1	146.8	153.6	160.4	167.1	173.9	12	4
12	5	141.4	143.0	145.4	148.4	150.6	152.4	154.1	155.8	157.6	159.8	162.7	165.2	166.8	133.8	140.6	147.3	154.1	160.8	167.6	174.3	12	5
12	6	141.9	143.5	145.9	148.9	151.0	152.9	154.6	156.3	158.1	160.2	163.2	165.6	167.2	134.4	141.1	147.8	154.6	161.3	168.0	174.8	12	6
12	7	142.4	144.0	146.4	149.4	151.5	153.3	155.0	156.7	158.6	160.7	163.7	166.1	167.7	134.9	141.6	148.3	155.0	161.8	168.5	175.2	12	7
12	8	142.9	144.5	146.9	149.8	152.0	153.8	155.5	157.2	159.0	161.1	164.1	166.5	168.1	135.4	142.1	148.8	155.5	162.2	168.9	175.6	12	8
12	9	143.3	144.9	147.3	150.3	152.4	154.2	155.9	157.6	159.4	161.6	164.5	166.9	168.5	135.8	142.5	149.2	155.9	162.6	169.3	176.0	12	9
12	10	143.8	145.3	147.8	150.7	152.8	154.6	156.3	158.0	159.9	162.0	164.9	167.3	168.9	136.3	143.0	149.7	156.3	163.0	169.7	176.4	12	10
12	11	144.2	145.8	148.2	151.1	153.2	155.1	156.7	158.4	160.2	162.4	165.3	167.7	169.3	136.7	143.4	150.1	156.7	163.4	170.1	176.8	12	11
13	0	144.6	146.2	148.6	151.5	153.6	155.4	157.1	158.8	160.6	162.7	165.7	168.1	169.7	137.1	143.8	150.5	157.1	163.8	170.5	177.1	13	0
13	1	144.9	146.5	148.9	151.9	154.0	155.8	157.5	159.2	161.0	163.1	166.0	168.5	170.0	137.5	144.2	150.8	157.5	164.2	170.8	177.5	13	1
13	2	145.3	146.9	149.3	152.2	154.3	156.1	157.8	159.5	161.3	163.4	166.4	168.8	170.4	137.8	144.5	151.2	157.8	164.5	171.2	177.8	13	2
13	3	145.6	147.2	149.6	152.6	154.7	156.5	158.2	159.8	161.7	163.8	166.7	169.1	170.7	138.2	144.8	151.5	158.2	164.8	171.5	178.1	13	3
13	4	145.9	147.5	149.9	152.9	155.0	156.8	158.5	160.2	162.0	164.1	167.0	169.4	171.0	138.5	145.1	151.8	158.5	165.1	171.8	178.5	13	4
13	5	146.2	147.8	150.2	153.2	155.3	157.1	158.8	160.4	162.3	164.4	167.3	169.7	171.3	138.8	145.4	152.1	158.8	165.4	172.1	178.7	13	5
13	6	146.5	148.1	150.5	153.4	155.5	157.3	159.0	160.7	162.5	164.6	167.6	170.0	171.6	139.0	145.7	152.4	159.0	165.7	172.4	179.0	13	6
13	7	146.8	148.3	150.8	153.7	155.8	157.6	159.3	161.0	162.8	164.9	167.8	170.3	171.8	139.3	146.0	152.6	159.3	166.0	172.6	179.3	13	7
13	8	147.0	148.6	151.0	153.9	156.0	157.8	159.5	161.2	163.0	165.1	168.1	170.5	172.1	139.5	146.2	152.9	159.5	166.2	172.9	179.5	13	8
13	9	147.2	148.8	151.2	154.1	156.3	158.1	159.8	161.5	163.3	165.4	168.3	170.7	172.3	139.8	146.4	153.1	159.8	166.4	173.1	179.8	13	9
13	10	147.4	149.0	151.4	154.4	156.5	158.3	160.0	161.7	163.5	165.6	168.5	171.0	172.5	140.0	146.6	153.3	160.0	166.7	173.3	180.0	13	10
13	11	147.6	149.2	151.6	154.6	156.7	158.5	160.2	161.9	163.7	165.8	168.7	171.2	172.7	140.1	146.8	153.5	160.2	166.9	173.5	180.2	13	11

Contd..

Contd...

Age Yrs	Mths	3rd	5th	10th	20th	30th	40th	50th	60th	70th	80th	90th	95th	97th	-3S.D.	-2S.D.	-1S.D.	Median	+1S.D.	+2S.D.	+3S.D.	Age Yrs	Mths
14	0	147.8	149.4	151.8	154.7	156.9	158.7	160.4	162.1	163.9	166.0	168.9	171.4	172.9	140.3	147.0	153.7	160.4	167.0	173.7	180.4	14	0
14	1	147.9	149.5	152.0	154.9	157.0	158.8	160.5	162.2	164.0	166.2	169.1	171.5	173.1	140.5	147.2	153.8	160.5	167.2	173.9	180.6	14	1
14	2	148.1	149.7	152.1	155.1	157.2	159.0	160.7	162.4	164.2	166.3	169.3	171.7	173.3	140.6	147.3	154.0	160.7	167.4	174.1	180.8	14	2
14	3	148.2	149.8	152.3	155.2	157.3	159.1	160.8	162.5	164.4	166.5	169.4	171.9	173.5	140.7	147.4	154.1	160.8	167.6	174.3	181.0	14	3
14	4	148.4	149.9	152.4	155.3	157.5	159.3	161.0	162.7	164.5	166.6	169.6	172.0	173.6	140.9	147.6	154.3	161.0	167.7	174.4	181.1	14	4
14	5	148.5	150.1	152.5	155.5	157.6	159.4	161.1	162.8	164.6	166.8	169.7	172.2	173.8	141.0	147.7	154.4	161.1	167.8	174.5	181.3	14	5
14	6	148.6	150.2	152.6	155.6	157.7	159.5	161.2	162.9	164.8	166.9	169.8	172.3	173.9	141.1	147.8	154.5	161.2	168.0	174.7	181.4	14	6
14	7	148.7	150.3	152.7	155.7	157.8	159.6	161.3	163.0	164.9	167.0	170.0	172.4	174.0	141.2	147.9	154.6	161.3	168.1	174.8	181.5	14	7
14	8	148.8	150.4	152.8	155.8	157.9	159.7	161.4	163.2	165.0	167.1	170.1	172.5	174.1	141.3	148.0	154.7	161.4	168.2	174.9	181.6	14	8
14	9	148.9	150.5	152.9	155.9	158.0	159.8	161.5	163.2	165.1	167.2	170.2	172.6	174.2	141.3	148.1	154.8	161.5	168.3	175.0	181.8	14	9
14	10	148.9	150.5	153.0	156.0	158.1	159.9	161.6	163.3	165.2	167.3	170.3	172.7	174.3	141.4	148.1	154.9	161.6	168.4	175.1	181.8	14	10
14	11	149.0	150.6	153.1	156.0	158.2	160.0	161.7	163.4	165.2	167.4	170.4	172.8	174.4	141.5	148.2	155.0	161.7	168.5	175.2	181.9	14	11
15	0	149.1	150.7	153.1	156.1	158.2	160.1	161.8	163.5	165.3	167.5	170.4	172.9	174.5	141.5	148.3	155.0	161.8	168.5	175.3	182.0	15	0
15	1	149.2	150.8	153.2	156.2	158.3	160.1	161.9	163.6	165.4	167.5	170.5	173.0	174.5	141.6	148.4	155.1	161.9	168.6	175.3	182.1	15	1
15	2	149.2	150.8	153.3	156.2	158.4	160.2	161.9	163.6	165.5	167.6	170.6	173.0	174.6	141.7	148.4	155.2	161.9	168.7	175.4	182.2	15	2
15	3	149.3	150.9	153.3	156.3	158.4	160.3	162.0	163.7	165.5	167.7	170.6	173.1	174.7	141.7	148.5	155.2	162.0	168.7	175.5	182.2	15	3
15	4	149.3	150.9	153.4	156.4	158.5	160.3	162.0	163.7	165.6	167.7	170.7	173.1	174.7	141.8	148.5	155.3	162.0	168.8	175.5	182.3	15	4
15	5	149.4	151.0	153.4	156.4	158.5	160.4	162.1	163.8	165.6	167.8	170.7	173.2	174.8	141.9	148.6	155.3	162.1	168.8	175.6	182.3	15	5
15	6	149.5	151.1	153.5	156.5	158.6	160.4	162.1	163.8	165.7	167.8	170.8	173.2	174.8	142.1	148.7	155.4	162.1	168.9	175.6	182.3	15	6
15	7	149.5	151.1	153.6	156.5	158.7	160.5	162.2	163.9	165.7	167.8	170.8	173.2	174.8	142.0	148.7	155.5	162.2	168.9	175.6	182.4	15	7
15	8	149.6	151.2	153.6	156.6	158.7	160.5	162.2	163.9	165.7	167.8	170.8	173.3	174.9	142.1	148.8	155.5	162.2	168.9	175.7	182.4	15	8
15	9	149.7	151.2	153.7	156.6	158.8	160.6	162.3	164.0	165.8	167.9	170.9	173.3	174.9	142.1	148.9	155.6	162.3	169.0	175.7	182.4	15	9
15	10	149.7	151.3	153.7	156.7	158.8	160.6	162.3	164.0	165.8	168.0	170.9	173.3	174.9	142.2	148.9	155.6	162.3	169.0	175.7	182.4	15	10
15	11	149.8	151.4	153.8	156.7	158.9	160.7	162.4	164.1	165.9	168.0	170.9	173.4	174.9	142.3	149.0	155.7	162.4	169.0	175.7	182.4	15	11

Percentiles — Standard Deviations

Contd...

Contd...

Age Yrs	Mths	3rd	5th	10th	20th	30th	40th	50th	60th	70th	80th	90th	95th	97th	-3S.D.	-2S.D.	-1S.D.	Median	+1S.D.	+2S.D.	+3S.D.	Age Yrs	Mths
						Percentiles											Standard Deviations						
16	0	149.9	151.4	153.9	156.8	158.9	160.7	162.4	164.1	165.9	168.0	171.0	173.4	175.0	142.4	149.1	155.7	162.4	169.1	175.7	182.4	16	0
16	1	150.0	151.5	153.9	156.9	159.0	160.8	162.5	164.1	165.9	168.1	171.0	173.4	175.0	142.5	149.2	155.8	162.5	169.1	175.8	182.4	16	1
16	2	150.0	151.6	154.0	156.9	159.0	160.8	162.5	164.2	166.0	168.1	171.0	173.4	175.0	142.6	149.3	155.9	162.5	169.1	175.8	182.4	16	2
16	3	150.1	151.7	154.1	157.0	159.1	160.9	162.6	164.2	166.0	168.1	171.0	173.4	175.0	142.8	149.4	156.0	162.6	169.2	175.8	182.4	16	3
16	4	150.2	151.8	154.2	157.1	159.2	160.9	162.6	164.3	166.1	168.2	171.0	173.4	175.0	142.9	149.5	156.0	162.6	169.2	175.8	182.3	16	4
16	5	150.3	151.9	154.3	157.2	159.2	161.0	162.7	164.3	166.1	168.2	171.1	173.4	175.0	143.0	149.6	156.1	162.7	169.2	175.8	182.3	16	5
16	6	150.4	152.0	154.4	157.2	159.3	161.1	162.7	164.4	166.1	168.2	171.1	173.5	175.0	143.2	149.7	156.2	162.7	169.2	175.8	182.3	16	6
16	7	150.6	152.1	154.5	157.3	159.4	161.1	162.8	164.4	166.2	168.2	171.1	173.5	175.0	143.3	149.8	156.3	162.8	169.3	175.8	182.3	16	7
16	8	150.7	152.2	154.5	157.4	159.4	161.2	162.8	164.5	166.2	168.3	171.1	173.5	175.0	143.4	149.9	156.4	162.8	169.3	175.8	182.2	16	8
16	9	150.8	152.3	154.6	157.5	159.5	161.3	162.9	164.5	166.3	168.3	171.1	173.5	175.0	143.6	150.0	156.5	162.9	169.3	175.8	182.2	16	9
16	10	150.9	152.4	154.7	157.6	159.6	161.3	162.9	164.6	166.3	168.3	171.2	173.5	175.0	143.7	150.1	156.5	162.9	169.3	175.8	182.2	16	10
16	11	151.0	152.5	154.8	157.6	159.7	161.4	163.0	164.6	166.3	168.4	171.2	173.5	175.0	143.9	150.3	156.6	163.0	169.4	175.7	182.1	16	11
17	0	151.1	152.6	154.9	157.7	159.7	161.5	163.1	164.7	166.4	168.4	171.2	173.5	175.0	144.1	150.4	156.7	163.1	169.4	175.7	182.1	17	0
17	1	151.3	152.7	155.0	157.8	159.8	161.5	163.1	164.7	166.4	168.4	171.2	173.5	175.0	144.2	150.5	156.8	163.1	169.4	175.7	182.0	17	1
17	2	151.4	152.9	155.1	157.9	159.9	161.6	163.2	164.8	166.5	168.5	171.2	173.5	175.0	144.4	150.6	156.9	163.2	169.4	157.7	182.0	17	2
17	3	151.5	153.0	155.2	158.0	160.0	161.7	163.2	164.8	166.5	168.5	171.2	173.5	175.0	144.5	150.8	157.0	163.2	169.5	175.7	181.9	17	3
17	4	151.6	153.1	155.3	158.1	160.0	161.7	163.3	164.9	166.5	168.5	171.2	173.5	174.9	144.7	150.9	157.1	163.3	169.5	175.7	181.9	17	4
17	5	151.7	153.2	155.4	158.1	160.1	161.8	163.3	164.9	166.6	168.5	171.3	173.5	175.0	144.8	151.0	157.2	163.3	169.5	175.7	181.9	17	5
17	6	151.8	153.3	155.5	158.2	160.2	161.8	163.4	165.0	166.6	168.6	171.3	173.5	174.9	145.0	151.1	157.3	163.4	169.5	175.7	181.8	17	6
17	7	152.0	153.4	155.6	158.3	160.3	161.9	163.5	165.0	166.7	168.6	171.3	173.5	174.9	145.1	151.2	157.3	163.5	169.6	175.7	181.8	17	7
17	8	152.1	153.5	155.7	158.4	160.3	162.0	163.5	165.0	166.7	168.6	171.3	173.5	174.9	145.3	151.4	157.4	163.5	169.6	175.7	181.7	17	8
17	9	152.2	153.6	155.8	158.5	160.4	162.0	163.6	165.1	166.7	168.6	171.3	173.5	174.9	145.4	151.5	157.5	163.6	169.6	175.7	181.7	17	9
17	10	152.3	153.7	155.9	158.5	160.5	162.1	163.6	165.1	166.8	168.7	171.3	173.5	174.9	145.6	151.6	157.6	163.6	169.6	175.6	181.7	17	10
17	11	152.4	153.8	156.0	158.6	160.5	162.1	163.7	165.2	166.8	168.7	171.3	173.5	174.9	145.7	151.7	157.7	163.7	169.7	175.6	181.6	17	11
18	0	152.5	153.9	156.1	158.7	160.6	162.2	163.7	165.2	166.8	168.7	171.4	173.5	174.9	145.8	151.8	157.7	163.7	169.7	175.6	181.6	18	0

APPENDIX 47.15

(NCHS/WHO) NORMALIZED REFERENCE VALUES FOR WEIGHT-FOR-HEIGHT AND WEIGHT-FOR-LENGTH

		Boys' weight (kg)			Length/Height* (cm)		Girls' weight (kg)			
−4 SD	−3 SD	−2 SD	−1 SD	Median		Median	-1 SD	-2 SD	-3 SD	-4 SD
1.8	2.1	2.5	2.8	3.1	49	3.3	2.9	2.6	2.2	1.8
1.8	2.2	2.5	2.9	3.3	50	3.4	3.0	2.6	2.3	1.9
1.8	2.2	2.6	3.1	3.5	51	3.5	3.1	2.7	2.3	1.9
1.9	2.3	2.8	3.2	3.7	52	3.7	3.3	2.8	2.4	2.0
1.9	2.4	2.9	3.4	3.9	53	3.9	3.4	3.0	2.5	2.1
2.0	2.6	3.1	3.6	4.1	54	4.1	3.6	3.1	2.7	2.2
2.2	2.7	3.3	3.8	4.3	55	4.3	3.8	3.3	2.8	2.3
2.3	2.9	3.5	4.0	4.6	56	4.5	4.0	3.5	3.0	2.4
2.5	3.1	3.7	4.3	4.8	57	4.8	4.2	3.7	3.1	2.6
2.7	3.3	3.9	4.5	5.1	58	5.0	4.4	3.9	3.3	2.7
2.9	3.5	4.1	4.8	5.4	59	5.3	4.7	4.1	3.5	2.9
3.1	3.7	4.4	5.0	5.7	60	5.5	4.9	4.3	3.7	3.1
3.3	4.0	4.6	5.3	5.9	61	5.8	5.2	4.6	3.9	3.3
3.5	4.2	4.9	5.6	6.2	62	6.1	5.4	4.8	4.1	3.5
3.8	4.5	5.2	5.8	6.5	63	6.4	5.7	5.0	4.4	3.7
4.0	4.7	5.4	6.1	6.8	64	6.7	6.0	5.3	4.6	3.9
4.3	5.0	5.7	6.4	7.1	65	7.0	6.3	5.5	4.8	4.1
4.5	5.3	6.0	6.7	7.4	66	7.3	6.5	5.8	5.1	4.3
4.8	5.5	6.2	7.0	7.7	67	7.5	6.8	6.0	5.3	4.5
5.1	5.8	6.5	7.3	8.0	68	7.8	7.1	6.3	5.5	4.8
5.3	6.0	6.8	7.5	8.3	69	8.1	7.3	6.5	5.8	5.0
5.5	6.3	7.0	7.8	8.5	70	8.4	7.6	6.8	6.0	5.2
5.8	6.5	7.3	8.1	8.8	71	8.6	7.8	7.0	6.2	5.4
6.0	6.8	7.5	8.3	9.1	72	8.9	8.1	7.2	6.4	5.6
6.2	7.0	7.8	8.6	9.3	73	9.1	8.3	7.5	6.6	5.8
6.4	7.2	8.0	8.8	9.6	74	9.4	8.5	7.7	6.8	6.0
6.6	7.4	8.2	9.0	9.8	75	9.6	8.7	7.9	7.0	6.2
6.8	7.6	8.4	9.2	10.0	76	9.8	8.9	8.1	7.2	6.4
7.0	7.8	8.6	9.4	10.3	77	10.0	9.1	8.3	7.4	6.6
7.1	8.0	8.8	9.7	10.5	78	10.2	9.3	8.5	7.6	6.7
7.3	8.2	9.0	9.9	10.7	79	10.4	9.5	8.7	7.8	6.9
7.5	8.3	9.2	10.1	10.9	80	10.6	9.7	8.8	8.0	7.1
7.6	8.5	9.4	10.2	11.1	81	10.8	9.9	9.0	8.1	7.2
7.8	8.7	9.6	10.4	11.3	82	11.0	10.1	9.2	8.3	7.4
7.9	8.8	9.7	10.6	11.5	83	11.2	10.3	9.4	8.5	7.6
8.1	9.0	9.9	10.8	11.7	84	11.4	10.5	9.6	8.7	7.7
7.8	8.9	9.9	11.0	12.1	85	11.8	10.8	9.7	8.6	7.6
7.9	9.0	10.1	11.2	12.3	86	12.0	11.0	9.9	8.8	7.7
8.1	9.2	10.3	11.5	12.6	87	12.3	11.2	10.1	9.0	7.9
8.3	9.4	10.5	11.7	12.8	88	12.5	11.4	10.3	9.2	8.1
8.4	9.6	10.7	11.9	13.0	89	12.7	11.6	10.5	9.3	8.2
8.6	9.8	10.9	12.1	13.3	90	12.9	11.8	10.7	9.5	8.4

Contd...

Contd...

		Boys' weight (kg)			Length/Height* (cm)		Girls' weight (kg)			
−4 SD	−3 SD	−2 SD	−1 SD	Median		Median	-1 SD	-2 SD	-3 SD	-4 SD
8.8	9.9	11.1	12.3	13.5	91	13.2	12.0	10.8	9.7	8.5
8.9	10.1	11.3	12.5	13.7	92	13.4	12.2	11.0	9.9	8.7
9.1	10.3	11.5	12.8	14.0	93	13.6	12.4	11.2	10.0	8.8
9.2	10.5	11.7	13.0	14.2	94	13.9	12.6	11.4	10.2	9.0
9.4	10.7	11.9	13.2	14.5	95	14.1	12.9	11.6	10.4	9.1
9.6	10.9	12.1	13.4	14.7	96	14.3	13.1	11.8	10.6	9.3
9.7	11.0	12.4	13.7	15.0	97	14.6	13.3	,12.0	10.7	9.5
9.9	11.2	12.6	13.9	15.2	98	14.9	13.5	12.2	10.9	9.6
10.1	11.4	12.8	14.1	15.5	99	15.1	13.8	12.4	11.1	9.8
10.3	11.6	13.0	14.4	15.7	100	15.4	14.0	12.7	11.3	9.9
10.4	11.8	13.2	14.6	16.0	101	15.6	14.3	12.9	11.5	10.1
10.6	12.0	13.4	14.9	16.3	102	15.9	14.5	13.1	11.7	10.3
10.8	12.2	13.7	15.1	16.6	103	16.2	14.7	13.3	11.9	10.5
11.0	12.4	13.9	15.4	16.9	104	16.5	15.0	13.5	12.1	10.6
11.2	12.7	14.2	15.6	17.1	105	16.7	15.3	13.8	12.3	10.8
11.4	12.9	14.4	15.9	17.4	106	17.0	15.5	14.0	12.5	11.0
11.6	13.1	14.7	16.2	17.7	107	17.3	15.8	14.3	12.7	11.2
11.8	13.4	14.9	16.5	18.0	108	17.6	16.1	14.5	13.0	11.4
12.0	13.6	15.2	16.8	18.3	109	17.9	16.4	14.8	13.2	11.6
12.2	13.8	15.4	17.1	18.7	110	18.2	16.6	15.0	13.4	11.9

SD: standard deviation score (or Z-score). Although the interpretation of a fixed percent-of-median value varies across age and height, and generally the two scales cannot be compared, the approximate percent-of-median values for -1 and -2 SD are 90% and 80% of median, respectively (Gorstein J et al issues in the assessment of nutritional status using anthropometry. *Bulletin of the World Health Organization* 1994; 72: 273-283).

*Length is measured for children below 85 cm. For children 85 cm or more, height is measured. Recumbent length is on average 0.5 cm greater than standing height; although the difference is of no importance to individual children, a correction may be made by subtracting 0.5 an from all lengths above 84.9 cm if standing height cannot be measured.

APPENDIX 47.16

**COMPREHENSIVE NCHS GROWTH RECORD FOR
1 TO 3 YEARS (WEIGHT, LENGTH, HC)**

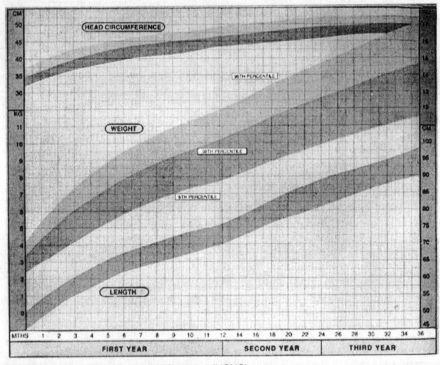

Source: National Centre for Health Statistics (NCHS)

APPENDIX 47.17

HEAD CIRCUMFERENCE

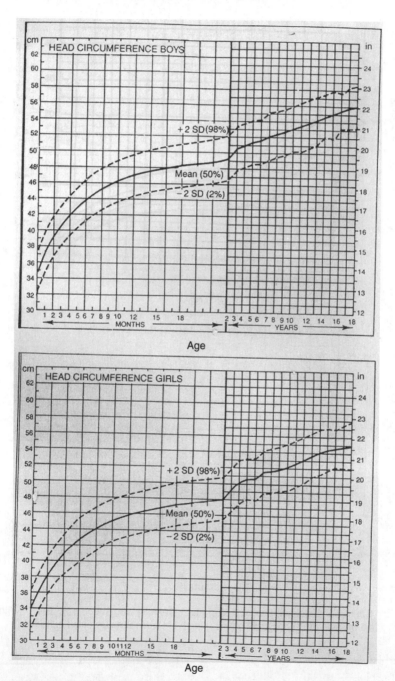

Source: Nellhaus, G: Pediatrics, 41:106, 1968. University of Colorado Medical Center Printing Services

APPENDIX 47.18

CHEST MEASUREMENTS

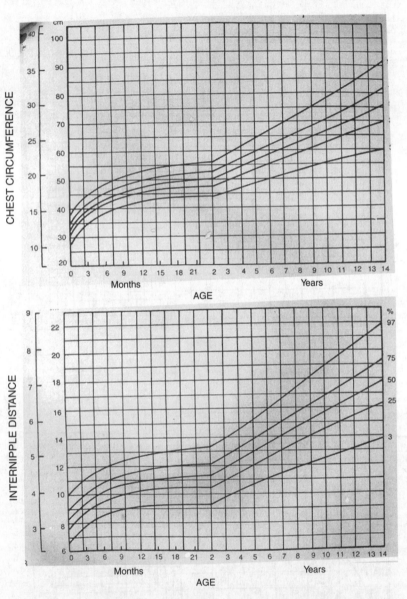

Source: Feingold M, Bossert WH: Birth Defects, 10 (Suppl. 13); 1947. With permission of the copyright holder, March of Dimes Birth Defects Foundation)

APPENDIX 47.19

HAND MEASUREMENTS (A, B, C, D)

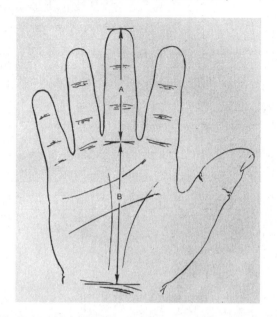

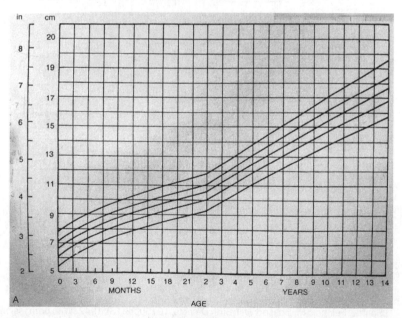

A. Middle finger length

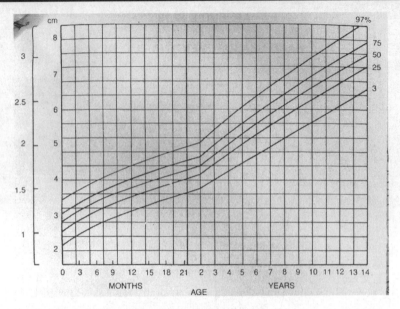

B. Palm length

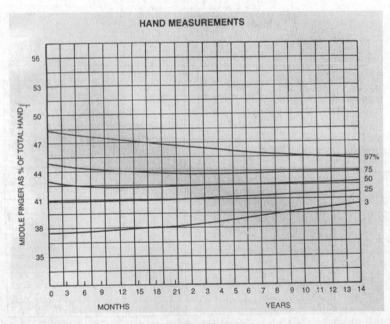

C. Total hand length

Source: Feingold M, Bossert WH: Birth Defects, 10 (Suppl. 13); 1947. With permission of the copyright holder, March of Dimes Birth Defects Foundation)

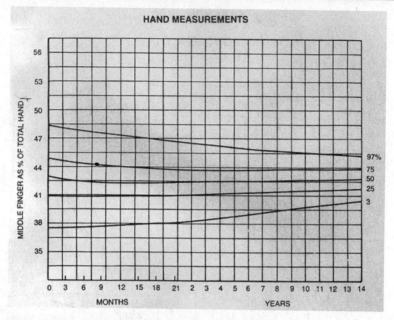

D

Proportion (per cent) of middle finger to hand length. (Source: Feingold M, Bossert WH: Birth Defects, 10(Suppl. 13): 1974. (With permission of the copyright holder, March of Dimes Birth Defects Foundation.)

APPENDIX 47.20

FOOT LENGTH

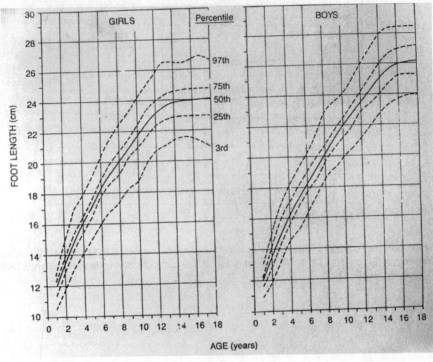

A

Mean and percentile values for foot length. Note: The adolescent growth spurt of the foot usually begins prior to the general linear growth spurt and ends before final height attainment. Thus, the foot growth spurt is a good early indicator of adolescence. Source: Blais MM, Green WT and Anderson M: J. Bone Joint Surg, 38-A:998, 1956, with permission.)

APPENDIX 47.21

FACIAL MEASUREMENTS

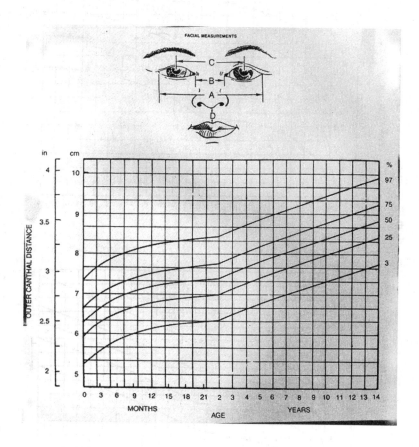

A

Outer canthal (A) inner canthal. (From Feingold M, Bossert WH: Birth defects, 10(Suppl 13): 1974. With permission of the copyright holder, March of Dimes Birth Defects Foundation)

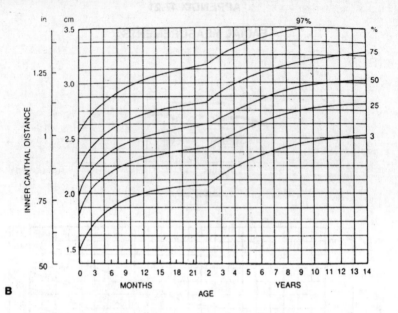

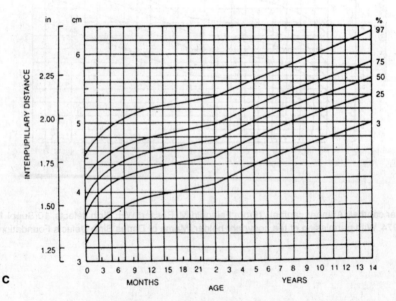

Outer canthal (B) interpupillary and (C) measurements. (From Feingold M, Bossert WH: Birth defects, 10(Suppl 13): 1974. With permission of the copyright holder, March of Dimes Birth Defects Foundation)

APPENDIX 47.22

EYE MEASUREMENTS

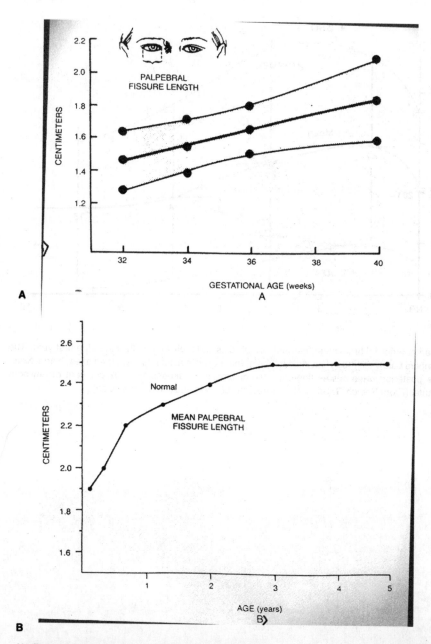

A

B

(A) Palpebral fissure length, 32-40 weeks. (From Jones KL et al: J Pediatr, 92:787, 1978, with permission.) (B) Palpebral fissure length, from inner to outer canthus, 1 to 5 years. (Data from Chouke KS: Am J Phys Antropol, 13:255;1929.

APPENDIX 47.23

FONTANEL MEASUREMENTS

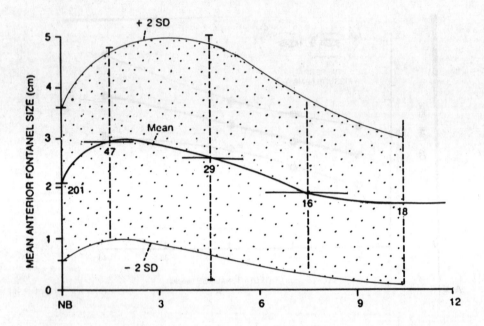

Mean anterior fontanel measurement (length plus width divided by 2) during the first year. The numbers below the mean line indicate the number of normal infants measured at each age. Note: The posterior fontanel was fingertip size or smaller in dimension in 97 per cent of newborn infants. (From Popich G, Smith DW: J Pediatr, 80:749;1972, with permission)

APPENDIX 47.24

EAR LENGTH

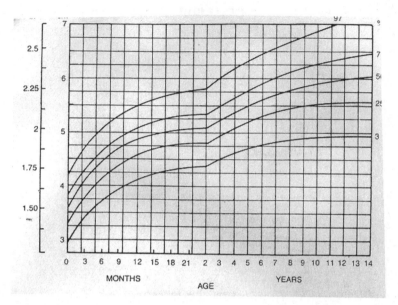

Maximum ear length. (From Feingold M, Bossert WH: Birth Defects, 10(Suppl. 13): 1974. With permission of the copyright holder, March of Dimes Birth Defects Foundation.)

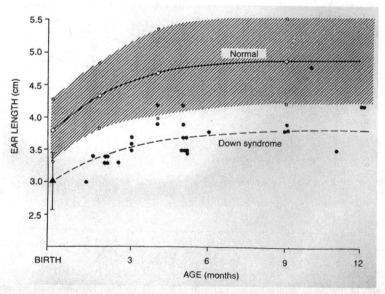

Ear length in normals during the first year, showing mean 2 standard deviations in hatched area, is contrasted with ear length in the Down syndrome, showing mean and 2 standard deviations for 26 affected newborns and individual values *(black dots)* during the first year. (From Aase JM et al: J Pediatr, 82:845, 1973, with permission.)

APPENDIX 47.25

PENILE LENGTH

PENILE LENGTH

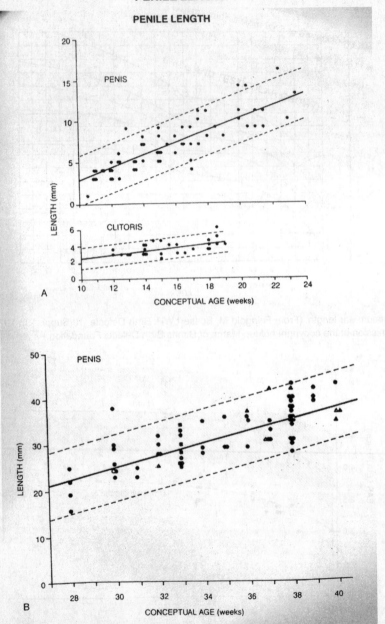

(A) Growth of the penis contrasted with growth of the clitoris from formalin-fixed fetuses (B) Penile stretched length (From public bone to tip of glans) in the newborn. The mean full-term length is 3.5 cm with a 2-standard deviation range, from 2.8 to 4.2 cm. The solid line approximates the mean values, and the broken lines the 2-standard deviation values. (From Feldman KW, Smith DW: J Pediatr, 86:395, 1975 with permission.)

APPENDIX 47.26

PENILE AND TESTICULAR GROWTH

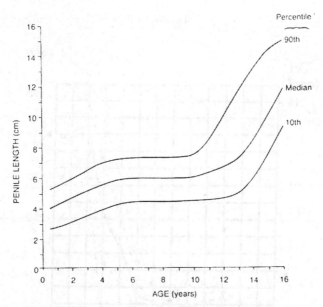

Penile growth in stretched length (From the pubic nramus to the tip of the glans) from infancy into adolescence. (From Schonfeld WA: Am J Dis Child 65:535, 1943, with permission)

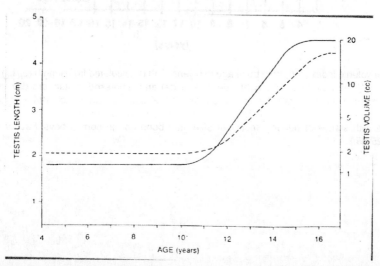

Testicular growth in length, adapted from normal standards of testicular volume. (Solid line from data of A Prader, Zurich; broken line from data of Laron A, Zilka E: J Clin endocrinol. Metab, 29:1409, 1969.)

APPENDIX 47.27

TESTICULAR VOLUME INDEX FROM BONE AGE OF 5 YEARS

$$TVI = \frac{(L_R \times W_R) + (L_L \times W_L)}{2}$$

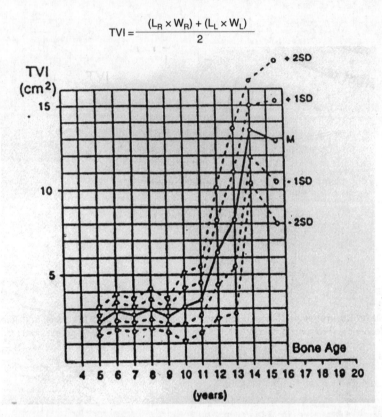

Testicular volume index (TVI) from bone age of 5 years. TVI is calculated from length (L_R L_L) and width (W_R W_L) of both testes (R, right side; L left side) and expressed in standard deviations (SD). M mean. (Adapted from Burr IM, Sizonenko PC, Kaplan SL, Crumbach MM. Hormonal changes during puberty: I Correlation of serum luteinizing hormone and follicle-stimulating hormone with stages of puberty, testicular size, and bone age in normal boys. Pediatr Res 1970;4:25-35.)

APPENDIX 47.28

NOMOGRAM FOR CALCULATION OF BODY SURFACE AREA (M²) FROM WEIGHT (KG) AND HEIGHT (CM)

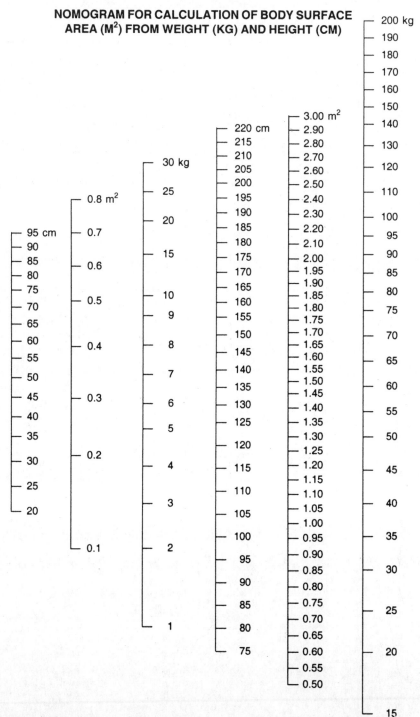

Nomogram for the calculation of body surface area (m²) from weigth (kg) and height (cm)

SECTION 7

Neonatology

CHAPTER

48

Neonatal History Taking

History taking, a special form of communication—is an art. The aim is to elicit an accurate account of all the events which could possibly determine the cause of the present conditions of the neonate.

The history taking for a neonate basically is communication between the doctor and the mother or a person in close relation with the mother.

The neonatal history comprises of the following parts. If the steps are followed as detailed below, important points in the neonatal history are likely to be picked up. They are:
- Antenatal history
- Natal history
- Neonatal history
- Family history

Points to Remember While Taking History

I. A detailed history should include:
   a. Obstetric history
   b. Maternal illness during or before pregnancy
   c. Maternal drug intake during pregnancy
   d. Antenatal, intranatal and postnatal history
   e. Intrapartum, postpartum events from obstetrician or birth attendant.
   f. Presenting complaints in newborn.
II. If it is a home delivery method of cord cutting, it should be enquired (Ex:- What instrument was used to cut, who had cut and when was it cut).

III. In the newborn confirm the passage of urine and meconium.

---

*For a detailed neonatal history taking refer to—Antenatal, Natal, Post-natal and Family History in Vol-I.

49 Physical Examination of Newborn

The examination of the newborn is carried out at 3 times, so as to make the process easy and also for early detection of abnormalities.

General Points to Remember During Examination of a Newborn
1. Examine 1 hour after feeding.
2. Examine in neutral thermal environment.
3. Examine in the presence of the mother.
4. Examine gently, methodically (from top to bottom)
5. Examine those systems which require a quiet child first (e.g. ascultation of heart, palpation of abdomen) and later do examinations that tend to distrub the child, e.g. reflex testing, ear examination.

FIRST EXAMINATION
This should be carried out immediately after birth, in the labor room, so as to establish a baseline for subsequent examination and to detect any life threatening congenital anomalies and to detect pathophysiological problems that may interfere with a normal cardiopulmonary and metabolic adaptation to extrauterine life.

Apgar Score
The traditional way of assessing the newborn is to use the Apgar score. The Apgar score was the first attempt at a systematic assessment of birth asphyxia. This was devised by Virginia Apgar (1953), and grades five clinical features with scores from 0 to 2 at 1 minute of age. In recent years, it is being assessed upto 20 minutes at an interval of 5 minutes each. There has been a tendency to be little with the Agpar score because it is a poor index of asphyxia. If a baby has a poor Apgar score, he has a problem. It may well not be asphyxia but sooner the problem is diagnosed and managed better is the outcome (Table 49.1).

Table 49.1: Apgar's evaluation of newborn

Sign	0	1	2
Heart rate	Absent	Below-100	Over 100
Respiratory effort	Absent	Slow, irregular	Good crying
Muscle tone	Limp	Some flexion of extremities	Active motion
Response to catheter in nostril	No response	Grimace	Cough or sneeze
Color	Blue or pale	Body pink, Blue extremities	Completely pink

A total score of 10 indicates that an infant is in the best possible condition.

An infant with a score of 0-3 requires immediate resuscitation. At the same time after evaluating the Apgar score are must detet the most common life threatening congenital anomalies which affect the newborn.

Table 49.2 Illustrates some life threatening congenital anomalies and their clinical manifestation

Table 49.2: Common life threatening congenital anomalies and their features

Names	Manifestations
Tracheoesophageal fistula (Fig. 49.1)	Polyhydramnios, choking with feeds and aspiration pneumonia, excessive drooling of saliva, inability to place nasogastric tube in stomach, suspect VATER association (vertebral anomalies, anal atresia, tracheoesophageal fistula and renal anomalies).

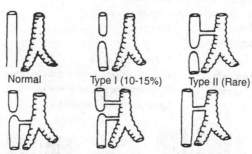

Fig. 49.1: Type of tracheoesophageal fistula

Diaphragmatic hernia (Fig. 49.2)	Respiratory distress and cyanosis Scaphoid abdomen Bowel sounds in the chest Dextroposition of heart

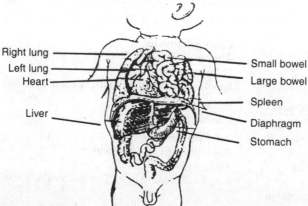

Fig. 49.2: Diaphragmatic hernia. The abdominal viscera have herniated into the thorax. The thoracic viscera have been displaced and compressed

Contd...

Contd...

Names	Manifestations
Choanal atresia	Respiratory distress in delivery room, Apnea, Inability to pass nasogastric tube through nostrils Suspect CHARGE association (coloboma, heart disease, atresia choanae, retarded mental development and growth, genital hypoplasia, ear anomalies and deafness).
Pierre-Robin syndrome	Micrognathia Cleft palate, glossoptosis (Posteriorly placed tongue), Airway obstruction
Ductal dependent Congenital heart disease* (e.g. Hypoplastic left heart syndrome)	Cyanosis Hypotension Murmur
Neural tube defects (Meningomyelocele and encephalocele) (Fig. 49.3)	Polyhydramnios Elevated alpha-fetoprotein levels in maternal serum during pregnancy (14-16 weeks) Decreased fetal activity

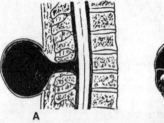 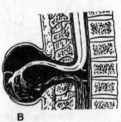

Fig. 49.3: (A) Section of spinal cord and vertebral column showing meningocele. Note that no nervous tissue protrudes through defect into sec. (B) Section of spinal cord and vertebral column showing a myelomeningocele. Nervous tissue if found in herniated meningeal sac

Renal agenesis, Potter's syndrome	Oligohydramnios Anuria Pulmonary hypoplasia Spontaneous pneumothorax, flat and squashed face.
Gastroschisis, omphalocele (Fig. 49.4)	Polyhydramnios Intestinal obstruction.
Intestinal obstruction, (volvulus, duodenal atresia, ileal atresia)	Polyhydramnios, Bile stained emesis in newborn, Abdominal distention, Suspect 21 trisomy, cystic fibrosis, cocaine abuse by mother
Birth trauma-recognition : Types of birth trauma : • Head and neck injuries	– Cephalhematoma – Caput succedaneum

Contd...

Contd...

Names	*Manifestations*

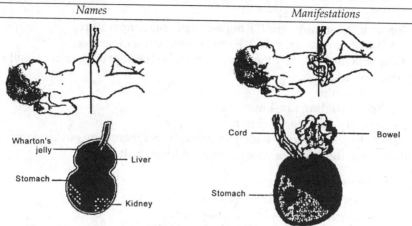

Fig. 49.4: Gastroschisis along the right anterior inferior aspect of the fetal abdomen lops of bowel emerge from the abdomen

	– Intracranial hemorrhage (ICH)
	– Skull fractures
	– Sternocleidomastoid tumour
	– Subgleal hematoma
	– Vaccum caput
	– Superficial head injury
	– Subaponeurotic hemorrhage
	– Mandibular fracture
	– Ocular injury/ear injury
• Nerve injuries	– Brachial plexus paralysis
	– Diaphragmatic paralysis
	– Facial paralysis
	– Median nerve paralysis
• Injuries to viscera	– Liver/spleen/kidney
• Bone injuries	– Clavical fractures
	– Humerus fractures
	– Femur fractures
• Skin and soft tissue injuries	– Abrasions
	– Petechiae and bruising
	– Subcutaneous fat necrosis

VITAL SIGNS MONITORING

Temperature

- Can be measured at several sites in the body via the oral, rectal, axillary, skin or tympanic memberane.
- Types of thermometers:
  - Mercury thermometer
  - Electronic thermometer
  - Tympanic membrane sensor

- Plastic strip
- Digital thermometer
- Rectal temperatures are 1°F higher than oral temperature,
- Axillary temperatures are 1°F lower than oral temperature,
- Length of time mercury thermometers should be kept in place are as follows, based on research:
  - Oral–7 min
  - Rectal reading for–4 min.
  - Axillary reading for–5 min.

These times may vary widely in practice and there may not be significant difference in the temperatures if recorded for a short time.

Child's Temperature
You should measure a child's temperature:
1. When the skin feels warm to your touch.
2. When the child is not acting like usual self.
3. Before seeing the doctor.

How to Read a Thermometer
- Before using the thermometer, make sure it reads 96°F or less. If not, holding the clear end, shake the thermometer sharply in the air, when it reads below 96°F, measure the temperature.
- Hold the clear end of the thermometer at the eye level, slowly turn it until you can see the silver line (mercury)
- Lower numbers will be on the left.
- The highest number that the silver line reaches is the temperature (Fig. 49.5).

How to Measure Axillary Temperature
1. Wash your hands
2. Have the thermometer and water ready.
3. Check that the thermometer is reading below 96°F.
4. Explain to the child/to the mother in case of newborns.
5. Place the thermometer under the child's arm the silver tip of the thermometer should rest in the center of the child's arm pit.
6. Hold the infant's arm firmly against his body.
7. Remove and read the thermometer after 3-4 minutes.
8. Note down the reading and the time of day.
9. Clean the thermometer with water and soap.

How to Measure Rectal Temperature
1. Rectal temperature should not be taken if the infant has diarrhoea.
2. Wash your hands.
3. Make sure thermometer reading is less than 96°F.
4. Measure 1 inch on the thermometer.
5. Place the child on his stomach, with one sides upper leg bent.
6. Dip the thermometer tip in vaseline.

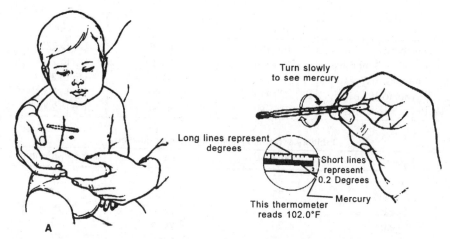

Fig. 49.5: (A) Position for measuring axillary temperature,
(B) Reading a thermometer

7. Place the silver end of the thermometer into the child's anus upto the 1 inch mark.
8. Check the reading after 2-3 minutes.
9. Wash your hands.

Pulse and Heart Rate

- Radial pulse—for children over 2 years of age
  Apical pulse—more reliable in infants and young children.
- Pulse is counted for one full minute in infants and young children.
- A comparison of radial and femoral pulse should be done atleast once during early childhood.
- Grading of pulses:
  O-Not palpable
  + 1 – Difficult to palpate, thready, weak, easily obliterated with pressure.
  + 2 – Difficult to palpate, may be obliterated with pressure.
  + 3 – Easy to palpate, not easily obliterated with pressure (normal).
  + 4 – Strong, bounding, not liberated with pressure.
  Table 49.3 depicts normal heart rates for infnats and children.
  - Normal heart rate is 120-160/min
  - Tachycardia is heart rate more than 160/min seen in cardiac disease, CCF, metabolic and infective causes.

Respiration

- Count by observing abdominal movements, in infants as the movement are primarily diaphragmatic.
- Count for one full minute for accuracy.
- Normal respiratory rates for children (Given in Table 49.4):

Table 49.3: Normal heart rates for infants and children

Rate/min

Age	Resting (awake)	Resting (sleeping)	Exercise (fever)
Newborn	100-180	80-160	Up to 220
1 week to 3 months	100-220	80-200	Up to 220
3 months to 2 years	80-150	70-120	Up to 220
2 years to 10 years	70-110	60-90	Up to 200
10 years to adults	55-90	50-90	Up to 200

Table 49.4: Normal respiratory rates for children

Age	Rate (Breaths/Min)	Age	Rate (Breaths/min)
Newborn	35		
1 to 11 months	35	10 years	20
2 years	30	12 years	19
4 years	25	14 years	18
6 years	23	16 years	17
8 years	21	18 years	16-18

- Normal variation 40-60/min
- Tachypnea is rate more than 60/min and indicates respiratory disease, cardiac disease and acidosis.
- Periodic breathing-periods of breathing interspersed with periods of apnea and lasting less than 10 seconds. It is normal in preterms.

Blood Pressure

Manual blood pressure monitoring is not routinely done in the neonatal nursery but in certain circumstances the blood pressure is usually recorded by blood pressure monitor. There are many normograms of newborns and older children. An example of normal blood pressure values for children is shown in Figure 49.6.

Anthropometric Measurements in the Newborn

The important anthropometric measurements that are recorded in the neonate are:
1. Birth weight, i.e. weight recorded within one hour of birth.
2. Length from crown to heel
3. Head circumference.
4. Mid arm circumference.
   The purpose of taking these measurements are:
a. To assess the baby's size against known standards for the population.
b. To compare the size with (especially the weight) with estimated period of gestation. Lubehenco's international standards or standards developed at AIIMS (New Delhi) are used for comparison (Figs 49.7 and 49.8).
c. To provide a base line against which subsequent progress can be measured.

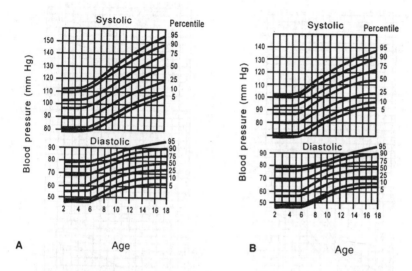

Fig. 49.6: (A) Percentiles of blood pressure measurement in boys (rights arm, seated),
(B) Percentiles of blood pressure measurement in girls (right arm, seated)

Birth Weight

True birth weight is one that is recorded within an hour of birth. Either a good spring weighing scale or preferably beam balance scale is used for the purpose. All the scales should be adjusted to zero before using. For weighing newborn in villages or homes, in clinics and hospitals, small weighing scales with a dial gives fairly good reading. Such a scale can be hung from a hook. Use a sling made from cloth or nylon to hold the child. Fix the scale at eye level for correct reading.

The beam balance scale is used in permanent clinics (Fig. 49.9).

It is accurate, must be kept clean and correctly adjusted. The other precaution to be taken while weighing children include;

a. Naked baby should be kept on a clean towel or paper on the scale pan.
b. The sick or premature infant can sometimes be weighed in an incubator using a spring balance.
c. In home delivery, weight should be taken by placing the baby in a sling using a simple spring balance.

Other Scales Used in the Comminuty

Color coded weighing scale:

It is a simple instrument to find out birth weight. It is a cylindrical instrument with a hook at lower end and a bar to hold the scale at the upper end. The weights are marked upto 5 kg with 100 gm divisions. A newborn weighing < 2.5 kg is low birth weight and hence the scale is colored yellow and red to indicate LBW.

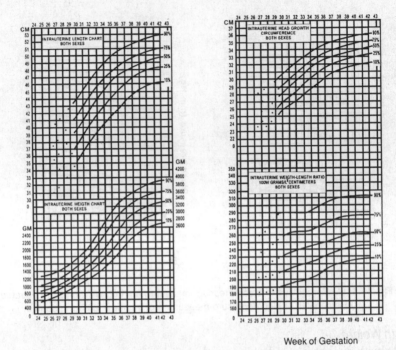

Fig. 49.7: Week of gestation—These data represent infants born in Denver at an altitude of 1 mole above sea level (From L.O. Lubcheno *et al*: Intrauterine growth in length and head circumference as estimated from live born birth weight data at 24 to 42 weeks of gestation. *Pediatrics* 37: 403, 1966)

Before using the scale, ensure that the pointer is at zero and if possible check against known weights. Fold the corners of a clean piece of cloth into a hammock.

Place the baby in the hammock, keeping your left hand underneath if baby slips. Hold the weighing scale by the right hand with the help of the bar. Check the weight by the color now visible on the color coded scale. If the weight falls in red or yellow color zone, the baby is of low birth weight and should be at your special attention. Always keep the scale at eye level while measuring the weight. Never hang weights heavier than 5 kg.

– A birth weight of < 10th or > 90th centile is abnormal. For this either the International (Lubehenco's) or Indians standards (AIIMS) are used.
– Recorded weight is plotted against gestational age and accordingly classified. Few of the definitions and terms are explained below.
– Preterm baby-born before 37 weeks of gestation.
– Term baby-born between 37-42 weeks of gestation.
– Post-term baby-born ofter 42 weeks of gestation.
  SFD (small for date) < 10th centile for the particular gestational age.
  AFG (appropriate for gestation) weight between 10th and 90th centile for that particular gestational.

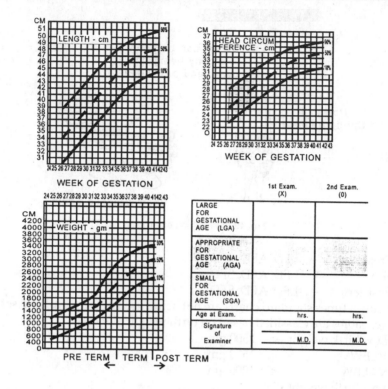

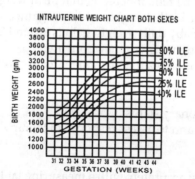

Fig. 49.8: Intrauterine weight chart for both sexes (AIIMS)

LFD (large for date) weight more than 90th centre for that particular gestation age.

Thus, there are nine different types of babies based on their gestational age and between weight.

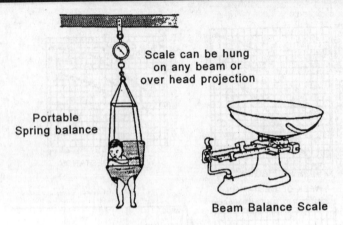

Fig. 49.9: Weighing small child

Preterm	–	LFD, AFD, SFD
Term	–	LFD, AFD, SFD
Post-term	–	LFD, AFD, SFD.

Many a times standard charts are not being used in the peripheral setting. Hence, babies are classified based on birth weight alone as
1. Low birth weight < 2500 gm
2. VLBW < 1500 gm
3. VVLBW < 1000 gm
4. Low birth weight babies requiring special care < 2000 gm.

An important part to be remembered is that birth weight falls in the first five days (not > 10% of birth weight) and is regained on the tenth day. Subsequently, in a term baby daily weight gain is around 25-30 gm.

Other uses of recording weight in newborn are:
a. Monitoring of weight is a sensitive parameter for assessment of nutritional status and its progress.
b. To assess fluid balance
c. To assess cardiopulmonary status
d. To assess renal status and to assess response to therapy.

Length

Length can be taken most accurately with a measuring table or a board with a fixed head piece on which the infant lies supine with his legs fully extended (Fig. 49.10). It is necessary to press the knees lightly back to ensure maximum length. The feet should be pressed against the movable foot piece with the ankles fixed to 90°. The length is recorded on a scale (infanto meter). Two persons are needed to hold the baby correctly (preferably not the mother) and take the measurement. This type of board is difficult to use in an incubator, so the length is measured with ruler or a tape. A specially designed measuring mat type infantometer may be used in peripheral setting.

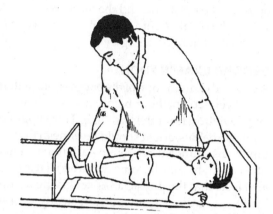

Fig. 49.10: Measuring length with an infantometer

Note: The length need not be taken immediately if the baby's condition gives rise to any anxiety but should be recorded certainly in the first 3 days.

Head Circumference

This measurement may change slightly during the first 3 days owing to moulding during labor, scalp edema or bruising and cephalhematoma. It is taken with a nonstretchable fiber glass tape at the occipitofrontal diameter. Other type of tapes may stretch after repeated measures and may also carry infection between infants hence the tapes should be frequently reversed or sterilized with antiseptic lotion, e.g. savlon, chlorhexidine. Dettol is not satisfactory as it is a weak antiseptic agent (Fig. 49.11).

Normally head circumference is 33-35 cm in a term baby. Head circumferences is usually 2-3 cm larger than the chest circumference. A head circumference less than 10th percentile or more than 90th centile (NCHS charts) is abnormal.

Chest Circumference

Chest circumference is measured at nipple line in mid expiration using nonstretchable fiberglass tape (Fig. 49.12). Normal chest circumference is 30-33 cm.

Mid Arm Circumference (MAC)

Studies have shown that the MAC values can be used as a surrogator for birth weight, because weighing children in remote places is difficult. A MAC of

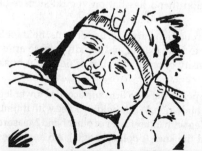

Fig. 49.11: Measuring head circumference

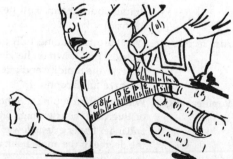

Fig. 49.12: Measuring chest circumference

< 8.5 cm is associated with increased risk of morbidity and mortality. It is measured using a nonstretchable fiber glass tape, conventionally on left arm, between the acromion and the olecranon process, when the arm is kept by the side of the trunk. A mid arm circumference of less than 8.7 cm is indicative of low birth weight (< 2.5 kg).

SECOND EXAMINATION

A detailed examination of the baby is done within 24 hours and the baby should have been fed one hour before the examination. This examination is to detect any deviation from the base line. This should be done in all but especially in high risk babies, and it should be done in the presence of mother and any even minor insignificant anatomic variations should be explained to the mother other wise she may become disturbed if it is found later by some body else and also feels that the physician is not giving accurate consideration to the child.

Examination of newborn basically requires patience, gentleness and procedural flexibility. If the infant is quiet and relaxed, palpation of the abdomen and auscultation of the heart should be performed first before other more disturbing manipulations are done.

Assessment of Gestational Age by Physical/Neurological Criteria

Using a combination of neuromuscular and external physical criteria, gestational age can be estimated indpendent of obstetric history. Accuracy is within 2 weeks for infants over 30 weeks of gestation. Assessment of gestational age in babies under 30 weeks is not very accurate (Table 49.5). Very immature babies are frequently assigned to high gestational age (Fig. 49.13).

Table 49.5: Description of tests used in assessing gestational age

Test	Assessment/Description
Posture	With the infant quiet and in a supine position, observe the degree of flexion in the arms and legs. Muscle tone and degree of flexion increase with maturity. Full flexion of the arms and legs = 4.
Square window	With the thumb supporting the back of the arm below the wirst, apply gentle pressure with index and third fingers on dorsum of hand without rotating the infant's wrist. Measure the angle between the base of the thumb and forearm. Full flexion (hand lies flat on ventral surface of forearm) = 4.
Arm recoil	With the infant supine, fully flex both forearms on upper arms, hold for 5 seconds; pull down on hands to fully extend and rapidly release arms. Observe the rapidity and intensity of recoil to a state of flexion. A brisk return to full flexion = 4.
Popliteal angle	With the infant supine and the pelvis flat on a firm surface, flex lower leg on thigh and then flex thigh on abdomen. While holding knee with thumb and index finger, extend lower leg with index finger of other hand. Measure the degree of the angle behind the knee (popliteal angle). An angle less than 90 degrees = 5.

Contd...

Contd...

Test	Assessment/Description
Scarf sign	With the infant supine, support the head in the midline with one hand; use other hand to pull infant's arm across the shoulder so that infant's hand touches the shoulder. Determine location of elbow in relation to midline. Elbow does not reach midline = 4.
Heel to ear	With the infant supine and the pelvis flat on a firm surface, pull the foot as far as possible up towards the ear on the same side. Measure the distance of the foot from the ear and degree of knee flexion (same as popliteal angle). Knees flexed with a popliteal angle less than 10 degrees = 4.

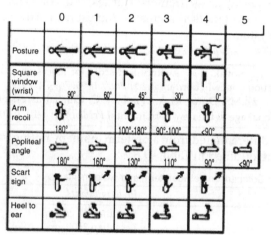

Fig. 49.13: Scoring system for clinical assessment of maturation in newborn infants (From Ballard *et al*)

Brazelton Neonatal Behavioral Assessment Scale (Neonatal Behaviors)

Habituation	– Ability of respond to and then inhibit responding to discrete stimulus (light, rattle, bell, pinprick) while asleep.
Orientation	– Quality of alert states and ability to attend to visual and auditory stimuli while alert.
Motor performance	– Quality of movement and tone.
Range of state	– measure of general arousal level or arousability of infant.
Regulation of state	– How infant responds when aroused.
Autonomic stability	– Signs of stress (tremors, startles, skin color) related to homeostatic (self-regulating) adjustment of the nervous system.
Reflexes	– Assessment of several neonatal reflexes.

REFERENCES
1. Ballard JL, Novak *et al:* A simplified score for assessment of fetal maturation of newly born infatns. *J Paediatr* **95**: 769-74, 1979.
2. Dubowitz LMS, Dutowitz V, Goldberg C: Clincial assessment of gestational age in the new born infant. *J Paediatr* **77**: 1-10, 1970.

A term infant can be differentiated from a preterm infant by noting various physical features that are outlined in Table 49.6.

Table 49.6: Comparison between term and preterm infants

	Term infants	*Preterm infants*
Length	50 cm	Less than 47 cm
Weight	2.5-4.0 kg	Less than 2500 gm
Proportions	Head circumference 33-35 cm	Less than 33 cm
	Chest circumference 33 cm	
	Umbilicus midway between symphysis pubis and xiphisternum	
Vitality	Strong and active	Weak and sluggish
	Wakes for feeds	Drowsy
	Lusty cry	Weak mewing cry
	Normal temperature and strong sucking	Subnormal temperature, sucking is feeble/absent
Skin	Pink and smooth	Red and wrinkled
	Subcutaneous fat present, nipples raised	Little fat present
		Nipples flat
Hair	Silky strands	Short and fuzzy
Ears	Ears firm and stand out	Ears soft and flat
Sole of feet	Complex series of criss crossed over the sole of feet	One or two transverse creases.
Nails	Hard	Soft
	Project beyond tips of fingers	Just to finger tips or not quite to finger tips
Genitals	Testis is descended into scrotum in males.	Testis not in scrotal sac in boys
	Labia minora covered by labia majora in females	Labia minora not covered by labia majora in females

HEAD TO FOOT EXAMINATION

Posture

Normal posture is that of universal flexion. Lack of this universal flexion is seen with hypotonicity or paralysis of limb. Excessive flexion indicates hypertonicity.

Skin

Pallor
- Anemia
- Edema
- Twin-twin transfusion (in donar)
- Shock
- Fetomaternal hemorrhage
- Hypoxia
- Hypotension
- Subcapsular hematoma of liver and spleen

Cyanosis
- Central cyanosis
- CHD
- Severe respiratory disease
- Peripheral cyanosis—may be a normal variant in otherwise normal baby.
- The causes of peripheral cyanosis are:
    - Hypothermia
    - Polycythemia
    - Shock
    - CCF
    - Infection
    - Hypoglycemia
    - Respiratory disease

Cyanosis may be confused with ecchymosis and it should be differentiated by blanching maneuver. When you apply pressure cyanosis disappear and reappear when pressure is taken off, where as ecchymosis does not disappear on pressure.

Jaundice
Appearing in the—First 24 hrs of life.
- Hemolytic disease of newborn
- Rh incompatibility
- ABO incompatibility
- TORCH infection
- G6PD, PK deficiency
- Drugs-sulfisoxozole
- Hereditary spherocytosis

Appearing—between 24-72 hours of life.
- Physiological
- Blood group incompatibility
- Polycythemia
- RBC enzyme deficiencies
- TORCH infections
- Hereditary spherocytosis
- Enclosed hemorrhage (cephalhematoma)

Appearing—after 72 hours
- Septicemia
- TORCH infection
- Extrahepatic biliary atresia
- Breast milk jaundice
- Metabolic disease and galactosemia
- Congenital hypertrophic pyloric stenosis
- Cretinism

Mongolian Spots
- Blue gray pigmentation over sacrum and buttocks.
- Caused by pigmentation in cells in deep layers of skin.
- They disappear maximum within 4 years or often much earlier.

Lanugo Hair
- Usually cover the forehead and brow and may also cover the scalp in premature infants.

Angiomatous Skin Lesions
Hemangioma is a developmental malformation of blood vessel rather than a rare tumour. Though it can occur in any tissue of the body, it is most common in skin and subcutaneous tissues.

It can be capillary, venous (cavernous) or arterial.
- Capillary hemangioma
    - Salmon patch: It is also called as stork bite. It is present at birth over the forehead, in the mid line, and over the occiput. It disappears by the age of 1 year.
    - Portwine stain: Present at birth, the color may alter a little and may become nodular in some areas.
    - Strawberry angioma: The baby is born normal at birth and at the age of 1 to 3 weeks noted to have a red mark which gradually increases until a strawberry or raspberry swelling is present. Then it ceases to grow and by the age of 7 years the involution is complete.
- Venous angioma:
    - Usually does not show tendency towards involution and may become larger.
- Arterial angioma
    - It is a type of congenital arteriovenous fistula.

In case of hemangiomas always suspect some underlying systemic diseases like Sturge-Weber syndrome, trisomy 13, Rubinstein Taybi syndrome, Beckwith Wideman syndrome.

Lymphangiomas
- Capillary Lymphangioma: Localized, brownish papules or wart like excrescences
- Cavernous lymphangioma: Consists of masses of lymphatic cysts particularly in neck or axilla, which is called as cystic hygroma.

Milia
- Minute white papules seen on the chin, nose, cheeks and forehead.
- Represent distended sebaceous glands and they disappear spontaneously in several days or weeks.

Erythema Toxicum
- Pink papular rash in which vesicles are superimposed and some times purulent.
- Appear 24-48 hr. after birth and spontaneously disappear. Etiology is unknown.

Sclerema
- Hardening of skin and subcutaneous tissue, often associated with shock, septicemia and severe cold stress.

Cafe Au Lait Spots
- Appear like a drop of coffee in milk and are seen in-Ataxia telangiectasia
- Bloom syndrome
- Chediak-Higashi syndrome,
- Fanconi's anemia
- McCune-Albright syndrome
- Multiple lentigenosis
- Neurofibromatosis and
- Russel-Silver syndrome

Vernix Ceseosa
- Sticky, white cheesy material seen in full term newborns, in axilla and groin at the time of birth.

Blisters
- These are seen in herpes simplex, varicella, syphilis, candidiasis, impetigo, SSS (Staphylococcal scalded skin syndrome), erythema toxicum and sepsis.

Petechiae
- Infection
- ITP
- von Willebrand's disease
- DIC

- Rh isommunization
- Wiskot-Aldrich syndrome
- Leukemia
- Hemangioma
- Vitamin K deficiency
- Birth injury.

Miliaria

Results from obstruction of eccrine sweat gland and is colloquially known as prickly heat. When it involves superficial layers, it is easily ruptured, non inflamed vesicles and is called as miliaria crystalina. When it involves deeper layer, it is called miliaria rubra.

Edema

Local — Caput succedaneum
Fracture femur, humerus
Vitamin E deficiency
Superior vena caval (SVC) syndrome
Turner syndrome (usually over dorsum of hands and feet in female infant).
Congenital lymphedema
Generalized — Anemia, Rh isoimmunization
CCF, SIADH, TORCH infection
Congenital nephrosis
Renal failure
Over hydration
Liver failure
Cystic adenomatous malformation of lungs
Congenital heart disease (CHD)
Urinary infection
Cold injury syndrome
Idiopathic respiratory distress.

Activity

Poor activity in all limbs — Severe asphyxia
— Hypotonia
— Sick baby
Single limb — Paralysis
— Fracture
— Neuropraxia
— Local injury
— Syphilis

Cry

Depressed — Maternal sedation
— Asphyxia neonatorum
— Sick baby

Highpitched – CNS involvement
Weak cry – Respiratory distress

Types of Cry
- Lusty and angry cry of the healthy newborn.
- Cry of hunger
- Cry of pain
- Grunting cry of baby with respiratory distress
- Feeble cry of preterm baby
- Shrill cry of brain damaged baby
- Hoarse cry of hypothyroid baby
- Cat cry (mewling of a cat)—Cat cry syndrome
- Moaning sick babies
- Bleeting cry (Goat's cry) in megaloblastic anemia and cornelia-de-Lange syndrome.

Head

Head Circumference
Head Circumference 33-35 cm in full term infants (Fig. 49.14).

Microcephaly – Head circumference < 2.5 standard deviation below the mean for gestational age.

Causes – Familial
Congenital
Down syndrome (21 trisomy)
Edward syndrome (18 trisomy)
Trisomy 13
Cri du chat (5p-)
Cornelia de Lange syndrome
Rubinstein Taybi syndrome
Smith Lemli Opitz syndrome
Radiation
Cytomegalovirus infection
Rubella
Toxoplasmosis
Fetal alcohol syndrome
Fetal hydantoin syndrome
Malnutrition
Hypoxic ischemic encephalopathy (HIE)
IUGR
Hyperthyroidism
Intracranial hemorrhage
Maternal phenylketonuria
Infant of diabetic mother (relatively small head)

Macrocephaly – Head circumference greater than 2 std deviation compared to mean for that particular gestational age.

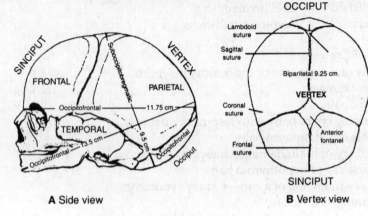

Fig. 49.14: Skull sutures and fontanelle

Causes   – Hydrocephalus
              Cerebral gigantism (Soto's syndrome)
              Hunter syndrome
              Morquios syndrome
              Weaver syndrome
              Hurler syndrome
              Cerebral edema
              Dwarfism
              Dysmaturity
              IUGR
              Hypothyroidism
              Osteopetrosis
              Familial
              Normal variant
              Beckwith-Wiedemann syndrome
              Large for gestational age baby (LGA)

Miss shaped head Caput succedaneum
              Cephalhematoma
              Subgleal hemorrhage
              Encephalocele
              Dolicocephalus
              Brachycephalus (e.g. in Down's syndrome)
              Anencephalus
              Depressed fracture

Craniosynostosis Scaphocephaly
              Trigonocephaly
              Plagiocephaly
              Turricephaly
              Oxycephaly
              Pachycephaly
              Triphyllocephaly

Sutures
- Sutures are palpable as cracks
- Coronal suture-2
- Metopic suture-1
- Sagittal suture -1
- Lamledoid suture-2

Widely separated sutures
- Preterm
- Hydrocephalus
- Cerebral edema
- Intracranial tumors
- Skeletal dysplasia
- Intracranial hemorrhage (ICH)
- Osteogenesis imperfecta
- Increased intracranial pressure
- Dysmaturity
- Growing premature infants.
- Congenital hypothyroidism
- Dwarfism
- Cleidocranial dysostosis
- Vitamin A toxicity
- Chronic pulmonary disorders.

Craniostenosis
- Premature fusion of one or more sutures
- Scaphocephalus
- Oxycephaly
- Turricephaly
- Clover leaf skull

Craniotabes
It is softening of skull bones,which is felt as 'ping pong ball' feel with a pressure exerted on skull 1" above and 1" behind the ear. The causes are:

Osteogenesis imperfecta, Down syndrome, cleidocranial dysostosis, cretinism, lacunar skull.

Craniotabes may be normal upto 2 months of age.

Fontanelles
Four lateral fontanelles are closed at birth. Anterior fontanelle: formed by sagittal and coronal sutures and is diamond shaped (Figs 49.15 and 49.16).

Closure   : 9-18 months.

Depressed : Dehydration

Bulging Fontanelle
- Subdural hemorrhage
- Subarachnoid, epidural hemorrhage

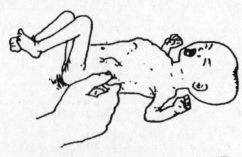

Fig. 49.15: Depressed anterior fontanelle (AF)

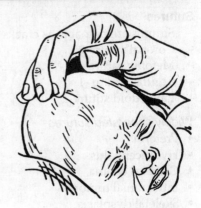

Fig. 49.16: Palpating anterior fontanele (AF)

- Cerebral contusion
- Craniosynostosis
- Hydrocephalus
- TORCH infection
- Turner syndrome
- AV malformation
- Dysmaturity
- Periventricular and or intraventricular hemorrhage (PV-IVH)
- Vitamin A intoxication
- Congestive heart failure (CHF)
- Chronic pulmonary disorder

Large anterior fontanelle
- Achondroplasia
- Apert syndrome
- Athyrotic hypothyroidism
- Cleidocranial dysostosis
- Hallermann-Streiff syndrome
- Hydrocephalus
- Hypophosphatasia
- IUGR
- Osteogenesis imperfecta
- Pyknodysostosis
- Prematurity
- Rubella syndrome
- Russel-Silver syndrome
- 13,18,21-Trisomy
- Vitamin D deficiency—Rickets.

Caput Succedaneum
Diffuse swelling of subcutaneous tissue over presenting part at birth, not restricted to suture lines.
    Decreases in 24-48 hours.
    Absent in breech presentation.

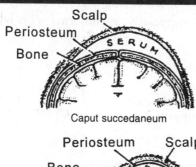

Caput succedaneum

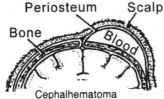

Cephalhematoma

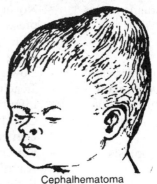

Cephalhematoma

Fig. 49.17: Clinical appearance of cephalhematoma

Cephalhematoma

Well demarcated subperiosteal hemorrhage over parietal bone, restricted by suture line. Appears 6-12 hours after birth. Absorbed or calcified in 4-6 weeks (Fig. 49.17).

Causes of cephalhematoma – Forceps application,
         – Vaccum extraction,
         – Difficult delivery, contribute to its occurrence.

Complications that might result from cephalhaematoma include:
– Anemia
– Jaundice
– Infection

Hair

Preterm baby   – Fuzzy hair
Low hair line   – Turner's syndrome
              Cornelia de Lange syndrome

Tufts of hair on lumbo sacral region suggests—spina bifida oculta.

Transillumination of Skull

It is done when a neurological disorder is suspected. In a dark room, devoid of light leaks, the examiner gets dark adapted (when light placed into the examiner palm, is transmitted through the hand so that shadows of the distal metacarpal bones are clearly visible as light penetrates the soft tissues). Then the flash light is snuggly applied to the skull to avoid light leaks. A flare of light greater than 1.5-2 cm beyond the rim of fitting is considered abnormal.

Causes of positive transillumination:
• Hydranencephaly
• Hydrocephalus

Eyes

To examine the eyes donot separate the eyes forcibly as it is very difficult. Hold the baby up and move gently forward and backward. This maneuver, as a result of labrynthine and neck reflexes, makes the baby's eyes open.

a. Edema of lids – Normally seen especially in preterms with face presentation.
   – CCF
   – Congenital nephrosis
b. Upward slant – Down syndrome
c. Down slant – Treacher-Collin syndrome
d. Buphthalmos – Infantile glaucoma
   Cloudy cornea
   Corneomegaly
e. Proptosis – Retrobulbar hematoma
   Neuroblastoma
   Retinoblastoma
   Craniostenosis
   Orbital encephalocele
f. Subconjunctival hemorrhages – Normal
   Severe asphyxia
g. Conjunctivitis – Chemical: Instillation of silver nitrate drops
   Purulent: Gonococcal, staphylococcal
h. A normal newborn should have pupillary reflex and blink response to bright light.
i. Brushfield spots over iris – Down syndrome
j. Cataracts – Congenital
   Familial
   Rubella
   Toxoplasmosis
   CMV
   Galactosemia
   Down's syndrome
   Hypothyroidism
k. Corneal opacities – Trauma
   Herpes virus
   Congenital rubella
l. Colobomas – Treacher-Collin syndrome
   Trisomy 13
m. White pupil – • TORCH infection
   • Galactosemia
   • Lowe's syndrome
   • Microophthalmia
   • Retinopathy of prematurity (ROP)
   • Retinoblastoma
   • Herpes simplex
   The presence of red reflex which is normal should always be looked for. A white reflex in pupil (Leucocoria) indicates-cataract, tumour, chorioretinitis, retinopathy of prematurity (ROP).
n. Blue sclera is seen in osteogenesis imperfecta and Ehler Danlos syndrome.

Nose

Neonates are obligatory nose breathers. Always check for patency. Sneezing is normal in newborns.

a. Oral breathing – Obstruction by mucus plug
Choanal atresia or stenosis
b. Snuffles/serosangeous discharge–congenital syphilis
c. Stuffy nose—reserpine given to mother.

Ears

The top of pinna is in line with the outer canthus of eye. The pinna is flexible and cartilage is present in term normal newborn. Infant normally shows Moro's or Startle reflex to a loud and sudden noise.

a. Ear tags – Renal anomalies, cardiac anomalies, verterbral anomalies, occular anomalies (Goldenhar syndrome) should be ruled out.
b. Preauricular sinus
c. Low set ears
d. Tympanic membrane – Dull grey in new born.

Mouth and Throat

a. Excessive salivation – Hare lip
Cleft palate
Tracheoesophageal fistula
b. Ranula – Benign swelling at the floor of the mouth.
c. Precocious teeth – Fall off normally (Neonatal teeth). Occurs once in 2000 births and often familial.
Should be removed when feeding difficulties occur. The child may aspirate these teeth. Pierre-Robin syndrome, Ellis van Creveld syndrome and Hallermann-Striff syndrome should be suspected in the presence of neonatal teeth.
d. Glossoptosis – Pierre Robin syndrome
e. Macroglossia – Hypothyroidism
Muscular macroglossia
Beckwith-Widemann syndrome
Hurler syndrome
Pompe's syndrome
Sublingual hemangioma
Lymphangioma
Trisomy 21
Hemangioma of tongue.
f. Tongue tie: Normal phenomenon
g. Cleft lip and cleft palate
h. High arched palate – Marfan syndrome
i. Epstein pearls – Small white papular structures on each side of mid line of hard palate due to accumulation of epithelial cells. Disappear within few weeks after birth.

j. Micrognathia   – Pierre Robin syndrome.
                                           Treacher Collin syndrome.
k. Deviation of angle of mouth – 7th nerve palsy.
i. Symmetrical facial palsy   – Moebius syndrome

Neck

Neonate's neck is usually short

a. Webbing of neck—Turner's syndrome
b. Swelling in neck—Sternomastoid tumor common in breech, forceps delivery and causes torticollis. Goiter (enlargement of thyroid), thyroglossal cysts.
       Cystic hygroma (Transillumination +ve)
c. Absence of clavicles: Cleidocranial dysostosis.
       Look for fracture of clavicles.

Thorax

a. Shape   – Normally barrel shaped
b. Supernumerary nipples   – In the mammary line vary from few mm. in size, no glandular tissue, harmless.
c. Gynecomastia   – Breast hypertrophy
                              – Due to maternal hormonal effect, secretion of milk may be evident (Witch's milk).
d. Breast abscess   – Asymmetric swelling around the areola with severe erythema of skin.
e. Respiratory rate   – Normal 40-60/min
f. Type of breathing   – Diaphragmatic is normal (abdomino-thoracic).
g. Emphysematous chest   – Meconium aspiration
h. Unilateral bulge   – Pneumothorax
i. Heart rate   – 120-160 beats/min
j. Dextrocardia   – Suspect diaphragmatic hernia
k. Murmurs   – Usually not present at birth, present later, only 1:12 chances the murmur heard at birth represents congenital heart disease (CHD).
l. Femoral pulses should be felt to detect coarctation of aorta.

Abdomen

a. Normally   – Protruberant
b. Scaphoid   – Diaphragmatic hernia, tracheoesophageal fistula.
c. Distended   – Ascites
                    Intestinal obstruction
                    Hydronephrosis
                    Meconium ileus
                    Paralytic ileus
                    Diastasis recti
                    Prune Belly syndrome
                    Exomphalos.
d. Umbilical cord: Color   – Blue to white at birth, green in meconium staining.
                  Structure – Normally 2 arteries, one vein are seen.

Single umbilical artery may be associated with cardiac anomalies, renal anomalies, intestinal malformations.

Types of Cords

Short cords	– Fetal hypotonia
Long cords	– Risk for true knots, wrapping around fetal parts (nuchal, arm).
Straight and untwisted cord	– Fetal distress
	– Anomalies, omphalocele
	– Intrauterine fetal demise.

Delayed Separation (> 1 month)

– Associated with neutropil chemotactic defects and
– Infection.

Purulent discharge from umbilicus	:	Umbilical sepsis
Mucoid, persistent	–	Patent vitellointestinal ducts
Watery, persistent	–	Patent urachus

Abdominal Mass

Upper abdominal

Liver	:	Hematoma
		Hepatoblastoma
		Neuroblastoma
		Choledochal cyst
		Distended gallbladder secondary to cystic fibroma.
Gastric	:	Bag and mask ventilation
		Duodenal obstruction
		Nasal CAP
Adrenal	:	Neuroblastoma
		Hemorrhage.

Middle abdominal/Flank

Kidney	:	Hydronephrosis
		Multiple cysts
		Polycystic disease
		Nephroblastoma
		Renal vein thrombosis
Adrenals	:	Neuroblastoma
		Hemorrhage
Retroperitoneal	:	Teratoma
		Vitellous cyst
		Urachal cyst

Lower abdominal/Pelvis

Hydrometrocolpos in female infants
Presacral teratoma
Neuroblastoma

Uretheral volvulus
Uretheral stenosis
Neurogenic bladder
Ectopic kidney

Variable : Mesenteric cyst
Omental cysts
Meconium ileus
Abscess.

Genitalia

a. Male : Normally perpuce covers the entire glans penis so that external meatus is not visible and sometimes prepuce cannot be retracted back upto 4-6 months, in normal babies.

   Abnormalities : Phimosis
   Hypospadiasis
   Epispadiasis

   Scrotum : Varies in size, rugated with descended testis, is seen in term babies.

   Abnormalities : Hydrocele congenital
   Hernia
   Transitory hydrocele

   Ambiguous genitalia : Adrenogenital syndrome
   Hermophrodite

b. Female : Normally labia majora covers the minora.
   Hymenal tag—protrudes from the floor of the vagina and disappears after few weeks.

Vaginal milky white secretion—maternal harmonal influence and disappears by 2 weeks.

Urine should be voided with in 24-48 hours after birth. Meconium should be passed within 24 hours.

Extremities

a. Single Palmar crease—Down's syndrome
b. Polydactly
c. Syndactly
d. Simian crease
e. Congenital ring construction—amniotic band syndrome and amputation.

Bone and Joints

Short limbs – Achondroplasia
Dwarfism
Phocomelia (thalidomide)

Amputation of finger – Amniotic band syndrome

Contractures of various joints – Congenital arthrogyposis multiplexa, myotonic dystrophy

Fractures – Breech presentation

Hemihypertrophy	– AV fistula
	Neurofibromatosis
	Wilm's tumor
Rib cage deformities	– Asphyxiating thoracic dystrophy
Spine	– Tuft of hair
	Pilonidal sinus
	Spina bifida
	Meningomyelocele
Hips	– Congenital dislocation of hip

PRIMARY NEONATAL REFLEXES

Primary Neonatal Reflexes

In total, there are about 73 reflexes, but a few are important which should be checked routinely.

Moro's Reflex

Elicited by raising the head of supine infant and allowing it to drop by 10° onto examiners supporting hand.

or

Hold the baby at an angle of 45° from the couch and then suddenly let the head fall back a short way into the palm (Fig. 49.18).

Response Abduction and extension of arms with open fingers, followed by adduction and anterior flexion of arms and closure of fists and cries.

Normal	28 weeks	— Only opening hands
	32 weeks	— Opening hands, extreme abduction, followed by anterior flexion, adduction.
Less prominent	–	Asphyxia
		Meningitis
		Septicemia
		Anaesthesia and narcotic effects
		Kernicterus
		Hypotonia
		Hypertonia
Assymetrical	–	Erb's palsy
		Fracture clavicle, humerus
		Hemiplegia

Disappears by-3-4 months
Persists > 6 months in spastic CP and other conditions with brain damage.

Rooting Reflex

Elicited by touching the corner of mouth lightly with finger (Fig. 49.19).

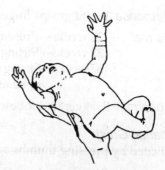

Fig. 49.18: Moro's response

Response Bottom lip is lowered on the same side and the tongue moves towards the point of stimulation as finger slides away, head turns to follow it.

Normal Present from 28 weeks but well elicited after 32 weeks. May not be elicited immediately after feeding. Disappears by 4 months (in awake state) 7 months (in sleeping state).

Abnormal Absence of rooting at birth or persistence beyond 7th month, indicates developmental defect

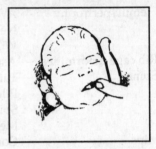

Fig. 49.19: Rooting reflex

Sucking Reflex
Elicited by introducing a clean finger into the mouth or better by putting the baby to breast.

Response Vigorous sucking

Normal Present from 28 weeks of gestation.
Disappears by 4 months (in awake state) and 7 months (in sleeping state)

Abnormal Absence of sucking at birth indicates sickness and persistance beyond 7 months indicates developmental defects.

Swallowing Reflex
Swallowing reflex is elicited by putting the baby to breast.

Response Rhythmical swallowing movements will be felt and can also be seen at neck.

Normal Present at birth and disappears by 6-9 months.

Abnormal Decreased or absent in general neurological depression, hypotonia, immaturity and bulbar palsy.

Palmar Grasp
Elicited by applying pressure with index finger over ulnar aspect of palm (Fig. 49.20).

Response Infant grasps finger tightly

Normal – 28 weeks—Present, but weak
           32 weeks—Strong
           37 weeks—Strong even involving upper limbs allowing the infants
                   to be lifted off the bed.

Abnormal Exaggerated following severe bilateral cerebral injury

Plantar Grasp
Elicited by pressing thumbs against the balls of the infants feet (Fig. 49.21).

Response Plantar flexion of toes and fingers.

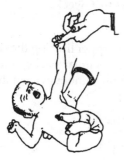

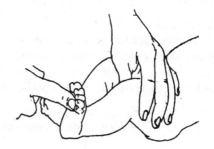

Fig. 49.20: Palmar grasp   **Fig. 49.21:** Plantar grasp

Normal Present at birth and disappears by 6-9 months.

Abnormal Absent—spinal cord defects
             Asymmetrical—CNS defects.

Placing Reflex
Elicited by bringing the anterior aspect of tibia against the edge of the table
(Fig. 49.22).

Response The baby lifts the leg up to step onto table.

Normal Present in full term at birth and preterms weighing more than > 1700
gm after 24 hours. Disappears at 5-6 weeks.

Walking Reflex (Stepping Reflex)
Elicited by holding the baby upright and holding over a table, so that sole
presses against table (Fig. 49.23).

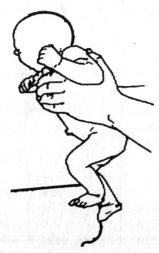

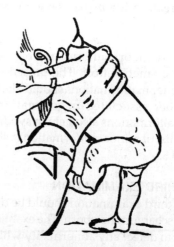

Fig. 49.22: Placing reflex   **Fig. 49.23:** Walking reflex

Response Simulates walking

Normal Present at birth in full term but disapperas by 6 weeks.

Tonic Neck Reflex
Elicited by rotation of head to one side. Extension of upper limb on the side to which face is rotated, flexion on side of occiput, less similar participation of lower limbs. Present from 35 weeks onwards most prominent in term infants and disappear by 5 months age (Fig. 49.24).

Abnormal – Exaggerated, stereotyped, non-habituating
– Severe bilateral cerebral injury

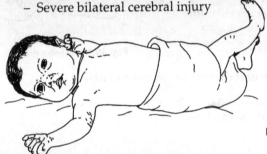

Fig. 49.24: Tonic neck reflex

Gallant's Reflex (Trunk Incurvation Reflex)
Elicited by ventrally suspending the baby and stroking on side of the spine.

Response Trunk comes to that side.

Normal Present at birth and disappears by 6 weeks.

Examination for Detection of Malformations
A thorough examination should be done to detect congenital malformations (i.e., a structural defect seen at birth). A major malformation is one which threatens life or has severe cosmetic effect (Fig. 49.26).

The examples are given in the Table 49.7.

A minor malformation has no life threatening or cosmetic effect. The presence of more than 3 minor malformations should alert one to search for other associated major malformations. Minor malformations also help in syndrome delineation. A list of minor malformation is shown in the Table 49.8.

THIRD EXAMINATION
A third examination should be done at the time of discharge of newborn. The examination at this time is to detect any abnormality which was missed in the initial examinations. Also sometimes the

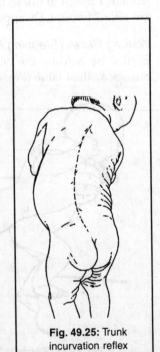

Fig. 49.25: Trunk incurvation reflex

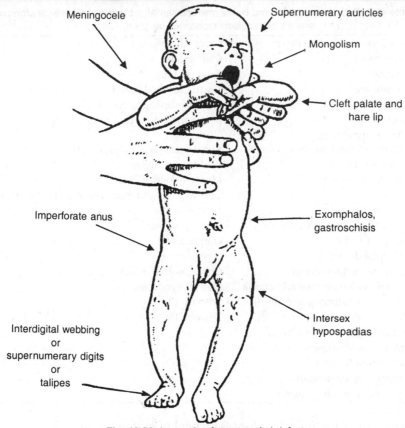

Fig. 49.26: Inspection for congenital defects

abnormalities which are not present at the time of initial examination, may appear at this time.

For example: Since there is high pulmonary vascular resistance at birth, shunt murmurs associated with congenital heart diseases are not frequently evident until a few days.

A careful general examination of a newborn baby provides more information of the condition of the baby, as compared to conventional systemic examination. However a quick systemic examination is important in confirming the abnormalities suspected on general examination.

The systems to be examined includes:
– Cardiovascular system (CVS)
– Respiratory system (RS)
– Central nervous system (CNS)
– Abdomen

CNS
1. Examination for newborn reflexes.
2. Conventional neurological examination.

Table 49.7: Birth defects monitored by the metropolitan Atlanta congenital defects program and the birth defects monitoring program, 1991

Central Nervous System defects	Orofacial defects
Anencephaly	Cleft palate
Spina bifida	Total cleft lip
Encephalocele	Gastrointestinal defects
Hydrocephaly	Tracheoesophageal anomalies
Microcephaly	Rectal and intestinal atresia
Genitourinary defects	
Anophthalmia and microphthalmia	Renal agenesis and dysgenesis
Congenital cataract	Bladder exstrophy
Coloboma of the eye	Musculoskeletal defects
Aniridia	Club foot without central nervous system defects
Cardiovascular defects	Limb reduction defects
Transposition of the great vessels	Arthrogryposis
Tetralogy of Fallot	Omphalocele
Atrial septal defect	Gastroschisis
Endocardial cushion defect	Chromosomal defects
Pulmonary valve stenosis and atresia	Down's syndrome
Tricuspid valve stenosis and atresia	Trisomy 13
Aortic valve stenosis	Trisomy 18
Hypoplastic left heart syndrome	
Patent ductus arteriosus	
Coarctation of the aorta	
Pulmonary artery stenosis	
Lung agenesis and hypoplasia	

3. Neurological examination for assessment of gestational age.
4. Examination for assessing wakeful stage.

Conventional Examination

Consciousness
Note for the following
- Immediate and delayed response to external stimuli
- Response to comforting
- Excessive crying
- Excessive quiteness

Involuntary Movements
- Jitteriness
- Convulsive movement
- Spasms of tetanus

Cranial Nerves
II   : i. Pupillary response
             ii. Visual acuity by dangling a bright red object infront of baby's eyes, when baby watches at an angle of 45°.
           iii. Flashing light causes blink, pupillary constriction.

Table 49.8: Examples of "common" minor malformations

Skull	Genitalia
Parietal foramina	Labial adhesions
Parietal bossing	Hydrocele
Prominent forehead	Mild hypospadias
	Undescended testis
Ears	
Preauricular pits	Anus and perineum
Preauricular tags	Anal tags
Anomalies of auricular cartilage	Anal stenosis
Eyes	Back
Heterochromia of the iris	Sacral dimples
Coloboma of the iris	
	Skin
Nose	Isolated pigmented nevi
Short columella	Small vascular nevi
Bulbous nasal tip	Skin dimples over lying bony prominences
Perioral zone	Hair
Smooth philtrum	Upswept posterior hairline
Narrow vermilion	Supernumerary scalp hair whorl
Angular lip pits	White forelock
Mouth	Nails
Palatal pits	"Spooned" nail
Torus palatinus	Nail grooves
Hypoplastic lateral incisors	Joint
Short lingual frenulum	Infantile bowleg
	Camptodactyly of fifth fingers
Neck	
Branchial arch remnants	Hands
	Clinodactyly of fifth fingers
Chest	"Potter's thumb"
Supernumerary nipples	
	Feet
Abdomen	Syndactyly of second and third toes
Single umbilical artery	Short fourth metatarsal
Umbilical hernia	

III, IV, V	:	(Oculomotor nerves) Doll's eye maneuver—Rotation of head stimulates semicircular canals, impulses travel through VIII nerve to brain stem, MLB, to III and VI nerve nucleus.
V	:	Rooting reflex and good sucking reflex indicates intactness of V nerve.
VII	:	Asymmetry of face indicates VII nerve paresis.
VIII	:	Response to sound, of various intensity.
IX, X, XII	:	Good swallowing without regurgitation and good voice indicate intactness of the nerves.

Motor

Power   – Watch active movements and movements on stimulation and posture of the neonate.

Tone   – Assessed by posture, posture in ventral suspension and in pull to sitting maneuver. Clonus is common.

Abnormal Movements

Jitteriness, tonic/clonic convulsion.

Sensory

Withdrawal and cry to pain, response

Superficial Reflex

Usually not done, plantar upgoing,

Deep Tendon Reflexes

Usually brisk (knee, ankle, biceps and triceps).

Examination of Abdomen

1. Normally slightly protruberant.
2. Scaphoid abdomen in the immediate neonatal period should arouse suspicion of diaphragmatic hernia.
3. Mild VP may be seen especially in low birth weight babies.
4. Gross distention is due to ascites, lower gut obstruction, paralytic ileus and mass.
5. Prune-Belly syndrome is a condition due to absence of abdominal muscles that gives wrinkled appearance to abdomen and is often associated with undescended testis and urinary anomalies.
6. Palpate kidney, by unidigital method, wherein the thumb of examiner is placed infront over lumbar region and index and middle fingers are kept on the posterior aspect of lumbar region and an attempt is made to approximate to the fingers. An enlarged kidney is palpable between the fingers. Normally right kidney may be palpable.
7. Liver is normally palpable 1-2 cm below right costal margin.
8. Splenic tip is occasionally palpable in normal newborn.
9. Umbilicus:
    - i. Umbilical vessels   – 2 arteries
                          – 1 vein
    - ii. Evidence of infection.
    - iii. Bleeding   – Infection
                          – Poor ligation of cord
                          – Factor 13 deficiency
    - iv. Granuloma
    - v. Early or late fall should arouse the suspicion of infection
    - vi. Exomphalos/hernia
    - vii. Polyp

Examination of Respiratory System

History of

Cough   –   Pneumonia

Diabetes mellitus	–	Respiratory distress syndrome
Gestation (preterm)	–	Respiratory distress syndrome
Polyhydramnios	–	Tracheo-oesophageal fistula
PROM, MAS, prolapse	–	Asphyxia, respiratory distress

Character

Dyspnea, tachypnea, apnea, grunting

Absence of movement   –   Pneumothorax, effusion and hypoplastic lungs.

Auscultation

Not very useful as conduction of sound is common. Absence of sounds indicates pneumothorax, effusion, hypoplastic lung.

Bowel sounds indicate—congenital diaphragmatic hernia.

Laryngoscopy is done to identify the cause of stridor.

Examination of CVS

History of

Drug and TORCH exposure

Anomalies—cleft lip/palate, cataract, polydactyly.

Respiratory rate—normal/increased or decreased/type of breathing.

Pulse—radial, femoral (coarctation of aorta), posterior tibial, dorsalis pedis.

Blood pressure—measured by sphygmomanometer, flush method and Doppler method.

Average BP in   Term baby 70/45 mm Hg

Preterm 60/20 mm Hg

Cry elevates BP by 20 mm Hg

Signs of congestive cardiac failure-enlarged liver, facial edema (increased JVP, edema, of feet rare).

Precordium: Apex, thrill, RV impulse, heart rate, sounds and murmurs.

Examination at the Time of Discharge

All babies should be examined. Note the weight on the day of discharge. This can be a superficial examination. The main purposes are:

a. To determine that nutrition is satisfactory.

b. To detect acquired abnormalities, e.g. skin lesions, discharge from eyes, nose, ear, vagina, oral infection especially trunk, umbilical sepsis, jaundice, cyanosis and anemia.

c. To test hip joint for instability.

d. To detect whether visceral abnormality and hernia are present by inspection and palpation of the abdomen.

e. To detect any abnormality of the heart which may not have been found during earlier examinations but which is sometimes detectable after 7-10 days by auscultation.

All mothers should be given a discharge card on which the gestational age, birth weight, type of delivery, neonatal problems, discharge weight and recommended method of feeding should be recorded in addition to the basic information like name of the mother, hospital number, etc.

Guidelines for Discharge Information

1. Significant perinatal history including maternal history, prenatal course, medications, drug exposures, social history, labor and delivery history, including birth weight, gestational age, appropriateness for gestational age, Apgars, and resuscitation efforts.
2. Summary of hospital course including:
   a. Respiratory course including ventilator support, oxygen needs, apnea and bradycardia, bronchopulmonary dysplasia.
   b. Neurological complications, including intraventricular hemorrhage, seizures hydrocephalus and ophthalmic evaluation.
   c. Cardiovascular needs.
   d. Nutrition history and present feeding regimen.
   e. Transfusions and central lines used.
   f. Surgical procedures and exchange transfusion.
   g. Infections.
   i. Any other major complications (such as necrotizing enterocolitis, osteopenia of prematurity, retinopathy of prematurity, anemia of prematurity.
3. Pertinent laboratories: Highest bilirubin, most recent hemoglobin and reticulocyte count, newborn screening, others as indicated.
4. Pertinent radiologic studies: X-rays, cranial ultrasound, echocardiogram, others.
5. Discharge medications and levels.
6. Immunizations.
7. Discharge physical, including weight, length, and head circumference.
8. Home nursing and therapies (occupational, physical, or speech therapy), home equipment needs.
9. Follow-up appointments with all services involved.

Follow-up Examination of Baby at Home

This should be the responsibility of the community health team during the first two weeks in particular. They should examine the baby to ascertain the following:

1. That it is vigorous as shown by muscle activity, good cry and good sucking.
2. The eyes, nose, skin, umbilicus and mouth shows no signs of deviation from normal that there is no discharge, rash, jaundice or oral thrush.
3. That stool consistency and colors are normal.
4. That there is no vomiting.
5. That weight gain is normal (this can be done by inspection, but it is preferable to use a sling balance when possible).

6. Ask mother to report to health worker/doctor if there are any danger signs (Refusal of feeds, increased drowsiness, cold to touch, convulsions, persistent vomiting, deep jaundice).

Daily Follow-up Examination in the Hospital

1. Color
2. Respiration
3. Activity
4. Jaundice
5. Eyes, mouth, skin, umbilicus for evidence of infection.
6. Stool, urine color, passage (time of passage and frequency).
7. Feeding behavior
8. Weight
9. Danger signs.

SUMMARY: PHYSICAL EXAMINATION OF NEWBORN

1st Examination (In labor room)

- Apgar score evaluation
- Identification of common life threatening congenital anomalies
- Recognition of birth injuries
- Vital signs monitoring—Temperature/RR/HR/BP
- Anthropometric measurements
    - Weight
    - Length
    - Head circumference
    - Chest circumference
    - MAC.

2nd Examination (< 24 hours)

- Assessment of gestational age
- Comparison between term/preterm
- Head to foot examination
    - Posture
    - Skin
    - Activity
    - Cry
    - Head
    - Eyes
    - Nose
    - Ears
    - Mouth and throat
    - Neck
    - Thorax/Chest
    - Abdomen

- Genitalia
- Extremities
- Bones and joints
- Primary neonatal reflexes
- Examination for detection of malformations

3rd Examination
- Central nervous system
- Per abdomen
- Respiratory system
- Cardiovascular system

Examination at the time of discharge

Follow-up examination of the baby at home

Daily follow-up examination in the hospital

50 Neonatal Records

1. Neonatal case records
2. Neonatal physical assessment record sheet
3. Monitoring in NICU setup
4. Referral sheet
5. Discharge summary sheet
6. Apgar score sheet
7. Blood gas record sheet
8. IAP card
9. Immunization card (Karnataka).

NEONATAL CASE RECORD

Infant of .... Hosp. No. .... Mother's Hosp. No. ....

Date of birth .... Time .... hrs. Sex ....

Father Age .... yrs.   Occupation ....

Town/Village .... District .... State .... Admission date ....

MATERNAL MEDICAL HISTORY

Age..... yrs. Gravida..... Parity..... Living..... Blood group..... Rh type...... Hb.....
Level of Education........................ Ht..........cm Wt................kg.wt.gain..........kg

Maternal History

		Family history			Family history
____	____	Consanguinity	____	____	Heart disease
____	____	Abortions/still births	____	____	Tuberculosis
____	____	Neonatal deaths	____	____	Asthma
____	____	Premature labor/delivery	____	____	Epilepsy
____	____	Previous C-section	____	____	UTI
____	____	Infant with cong anomaly	____	____	Thyroid disease
____	____	Hypertension	____	____	Others ____

Notes _____

_____

_____

PRESENT PREGNANCY

LMP........... EDD.......... VDRL........... HBsAg............. HIV............ ANC...........

US.............. X-ray............................. NST................. OCT...........

___ Hyperemesis

___ Hypertension/PIH/eclampsia

___ Anemia

___ Infection

___ Jaundice

___ Diabetes

___ Urinary infection

___ Drugs _____

___ Oligohydramnios/polyhydramnios

___ Vaginal bleeding

___ Heart disease

___ Seizure disorder

___ Premature labor/ROM

___ Placental insufficiency

___ Post-term

___ Drugs _____

LABOR

Spontaneous/induced.............. Duration: 1st stg............hrs 2nd stg.............mts

Drugs _____ IV fluids

_____ Oxytocin

_____ Pethidine

_____ Tocolytic agents

_____ Others _____

RMDI _____ 1-2 hours

_____ 12-24 hours

_____ 24 hours

_____ Meconium

DELIVERY TYPE

_____ Normal vaginal

_____ Instrumental

_____ C-section

Presentation

_____ Vertex

_____ Breech

_____ Other

Place

_____ BH

_____ PHC

_____ Outreach centre

_____ Other hospitals

_____ Home

Mat.indications	Fetal indications	Drugs	FHR
__ Repeat C-section	__ Fetal distress	__ Gen.anesthesia	__ 100
__ CPD	__ IUGR	__ Spinal/epidural	__ 100-160
__ Prolonged labor	__ Breech/malpres	__ Pethidine	__ 160
__ PIH/PET/eclampisa	__ Multiple preg.	__ Other _____ decelerations	

Liquor—Clear/foul smelling/meconium stained

Placenta   – Wt.

           – Description

POST DELIVERY

Apgar score	HR	Resp. effort	Tone	Reflex response	Color	Total
1 minute	____	____	____	____	____	____
5 minute	____	____	____	____	____	____
10 minute	____	____	____	____	____	____
20 minute	____	____	____	____	____	____

Resuscitation method: Drugs

_____ Oxygen flow by   _____ Sodium bicarbonate

_____ Mask and ambu bag   _____ Dextrose

_____ Intubation   _____ Adrenaline

_____ Umbilical catheter   _____ Nalorphine

                                              _____ Other _____

PHYSICAL EXAMINATION

Single/twin....... 1st/2nd twin....... AGA:by dates....... weeks;by exa.......weeks;

Length............cm. Birth weight..............gm. MAC............cm. Cord............cm.

General and systemic examination: HC...........cm. AF:AP...........cm. Tr........cm.

Vital signs:

Skin: Color............................... Pallor........................ Jaundice...........................

Scalp.. Fontanelle................. Oral cavity......................

Palate.. Eyes................... Ears................. Nose..............

Chest:

CVS:

Lungs:

Abdomen: Umbilical stump........................... Umbilical vessels........................

               Liver................. Spleen............ Any other mass..........................

Genitalia:

Extremities:

Back:

CNS: Activity   Tone   Movements   Deep tendon reflexes

               N reflexes-Moro's   Rooting   Suck   Grasp

               Urine 1st passed at-

               Meconium 1st passed at-

Impression: Plan:

Name: _____   Signature _____

PROBLEM LIST

Date	Age	Feeding	Stool	Color	Jaundice	Umbilical stump	Problem	Treatment

Procedures

_____ Umbilical catheter
_____ Spinal tap
_____ Head ultrasound
_____ X-rays
_____ ECG
_____ Abdominal US
_____ Postmortem
_____ Development assessment
_____ Other

Drugs/Therapy

_____ Artificial feedings
_____ TV fluids
_____ Phototherapy
_____ Antibiotics
_____ Calcium
_____ Steroids
_____ Diuretics
_____ Blood transfusion
_____ Other _____

Discharge date _____

Baby: Status_____ Bed category_____ Blood group_____ Rh type_____

Weight_____gm. HC_____cm. Hb_____gm. Discharge date_____

Immunizations: BCG____ OPV_____ Age_____ Days_____ HBV_____

Course in hospital:

Impression:

Discharge plan:

1. Feeding :
2. Medication :
3. Follow-up visit :

Name of the Doctor :   Signature :

A DETAILED NEONATAL PHYSICAL ASSESSMENT SHEET

Date _____

Name of infant_____ Sex _____

Date and time of delivery _____ Age now _____

Admission data:

Time of admission _____

Placed in warmer? _____ Isolette _____ Servo temp _____

Eye prophylaxis _____

Vitamin K _____ Time _____

Location _____

Cord blood:

Blood type and Rh _____

Direct Coomb's test _____

VDRL (Serology) _____

HBsAg_____

HIV _____

Initial physical examination:

Date_____ Time_____ Age of infant_____

Findings:

General

Vital signs: Temperature_____ Pulse_____ Respirations_____ BP_____

Weight_____ Height____ Head circumference____ Chest circumference____

Color_____ Activity_____

State_____ Cry_____

Skin

    Color _____ Lesions _____

    Desquamation _____ Vernix caseosa _____

    Hair distribution _____

    Petechiae/ecchymosis/trauma _____

    Nails (length) _____

    Turgor (evidence of subcutaneous loss) _____

    Other _____

Head

    Circumference _____ Shape _____

    Moulding _____

    Fontanels/sutures (size, placement, fullness) _____

    Birth trauma _____ Forceps marks _____

    Caput succedaneum _____ Cephalhematoma _____

    Facial symmetry _____ Other _____

Ears

    Position _____ Size _____

    Cartilage formation _____ Other _____

Eyes

    Position (slant, hypertelorism) _____

    Size _____ Iris _____

    Sclerae _____ Discharge _____

    Other _____

Nose

    Patency _____ Flaring _____

    Nasolabial folds _____ Other _____

Throat and Mouth

    Lips (color, formation) _____ Symmetrical facial movement _____

    Palate _____ Gums/teeth (neonatal) _____

    Tongue (midline, gap) _____ Secretions _____

    Other _____

Neck

    Webbing _____ Masses _____

    Range of motion _____ Other _____

Chest

    Circumference _____

    Respiratory rate and quality (retractions/grunting) _____

    Breath sounds _____

    Thorax (symmetry of movement anterior posterior diameter, bulging) _

    _____

    Breast tissue/areola _____ Other _____

Cardiovascular

    Color: Cyanosis (location), pallor, plethora _____

    Heart rate _____ unusual rhythm/murmurs _____

    Location of PMI _____

    Pulses: Brachial _____ Femoral _____

    Capillary filling _____ Cyanosis/pallor/rudiness _____

    Hct (if done) _____ Other _____

Abdomen

    Shape _____

    Umbilical cord/vessels/color/size/drainage _____

    Liver _____ Spleen _____

    Kidneys _____ Anus (patency, location) _____

    Other _____

Extremities and Back

    Spine _____

    Upper extremities (digits, symmetry of size, movement, tone) _____

    _____

    Lower extremities (digits, symmetry of size, movement, tone) _____

    _____

    Palmar/plantar, gluteal and thigh creases _____

    Ortolani's maneuver _____

    Other _____

Genitalia

    Female

    Labia major/minor/clitoris/vagina _____

    Discharge _____ Edema/ecchymosis _____

    Placement of urinary meatus and anus _____ Patency of anus _____

    Other _____

Neurologic/behavioral

    Reflexes

    Moro _____ Tonic neck _____

    Neck righting _____ Stepping _____

    Babinski _____ Palmar grasp _____

    Traction response _____ Plantar grasp _____

    Rooting _____ Sucking _____

    Swallowing _____ Other _____

Behavioral

State _____

Visual following _____ Auditory following _____

Consolableness _____ Hand-to-mouth activity _____

Tremors

Description (location, type) _____

Stimulus related _____

Assessment of gestational age:

Via dates _____ Via ultrasound _____

Via examination: Initial _____ After 24 hours _____

Classification:

Preterm	Term	Post term	SGA
			AGA
			LGA

MONITORING IN NICU SET UP

Name   :   I.P.No.   :

Age   :   Unit   :

Weight   :   Diagnosis :

                                 Dates   :

Neurological Monitoring

Level of Consciousness :

Newborn Reflexes-Moro's :

Hie staging-   Stage I   Stage II   Stage III   Stage IV

Respiratory Monitoring

Resp. rate
Oral/tracheal secretions
Air ways patency
Retraction
Grunting
Color
Air entry
Chest
Breath sounds
RDS grading
Stridor
Wheeze
Chest X-ray
Blood gas analysis
$$PaO_2$$
$$PCO_2$$
$$PH$$
$$HOC_3$$

Cardiac Monitoring

Heart rate
Pulse
BP
CVP
Peripheral pulses
Capillary filling time
Skin temperature
Skin color
Cardiac size
Peripheral signs of shock
Signs of CCF

Renal Monitoring

Urine output
Fluid intake
Weight
Sp. gravity of urine
Albumin in urine
Serum Na
Serum K
Serum   Creatinine
           Bun
           Glucose
           Calcium

GIT Monitoring

Abdomen girth
Stool, blood
Gastric content
Feeding

Hematological Monitoring

Hematocrit
Platelets
Bleeding time
Clottting time
PT/APTT

Biochemical Monitoring

Blood glucose
Serum calcium
Serum sodium
Serum potassium

Bilirubin Levels   :

Septic Screening

Absolute neutrophilic count
Band forms
C-Reactive protein
Blood culture and sensitivity

Pharmacological Monitoring

Drugs-Dose Frequency

Drug Toxicity

REFERRAL SHEET

Name of the Hospital : .... Name of the child : ....
OP/IP No.: ....
Address of the Hospital : .... Date of birth : ....
.... Time of birth : ....
.... Age of the child : ....

Address of the patient : ....
....

Telephone: .... Unit : .... Date of discharge : ....
Family names: Mother .... Father ....
Grand parents ....
Diagnosis :...
....
....
....

Information given to family regarding prognosis : ....
Reasons for referral : ....
....
....
....

Problems	Plan
....	....
....	....
....	....
....	....
....	....
....	....
....	....

Patients discharge information including procedures, medications, treatments,
referrals and individualized care plan   ☐ is attached
(please tick right in the box)   ☐ will be sent later
Name of the referring Doctor : ....
Signature :...
Additional refferals made to: ....
Report to be sent back to : ....
Referral given to : ....
Name of the Hospital : .... Address: ....
Name of the Doctor : .... Telephone number: ....

DISCHARGE SUMMARY SHEET

Name : ....

Date of birth .... Date of discharge .... Hosp. No. ....

Birth weight .... Wt. at discharge .... Length ....

Suggested diet ....

Medications ....

....

....

Return visit: Date .... Time ....

            Place .... Phone ....

Pediatricians name : ....

Relevant antenatal history : ....

....

....

....

Complete diagnosis of all problems in chronological order : ....

....

....

....

....

....

Details of each diagnosis : ....

....

....

....

....

....

....

....

Hospital course: (this should also include duration of IV fluids, duration, dose and complications if any of parenteral nutrition, age at which feeds started, type and method of feeding, maximum weight loss) .... on day ...., birth weight regained on .... day, doses and duration of drugs, phototherapy, blood, plasma and exchange transfusion).

....

....

....

....

Special instructions : ....

....

Other instructions : ....

....

....

APGAR SCORE SHEET

Name .... Date			Time from birth minutes		
	0	1	2	1	2
Heart rate	Absent	Below 100	Above 100		
Respiratory effort	Absent	Slow Irregular	Good crying		
Muscle tone	Limp	Some flexion of extremities	Active Good tone		
Response to catheter	No Response	Grimace	Cough or sneeze		
Color	Blue Pale Blue	Body pink Extremities	Completely pink		
			Total		

BLOOD GAS RECORD SHEET

Start _____

     Date   Time

Finish _____

     Date   Time

ACTIVITY

++ = Active
+ = Active (stimulated)
− = Limp
A = Irritable
S = Twitchy

COLOR

P = Pink   R = Rectal
W = Pale   M = Mean
D = Dusky
B = Blue
S = Skin

	Time	Age (Hrs.)	O_2 conc.	Hood Inc.	S R	BP (M)	P.	R.	Hct, Hgb	Dext. Sug.	Bil	#	pH	pO_2	pCO_2	ACT. HCO_2
Example case one		8	70	34 / 34	36^6 / 37^1							5	7.16	50	60	21

Temperature (°C) — Vital signs — Lab. Work — Blood Gases

IAP CARD

Indian Academy of Pediatrics
Immunization & Health Record

Step by step protection against childhood infections is what your child needs. Follow the steps of vaccination your Doctor advises you.

Name of the child

Date of birth

Home address

Doctor's name

Clinic address

BIRTH RECORD

Time of Birth :

Sex: Male / Female

Delivery: Normal / Vacuum / Forceps/ Caesarean

Neonatal Status :

Birth Weight :

Length :

Head Circumference :

Blood Group :

Remarks :

Name of The Mother

Name of The Father

Mother's Blood Group

Father's Blood Group

Details of Siblings

DEVELOPMENT CARD

Make sure your child sees, hears and listens.

Points to parts of doll (paris)
Walks upstairs with help
Walks Backwards
Says Two Words
Walks Alone
Throws ball
Walks with help
Pats a cake
Fine prehension pellet
Standing up by Furniture
Raises self to sitting position
Transfers objects hand to hand
Turns head to sound of bell / rattle
Rolls from back to stomach
Holds head steady
Eyes follow pen/pencil
Social Smile

1 2 3 4 5 6 7 8 9 10 11 12 13 14 15 16 17 18 19 20 21 23 23 24 months

Note :To use this chart, keep a pencil vertically on the age of the child all milestones falling to the left of the pencil should have been achieved by the child

Based on BSID Baroda norms & Trivandrum Developmental Screening Chart (TDSC)

HEALTH RECORD

Date	AGE	WEIGHT	HEIGHT	HEAD CIRCUM.	REMARKS

THIRD YEAR — DENTAL / BP/ HEARING

FOURTH YEAR — DENTAL / BP/ VISION /HEARING

FIFTH YEAR — DENTAL / BP/ VISION /HEARING

SIXTH YEAR

IMMUNIZATION CARD (KARNATAKA)

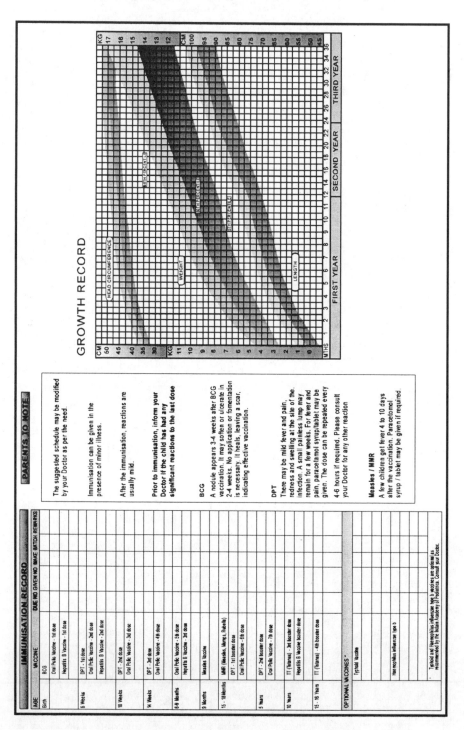

GROWTH RECORD

PARENTS TO NOTE

The suggested schedule may be modified by your Doctor as per the need.

Immunisation can be given in the presence of minor illness.

After the immunisation, reactions are usually mild.

Prior to immunisation, inform your Doctor if the child has had any significant reactions to the last dose

BCG

A nodule appears 3-4 weeks after BCG vaccination. It may soften or ulcerate in 2-4 weeks. No application or fomentation is necessary. It heals, leaving a scar, indicating effective vaccination.

DPT

There may be mild fever and pain, redness and swelling at the site of the infection. A small painless lump may remain for a few weeks. For fever and pain, paracetamol syrup/tablet may be given. The dose can be repeated every 4-6 hours if required. Please consult your Doctor for any other reaction

Measles / MMR

A few children get fever 4 to 10 days after the vaccination. Paracetamol syrup / tablet may be given if required.

IMMUNISATION RECORD

AGE	VACCINE	DUE	NO GIVEN	NO MAKE	BATCH	REMARKS
Birth	BCG					
	Oral Polio Vaccine - 1st dose					
	Hepatitis B Vaccine - 1st dose					
6 Weeks	DPT - 1st dose					
	Oral Polio Vaccine - 2nd dose					
	Hepatitis B Vaccine - 2nd dose					
10 Weeks	DPT - 2nd dose					
	Oral Polio Vaccine - 3rd dose					
14 Weeks	DPT - 3rd dose					
	Oral Polio Vaccine - 4th dose					
6-9 Months	Oral Polio Vaccine - 5th dose					
	Hepatitis B Vaccine - 3rd dose					
9 Months	Measles Vaccine					
15 - 18 Months	MMR (Measles, Mumps, Rubella)					
	DPT - 1st booster dose					
	Oral Polio Vaccine - 6th dose					
5 Years	DPT - 2nd booster dose					
	Oral Polio Vaccine - 7th dose					
10 Years	TT (Tetanus) - 3rd booster dose					
	Hepatitis B Vaccine booster dose					
15 - 16 Years	TT (Tetanus) - 4th booster dose					

OPTIONAL VACCINES *

	Typhoid Vaccine					
	Haemophilus influenzae type b					

* Typhoid and Haemophilus influenzae type b vaccines are optional as recommended by the Indian Academy of Pediatrics. Consult your Doctor.

SECTION 8

Author's Tips

51 Author's Tips for Good Pediatric Examination

1. Keep your head cool. More the child cries, more cool your head should be!

   Children deserve sympathy specially when they do not deserve it!

2. Take a diagnostic challenge every time you see a patient.

3. Feel yourself "charged" before you approach a child. (Like charging your cell phone before using!)

4. Always have a professional approach but flexibility is also important.

5. Approach the child depending on his development, temperament and situation at adjustment. Be an opportunist.

6. Come down to the patients level, both physically and mentally.

7. Always anticipate and examine (i.e., anticipation of features of a disease, its association, progress and complications).

8. If you think of common conditions you will be commonly right. If you think of a rare condition, rarely you will be right.

   In an unusual presentation, think of, in the following order:

   a. Rare manifestations of a common condition.

   b. Common manifestations of a rare condition and

   c. Rare manifestations of a rare condition.

9. In a diagnostic process the process of exclusion of certain conditions helps in narrowing down the diagnostic possibilities.

10. Retrospective history (i.e., after finding something on examination) and repeated and periodic examinations are important factors in a diagnostic challenge.

11. Reconsideration of a diagnosis, taking a second opinion from a colleague, cross consultation with another specialist, not only yields valuable informations but also helps you learn more and keeps you safe in the event of a consumer protection problem.

12. Do not be misled by a patient diagnosis, reports of investigations (specially computer generated!), another specialists' diagnosis, even if it is from a Big Doctor (This is not intended to teach arrogance to students but to make them exercise their clinical skills in an orderly fashion).

13. Love children, respect parents, talk to them softly, try to understand their concerns and apprehensions.

14. Develop a powerful observational skill that has depth, breadth, insight, intellect and gentleness.

15. Your successful diagnosis should boost your morale and make you happier but a failed diagnosis should make you wiser and humble.

16. Sympathize with patient (feel for) but do not empathize with patient (feel with).

17. Practice clinical medicine not clerical medicine.

18. Evolve over the ladder of:
    - Knowledge
    - Wisdom (knowledge + experience)
    - Philosophy (wisdom + insight).

Index